Cases and Concepts Step 1:
Pathophysiology Review

Cases and Concepts Step 1:
Pathophysiology Review

Aaron B. Caughey, MD, MPP, MPH, PhD
Associate Professor, Fellowship Program Director
Division of Maternal-Fetal Medicine
Department of Obstetrics, Gynecology, and Reproductive Services
University of California at San Francisco
San Francisco, California

Christie del Castillo-Hegyi, MD
Attending Emergency Physician
Presbyterian Hospital
University of New Mexico
Albuquerque, New Mexico

Michael Filbin, MD
Clinical Instructor, Department of Emergency Medicine
Harvard Affiliated Emergency Medicine Residency
Massachusetts General Hospital
Boston, Massachusetts

Holbrook E. Kohrt, MD
Fellow, Hematology-Oncology
Stanford University School of Medicine
Stanford, California

Lisa M. Lee, MD
Gynecologic Oncologist
Department of Obstetrics and Gynecology
Santa Clara Valley Medical Center
Santa Clara, CA

Gordon Leung, MD
Cardiologist
San Francisco, California

Sarah Little, MD
Resident
Department of Obstetrics and Gynecology
Brigham and Women's Hospital
Boston, Massachusetts

Jillian S. Main
Class of 2009
Chicago Medical School
Chicago, Illinois

Alexander M. Morss, MD
Resident, Department of Neurology
Resident, Department of Medicine
Massachusetts General Hospital/Brigham and Women's Hospital
Boston, Massachusetts

Nancy Palmer, MD
Class of 2003
University of California at San Francisco School of Medicine
San Francisco, California

Brian L. Shaffer, MD
Fellow, Maternal-Fetal Medicine and Clinical Genetics
Department of Obstetrics, Gynecology, and Reproductive Sciences
University of California at San Francisco
San Francisco, California

Laetitia Poisson de Souzy, MD
Resident
Department of Obstetrics and Gynecology
University of California at San Francisco
San Francisco, California

Teresa Sparks
Class of 2009
UCSF School of Medicine
San Francisco, California

Karen Spizer, MD
Chief Resident
California Pacific Medical Center
San Francisco, California

Tina O. Tan, MD
Attending Physician
Department of Obstetrics and Gynecology
Santa Clara Valley Medical Center
South San Francisco, California

Susan H. Tran, MD
Fellow, Maternal-Fetal Medicine and Clinical Genetics
Department of Obstetrics, Gynecology,
    and Reproductive Sciences
University of California at San Francisco
San Francisco, California

Dana Tuttle, MD
Development Project Management
Product Development
Genentech, Inc.
South San Francisco, California

Robert T. Wechsler, MD, PhD
Epilepsy and Clinical Neurophysiology Fellow
Stanford Comprehensive Epilepsy Center
Stanford University School of Medicine
Palo Alto, California

Jed T. Wolpaw, M.Ed.
Class of 2010
UCSF School of Medicine
San Francisco, California

Kelly N. Wright, MD
Resident
Department of Obstetrics, Gynecology, and Reproductive Biology
Brigham and Women's Hospital
Boston, Massachusetts

Courtney J. Wusthoff, MD
Resident-Department of Neurology
University of Pennsylvania
Philadelphia, Pennsylvania

Series Editor: Aaron B. Caughey, MD, MPP, MPH, PhD

Wolters Kluwer | Lippincott Williams & Wilkins
Health
Philadelphia · Baltimore · New York · London
Buenos Aires · Hong Kong · Sydney · Tokyo

Acquisitions Editor: Charles W. Mitchell
Senior Managing Editor: Stacey L. Sebring
Managing Editor: Nancy Hoffmann
Marketing Manager: Emilie J. Moyer
Production Editor: John Larkin
Creative Director: Doug Smock
Compositor: International Typesetting and Composition

First Edition

Library of Congress Cataloging-in-Publication Data

Cases and Concepts Step 1: Pathophysiology Review / Aaron B. Caughey . . . [et al.].
    p. ; cm.
  Includes index.
  ISBN-13: 978-0-7817-8254-8
  ISBN-10: 0-7817-8254-6
 1. Physiology, Pathological—Case studies.   I. Caughey, Aaron B.
II. Title: Pathophysiology review.
  [DNLM: 1. Pathology—Case Reports.   2. Pathology—Examination Questions.
3. Clinical Medicine—methods—Case Reports.   4. Clinical
Medicine—methods—Examination Questions.   5. Physiology—Case Reports.
6. Physiology—Examination Questions.   WB 293 C3384 2009]
  RB123.C37 2009
  616.07—dc22

                                            2008044381

DISCLAIMER

Care has been taken to confirm the accuracy of the information present and to describe generally accepted practices. However, the authors, editors, and publisher are not responsible for errors or omissions or for any consequences from application of the information in this book and make no warranty, expressed or implied, with respect to the currency, completeness, or accuracy of the contents of the publication. Application of this information in a particular situation remains the professional responsibility of the practitioner; the clinical treatments described and recommended may not be considered absolute and universal recommendations.

The authors, editors, and publisher have exerted every effort to ensure that drug selection and dosage set forth in this text are in accordance with the current recommendations and practice at the time of publication. However, in view of ongoing research, changes in government regulations, and the constant flow of information relating to drug therapy and drug reactions, the reader is urged to check the package insert for each drug for any change in indications and dosage and for added warnings and precautions. This is particularly important when the recommended agent is a new or infrequently employed drug.

Some drugs and medical devices presented in this publication have Food and Drug Administration (FDA) clearance for limited use in restricted research settings. It is the responsibility of the health care provider to ascertain the FDA status of each drug or device planned for use in their clinical practice.

To purchase additional copies of this book, call our customer service department at **(800) 638-3030** or fax orders to **(301) 223-2320.** International customers should call **(301) 223-2300.**

Visit Lippincott Williams &Wilkins on the Internet: http://www.lww.com. Lippincott Williams &Wilkins customer service representatives are available from 8:30 am to 6:00 pm, EST.

PREFACE

The first two years of medical school are a demanding time for medical students. Whether the school follows a traditional curriculum or one that is case based, every student is expected to learn and be able to apply basic science information in a clinical situation.

Medical schools are increasingly using clinical presentations as the background to teach the basic sciences. Case-based learning has become more common at many medical schools, as it offers a way to catalogue the multitude of symptoms, syndromes, and diseases in medicine.

Cases and Concepts is a new series by Lippincott Williams & Wilkins designed to provide students with a textbook to study the basic science topics combined with clinical data. This method of learning is also the way to prepare for the clinical case format of USMLE questions. The books in this series will make the basic science topics not only more interesting but also more meaningful and memorable. Students will be learning not only the why of a principle but also how it might commonly be seen in practice.

The books in the *Cases and Concepts* series feature a comprehensive collection of cases that are designed to introduce one or more basic science topics. Through these cases, students gain an understanding of the coursework as they learn to:

- Think through the cases
- Look for classic presentations of most common diseases and syndromes
- Integrate the basic science content with clinical application
- Prepare for course exams and Step 1 USMLE
- Be prepared for clinical rotations

This series covers all the essential material needed in the basic science courses. Where possible, the books are organized in an organ-based system. Clinical cases lead off and are the basis for discussion of the basic science content. A list of thought questions follows the case presentation. These questions are designed to challenge the reader to begin to think about how basic science topics apply to real-life clinical situations. The **answers to these questions** are integrated within the **basic science review and discussion** that follows. This offers a clinical framework from which to understand the basic content.

The discussion section is followed by a high-yield **Thumbnail table and Key Points box** that highlight and summarize the essential information presented in the discussion. The cases also include two to four multiple-choice questions that allow readers to check their knowledge of that topic. Many of the answer explanations provide an opportunity for further discussion by delving into more depth in related areas. Full answer explanations can be found at the end of the book.

This series was designed to provide comprehensive content in a concise and templated format for ease in learning. A dedicated attempt was made to include sufficient art, tables, and clinical treatment information, all while keeping the books from becoming too lengthy. We know you have much to read and that what you want is high-yield, vital facts.

Lippincott Williams & Wilkins and the authors wish you success in your studies and in your future medical career. Please feel free to offer us any comments or suggestions on these books at **www.lww.com**.

CONTENTS

Contents

ABBREVIATIONS

17-OHP	17-OH progesterone
[CO$_2$]	concentration of dissolved CO$_2$ in serum measured by partial pressure PCO$_2$
[HCO$_3^-$]	concentration of serum HCO$_3^-$
°C	degrees Celsius
°F	degrees Fahrenheit
2°	"due to" or "secondary to"
3bHSD	3b-hydroxysteroid dehydrogenase
5-HIAA	5-hydroxyindole acetic acid
5-HT	5-hydroxytryptamine (serotonin)
α-IFN	alpha interferon
A	adenine
A-a gradient	difference in partial pressure of oxygen between alveoli and arterial blood
Ab	antibody
Abd	abdomen
ABG	arterial blood gas
ABO	blood types with surface antigens A, B, and O
abx	antibiotics
ACA	anterior cerebral artery
ACD	anemia of chronic disease
ACE	angiotensin-converting enzyme
ACEI	angiotensin-converting enzyme inhibitor
ACh	acetylcholine
ACom	anterior communicating artery
ACS	acute coronary syndrome
ACTH	adrenocorticotropic hormone
AD	autosomal dominant
ADH	antidiuretic hormone
ADP	adenosine diphosphate
ADPKD	autosomal dominant polycystic kidney disease
AF	atrial fibrillation
AFP	alpha-fetoprotein
AG	anion gap
Ag-Ab	antigen-antibody
AICA	anteroinferior cerebellar artery
AIDS	acquired immunodeficiency syndrome
AIHA	autoimmune hemolytic anemia
AII	angiotensin II
AIN	acute interstitial nephritis
AJCC	American Joint Committee on Classification (of colorectal cancer)
alk phos	alkaline phosphate
ALL	acute lymphocytic leukemia
ALT	alanine aminotransferase
AML	acute myelogenous leukemia
AMP	adenosine monophosphate (adenylic acid)
AMPA	a-amino-3-hydroxyl-5-methyl-4-isoxazole-propionate
ANA	antinuclear antibody
ANC	absolute neutrophil count
ANCA	antineutrophil cytoplasmic antibody
ANS	autonomic nervous system
anti-dsDNA	anti–double-stranded DNA
anti-Sm	anti-Smith [as in anti-Smith antibody]
aPC	activated protein C
APC	adenomatous polyposis coli
APC	antigen-presenting cell
APSAC	acylated plasminogen streptokinase activator complex
AR	aortic regurgitation
AR	autosomal recessive
ARB	angiotensin receptor blocker
ARDS	acute respiratory distress syndrome
ARF	acute renal failure
AS	aortic stenosis
ASA	acetylsalicylic acid
ASCUS	atypical squamous cells of undetermined significance
ASD	atrial septal defect
ASO	antistreptolysin O (streptococcal antigen)
AST	aspartate aminotransferase
ATL	adult T-cell leukemia/lymphoma
ATM	acute transverse myelitis
ATM	ataxia-telangiectasia
ATN	acute tubular necrosis
ATP	adenosine triphosphate
ATPase	enzyme that uses adenosine triphosphate
AV	atrioventricular
AVA	aortic valve area
AVNRT	atrioventricular nodal re-entrant tachycardia
AVP	arginine vasopressin
AVRT	atrioventricular re-entrant tachycardia
AZT	zidovudine
B19	parvovirus B19
BC	Bowman capsule
BCC	basal cell carcinoma
bFGF	basic fibroblast growth factor
BM	basement membrane
BM	bone marrow
BP	blood pressure
BPH	benign prostatic hypertrophy
B-PLL	B-cell prolymphocytic leukemia
BPV	benign positional vertigo
BRCA	breast cancer
BS	barium swallow
BS	bowel sounds
BS	breath sounds
BUN	blood urea nitrogen
C	cytosine
C1–C4	complement 1–4
C1–C8	cervical spinal cord levels 1–8
CA	cancer
CA	carbonic anhydrase
CA1–CA4	cornu ammonis regions of the hippocampus
Ca2$^+$	calcium
CABG	coronary artery bypass graft
CAD	coronary artery disease
CAH	congenital adrenal hyperplasia
cAMP	cyclic adenosine monophosphate
CaO$_2$	arterial oxygen content
CAT	computed axial tomography
CBC	complete blood count
CCB	calcium channel blockers
CCK	cholecystokinin
CD	cluster of differentiation (leukocyte surface markers)
CD	collecting duct
CDI	central diabetes insipidus
CDK	cyclin-dependent kinase
CEA	carcinoembryonic antigen
CF	cystic fibrosis
CFTR	cystic fibrosis transmembrane regulator
CFU	colony-forming unit
CHF	congestive heart failure
CIN	cervical intraepithelial neoplasia
CK	creatinine kinase
CK MB	creatinine kinase myocardial band fraction
Cl	chloride
CLL	chronic lymphocytic leukemia
CML	chronic myeloid (myelogenous) leukemia
CMV	cytomegalovirus
CN	cranial nerve
CN I–XII	cranial nerves I–XII
CNS	central nervous system
CO	carbon monoxide
CO	cardiac output
CO$_2$	carbon dioxide
COHb	carboxy-hemoglobin
COPD	chronic obstructive pulmonary disease
COWS	cold opposite, warm same
CPM	central pontine myelinosis
Cr	creatinine

Abbreviations

CREST syndrome	calcinosis, Raynaud phenomenon, esophageal disease, sclerodactyly, telangiectasia
CRF	chronic renal failure
CRH	corticotropin-releasing hormone
CSF	cerebrospinal fluid
CT	computed tomography
CV	cardiovascular
CVA	cerebrovascular accident
CVA	costovertebral angle
CVAT	costovertebral angle tenderness
CVD	collagen vascular disease
CVS	chorionic villus sampling
CVS	cardiovascular system
CX	dissolved gas
CXR	chest x-ray
D&C	dilatation and curettage
D&E	dilatation and evacuation
DCIS	ductal carcinoma in situ
DCT	distal convoluted tubule
DDAVP	deamino-8-D-arginine vasopressin
DES	diethylstilbestrol
DHEA	dehydroepiandrosterone
DHEA-S	dehydroepiandrosterone sulfate
DHT	dihydrotestosterone
DI	diabetes insipidus
DIC	disseminated intravascular coagulation
DIP	distal interphalangeal
DKA	diabetic ketoacidosis
dL	deciliter
DLCO	diffusion capacity of gas across the alveolar-capillary membrane
DM	diabetes mellitus
DMPA	depot medroxyprogesterone acetate
DNA	deoxyribonucleic acid
DOD450	light absorption by bilirubin
DOPA	dihydroxyphenylalanine
DRE	digital rectal exam
dsDNA	double-stranded DNA
DTR	deep tendon reflex
DVT	deep vein thrombosis
EBV	Epstein-Barr virus
ECA	external carotid artery
ECF	extracellular fluid
ECF-A	eosinophil chemotactic factor of anaphylaxis
ECG	electrocardiogram
ECM	extracellular matrix
ED	emergency department
EDGF	epidermal-derived growth factor
EE	refers to cortical neurons that respond to sound heard best in both ears

EEG	electroencephalogram; electroencephalography
EF	ejection fraction
EGFR	epidermal growth factor receptor
EHL	extensor hallucis longus
EI	cortical neurons that respond to sound heard best in the contralateral ear
ELISA	enzyme-linked immunosorbent assay
EM	electron microscopy
EMB	eosin methylene blue agar
EMG	electromyography
EOMI	extraocular movements intact
Epo	erythropoietin
EPP	endplate potential
EPSP	excitatory postsynaptic potential
ER	emergency room
ERCP	endoscopic retrograde cholangiopancreatography
ERPF	effective renal plasma flow
ESPVR	end-systolic pressure-volume loop
ESR	erythrocyte sedimentation rate
ESRD	end-stage renal disease
ESS	endometrial stromal sarcoma
ET	endothelin
ET	essential thrombocytopenia
EtOH	alcohol
Ext	extremities
F	factor
FamHx	family history
FAP	familial adenomatous polyposis
Fc	constant fragment of immunoglobulin
$Fc\gamma R$	receptor recognizing the constant fragment of immunoglobulin G
$Fc\epsilon R$	receptor recognizing the constant fragment of immunoglobulin E
Fe	iron
$FENa^+$	fractional excretion of sodium
FEV	forced expiratory volume
FEV_1	forced expiratory volume in 1 second
FGF	fibroblast growth factor
FIGO	International Federation of Gynecology and Obstetrics
FiO_2	fractional percentage of oxygen in inspired air
fL	fluid liters
FNA	fine needle aspiration
FNHTR	febrile nonhemolytic transfusion reaction
FOBT	fecal occult blood test
FRC	functional residual capacity
FS	flexible sigmoidoscopy
FSGS	focal segmental glomerulosclerosis

FSH	follicle-stimulating hormone
FT4	free thyroxine (T4)
FVC	functional vital capacity
g	grams
G	gravida (pregnancies)
G	guanine
G − or +	Gram stain − or +
G# P#	gravida (pregnancies) and para (deliveries)
G6PD	glucose-6-phosphate dehydrogenase
GA	gestational age
GABA	γ-aminobutyric acid
GAS	group A streptococcus
GBM	glioblastoma multiforme
GBM	glomerular basement membrane
GC	gonococcal
G-CSF	granulocyte colony-stimulating factor
Gen	general
GERD	gastroesophageal reflux disease
GFR	glomerular filtration rate
GGT	gamma-glutamyltransferase
GH	growth hormone
GHRH	growth hormone-releasing hormone
GI	gastrointestinal
GM-CSF	granulocyte-macrophage colony-stimulating factor
GMP	guanylic acid
GN	glomerulonephritis
GnRH	gonadotropin-releasing hormone
GTD	gestational trophoblastic disease
GTT	gestational trophoblastic neoplasia
GU	genitourinary
GVHD	graft-versus-host disease
H2	histamine-2
H&E	hematoxylin and eosin
H/N	head and neck
H+	proton/hydrogen ion
H_2CO_3	carbonic acid
H_2O	water
H4 folate	tetrahydrofolate
HAV	hepatitis A virus
Hb S	hemoglobin S
HbA1c	hemoglobin A1c
HBAb	hepatitis B surface antibody
HBcAb	hepatitis B core antibody
HBcAg	hepatitis B core antigen
HBeAb	hepatitis B envelope antibody
HBeAg	hepatitis B envelope antigen
HBsAg	hepatitis B surface antigen
HBV	hepatitis B virus
HCC	hepatocellular carcinoma
hCG	human chorionic gonadotropin
HCl	hydrochloric acid
HCL	hairy cell leukemia
HCO_3	bicarbonate

Hct	hematocrit	INO	internuclear ophthalmoplegia	LUQ	left upper quadrant
HCV	hepatitis C virus	INR	international normalized ratio	LV	left ventricle
HCVAb	hepatitis C antibody	IPF	idiopathic pulmonary fibrosis OR	LVEDP	left ventricular end-diastolic
HD	Hodgkin disease		interstitial pulmonary fibrosis		pressure
HD	Huntington disease	IPSP	inhibitory postsynaptic potential	M/S	musculoskeletal
HDV	hepatitis D virus	ITP	idiopathic thrombocytopenic	MAHA	microangiopathic hemolytic
HEENT	head, eyes, ears, nose, and throat		purpura		anemia
HEV	hepatitis E virus	IUD	intrauterine device	MAOI	monoamine oxidase inhibitor
Hgb	hemoglobin	IV	intravenous	MCA	middle cerebral artery
HGPRT	hypoxanthine-guanine	IVC	inferior vena cava	MCHC	mean corpuscular hemoglobin
	phosphoribosyltransferase	IVDA	intravenous drug abuse		concentration
HGSIL	high-grade squamous	IVDU	intravenous drug use	MCP	metacarpophalangeal
	intraepithelial lesion	IVF	in vitro fertilization	MCV	mean corpuscular volume
HIT	heparin-induced	IVIG	intravenous immunoglobulin	MDS	myelodysplastic syndrome
	thrombocytopenia	IVP	intravenous pyelogram	Meds	medications
HIV	human immunodeficiency virus	J receptors	juxtacapillary receptors	MEN	multiple endocrine neoplasia
HLA	human lymphocytic antigen	JG	juxtaglomerular	MEPP	miniature endplate potential
HNPCC	hereditary nonpolyposis colon	JGA	juxtaglomerular apparatus	mEq	milliequivalents
	cancer	JVD	jugular venous distension	MF	myelofibrosis
hpf	high-power field	JVP	jugular venous pressure	mg	milligrams
HPI	history of present illness	K, K+	potassium	MGN	medial geniculate nucleus
HPV	human papilloma virus	KD	Kawasaki disease	MHC	major histocompatibility complex
HR	heart rate	KOH	potassium hydroxide	MI	myocardial infarction
HRT	hormone replacement therapy	KUB	kidneys, ureters, bladder	MIS	müllerian-inhibiting substance
HS	hereditary spherocytosis	L	left	mL	milliliter
HSM	hepatosplenomegaly	L + H cells	lymphohistiocytic cells	MLF	medial longitudinal fasciculus
HSV	herpes simplex virus		("popcorn cells")	mm	millimeters
HSV-1	herpes simplex virus type 1	L1–L5	lumbar spinal cord levels 1–5	MM	multiple myeloma
HSV-2	herpes simplex virus type 2	LA	left atrium, left atrial	mm Hg	millimeters of mercury
HTLV-1	human T-cell leukemia virus	LAD	left anterior descending	MMM	myelofibrosis with myeloid
HTN	hypertension	LAD	leukocyte adhesion deficiencies		metaplasia
HUS	hemolytic-uremic syndrome	LAD	lymphadenopathy	MMT	mixed müllerian tumor
HVA	homovanillic acid	LCIS	lobular carcinoma in situ	mOsm	milliosmoles
Hx	history	LCV	lymphocyte choriomeningitis	MPO	myeloperoxidase
IBD	inflammatory bowel disease	LDH	lactate dehydrogenase	MPTP	1-methyl-4-phenyl-1,2,5,
IBS	irritable bowel syndrome	LDL	low-density lipoproteins		6-tetrahydropyridine
ICA	internal carotid artery	LEEP	loop electrosurgical excision	MR	mitral regurgitation
ICAM-1	intracellular adhesion molecules-1		procedure	MRG	murmurs, rubs, gallops
ICF	intracellular fluid	LES	lower esophageal sphincter	MRI	magnetic resonance imaging
ICP	intracranial pressure	LFS	Li-Fraumeni syndrome	MS	mitral stenosis
ICSI	intracytoplasmic sperm injection	LFT	liver function test	MS	multiple sclerosis
ICU	intensive care unit	LGL	large granular lymphocytic	MSA	multiple system atrophy
IE	infective endocarditis		leukemia	MSH	melanocyte-stimulating hormone
IF	immunofluorescence	LGN	lateral geniculate nucleus	MTS	mesial temporal sclerosis
IF	intrinsic factor	LGSIL	low-grade squamous	MV	minute ventilation
IFN	interferon		intraepithelial lesion	MW	molecular weight
Ig	immunoglobulin	LH	loop of Henle	N/V	nausea and vomiting
IgA	immunoglobulin A	LH	luteinizing hormone	Na, Na+	sodium
IgD	immunoglobulin D	LLQ	left lower quadrant	NaCl	sodium chloride
IgE	immunoglobulin E	LM	light microscopy	NAD+	nicotine adenine dinucleotide,
IGF	insulin-like growth factor	LMN	lower motor neuron		oxidized form
IGF-1	insulin-like growth factor 1	LMP	last menstrual period	NADH	nicotine adenine dinucleotide,
IgG	immunoglobulin G	LMW	low molecular weight		reduced form
IgM	immunoglobulin M	LPS	lipopolysaccharide (component	NADPH	reduced nicotinamide adenine
IHD	ischemic heart disease		of endotoxin of gram-negative		dinucleotide phosphate
IL	interleukin		bacteria)	NDI	nephrogenic diabetes insipidus
IM	intramuscular	LSB	left sternal border	NE	norepinephrine
IMP	inosine monophosphate	LT	labile toxin	NEC	necrotizing enterocolitis

Abbreviations

Neuro	neurologic	PE	pulmonary embolism	PVN	paraventricular nucleus
NF	neurofibromatosis	PEEP	positive end-expiratory pressure	PVO$_2$	partial pressure of oxygen in venous blood
ng	nanogram	PERRLA	pupils equally round and reactive to light and accommodation		
NG	nasogastric (decompression)			Px	partial pressure
NHL	non-Hodgkin lymphoma	PFO	patent foramen ovale	Q	perfusion
NIH	National Institutes of Health	PFT	pulmonary function test	QID	four times a day
NK	natural killer	pg	picogram	R	right
Nl, nl	normal	PG	prostaglandin	RA	right atrium
NMDA	N-methyl d-aspartate	PGE2	prostaglandin E2	RA	rheumatoid arthritis
NMJ	neuromuscular junction	pi	interstitial oncotic pressure	RA	room air
NPH	normal-pressure hydrocephalus	Pi	interstitial hydrostatic pressure	RAA	renin-angiotensin-aldosterone
NPPV	noninvasive positive-pressure ventilation	PICA	posteroinferior cerebellar artery	RAI	radioactive iodine
		PID	pelvic inflammatory disease	RAS	renin-angiotensin system
NSAID	nonsteroidal anti-inflammatory drug	PIO$_2$	partial pressure of inhaled oxygen	RBBB	right bundle branch block
		PIP	proximal interphalangeal	RBC	red blood cell
NSE	nonspecific esterase	PKD1	polycystic kidney disease 1 gene	RBF	renal blood flow
NST	no special type	PKD2	polycystic kidney disease 2 gene	RCA	right coronary artery
NSTEMI	non-ST segment elevation myocardial infarction	Plt	platelets	Re	Reynold number
		PMD	primary medical doctor	RE	reticuloendothelial
O$_2$	oxygen	PMH, PMHx	past medical history	REM	rapid eye movement
O$_2$Sat	hemoglobin oxygen saturation	PmHx	previous medical history	RF	rheumatic fever
OCP	oral contraceptive pill	PMI	point of maximum impulse	RFLP	restriction fragment length polymorphism
OR	operating room	PMN	polymorphonuclear cell (neutrophil)		
ORF	open reading frame			Rh	rhesus factor
OS	opening snap	PNH	paroxysmal nocturnal hemoglobinuria	RLQ	right lower quadrant
OTC	over the counter			RNA	ribonucleic acid
P	plasma concentration	PNMT	phenylethanolamine-N-methyltransferase	RNP	ribonucleoprotein
P	pulse			ROS	review of systems
P#	para (deliveries)	PNS	peripheral nervous system	RPR	rapid plasma reagent
P2	pulmonic component to second heart sound	PO$_2$	pressure of oxygen	RR	respiratory rate
		PO42-	phosphate	RRR	regular rate and rhythm
P50	oxygen tension that produces 50% hemoglobin saturation	POMC	pro-opiomelanocortin	RS cells	Reed-Sternberg cells
		pp	capillary oncotic pressure	RTA	renal tubular acidosis
PaCO$_2$	partial pressure of carbon dioxide in arterial blood	Pp	capillary hydrostatic pressure	RUQ	right upper quadrant
		PPD	purified protein derivative (tuberculin antigen)	RV	residual volume
PAH	para-aminohippuric acid			RV	right ventricle
PAMP	pathogen-associated molecular pattern	PPRF	para-pontine reticular formation	RVH	right ventricular hypertrophy
		PRL	prolactin	Rx	medications
PaO$_2$	partial pressure of oxygen in arterial blood	PRPD	5-phosphoribosyl-1-pyrophosphate	S/Sx	signs and symptoms
				S1	first heart sound (closure of mitral and tricuspid valve)
Pap smear	Papanicolaou smear	PSA	prostate serum antigen		
PAS	periodic acid Schiff	PSC	primary sclerosing cholangitis	S1–S5	sacral spinal cord levels 1–5
PBC	primary biliary cirrhosis	PSH, PSHx	past surgical history	S2	second heart sound (closure of aortic and pulmonic valve)
PBS	peripheral blood smear	PSTT	placental site trophoblastic tumor		
PCA	patient-controlled analgesia	PT	prothrombin time	s3	abnormal heart sound heard right after s2; sound of ventricle filling
PCA	posterior cerebral artery	PTH	parathyroid hormone		
PCO$_2$	partial pressure of carbon dioxide as measured by blood gas analysis	PTHrP	parathyroid hormone-related protein	s4	abnormal heart sound heard right before s1; atrial kick
		PTSD	posttraumatic stress disorder	SA	sinoatrial
PCom	posterior communicating artery	PTT	partial thromboplastin time	SaO$_2$	arterial oxygen saturation
PCOS	polycystic ovarian syndrome	PTU	propylthiouracil	SCA	superior cerebellar artery
PCR	polymerase chain reaction	PUBS	percutaneous umbilical cord sampling	SCC	squamous cell carcinoma
PCRV	polycythemia rubra vera			SCD	sickle cell disease
PCT	proximal convoluted tubule	PUD	peptic ulcer disease	SCSD	subacute combined systems degeneration
PD	Parkinson disease	PV	polycythemia vera		
PDA	patent ductus arteriosus	PVC	premature ventricular contraction	SCU-PA	single-chain urokinase-type plasminogen activator
PDGF	platelet-derived growth factor				
PE	physical exam				

SERM	selective estrogen receptor modulators	TdT	terminal deoxynucleotidyl transferase	UMN	upper motor neuron
SGOT	serum glutamic oxaloacetic transferase	TF	tubular fluid	UPEP	urine protein electrophoresis
		TFPI	tissue factor pathway inhibitor	URI	upper respiratory infection
SGPT	serum glutamic pyruvic transaminase	TFT	thyroid function test	US	ultrasound
		TGA	transposition of great arteries	USA	unstable angina
SH	social history	TGF-α	transforming growth factor-alpha	UTI	urinary tract infection
SIADH	syndrome of inappropriate antidiuretic hormone	TGF-β	transforming growth factor-beta	UV	ultraviolet
		TH	thyroid hormone	V	ventilation
SLE	systemic lupus erythematosus	Th-cell	T-helper cell (type 1 or 2)	V/Q ratio	ventilation/perfusion ratio
SON	supraoptic nucleus	TIMI study	Thrombolysis in Myocardial Infarction study	V1–V3	ophthalmic, maxillary, and mandibular divisions of the trigeminal nerve
SPEP	serum protein electrophoresis				
SRS-A	slow-reacting substance of anaphylaxis	Tis	Tumor in situ	V1–V5	refers to visual cortex regions
		TLC	total lung capacity	VA	alveolar ventilation
SRY	sex-determining region of the Y chromosome	TLR	toll-like receptor	VA	Veterans Administration
		T_{max}	maximum temperature	VC	vital capacity
SSRI	selective serotonin reuptake inhibitor	TNF	tumor necrosis factor	VCO_2	carbon dioxide produced by peripheral tissue
		TNM	tumor, node, metastasis (classification system)		
SSS	sick sinus syndrome			VEGF	vascular endothelial growth factor
ST	stable toxin	TOF	tetralogy of Fallot	VF	ventricular fibrillation
STD	sexually transmitted disease	tPA	tissue plasminogen activator	VGEF	vascular endothelial growth factor
STEMI	ST elevation myocardial infarction	T-PLL	T-cell prolymphocytic leukemia	VHL	von Hippel-Lindau
		TPO	thyroid peroxidase	VIP	vasoactive intestinal polypeptide
SUNCT	short-lasting, unilateral, neuralgiform headaches with conjunctival injection and tearing	TR	tricuspid regurgitation	VLDL	very low-density lipoprotein
		TRH	thyroid-releasing hormone	VMA	vanillylmandelic acid
		TRUS	transrectal ultrasound	VOR	vestibulo-ocular reflex
SV	stroke volume	TSH	thyroid-stimulating hormone	VPL	ventral posterolateral nucleus (of thalamus)
SVC	superior vena cava	TSS	toxic shock syndrome		
SVR	systemic vascular resistance	TT	thrombin time	VS	vital signs
SVT	supraventricular tachycardia	TTP	thrombotic thrombocytopenic purpura	VSD	ventricular septal defect
T	temperature			VT	ventricular tachycardia
T	thymine	TURP	transurethral radical prostatectomy	vWD	von Willebrand disease
t(x,y)	translocation between chromosome x and chromosome y			vWF	von Willebrand factor
		U	urine concentration	WAGR	Wilms tumor, aniridia, genital anomalies, mental retardation syndrome
T1–T12	thoracic spinal cord levels 1–12	UA	urine analysis		
T_3	tri-iodothyronine	UC	ulcerative colitis		
T_4	thyroxine	UDC	uridine diphosphate	WBC	white blood cell count
TAH-BSO	total abdominal hysterectomy and bilateral salpingo-oophorectomy	UDP	uridinediphosphate	WHI	Women's Health Initiative
		UES	upper esophageal sphincter	WHO	World Health Organization
TB	tuberculosis	UG	urogenital	WPW	Wolff-Parkinson-White syndrome
TBW	total body water	UGT	UDP-bilirubin glucuronosyltransferase	WT-1	Wilms tumor 1 gene (11p13)
TCA	tricyclic antidepressant			WT-2	Wilms tumor 2 gene

BLOOD, PLASMA, SERUM

Alanine aminotransferase (ALT, GPT at 30°C)	8–20 U/L
Amylase, serum	25–125 U/L
Aspartate aminotransferase (AST, GOT at 30°C)	8–20 U/L
Bilirubin, serum (adult) Total // Direct	0.1–1.0 mg/dL // 0.0–0.3 mg/dL
Calcium, serum (Ca^{2+})	8.4–10.2 mg/dL
Cholesterol, serum	Rec: <200 mg/dL
Cortisol, serum	0800 h: 5–23 g/dL // 1600 h: 3–15 g/dL
	2000 h: 50% of 0800 h
Creatine kinase, serum	Male: 25–90 U/L
	Female: 10–70 U/L
Creatinine, serum	0.6–1.2 mg/dL
Electrolytes, serum	
Sodium	(Na^+) 136–145 mEq/L
Chloride	(Cl^-) 95–105 mEq/L
Potassium	(K^+) 3.5–5.0 mEq/L
Bicarbonate	(HCO_3^-) 22–28 mEq/L
Magnesium	(Mg^{2+}) 1.5–2.0 mEq/L
Ferritin, serum	Male: 15–200 ng/mL
	Female: 12–150 ng/mL
Follicle-stimulating hormone, serum/plasma	Male: 4–25 mIU/mL
	Female: premenopause 4–30 mIU/mL
	midcycle peak 10–90 mIU/mL
	postmenopause 40–250 mIU/mL
Gases, arterial blood (room air)	
pH	7.35–7.45
PCO_2	33–45 mm Hg
PO_2	75–105 mm Hg
Glucose, serum	Fasting: 70–110 mg/dL
	2-h postprandial: <120 mg/dL
Growth hormone—arginine stimulation	Fasting: <5 ng/mL
	provocative stimuli: >7 ng/mL
Iron	50–70 g/dL
Lactate dehydrogenase, serum	45–90 U/L
Luteinizing hormone, serum/plasma	Male: 6–23 mIU/mL
	Female: follicular phase 5–30 mIU/mL
	midcycle 75–150 mIU/mL
	postmenopause 30–200 mIU/mL
Osmolality, serum	275–295 mOsmol/kg
Parathyroid hormone, serum, N-terminal	230–630 pg/mL
Phosphate (alkaline), serum (p-NPP at 30°C)	20–70 U/L
Phosphorus (inorganic), serum	3.0–4.5 mg/dL
Prolactin, serum (hPRL)	<20 ng/mL
Proteins, serum	
Total (recumbent)	6.0–7.8 g/dL
Albumin	3.5–5.5 g/dL
Globulin	2.3–3.5 g/dL
Thyroid-stimulating hormone, serum or plasma	0.5–5.0 U/mL
Thyroidal iodine (123^I) uptake	8–30% of administered dose/24 h
Thyroxine (T_4), serum	5–12 g/dL
Transferrin	221–300 g/dL
Triglycerides, serum	35–160 mg/dL
Triiodothyronine (T_3), serum (RIA)	115–190 ng/dL
Triiodothyronine (T_3), resin uptake	25–35%
Urea nitrogen, serum (BUN)	7–18 mg/dL
Uric acid, serum	3.0–8.2 mg/dL

CEREBROSPINAL FLUID

Cell count	0–5 cells/mm^3
Chloride	118–132 mEq/L
Gamma globulin	3–12% total proteins
Glucose	40–70 mg/dL
Pressure	70–180 mm H$_2$O
Proteins, total	<40 mg/dL

HEMATOLOGIC

Bleeding time (template)	2–7 minutes
Erythrocyte count	Male: 4.3–5.9 million/mm^3
	Female: 3.5–5.5 million/mm^3
Erythrocyte sedimentation rate (Westergren)	Male: 0–15 mm/h
	Female: 0–20 mm/h
Hematocrit	Male: 41–53%
	Female: 36–46%
Hemoglobin A1C	6%
Hemoglobin, blood	Male: 13.5–17.5 g/dL
	Female: 12.0–16.0 g/dL
Leukocyte count and differential	
Leukocyte count	4500–11,000/mm^3
Segmented neutrophils	54–62%
Bands	3–5%
Eosinophils	1–3%
Basophils	0–0.75%
Lymphocytes	25–33%
Monocytes	3–7%
Mean corpuscular hemoglobin	25.4–34.6 pg/cell
Mean corpuscular hemoglobin concentration	31–36% Hgb/cell
Mean corpuscular volume	80–100 μm^3
Partial thromboplastin time (activated)	25–40 seconds
Platelet count	150,000–400,000/mm^3
Prothrombin time	11–15 seconds
Reticulocyte count	0.5–1.5% of red cells
Thrombin time	<2 seconds deviation from control
Volume	
Plasma	Male: 25–43 mL/kg
	Female: 28–45 mL/kg
Red cell	Male: 20–36 mL/kg
	Female: 19–31 mL/kg

SWEAT

Chloride	0–35 mmol/L

URINE

Calcium	100–300 mg/24 h
Chloride	Varies with intake
Creatine clearance	Male: 97–137 mL/min
	Female: 88–128 mL/min
Osmolality	50–1400 mOsmol/kg
Oxalate	8–40 g/mL
Potassium	Varies with diet
Proteins, total	<150 mg/24h
Sodium	Varies with diet
Uric acid	Varies with diet

PART I

Cardiovascular

CASE 1-1 Systolic and Diastolic Dysfunction

HPI: AHF is a 79-year-old man with a long-standing history of poorly controlled hypertension (HTN), stable coronary artery disease, and diabetes who presents to the emergency department with acute onset of shortness of breath but no chest pressure. He complains of increasing peripheral edema for several weeks, orthopnea, right upper quadrant (RUQ) pain, and increasing fatigue.

PE: Vitals: Blood pressure (BP) 160/50 mm Hg, heart rate (HR) 90 beats/min, respiratory rate (RR) 26 breaths/min, and maximum temperature (Tmax) 37°C. **General:** Tachypneic, uncomfortable appearing. **Head and Neck (H/N):** Jugular venous pressure (JVP) is 12 cm, pulses reduced in volume and upstroke. **Chest:** Crackles present one third of the way up bilaterally. **Cardiac:** Point of maximum impulse (PMI) displaced laterally and diffuse; S_3 and S_4 present. **Abdomen:** Mild pain in RUQ and mild hepatomegaly. **Extremity:** 3+ bilateral peripheral edema to knees. **Electrocardiography (ECG):** Normal sinus rhythm with nonspecific ST changes.

Labs: Creatinine 1.6 mg/dL, blood urea nitrogen (BUN) 24 mg/dL, troponin I < 0.05 mg/dL.

THOUGHT QUESTIONS

- What is heart failure?
- What are the causes of heart failure?
- What are the key mediators of cardiac output?
- How are pressure-volume loops affected in heart failure secondary to systolic dysfunction?
- What are the differences between systolic and diastolic dysfunction?
- What are the different causes for diastolic heart failure?
- How are pressure-volume loops affected in diastolic heart failure?

BASIC SCIENCE REVIEW AND DISCUSSION

Systolic Dysfunction

Heart failure is defined as the inability of the heart to meet the metabolic demands of the tissues. The most common cause of heart failure is ischemic heart disease followed by dilated cardiomyopathy.

Cardiac output is the product of the heart rate times the stroke volume ($CO = HR \times SV$). The stroke volume is determined by three parameters: (1) contractility, (2) preload, and (3) afterload. Contractility is the amount of force exerted at a given muscle fiber length. Preload is defined as the ventricular wall tension at the end of diastole and is quantified by the left ventricular end-diastolic pressure (LVEDP). Afterload is the ventricular wall tension during systole and is determined by the mean arterial pressure.

Another important equation is blood pressure equals cardiac output multiplied by the systemic vascular resistance ($BP = CO \times SVR$).

Systolic dysfunction is the result of impaired left ventricle (LV) contraction. The two major contributors to systolic dysfunction include impaired contractility and pressure overload (Table 1-1).

In systolic dysfunction, the normal pressure-volume loop is changed in the following fashion: (*a*) the end-systolic pressure volume loop (ESPVR) is shifted downward and rightward, resulting in a decreased stroke volume; and (*b*) the end-diastolic volume is increased with a resultant increase in the end-diastolic pressure. The decreased stroke volume precipitates decreased cardiac output. The increased LVEDP is transmitted into the pulmonary bed, resulting in pulmonary edema (Fig. 1-1).

Systolic dysfunction is compensated by three mechanisms:

1. *Ventricular hypertrophy:* Increased ventricular wall stress results in production of new myocardial sarcomeres and increased ventricular mass. Ventricular mass increases in two different patterns. **Pressure overload** causes synthesis of sarcomeres in parallel with previous sarcomeres, resulting in increased wall thickness without chamber dilatation. **Volume overload** stimulates sarcomere production in series with the previous sarcomeres, resulting in ventricular dilatation and enlargement.

2. *Neuroendocrine response:* When cardiac output declines, three neuroendocrine systems are activated to increase cardiac output. First, sympathetic tone increases, which then results in increased heart rate, increased contractility, and vasoconstriction. Second, the renin-angiotensin-aldosterone system is activated, which results in vasoconstriction and fluid retention to increase circulating volume and thereby **preload.** Third, increased antidiuretic hormone production promotes fluid retention.

3. *Frank-Starling response:* The increase in LV end-diastolic volume during systolic dysfunction results in an increase in preload. The **Frank-Starling response** to an increase in preload is a greater stroke volume on the subsequent systolic contraction. In effect, increased filling/preload causes an augmentation of cardiac output. In normal individuals, cardiac output increases as a function of end-diastolic volume. In systolic dysfunction, the cardiac output does not increase proportionally to an increase in end-diastolic volume. Pulmonary edema occurs as a result of the supranormal LVEDP necessary to maintain an adequate cardiac output (Fig. 1-2).

Systolic dysfunction is associated with the following symptoms:

1. Fatigue: most common presenting symptom secondary to decreased cardiac output to skeletal muscle
2. Dyspnea: secondary to pulmonary congestion when pulmonary venous pressure is greater than 20 mm Hg, which results in transudative leakage of fluid into the pulmonary parenchyma
3. Decreased mental acuity and urine output: result of diminished forward flow to cerebral and kidney circulation
4. Paroxysmal nocturnal dyspnea and orthopnea: fluid from gravity-dependent portions of the body are redistributed

TABLE 1-1 Major Contributors to Systolic Dysfunction

Impaired Contractility	Pressure Overload
Ischemic heart disease	Uncontrolled hypertension
Myocardial infarction	Aortic stenosis
Chronic volume overload	
Aortic regurgitation	
Mitral regurgitation	
Ventricular septal defect	
Arteriovenous shunting	
Dilated cardiomyopathy	
Viral myocarditis	
Cocaine, alcohol abuse	
Toxins, chemotherapy	
Idiopathic	
Chronic high-output states	
Anemia	
Thyrotoxicosis	
Beri-beri	

into intravascular circulation when recumbent, resulting in increased intracardiac filling pressures

5. Abdominal distension: elevated right-sided filling pressures cause hepatic swelling and intestinal edema
6. Peripheral edema and weight gain: fluid retention due to neuroendocrine mechanisms and elevated right-sided pressures cause accumulation of interstitial fluid

Physical findings of systolic dysfunction are different for left- and right-sided heart failure:

Left-sided heart failure:

1. Enlarged point of maximal impulse in dilated cardiomyopathy
2. Sustained point of maximal impulse in pressure-overloaded states (aortic stenosis or HTN)
3. Cool extremities, mild cyanosis, and poor capillary refill secondary to poor cardiac output
4. Tachycardia and tachypnea due to high sympathetic tone
5. Cheyne-Stokes breathing: hyperventilation followed by temporary cessation of breathing due to increased circulation time between lungs and central nervous system (CNS) respiratory centers.
6. Pulmonary rhonchi and rales occur if left atrial pressure is greater than 20 mm Hg
7. Third heart sound occurs during early diastole, during rapid ventricular filling phase: suggestive of pathologic increase in diastolic ventricular filling due to fluid overload
8. Fourth heart sound: produced by contraction of atria in late diastole and occurs when the atrial-augmented filling enters a pathologically stiffened ventricle

Right-sided heart failure:

1. Elevated jugular venous pulsation with prominent V wave and steep Y descent
2. Peripheral edema
3. Enlarged liver span from hepatic enlargement
4. Ascites
5. Hepatojugular reflux

Treatment of systolic dysfunction involves the following:

1. Diuretics reduce intravascular volume, which results in a decreased LV preload. Decreased LV preload results in a lower LVEDP, which then falls below the range that can cause pulmonary congestion and edema.

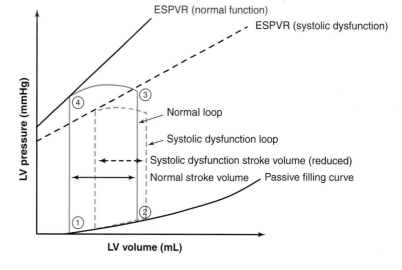

Figure 1-1. A pressure-volume loop is a plot of the LV pressure versus the LV volume and represents the cardiac cycle in a counter-clockwise direction. The width between the two vertical lines of the loop represents the stroke volume, and the area enclosed by the loop represents the cardiac output. In systolic dysfunction, the end-systolic pressure volume relationship is shifted downward and the end-diastolic volume as well as pressure (represented by point 2) increases. Both of these changes decrease the stroke volume as well as cardiac output. *ESPVR,* end-systolic pressure volume loop.

① Mitral valve opens
① → ② Diastolic filling
② Mitral valve closes (end-diastolic volume/pressure)
② → ③ Isovolumic LV contraction
③ Aortic valve opens
④ Aortic valve closes (end-systolic volume)
④ → ① Isovolumic LV relaxation

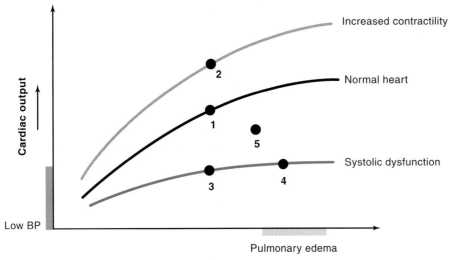

1 Normal patient
2 Normal patient on dopamine (↑ cardiac output at same LVEDP)
3 Systolic dysfunction patient with hypotension
4 Systolic dysfunction patient with fluid overload (↑ LVEDP)
   but no ↑ in cardiac output: patient remains hypotensive with
   pulmonary edema
5 Systolic dysfunction patient on positive inotropes and diuresis

• **Figure 1-2.** The Frank-Starling response is the observation that the cardiac output increases as a function of the LV end-diastolic pressure. The response to an increase in preload is a greater stroke volume on the subsequent systolic contraction. Positive inotropes, such as dopamine, shift the Frank-Starling response curve upward so that a given LV end-diastolic pressure produces a greater cardiac output. In systolic dysfunction, the Frank-Starling curve is shifted downward so that a given LV end-diastolic pressure results in a lesser cardiac output. *LVEDP*, left ventricular end-diastolic pressure.

2. Inotropes: Digoxin, beta-agonists (dopamine, dobutamine), and phosphodiesterase inhibitors (milrinone) increase the stroke volume, cardiac output, and actual contractility at any given preload.
3. Nitrates: Venous vasodilators decrease LV preload by increasing venous capacitance.
4. Angiotensin-converting enzyme (ACE) inhibitors reduce systemic vascular resistance by inhibiting the formation of vasoconstrictor angiotensin II, and thereby decreasing LV afterload. Decreased afterload results in increased stroke volume at any given end-diastolic volume. ACE inhibitors also affect the neuroendocrine response by decreasing the formation of aldosterone, which then accelerates the elimination of sodium with a concomitant reduction in intravascular volume.
5. Angiotensin receptor blockers (ARBs) reduce systemic vascular resistance by blocking the angiotensin receptor, and thereby decreasing LV afterload.
6. Hydralazine and nitroprusside are both direct-acting arterial vasodilators that decrease LV afterload, resulting in an augmented stroke volume for a given preload.

Diastolic Dysfunction

Left ventricular diastolic dysfunction is present when there is clinical evidence of heart failure in the presence of normal ejection fraction. Up to one third of patients with heart failure symptoms have preserved systolic function and present with heart failure secondary to diastolic dysfunction.

Pathophysiologic conditions associated with diastolic dysfunction include ischemic conditions such as myocardial ischemia, LV hypertrophy secondary to HTN or aortic stenosis, hypertrophic cardiomyopathy, diabetes, restrictive processes such as endocardial fibrosis or external radiation, or infiltrative processes such as sarcoidosis, amyloidosis, or hemochromatosis. In diastolic heart failure, the LV has decreased compliance (increased chamber stiffness) and cannot fill at normal diastolic pressures. As a result, there is reduced LV volume, leading to decreased stroke volume and cardiac output. In addition, the greater than normal LV diastolic filling pressure results in pulmonary and systemic congestion (Fig. 1-3).

Initial treatment of congestive heart failure (CHF) secondary to diastolic dysfunction is similar to that of patients with systolic dysfunction. Treatments include supplemental oxygen, diuresis, intravenous (IV) nitroglycerin, and morphine. Long-term treatment of diastolic heart failure is aimed at (*a*) reducing afterload by controlling HTN; (*b*) preventing myocardial ischemia; (*c*) avoiding tachycardia and promoting bradycardia; (*d*) improving ventricular relaxation; and (*e*) decreasing activation of the renin-angiotensin-aldosterone system.

Unlike with systolic dysfunction, patients with heart failure secondary to diastolic dysfunction do not tolerate positive inotropic drugs such as milrinone, beta-agonists (dobutamine, dopamine), and digoxin. Because the ejection fraction is already preserved, positive inotropes have little benefit and may worsen underlying myocardial ischemia. In addition, beta-agonists promote tachycardia that can worsen diastolic dysfunction. The benefits of bradycardia include (*a*) increased coronary perfusion time; (*b*) decreased myocardial oxygen requirements; and (*c*) lower ventricular diastolic pressure and improved filling from more complete relaxation between beats.

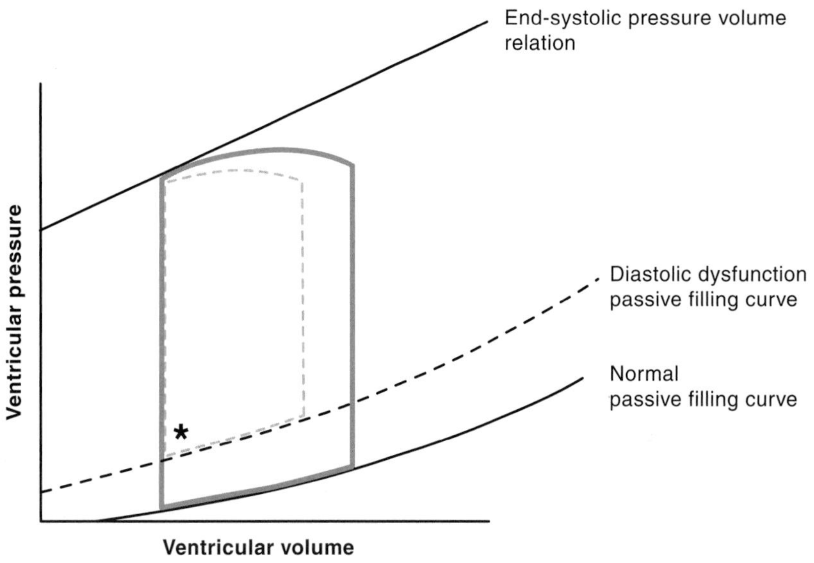

Figure 1-3. Diastolic dysfunction loop. Normal pressure volume loop is indicated by the *thick black loop,* while the pressure volume loop of diastolic dysfunction is indicated by the *dotted loop.* In diastolic dysfunction, the passive filling curve of the left ventricle is shifted upward so that at any diastolic volume, the ventricular pressure is greater than normal. As a result, the end-diastolic volume (*star*) is also reduced due to the reduced filling of the ventricle during diastole.

CASE CONCLUSION

AHF presents with systolic heart failure and dilated cardiomyopathy secondary to poorly controlled HTN. In addition, preexisting coronary artery disease contributes to decreased LV compliance and elevated diastolic filling pressures. His weight gain is secondary to fluid retention and his RUQ pain/hepatomegaly is the result of hepatic congestion from elevated right-sided filling pressures. His fatigue is the result of decreased cardiac output, and his orthopnea is secondary to redistribution of fluid from the extremities to the intravascular compartment. His elevated JVP is suggestive of a fluid-overloaded state. The elevated creatinine is secondary to inadequate renal perfusion secondary to poor cardiac output. His hyperadrenergic state leading to increased SVR and fluid overload contributes to his hypertensive presentation (remember BP = CO × SVR). His normal troponin and ECG without ischemia suggest that acute ischemia is an unlikely cause for his CHF exacerbation. After aggressive diuresis and afterload reduction with ACE inhibitors, his symptoms markedly improve.

THUMBNAIL: Pharmacologic Management of Systolic Heart Failure

Drug Class	Examples
Renin-angiotensin aldosterone inhibitors	ACE inhibitors → captopril Angiotensin receptor blockers → losartan Aldosterone antagonists → spironolactone
Beta-blockers	Cardioselective → metoprolol Nonselective with vasodilating properties → carvedilol
Digitalis	Digoxin
Vasodilators	Calcium channel blockers → amlodipine Nitrates Hydralazine Nitroprusside
Positive inotropic agents	Dobutamine, dopamine Phosphodiesterase inhibitors → milrinone
Diuretics	Thiazide diuretics → hydrochlorothiazide, metolazone Loop diuretics → furosemide Aldosterone antagonists → spironolactone

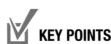 **THUMBNAIL:** Treatment of Left-Sided Diastolic Dysfunction

Goals of Therapy	Therapeutic Intervention
Prevent ischemia	Bypass surgery, angioplasty, nitrates, beta-blockers
Reduce fluid overloads	Diuretics, salt restriction, dialysis
Control HTN	Beta-blockers, ACE inhibitors, angiotensin II, receptor blockers, calcium channel blockers
Decrease neurohormonal activation	Beta-blockers, ACE inhibitors, spironolactone
Improve ventricular relaxation	Beta-blockers, calcium channel blockers
Prevent tachycardia	Beta-blockers, calcium channel blockers

KEY POINTS

- Cardiac output = heart rate × stroke volume
- Blood pressure = cardiac output × systemic vascular resistance
- Most common causes of systolic dysfunction in the United States are uncontrolled HTN, ischemic heart disease, and alcoholic cardiomyopathy
- Three compensatory mechanisms for systolic dysfunction are ventricular hypertrophy, neuroendocrine response, and the Frank-Starling response

- Diastolic dysfunction is defined as clinical evidence of heart failure in patients with normal systolic ejection fraction
- Decreased LV compliance in diastolic dysfunction is the underlying abnormality in diastolic dysfunction
- Although the treatments for systolic dysfunction and diastolic dysfunction are similar, the major difference is that the use of positive inotropes in diastolic dysfunction is relatively contraindicated

QUESTIONS

1. Which of the following pathophysiologic processes results in a concentric hypertrophy rather than eccentric hypertrophy?

   A. Aortic regurgitation
   B. Mitral regurgitation
   C. Aortic stenosis
   D. Ventricular septal defect
   E. Atrial septal defect

2. The most effective agent for acutely decreasing LV preload is:

   A. ACE inhibitors
   B. Hydralazine
   C. Nitroprusside
   D. IV nitrates
   E. Angiotensin receptor blockers

3. A 74-year-old man with a history of hypertensive heart disease will be discharged today after a 2-day stay for management of his CHF secondary to presumptive diastolic dysfunction. Which one of the following treatments would

be least effective in the long-term management of his heart failure?

   A. Furosemide
   B. Digoxin
   C. Verapamil
   D. Atenolol
   E. Lisinopril

4. Although beta-blockers are traditionally contraindicated in heart failure secondary to systolic dysfunction, this class of medications is considered beneficial in diastolic dysfunction. The modification of which parameter does not contribute to the beneficial effects of beta-blockers in diastolic dysfunction?

   A. Increasing diastolic filling time
   B. Decreasing myocardial oxygen demand
   C. Improved LV filling secondary to improved relaxation
   D. Decreasing risk of myocardial ischemia
   E. Increasing LV outflow gradient

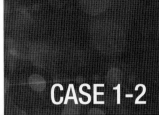

CASE 1-2 Acute Coronary Syndromes

HPI: JM is a 67-year-old man with cardiac risk factors of cigarette smoking, diabetes, and positive family history. He called 911 after 2 hours of prolonged chest pain associated with dyspnea and diaphoresis. In the emergency department, he is profoundly hypotensive and hypoxic. He is emergently intubated and started on IV dopamine for BP support.

PE: Vitals: BP 80/50 mm Hg, HR 130 beats/min, Tmax 38.1°C, RR 24 breaths/min (on ventilator). **General:** Cool, clammy, cyanotic, intubated. **H/N:** JVP 12 cm, markedly decreased carotid upstroke. **Chest:** Bilateral crackles diffusely. **Cardiac:** Dyskinetic apical impulse with positive S_3 and S_4, 4/6 systolic murmur at base radiating laterally. **Extremities:** Cool with decreased peripheral pulses, mild peripheral edema. **Chest x-ray (CXR):** Endotracheal tube in good position, marked CHF, normal cardiac silhouette. **ECG:** 4 mm ST elevation in V_1 to V_4.

Labs: Hematocrit (Hct) 41.0, white blood cell count (WBC) 11 K/mm^3, total creatinine kinase (CK) 40 U/L, creatinine kinase myocardial band fraction (CK MB) 1%, troponin I <0.05 mg/mL.

THOUGHT QUESTIONS

- What are the differences between unstable angina, non-ST elevation myocardial infarction (MI), and ST elevation MI?
- What are the pathologic differences between non-ST elevation MI and ST elevation MI?
- What are nonatherosclerotic causes for myocardial ischemia and infarction?
- What are common complications of MI?

BASIC SCIENCE REVIEW AND DISCUSSION

Acute coronary syndrome (ACS) is a broad term that describes all conditions that result from a sudden impairment in blood flow leading to myocardial ischemia. ACS can be subdivided into three categories of increasing severity: (1) unstable angina (USA); (2) non-ST elevation myocardial infarction (NSTEMI); and (3) ST elevation myocardial infarction (STEMI). In contrast to NSTEMI and STEMI, biochemical markers (troponin, CK MB) remain negative in USA because no irreversible myocardial necrosis has occurred. STEMI is clinically differentiated from NSTEMI by the ECG pattern; STEMI is associated with ST elevation and/or new Q waves, while NSTEMI is associated with ST depressions and/or T wave inversions (Fig. 1-4).

NSTEMI and STEMI also relate pathologically to the degree of necrosis within the myocardial wall. NSTEMI is limited to subendocardial infarcts that involve the innermost layers of the myocardium. These inner layers of myocardium are the most susceptible to ischemia because they have the fewest collateral vessels and are subjected to the highest left ventricular wall pressure. STEMI is the most emergent ACS condition because persistent total occlusion results in transmural infarction spanning the entire thickness of the myocardium.

Although ACS is clinically subclassified into three categories, ACS also can be regarded as a clinical continuum, with all three syndromes sharing the underlying pathophysiology of compromised blood flow secondary to plaque disruption and thrombus formation. Over 85% of ACS is secondary to formation of an acute thrombus obstructing an atherosclerotic artery. The remaining 15% of ACS is secondary to nonatherosclerotic causes, including (a) coronary artery spasm (primary, such as Prinzmetal angina or cocaine induced); (b) markedly increased myocardial oxygen demand (e.g., aortic stenosis); (c) increased blood viscosity (e.g., polycythemia vera); (d) vasculitis; and (e) anomalous coronary anatomy.

In atherosclerotic ACS, the 75% of thrombi are precipitated by mechanical rupture of the plaque, and 25% are secondary to superficial erosion of the endothelium covering the plaque. Once a plaque ruptures, subendothelial collagen activates platelet aggregation and the coagulation cascade via the extrinsic pathway. Activated platelets release (a) adenosine diphosphate (ADP), which promotes further platelet aggregation; and (b) thromboxane A_2, which can induce vasospasm and further decrease in blood flow. Vasospasm is further potentiated by damaged endothelium that is unable to produce vasodilating substances, such as nitric oxide and prostacyclin.

Cellular and histopathologic changes occur immediately with the onset of oxygen deprivation as outlined in Table 1-2.

Clinical Presentation and Diagnosis of Acute Coronary Syndrome

The clinical presentation of ACS includes the typical substernal chest pressure that is often referred to the C7–T4 dermatomes, which includes the neck, shoulders, and arms. However, up to 20% of patients remain asymptomatic during ACS. Atypical or asymptomatic presentations are more common in diabetics secondary to their peripheral neuropathy, as well as in elderly patients and women. Other symptoms and physical findings are summarized in Table 1-3.

In addition to the clinical signs/symptoms and ECG findings, serum biochemical markers are released into the circulation in STEMI and NSTEMI (but not in USA). The two most widely used biochemical markers include (a) CK and the cardiac-specific isoenzyme CK MB; and (b) troponin. Both markers begin to rise at 4 to 6 hours and peak at 24 hours, but troponin remains elevated for up to 10 days while CK returns to baseline after 48 hours. Other noncardiac specific markers that are elevated in STEMI and NSTEMI include serum glutamic oxaloacetic transaminase (SGOT), lactate dehydrogenase (LDH), and myoglobin (Fig. 1-5).

Complications of Acute Coronary Syndrome

Complications of ACS can be subdivided into arrhythmic and nonarrhythmic categories as outlined in Table 1-4. Ventricular fibrillation is the most common reason for sudden cardiac death associated with MI.

Nomenclature of Acute Coronary Syndrome (ACS)

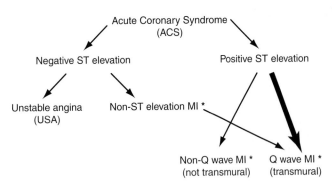

* = positive cardiac marker

• **Figure 1-4.** Acute coronary syndrome is divided into three categories: (1) unstable angina (USA), (2) non-ST elevation myocardial infarction (NSTEMI), and (3) ST-elevation myocardial infarction (STEMI). In USA, no myocardial necrosis has occurred and biochemical markers (troponin, CK MB) remain negative. In NSTEMI and STEMI, myocardial necrosis has occurred and biochemical markers are released. The majority of NSTEMI become non-Q wave MI, which is limited to partial myocardial thickness (nontransmural), but a minority of NSTEMI evolve into Q wave MI, which involve the entire myocardial thickness (transmural). Conversely, the majority of STEMI become Q wave MI, involving the entire thickness of the myocardium, but a small fraction evolve into non-Q wave MI, which involve only a partial thickness of the myocardium.

Treatment of Acute Coronary Syndromes

Patients with USA or NSTEMI should be stratified using TIMI (Thrombolysis in Myocardial Infarction study) risk scores, to assess risk for MI, urgent revascularization, or death. The TIMI

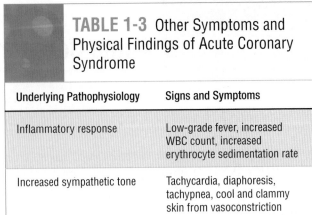

TABLE 1-3 Other Symptoms and Physical Findings of Acute Coronary Syndrome

Underlying Pathophysiology	Signs and Symptoms
Inflammatory response	Low-grade fever, increased WBC count, increased erythrocyte sedimentation rate
Increased sympathetic tone	Tachycardia, diaphoresis, tachypnea, cool and clammy skin from vasoconstriction
Increased vagal tone (more common in inferior MI)	Nausea and vomiting, weakness, sinus bradycardia
Decreased LV contractility and compliance	Pulmonary rales and CHF Elevated jugular venous pressure Dyskinetic cardiac impulse S_4 from atrial contraction into noncompliant ischemic LV S_3 from rapid filling in failing LV
Ischemia-induced papillary muscle dysfunction	Ischemia-induced mitral regurgitation

WBC, white blood cell; *MI*, myocardial infarction; *LV*, left ventricular; *CHF*, congestive heart failure

risk score takes into account known coronary artery disease (CAD), CAD risk factors, age, recent acetylsalicylic acid (ASA) use, elevated cardiac markers, recent severe angina, and ST deviation on ECG. In general, the treatment for USA and NSTEMI is medical and includes beta-blockers, aspirin, nitrates, and heparin. However, in STEMI with complete and prolonged occlusion of a coronary artery, the goal of treatment is reperfusion by means of angioplasty or thrombolysis (Table 1-5).

TABLE 1-2 Cellular and Histopathologic Changes with the Onset of Oxygen Deprivation

Feature	Time after MI
Onset of ATP depletion	seconds
Loss of contractility	<2 min
Irreversible cell injury	20–40 min
Microvascular injury (seen in light microscope)	1–2 h
Beginning of coagulation necrosis, edema, focal hemorrhage	6 h
Hyperemic border with central yellow-brown softening	3–7 days
Fibrosis and scarring	7 wk

ATP, adenosine triphosphate

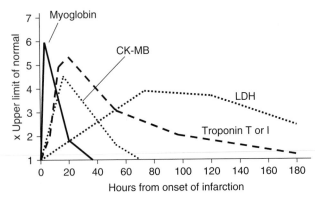

• **Figure 1-5.** Serum markers of myocardial injury. (Reprinted with permission from Awtry EH, Gururaj AV, Maytin M, et al. Blueprints in Cardiology. Malden, MA: Blackwell Science, 1003:69.)

TABLE 1-4 Complications of Acute Coronary Syndrome

Arrhythmia	Pathophysiology
Ventricular fibrillation Ventricular tachycardia	Electrical instability secondary to ischemia
Sinus bradycardia	Excessive vagal output Ischemia of SA node
Sinus tachycardia	Increased sympathetic output, pain, CHF
Atrial fibrillation	Atrial ischemia, CHF-induced atrial stretch
1st-, 2nd-, or 3rd-degree heart block	Ischemia of SA node Ischemia of AV node (usually seen in inferior MI with occlusion of right coronary artery) Excessive vagal output

Nonarrhythmic Complication	Pathophysiology
Cardiogenic shock	Decreased cardiac output secondary to ischemia-induced decrease in contractility
CHF	Decreased contractility → systolic dysfunction Increased myocardial stiffness → diastolic dysfunction
Pericarditis	Occurs in 10% of patients post-MI Inflammation extending to pericardium and epicardium
Mitral regurgitation	Ischemia-induced papillary muscle dysfunction
Ventricular septal defect	Myocyte necrosis/softening of ventricular septum
Rupture of LV free wall	Myocyte necrosis/softening of LV wall with hemorrhage into pericardial space and tamponade
Pseudoaneurysm of LV free wall	Myocyte necrosis/softening of LV free wall with incomplete rupture secondary to thrombus formation within transmural defect
Aneurysm of LV	Myocyte necrosis and fibrosis with bulging of LV wall Akinetic aneurysm predisposes patient to formation of mural thrombus and subsequent systemic embolization

SA, sinoatrial; *CHF,* congestive heart failure; *AV,* atrioventricular; *MI,* myocardial infarction; *LV,* left ventricular

TABLE 1-5 Etiology and Treatment

Pathophysiologic Etiology	Treatment
Mechanical obstruction	Angioplasty/stenting or coronary bypass surgery Thrombolysis
Dynamic obstruction/spasm (Prinzmetal angina)	Nitrates Calcium channel blockers
Thrombosis	Heparin, low molecular-weight heparin Direct thrombin inhibitors Aspirin, clopidogrel (ADP receptor inhibitor) IIb/IIIa receptor antagonists
Increased oxygen demand	Beta-blockers, supplemental oxygen Nitrates, morphine, transfusion if anemic
Inflammation	Statins, aspirin

CASE CONCLUSION

JM is in cardiogenic shock from an ST elevation MI secondary to an occlusion of his proximal left anterior descending (LAD) artery (ST elevation is in LAD distribution). His profound hypotension and CHF is secondary to two processes: (1) ischemic systolic dysfunction; and (2) ischemia-induced papillary muscle rupture, resulting in a flail mitral leaflet (4/6 murmur on exam). Although his clinical presentation, low-grade fever, leukocytosis, and ECG are consistent with ST elevation MI, the troponin and CK were negative on admission because 4 to 6 hours must elapse from infarction onset before significant elevation of these biochemical markers may be observed. JM subsequently developed ventricular fibrillation requiring electrical defibrillation before he was brought to the cardiac catheterization laboratory, where his LAD artery was successfully opened with angioplasty and stenting.

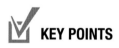

THUMBNAIL: Summary of Acute Coronary Syndromes

Syndrome	ECG Findings	Biochemical Markers	Treatment	Coronary Lesion	Myocardial Lesion
ST elevation MI	ST elevation New Q waves	Positive troponin or CK MB	Angioplasty Thrombolysis Aspirin Oxygen Beta-blockers Nitrates	Persistent thrombotic total occlusion	Transmural MI
Non-ST elevation MI	ST depression wave inversion No ST elevation No new Q wave	Positive troponin or CK MB	Aspirin, Heparin Beta-blockers Oxygen Nitrates	Transient thrombotic total occlusion or thrombotic severe stenosis	Partial-thickness MI
Unstable angina	ST depression T wave inversion No ST elevation No new Q wave	Negative troponin or CK MB	Aspirin, Heparin Beta-blockers Oxygen, Nitrates	Transient thrombotic total occlusion or thrombotic severe stenosis	Myocardium at ischemic risk

KEY POINTS

- All three subcategories of ACS (USA, NSTEMI, and STEMI) share the same underlying pathophysiology (rupture or erosion of a vulnerable plaque)
- Biochemical markers (troponin and CK) are not elevated in USA but are elevated in MI (NSTEMI and STEMI)
- Patients with USA or NSTEMI should be stratified using TIMI risk scores

- While the treatment for USA and NSTEMI is medical stabilization with aspirin, heparin, beta-blockers, oxygen, and nitrates, the management of STEMI is immediate reperfusion with angioplasty or thrombolysis
- Ventricular fibrillation is the most common cause of sudden cardiac death within the first 24 hours of myocardial ischemia: therefore, telemetry (constant ECG monitoring) is essential for all patients admitted for acute coronary syndromes

QUESTIONS

1. JF is an 80-year-old male diabetic who is a very poor historian. His family escorts him to your emergency room because he complained of an episode of acute dyspnea 8 days ago. His ECG is now normal, but you are concerned that JF may have had an NSTEMI-induced CHF episode 8 days ago. Which biochemical test would be the most helpful to determine whether or not he had an infarct 8 days ago?

   A. CK
   B. SGOT
   C. Troponin I
   D. LDH
   E. Myoglobin

2. A 58-year-old man presents with chest pain, severe nausea, elevated JVP, pulsatile liver, severe bradycardia degenerating into third-degree heart block, with ST elevation in the inferior leads (II, III, aVF). Despite his severe hypotension with a blood pressure of 70/30 mm Hg, his lungs are clear and there is no evidence of heart failure. On angiography, which vessel is the most likely culprit vessel?

   A. LAD artery
   B. Circumflex artery
   C. Diagonal artery
   D. Right coronary artery
   E. Obtuse marginal artery

CASE 1-3　Valvular Heart Disease

HPI: AB is a 76-year-old Asian man who presents with new-onset syncope. He denies palpitations or angina but experiences dyspnea with mild exertion and early fatigue. His past medical history is notable for diabetes, HTN, and a severe childhood febrile illness with associated sore throat. AB has also experienced a persistent cardiac murmur since the childhood illness.

PE: Vitals: Temperature (T) 37.0°C; HR 70 beats/min; BP 160/80 mm Hg; RR 16 breaths/min, JVP 7 cm with slow carotid upstroke and decreased carotid volume. **Chest:** Clear to auscultation. **Cardiac:** Sustained enlarged PMI with late-peaking 4/6 systolic murmur at right sternal border radiating into the neck and single second heart sound. Opening snap (OS) present after S_2 with a 2/4 diastolic decrescendo murmur. **Extremities:** No edema. **CXR:** Mild cardiomegaly. **ECG:** Normal sinus rhythm with LV hypertrophy.

THOUGHT QUESTIONS

- How is the diagnosis of rheumatic fever (RF) established?
- What are the three symptoms typically associated with aortic stenosis (AS)?
- How does the left ventricle (LV) adapt to AS versus aortic regurgitation (AR)?
- What physical findings are associated with severe AR?
- What are the hemodynamic consequences of acute versus chronic mitral regurgitation (MR)?

BASIC SCIENCE REVIEW AND DISCUSSION

Rheumatic Heart Disease

RF is secondary to untreated group A streptococcus (GAS) pharyngitis. RF is an inflammatory condition involving primarily the connective tissue of the heart, joints, and CNS. The pathogenesis is unclear but is thought to be secondary to an autoimmune response between rheumatogenic streptococcal antigens and human tissue epitopes. The diagnosis of an acute initial attack is summarized in Table 1-6. After establishing evidence of a previous GAS infection by throat culture or rising GAS antibody titers, the presence of two major manifestations or one major and two minor manifestations suggests diagnosis of RF.

RF carditis involves all three layers of the heart (endocardium, myocardium, and pericardium) and is almost always associated with a valvulitis involving the mitral and aortic valves. The median age for RF is 9 to 11 years. During the initial RF attack, MR is the most common valvular manifestation, with AR the second most common. The pulmonic and tricuspid valves are rarely involved. The symptoms of rheumatic valve scarring do not usually become apparent until 10 to 30 years after the initial RF episode.

Although the prevalence is only 0.6 per 1000 U.S. school-aged children, it is the most common acquired heart disease in children and young adults worldwide (up to 21 per 1000 Asian school-aged children). Treatment of GAS pharyngitis virtually eliminates the risk for progression to RF, but up to 3% of untreated GAS pharyngitis may progress to RF after a 3-week latency period. Treatment of the acute RF episode is largely supportive, with salicylates or steroids to decrease inflammation and penicillin to treat residual GAS. After the initial attack of RF, the patient is at risk for recurrent RF attacks and therefore requires long-term continuous antibiotic prophylaxis (10 years to lifelong depending on residual valvular disease).

Aortic Stenosis

AS is the most common valve lesion in the United States. There are three forms of AS: (1) congenital/bicuspid; (2) rheumatic/postinflammatory; and (3) senile/degenerative. The etiology of AS depends on the patient's age group (Table 1-7). Both diabetes and hypercholesterolemia are risk factors for degenerative AS, and degenerative AS is associated with HTN and smoking.

In AS, the increased resistance across the aortic valve imposes a chronic pressure overload on the LV. To compensate for the pressure overload, the LV hypertrophies (increases in thickness) in order to decrease LV wall stress according to the law of Laplace:

$$\text{Stress} = \frac{\text{Pressure} \times \text{Radius}}{2 \times \text{Thickness}}$$

However, with progressive LV hypertrophy, abnormal pathophysiologic mechanisms set in with resulting reduced LV compliance and increased left ventricular end-diastolic pressure (LVEDP), left atrial (LA) hypertrophy, decreased coronary blood flow, and increased myocardial oxygen demand (from increased muscle mass, increased wall stress, and decreased perfusion pressure gradient between the aorta and subendocardium). Eventual CHF may result secondary to insurmountable afterload and subsequent LV dilatation and systolic dysfunction.

AS presents as a gradual disease and, unlike with mitral stenosis (MS), patients usually remain well compensated and asymptomatic for many years. The four common AS-associated clinical presentations are angina secondary to increased oxygen demand, syncope during exercise due to reduced cerebral perfusion in the setting of fixed cardiac output and increased systemic vasodilatation, heart failure secondary to LV dilatation and decreased systolic function, and gastrointestinal (GI) bleeding (idiopathic or angiodysplasia of the right colon). The latency period from the onset of severe symptoms to the average age of death is approximately 5 years for angina, 3 years for syncope, and 2 years for CHF.

On physical exam, arterial pulse rises slowly, is sustained, and is small in volume. Cardiac impulse is sustained and will become inferolaterally displaced with LV dilatation and failure. A systolic thrill may be appreciated upon palpation of the precordium. Upon auscultation, S_1 is normal and S_2 may be single, although a prolonged LV systolic phase may also result in paradoxical splitting with P_2 before A_2. S_4 may also be present because atrial contraction is increased. The systolic AS murmur is mid-peaking, loudest at the base, and transmitted cranially along both carotid

TABLE 1-6 Diagnosis of an Acute Initial Attack

Major Manifestations	Minor Manifestations
Carditis	Arthralgias
Polyarthritis	Fever
Chorea marginatum	Increased acute phase reactants (ESR, C-reactive erythema protein)
Subcutaneous nodules	Prolonged PR interval

ESR, erythrocyte sedimentation rate

TABLE 1-8 Etiology of Aortic Regurgitation

Causes of Acute AR	Causes of Chronic AR
Bacterial endocarditis Blunt chest trauma Aortic dissection	Connective tissue disorders (most common causes of chronic AR): Marfan, Ehlers-Danlos, osteogenesis imperfecta Blunt chest trauma Aortic dissection Bacterial endocarditis Congenital (bicuspid aortic valve, coarctation) Degenerative calcific disease of aortic valve Antiphospholipid syndrome Drugs (dexfenfluramine/phentermine)

vessels. Occasionally, high-frequency components radiate to the apex and may be confused for MR (Gallavardin phenomenon).

Symptomatic candidates with severe AS should avoid vigorous physical activity and should be referred to surgery because medical management has little influence on the disease course. Indications for surgery are severe AS (aortic valve area [AVA] ≤0.9 cm²) with symptoms secondary to AS or asymptomatic patients with progressive LV dysfunction or hypotensive response to exercise. In asymptomatic patients without indications for surgery, the three components of medical therapy include digoxin, diuretics, and beta-blockers.

Aortic Regurgitation

The etiology of AR can be classified into acute versus chronic processes (Table 1-8). In acute-onset AR, the LV is unable to adapt to the sudden increase in volume. As a result, there is an immediate rise in LVEDP and premature mitral valve closure. Premature mitral valve closure prevents LA emptying, and the increased LVEDP is transmitted to the atrium and pulmonary vasculature, resulting in dyspnea and pulmonary edema.

In chronic AR, the LV undergoes both dilatation (in response to volume overload) and hypertrophy (in response to pressure overload). Dilatation increases LV compliance and permits the LV to accommodate a large regurgitant fraction and increasing preload. With the increased LV stroke volume and large regurgitant fraction, patients with AR have a large difference between systolic and diastolic pressure (pulse pressure). While chronic AR is well tolerated, prolonged exposure of the LV to pressure and fluid overload leads to LV dilatation, myocardial fibrosis, systolic dysfunction, and CHF symptoms. Angina occurs secondary to decreased aortic perfusion pressure and increased myocardial oxygen demand.

Physical findings are notable for the following:

1. Auscultation—diastolic high-pitched murmur is loudest over the third intercostal space along the left sternal border (LSB). The murmur radiates apically and is loudest with the patient in an upright position. The Austin-Flint murmur (secondary to vibration of a prematurely and partially closed mitral valve by rapid LA inflow) is a mid- to late-diastolic rumble that is observed in moderate to severe, chronic AR and can mimic MS.
2. "Waterhammer" or Corrigan pulse—widened pulse pressure.
3. Traube sign—auscultation of femoral artery reveals "pistol shot" sounds secondary to arterial wall vibrations.
4. Duroziez sign—auscultation of partially compressed femoral artery reveals a systolic and diastolic "to and fro" murmur secondary to the regurgitant volume.
5. Quincke sign—alternating capillary filling and emptying of the nail beds with partial compression.
6. Bisferiens morphology of carotid pulse—a slight dip during the carotid upstroke secondary to a Venturi effect-induced temporary depression of the systolic pressure.
7. Hyperdynamic LV apical impulse.

In chronic asymptomatic AR, the goal of treatment is to decrease afterload with vasodilators such as hydralazine, nifedipine, or ACE inhibitors. Adjunctive therapy for CHF symptoms includes digitalis, nitrates, and diuretics. Aortic valve replacement should be considered for the following indications: (a) onset of angina or dyspnea; (b) objective evidence of decreased exercise tolerance; and (c) in asymptomatic patients, evidence of LV dysfunction at rest (decreased LV ejection fraction or progressive LV chamber dilatation).

Pulmonic Stenosis

Pulmonic stenosis is usually a congenital malformation or secondary to carcinoid syndrome. The stenotic pulmonic valve causes right ventricle (RV) pressure overload and hypertrophy. Associated

TABLE 1-7 Causes of Aortic Stenosis

Younger Than 70 Years	Older Than 70 Years
50% Bicuspid	48% Degenerative
25% Postinflammatory	27% Bicuspid
18% Degenerative	23% Postinflammatory
3% Unicommissural	2% Unknown
2% Hypoplastic	
2% Unknown	

symptoms include angina, dyspnea, and syncope (if forward flow is severely impeded). Patients usually become symptomatic with gradients of >50 mm Hg. Signs of pulmonic stenosis on physical exam include RV lift secondary to right ventricular hypertrophy (RVH) and a loud systolic ejection murmur preceded by an ejection click (which decreases with inspiration because the valve is passively opened). Percutaneous balloon valvotomy is the procedure of choice in the symptomatic patient or when the gradient exceeds 75 mm Hg.

Pulmonic Regurgitation

Pulmonic regurgitation is often present in severe pulmonary HTN. The classic murmur is a decrescendo murmur at the LSB that is similar to an AR murmur. Treatment is directed toward the underlying cause of pulmonary HTN.

Mitral Stenosis

More than 90% of MS cases are secondary to RF. Other rare causes include systemic lupus erythematosus and carcinoid tumors. Complications of untreated MS include systemic embolism from thrombus, severe pulmonary HTN, endocarditis, and pulmonary edema.

Narrowing of the mitral valve results in increased LA pressure, which is then transmitted retrograde to the pulmonary and right heart circulation. LA HTN results in several pathophysiologic effects:

1. LA enlargement, which increases the risk of atrial fibrillation.
2. Reduced ability of the LA to empty during diastole results in increased stasis of blood within the atrium. Twenty percent of patients diagnosed with MS and not on anticoagulation present with an LA thrombus.
3. Cardiac output is reduced in severe MS and is inversely related to heart rate.
4. Reduced ejection fraction (EF) is noted in one third of patients with MS, due to reduced preload of the left ventricle (LV), scarring of the LV secondary to the rheumatic carditis, and increased afterload from vasoconstriction and neurohormonal activation.
5. In acute, severe MS, elevated pulmonary pressures result in pulmonary edema once LA pressures exceed 25 to 28 mm Hg. With chronic pulmonary HTN, there is reactive narrowing and intimal hyperplasia of the pulmonary circulation, and LA pressures must be much higher than 28 mm Hg to cause pulmonary edema. Prolonged pulmonary HTN results in RVH, RV dilatation, and right-heart failure.

Although severe MS can appear as early as 5 years after an acute RF episode, symptomatic MS usually does not present until several decades after. Dyspnea and fatigue occur secondary to pulmonary edema and decreased cardiac output, respectively. Chest fullness or atypical chest pain may result from pulmonary HTN. RVH and RV failure can lead to peripheral edema. LA enlargement can compress the left main bronchus and induce a cough. Systemic embolization from intra-atrial thrombus and atrial fibrillation are additional presentations.

Physical exam is notable for:

1. RV heave associated with pulmonary hypertension, RVH, and RV dilatation
2. Peripheral edema from right-sided heart failure
3. Malar flush ("mitral valve facies") secondary to systemic vasoconstriction and decreased cardiac output
4. Characteristic auscultation findings include (a) accentuated P_2 associated with pulmonary HTN; (b) loud S_1 secondary

TABLE 1-9 Severity of Mitral Stenosis

Stage	Cross-Sectional Area (cm²)	Symptoms
Minimal	>2.5 cm	None
Mild	1.4–2.5	Minimal dyspnea on exertion, mild fatigue
Moderate	1.0–1.14	Moderate dyspnea on exertion, orthopnea
Severe	<1.0	Dyspnea at rest

to abrupt closure of the mitral valve leaflets that were held wide open by the prolonged transmitral pressure gradient; (c) OS after S_2 secondary to abrupt deceleration of the mitral valve leaflets; and (d) diastolic, rumbling, decrescendo murmur starting with the OS.

Patients should limit exercise to minimize the hemodynamic consequences of MS and may be started on beta-blockers, calcium channel blockers, and/or digoxin to maintain relative bradycardia. Medical treatment also includes anticoagulation for patients with a history of recurrent atrial fibrillation and antibiotic prophylaxis to prevent endocarditis and recurrent RF.

Percutaneous mitral balloon valvotomy is indicated in patients without severe MR, severe mitral valve calcification, and/or thickening (Table 1-9). Surgical options include commissurotomy or mitral valve replacement. Mitral valve replacement is indicated for patients with MS compounded by MR and for patients with severely deformed valves.

Mitral Regurgitation

MR is the second most common valvular lesion in the United States. The mitral valve apparatus includes not only the valve itself but also the chordae tendineae, papillary muscles, and the mitral valve annulus. Malfunction of any of these components can lead to mitral valve regurgitation. The most common cause of MR is myxomatous degeneration mitral valve prolapse followed by ischemic heart disease. Other causes of MR include endocarditis, rheumatic heart disease, collagen vascular disease, chordal rupture, and dexfenfluramine and fenfluramine use.

In acute-onset MR, there is an acute increase in LV preload from both the pathologic regurgitant fraction and the physiologic pulmonary venous inflow. With increased preload, stroke volume is increased by the Frank-Starling mechanism, but because a large fraction of the stroke volume is retrograde, the effective forward cardiac output is decreased. The sudden volume overload within the LV also increases LVEDP, which in turn raises LA pressure and pulmonary artery pressure. Pulmonary edema and dyspnea ensue when LA pressures exceed 25 to 28 mm Hg.

In chronic, compensated MR, the LV adapts to the volume overload by eccentric LV hypertrophy. Thinning of the LV wall also increases LV compliance, permitting the dilated LV to fill during diastole while maintaining a relatively normal LVEDP. LA dilatation also occurs in response to MR. The dilated LA is also more compliant and allows for increased regurgitant volume, but it predisposes to atrial fibrillation. Chronic, compensated MR can degenerate into decompensated MR with LV dilatation and decreased wall thickness, increased LV end-diastolic volume and pressure, and pulmonary congestion and dyspnea.

TABLE 1-10 Provocative Maneuvers		
Maneuver	Hemodynamic Effect	Effect on Murmur Intensity
Handgrip	Increases afterload	MR increases but no change in AS
Premature ventricular contractions	Increased stroke volume	AS increases but no change in MR

MR, mitral regurgitation; *AS*, aortic stenosis

TABLE 1-11 Causes of Tricuspid Regurgitation	
Primary Etiologies	Secondary Etiologies
Bacterial endocarditis	Pulmonary HTN
Trauma	Mitral stenosis
RV infarction	Atrial septal defect/intracardiac shunts
Myxomatous degeneration	LV failure

HTN, hypertension; *RV*, right ventricular; *LV*, left ventricular

Mild to moderate MR or chronic, severe MR may not be symptomatic. On the other hand, in acute MR or chronic, decompensated MR, there is a rise in pressures within the left-sided heart chambers and patients present with symptoms of CHF (dyspnea, orthopnea, and fatigue) secondary to pulmonary congestion and decreased cardiac output.

An apical holosystolic murmur radiates to the axilla in MR and is usually accompanied by S_3. In acute, severe MR the systolic murmur is short and soft because the pressure in the small, noncompliant atrium rises quickly and reduces/shortens the pressure gradient between the LV and LA during systole. The provocative maneuvers outlined in Table 1-10 can be performed to differentiate between AS and MR (both systolic murmurs).

In the hemodynamically stable patient, the medical treatment of choice for acute MR is sodium nitroprusside. As a vasodilator, nitroprusside lowers the afterload, which improves forward cardiac output and decreases the regurgitant fraction. In the hemodynamically unstable patient with severe MR, intra-aortic balloon counterpulsation decreases afterload and helps maintain the diastolic blood pressure. In chronic MR, vasodilator therapy (ACE inhibitors, angiotensin receptor blockers) is also used to augment forward cardiac flow. With the onset of heart failure symptoms, standard CHF therapy is initiated (diuretics and digoxin).

Surgical treatment includes three alternatives: (*1*) mitral valve repair; (*2*) mitral valve replacement with conservation of the mitral valve apparatus; and (*3*) standard mitral valve replacement with no conservation of the mitral valve apparatus. Mitral valve repair is the preferred method of treatment since repair preserves the mitral valve apparatus and obviates the need for anticoagulation or a prosthetic valve. Mitral valve replacement with chordal preservation is preferred if mitral valve function cannot be restored by repair alone (severely deformed rheumatic mitral valve). Although valve competence is ensured, removal of the subvalvular structures damages the LV, with a resultant decrease in LV performance. Surgery should be considered for acute, severe MR or chronic, stable MR

when patients become symptomatic, LV EF is <60%, end-systolic LV dimension is >45 mm, or pulmonary HTN is present.

Tricuspid Stenosis

Tricuspid stenosis is a rare condition caused by rheumatic heart disease or carcinoid syndrome. The stenotic tricuspid valve results in a diastolic rumble across the LSB that increases with inspiration due to increased right heart flow, right atrial (RA) HTN, right-sided failure signs and symptoms (ascites, peripheral edema), and distended neck veins with a large "a" wave because of RA contraction against a stenotic tricuspid valve. A gradient of greater than 5 mm Hg is considered severe, and therapy is required. If diuretics are not effective in relieving the right-sided failure symptoms, tricuspid valvulotomy or surgical valve replacement should be considered.

Tricuspid Regurgitation

The etiologies for **tricuspid regurgitation (TR)** are divided between primary causes and secondary causes (Table 1-11). The most common cause of TR is pulmonary HTN. The most common cause of primary TR is bacterial endocarditis.

Signs and symptoms of TR are fatigue, dyspnea, ascites, peripheral edema, RUQ tenderness and increased liver span from hepatic congestion, soft holosystolic murmur over the LSB that increases with inspiration, RV heave/lift secondary to the enlarged RV, accentuated P_2 if pulmonary HTN is present, and distended neck veins with a prominent V wave (secondary to the regurgitant fraction of blood during systole that is transmitted retrograde from the RV to the RA and then to jugular veins).

Because TR is most often secondary to another cause, treating the underlying cause is the mainstay of therapy. Medical therapy with vasodilators for primary TR has minimal effect since the pulmonary vascular resistance is already low. Tricuspid valve replacement/repair should be considered if the patient has RV failure.

CASE CONCLUSION

AB was admitted, and transthoracic echocardiography documented severe AS with a calculated valve area of 0.6 cm^2 and a peak gradient of 80 mm Hg. Mild MS was also present with a calculated valve area of 1.4 cm^2. Severe LV hypertrophy and mild LV enlargement was also noted. Further questioning determined that he most likely had an episode of acute RF that resulted in both aortic and mitral stenosis. Syncope is one of the three symptoms of critical AS and predicts a 3-year survival period. AB underwent successful aortic valve replacement and mitral valve repair.

THUMBNAIL: Physical Findings in Valvular Heart Disease

Valvular Abnormality	Physical Findings	Auscultation
AS	Sustained apical impulse Nondisplaced apical impulse Delayed upstroke, low volume	Mid-systolic murmur Murmur radiates to neck Single or paradox, split S_2 3rd or 4th heart sounds 2nd right intercostal space Late peaking → more severe
AR	Corrigan's/Waterhammer pulse "Pistol shot" femoral arteries Duroziez's sign (femoral murmur) Quincke's sign (capillary pulsations) Widened pulse pressure	Diastolic regurgitant murmur LSB Radiates to xiphoid Intensity of murmur varies directly with BP Longer murmur lasts in diastole → more severe Best heard with patient upright
Pulmonic stenosis	RVH → RV heave over sternum	Loud systolic ejection click Systolic murmur over LSB
Pulmonic regurgitation	RVG → RV heave over sternum	Decrescendo murmur over LSB
Mitral stenosis	Malar erythema Atrial fibrillation RV lift Peripheral edema	Loud S_1 and OS Diastolic rumble S_2–OS interval shortens with progression of MS Accentuated P_2 in pulmonary HTN
MR	if acute → pulmonary edema if chronic → PMI enlarged and displaced	Holosystolic murmur at apex radiating to axilla S_3 present
Tricuspid stenosis	Ascites Peripheral edema	Diastolic rumbling at LSB Murmur increased with inspiration
Tricuspid regurgitation	Prominent V waves of neck veins Enlarged, pulsatile liver Possible ascites and edema RV sternal lift	Holosystolic murmur at LSB Murmur increased with inspiration

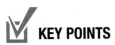 **KEY POINTS**

- Rheumatic heart disease is the most common acquired heart disease in children and young adults worldwide, and it primarily affects the aortic and mitral valves

- In AS, latency period from the onset of severe symptoms to the average age of death is approximately 5 years for angina, 3 years for syncope, and 2 years for CHF

- Acute AR presents as a volume overload phenomenon, while chronic AR is a volume as well as pressure overload situation

- In addition to the hemodynamic consequences, MS places the patient at much higher risk for endocarditis and systemic thromboembolic disease

- MR can result from a defect of not only the valve itself but also from any other components of the mitral valve apparatus (chordae, papillary muscles, or mitral valve annulus)

- The most common cause of TR is pulmonary HTN

QUESTIONS

Please refer to Figures 1-6 through 1-10 for Question 1.

1. A 70-year-old man presents with progressive fatigue and new-onset syncope. On exam, he has a 3/6 mid-peaking systolic murmur at the base that radiates upward but also apically. The second heart sound is paradoxically split, and the murmur does not change with handgrip. The ECG is notable for LV hypertrophy. Cardiac catheterization is performed and two intravascular pressure transducers are placed, one in the LV and one in the ascending aorta. Which of the following hemodynamic tracings is most consistent with the patient's diagnosis?

   A. Tracing 1
   B. Tracing 2
   C. Tracing 3
   D. Tracing 4
   E. Tracing 5

2. An 84-year-old patient has increasing CHF symptoms, angina, and a diastolic, decrescendo murmur. A widened pulse pressure and a "waterhammer" pulse are detected on exam. A transthoracic echocardiogram reveals severe aortic insufficiency with moderate LV enlargement and moderate systolic dysfunction. A recent cardiac catheterization revealed no significant epicardial coronary disease. Which of the following interventions would worsen the patient's condition?

   A. ACE inhibitors
   B. Diuresis
   C. Digoxin
   D. Hydralazine
   E. Beta-blockers

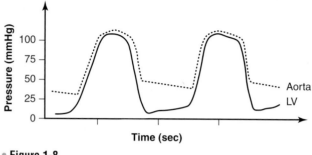

• **Figure 1-8.**

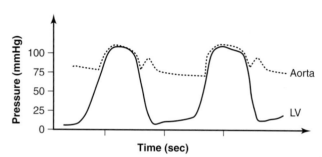

• **Figure 1-9.**

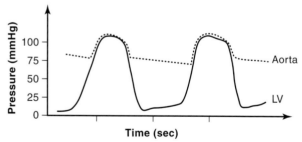

• **Figure 1-6.**

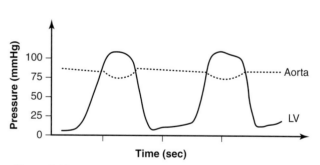

• **Figure 1-10.**

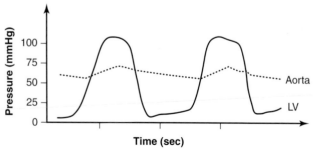

• **Figure 1-7.**

Please refer to Figures 1-11 through 1-15 to answer the following questions.

3. An 80-year-old woman with a history of rheumatic heart disease presents with progressive fatigue and dyspnea on exertion. On exam, she has an RV lift, a diastolic decrescendo murmur, and an extra "snapping" sound after S_2. Her ECG is notable for atrial fibrillation, RVH, and LA enlargement. She appears to have an erythematous rash on her face and peripheral edema. Cardiac catheterization is performed and two intracardiac pressure transducers are placed, one in the LV and one in the LA. Which of the following hemodynamic tracings is most consistent with the patient's diagnosis?

   A. Tracing 1
   B. Tracing 2
   C. Tracing 3
   D. Tracing 4
   E. Tracing 5

4. The patient above underwent a percutaneous procedure to repair the affected valve. After 2 days, she becomes more short of breath and a holosystolic murmur radiating laterally is detected. Cardiac catheterization with two transducers, one in the LV and one in the LA, is performed again. Which of the following hemodynamic tracings is consistent with the patient's diagnosis?

   A. Tracing 1
   B. Tracing 2
   C. Tracing 3
   D. Tracing 4
   E. Tracing 5

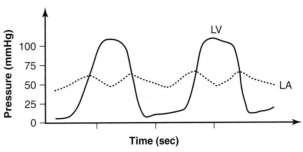

• Figure 1-13.

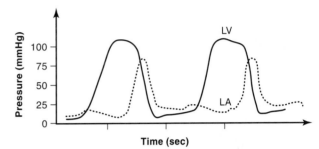

• Figure 1-14.

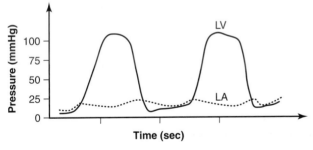

• Figure 1-11.

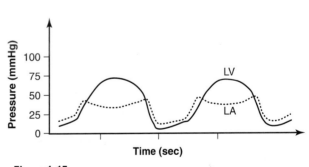

• Figure 1-15.

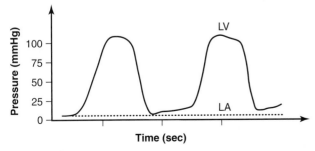

• Figure 1-12.

Infective Endocarditis

HPI: JC is a 26-year-old man with a history of hepatitis C and IV drug use who was in good health until 3 days ago when he noted the acute onset of fevers, chills, and myalgias. Three hours prior to admission, he became increasingly short of breath and was unable to move his right arm.

PE: Vitals: T 39.4°C; HR 110 beats/min; BP 90/50 mm Hg; RR 22 breaths/min. **H/N:** Small retinal hemorrhages, JVP 7 cm. **Chest:** Few basilar crackles. **Cardiac:** Hyperdynamic PMI with III/VI systolic murmur at apex radiating laterally. **Abdomen:** Splenomegaly. **Extremities:** IV needle markings, painless erythematous macules on palms. **ECG:** Sinus tachycardia with nonspecific changes. **CXR:** Multiple 1-cm opacifications throughout both lung fields.

Labs: WBC 16 K/mm³, HCT 29.0, platelets 400 K/mm³. **Urinalysis:** 3+ red blood cells (RBCs), 3+ WBC, >100,000 bacteria all per high-porous field.

THOUGHT QUESTIONS

- What are the common organisms that cause infective endo-carditis (IE)?
- What criteria are used for the diagnosis of IE?
- What are the sequelae of IE?
- What preexisting medical conditions and procedures require antibiotic prophylaxis for IE?

BASIC SCIENCE REVIEW AND DISCUSSION

IE is an infection of the endocardium by microorganisms. Despite the decrease of rheumatic heart disease, IE has been stable or increasing because of (a) the increase of age-related degenerative valve disease; (b) an increase in nosocomial endocarditis in the elderly; and (c) increased diagnosis with echocardiography. IE is a major cause of severe valvular lesions and is responsible for 10 to 25% of mitral and aortic regurgitation requiring surgical intervention. Despite early medical and surgical therapy, the **mortality rate for IE remains 20%.**

IE usually affects the left-sided heart chambers and valves (85% of total) over the right-sided heart chambers and valves (15% of total). The aortic valve alone is affected in 60% of cases, the mitral valve alone is affected in 35% of cases, and simultaneous involvement of both valves occurs in 10% of cases.

Although bacteremia is found in up to 70% of IE cases, the undamaged endothelium is resistant to infection. In addition to bacteremia, two other prerequisites for IE include an aseptic, fibrinoplatelet thrombus formation or damaged endothelium. The damaged endothelium may be secondary to rheumatic heart disease or valvular heart disease that can lead to aberrant blood flow, traumatizing the endothelium. Preexisting rheumatic/valvular/congenital disease is detected in up to 75% of cases of left-sided endocarditis.

IE manifests as valvular vegetations, valvular degeneration, myocardial abscesses, and extracardiac embolic phenomena. After the formation of the aseptic, fibrinoplatelet thrombus, transient bacteremia infects the thrombus to form a valvular vegetation. The **vegetation** is a sessile lesion composed of fibrin, platelets, WBCs, and microorganisms.

After localized valvular infection and vegetation formation, the affected valve can degenerate and cause severe regurgitation and heart failure. The valvular infection can then spread locally to form fistulae, aortic aneurysms, conduction disease, and septic pericarditis. Embolization of vegetations to other organs such as kidneys, spleen, liver, coronary arteries, and brain can cause septic infarction of the target organ (e.g., brain emboli leading to stroke, coronary artery emboli leading to MI) and distant abscesses. Finally, stimulation of the immune system can result in glomerulonephritis and arthritis.

Clinical Presentation

The clinical symptoms and signs of IE are fairly nonspecific, but the most common finding is fever. Other associated symptoms included sweating, chills, fatigue, and arthralgias. On exam, a murmur is detected in 30 to 50% of patients. Other signs include splenomegaly, hematuria, proteinuria, anemia, and retinal hemorrhages (**Roth spots**), **Janeway lesions** (small, nontender, erythematous macules on the palms and soles), nail beds with splinter hemorrhages, and **Osler nodes** (painful 1- to 3-mm erythematous nodules on the fingertips or toe pads). The majority of IE patients (90%) present subacutely, with symptoms occurring within 2 weeks of the initial bacteremia. Ten percent of patients present acutely, with a sudden onset of high fever. Acute-onset IE is usually associated with beta-hemolytic streptococcus, *Staphylococcus aureus*, or *Pseudomonas aeruginosa*.

Although IE predominantly affects the left-sided cardiac structures, 15% of IE involves the right-sided valves. Right-sided IE is associated with IV drug use, and the tricuspid valve is the most frequently affected valve (80% of cases). In addition to traditional symptoms, right-sided IE is complicated by septic pulmonary emboli. The most common cause of right-sided IE is *S. aureus* or *S. epidermidis*.

The diagnosis of IE is based on the **Duke criteria** (Box 1-1). Endocarditis is diagnosed when a patient's clinical presentation fulfills two major criteria, one major and three minor criteria, or five minor criteria.

Given that endocarditis usually follows bacteremia, **antibiotic prophylaxis** is justified for several clinical procedures. All patients with prosthetic heart valves, congenital heart disease [ventricular septal defect (VSD), bicuspid aortic valve, patent ductus arteriosus (PDA)], valvular heart disease (AS, AR, MR, mitral valve prolapse), and previous history of IE require antibiotic prophylaxis. Procedures that require antibiotic prophylaxis for the aforementioned patients include all dental, GI, urologic, upper respiratory tract, and genital procedures.

Medical therapy for endocarditis is long-term IV antibiotics for 2 to 6 weeks. The particular regimen and duration of antibiotic therapy depends on the particular microorganism and location of the IE. **Indications for surgery** include CHF secondary to valve dysfunction, persistent sepsis, recurrent embolism, intracardiac abscess, or fungal endocarditis.

BOX 1-1 Duke Criteria

Major Criteria

1. Positive blood cultures
2. New murmur, positive echo finding

Minor Criteria

1. Fever
2. Predisposing cardiac condition, IV drug abuse
3. Vascular phenomena (emboli, petechiae)
4. Immunologic findings (Roth spots, Osler nodes, glomerulonephritis)
5. Echo findings consistent with endocarditis but not meeting major criteria
6. Positive blood cultures not meeting major criteria

CASE CONCLUSION

JC presents with acute-onset endocarditis secondary to his IV drug use. His IV drug use has resulted in right-sided endocarditis involving the tricuspid valve with septic pulmonary emboli as detected by chest x-ray. His shortness of breath is secondary to acute MR from mitral valvular degeneration. His hypotension and tachycardia are secondary to sepsis syndrome. The small retinal hemorrhages, glomerulonephritis, and neurologic complications are the result of systemic arterial embolization of vegetations to the eyes, kidneys, and brain.

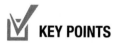

THUMBNAIL: Microbiology of Infectious Endocarditis

Causes of Bacteremia	Percentage of Cases	Microbiology
Dental procedures	20	Penicillin-sensitive streptococcus
Respiratory tract infection	5	Penicillin-sensitive streptococcus
Respiratory/oropharyngeal surgery	20	Penicillin-sensitive streptococcus
GI interventions/GI tumors/GI disease	15	Enterococci, *Streptococcus bovis,* gram-negative bacilli, staphylococcus
Urosepsis	10	Enterococci, gram-negative bacilli, *S. aureus*
Gynecologic infection/surgery	5	Streptococci, enterococci
Other causes: wound infections, in-dwelling catheters, IV drug use, osteomyelitis, cardiac procedures	25	*S. aureus, S. epidermidis,* gram-negative bacilli, fungi

KEY POINTS

- IE predominantly affects the left-sided heart chambers and valves, and the aortic valve is the most commonly affected valve
- The two precipitating factors for endocarditis are transient bacteremia and damaged endothelium, leading to aseptic, fibrinoplatelet thrombus formation
- Right-heart valve endocarditis is predominantly the result of IV drug use
- Heart failure is the principal cause of mortality in IE, and systemic embolization is the major cause of extracardiac complications

QUESTIONS

1. A 68-year-old man is admitted with 3 weeks of abdominal pain, fevers, chills, sweats, and a new systolic murmur. A transthoracic echocardiogram shows mitral valve vegetations, and 3/3 blood cultures are subsequently positive for *Streptococcus bovis.* After successfully completing his 4 weeks of IV penicillin treatment, he undergoes a whole-body computed tomography scan to evaluate his 25-pound weight loss. Which of the following tumors is most likely to be found?

   A. Thyroid carcinoma
   B. Squamous cell lung cancer
   C. Adenocarcinoma of the colon
   D. Transitional cell carcinoma of the bladder
   E. Small cell lung cancer

2. A 24-year-old woman complains of palpitations and occasional dyspnea on exertion. Which one of the following conditions would not require antibiotic prophylaxis for dental procedures?

   A. Mitral valve prolapse with MR
   B. Bicuspid aortic valve
   C. Mitral valve prolapse without MR
   D. PDA
   E. Prosthetic heart valve

CASE 1-5 Arrhythmias

HPI: JS is a 48-year-old woman with no significant past medical history who notes 3 months of palpitations, weight loss, and heat intolerance. The palpitations occur once or twice per week, last several minutes before self-terminating, and are not associated with chest pain or presyncope. A Holter monitor records several episodes of a regular narrow complex tachycardia at 160 beats/min. Review of the event monitor diary is notable for the association between coffee intake and tachycardia initiation. The patient is instructed to splash cold water on her face during palpitations. When she does so, the palpitations promptly terminate.

PE: Vitals: T 37.8°C; HR 110 beats/min; BP 90/50 mm Hg; RR 22 breaths/min. **H/N:** JVP 6 cm, 1-cm nodule in left thyroid lobe. **Chest:** Clear to exam. **Cardiac:** Tachycardic with normal impulse, normal S_1 and S_2 with no murmurs. **Abdomen:** Soft, no masses. **Extremities:** Hyperreflexic in upper and lower extremities. **ECG:** Sinus tachycardia with nonspecific changes.

THOUGHT QUESTIONS

- What are the two basic mechanisms that result in supraventricular tachycardias (SVTs)?
- How do antiarrhythmics suppress abnormal automaticity and re-entry?
- Which SVTs are terminated with adenosine or vagal maneuvers and why?
- What are the five phases of the cardiac action potential and how are they modified by antiarrhythmics?
- What are the different classes of antiarrhythmics and what are their mechanisms of action?
- What is the relationship between premature ventricular contractions (PVCs) and ventricular fibrillation (VF) and ventricular tachycardia (VT)?
- What is the most common cause of VF and VT?
- What are the two mechanisms responsible for bradyarrhythmias?
- What are the classic ECG findings of each bradyarrhythmia?

BASIC SCIENCE REVIEW AND DISCUSSION

Supraventricular Arrhythmias

Whenever the HR is greater than 100 beats/minute for three beats or more, a tachyarrhythmia is present. Tachyarrhythmias can originate either above the ventricles (supraventricular) or within the ventricles (ventricular). An SVT is any tachycardia that originates in the atria or that uses the atrium or atrioventricular (AV) junction and involves the tissue above the bifurcation of the bundle of His to propagate the tachycardic circuit.

SVTs are classified according to whether or not the tachycardia circuit involves the AV node. AV node-dependent tachycardias include AV nodal re-entrant tachycardia (AVNRT), AV re-entrant tachycardia (AVRT), and junctional tachycardia. AV node-independent tachycardias include sinus tachycardia, sinus node re-entry tachycardia, atrial tachycardia, atrial flutter, and atrial fibrillation (AF). An SVT can be classified as AV node dependent if the tachycardia can be terminated by blocking the AV node with a vagal maneuver such as a carotid sinus massage or with use of an AV node-blocking agent (adenosine).

The cardiac action potential is divided into five phases and is detailed in Table 1-12 and Figure 1-16.

All SVTs result from a disorder of either impulse formation or impulse conduction. Normal impulse formation depends on the intrinsic automaticity that is present in the SA node, some areas of the atria, the AV node, and the bundle of His. Intrinsic automaticity depends on unique pacemaker channels that open to Na^+ or K^+ when the membrane potential increases to –60 mV. The slow influx of cations during phase 4 depolarization drives the membrane potential closer to zero. When the membrane reaches the –40 mV threshold potential, voltage-gated Ca^{2+}/Na^+ channels open (phase 0 of the action potential), creating the upstroke of the action potential. Potassium efflux is then responsible for the repolarization of the pacemaker cell.

Abnormal Impulse Formation Secondary to Abnormal Automaticity

Altered impulse formation manifesting as increased automaticity can result in sinus tachycardia or ectopic atrial tachycardia. In ectopic (unifocal/multifocal) atrial tachycardia, foci of increased automaticity external to the SA node can override the intrinsic SA node pacemaker, resulting in an ECG with multiple P-wave morphologies. Each P-wave morphology corresponds to a different focus of increased automaticity.

Antiarrhythmics suppress automaticity by one of three mechanisms:

1. Decreasing the slope of phase 4 spontaneous depolarization
2. Shifting the threshold voltage at which Na^+/Ca^{2+} influx occurs to a more positive level
3. Hyperpolarizing the resting membrane potential

Abnormal Impulse Formation Secondary to Re-Entry

The second mechanism contributing to SVTs is aberrant impulse conduction manifested as re-entry. A re-entrant loop is a self-sustaining electrical pathway that repeatedly depolarizes the surrounding myocardium. For a re-entrant circuit to be established, both a unidirectional block and slowed retrograde conduction are necessary. Re-entry is the underlying mechanism for AVNRT, AVRT, re-entrant atrial tachycardia, atrial flutter, and AF.

In AVNRT, the re-entrant circuit is localized in the AV node. Once re-entry is established, the impulse not only depolarizes the ventricle via the bundle of His in an anterograde direction but also depolarizes the atrium via retrograde conduction. Because these depolarizations occur nearly simultaneously, the small P wave occurs at the same time as the much larger QRS depolarization, and the P wave therefore may not be visible on the ECG. AVRT is similar to AVNRT except that in AVRT, one limb of the re-entrant circuit is an accessory bypass tract external to the AV node (Fig. 1-17).

In typical atrial flutter, the re-entrant circuit is usually localized within the right atrium and propagates in a counter-clockwise

TABLE 1-12 Depolarization Phases		
Phase	Description	Mechanism
0	Upstroke/rapid depolarization	Opening of Na^+ channels
1	Early rapid repolarization	Inactivation of Na^+ channels and activation of K^+ and Ca^{2+} outward currents
2	Plateau	Conductance decreases for all ions
3	Final rapid repolarization	Inactivation of Ca^{2+} inward current and activation of K^+ outward current
4	Resting membrane potential/diastolic depolarization	Membrane potential maintained −50 to −80 mV due to inward K^+ current: if tissue has pacemaker channels, slow influx of cations can cause diastolic depolarization and automaticity

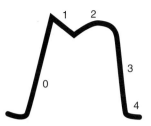

• **Figure 1-16.** Depolarization phases.

The termination of the SVT with adenosine or vagal maneuvers suggests that the arrhythmia is AV node dependent.

Sinus Tachycardia ECG demonstrates normal P waves followed by a QRS complex (Fig. 1-18). Sinus tachycardia is defined as an HR of 100 beats/minute or greater. Sinus tachycardia is usually secondary to increased sympathetic tone from physiologic (exercise) or pathophysiologic (fever, stress, pain, hyperthyroidism, hypovolemia, hypoxemia, anemia, etc.) causes. Addressing the precipitating stressor is the focus of treatment.

AVNRT/AVRT ECG demonstrates a very regular, narrow QRS complex tachycardia of 100 to 250 beats/minute. P waves may or may not be present (Fig. 1-19). In general, AVRT presents in adolescents and young adults, while AVNRT is more common in middle-aged adults with no history of structural heart disease. Because these SVTs involve the AV node, adenosine or vagal maneuvers are effective at terminating AVNRT/AVRT. Pharmacologic treatment is with calcium channel blockers (CCBs) (class IV), beta-blockers (class II), digoxin, and class Ia and Ic medications. However, catheter-based radiofrequency ablation is the mainstay of therapy for these arrhythmias.

Atrial Tachycardia This term refers to a number of different types of tachycardia that originate in the atria. The P-wave axis or morphology is different, and the QRS is usually the same as sinus rhythm. Because these tachycardias do not involve the AV node, vagal maneuvers or AV nodal blockers are usually ineffective at terminating the tachycardia. Most atrial tachycardias, with the exception of multifocal atrial tachycardia, are treated using radiofrequency ablation. Therapy for multifocal atrial tachycardia is directed at the underlying pulmonary illness. The subclassification of atrial tachycardia is based on mechanism.

Increased Automaticity Multifocal atrial tachycardia is associated with chronic pulmonary disease and presents with an atrial rate of 100 to 130 beats/minute and the P wave has three or more morphologies (Fig. 1-20). Treatment is based on the underlying

fashion when viewed from the cardiac apex. Atypical atrial flutter re-entrant circuits can also be established in other parts of the atrium or localized around scar tissue. In AF, the exact pathophysiologic mechanism is unclear, but one widely accepted theory suggests that multiple wave fronts of electrical activity sweep through the atria in a re-entrant but random fashion.

Antiarrhythmics suppress re-entry by slowing conduction or increasing refractoriness enough to essentially convert unidirectional block to bidirectional block.

Clinical Presentations

All SVTs present with a narrow QRS complex pattern by ECG (unless aberrant conduction of the supraventricular impulse is present). Typical manifestations of SVT include recurrent palpitations, chest fullness, "skipped" beats associated with lightheadedness, or presyncope. It is difficult to clinically differentiate between the different types of SVT based on clinical symptoms.

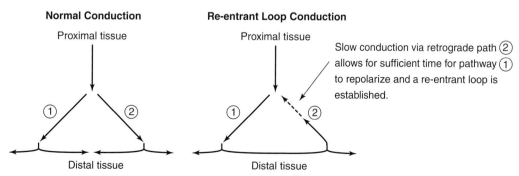

• **Figure 1-17.** Re-entry loops.

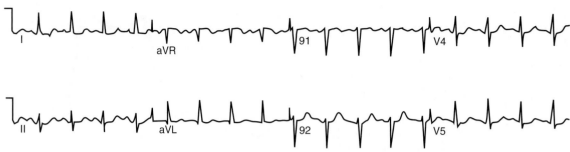

● **Figure 1-18.** Sinus tachycardia.

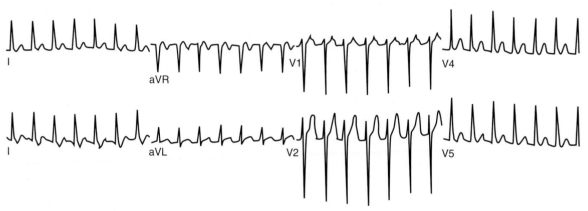

● **Figure 1-19.** AVNRT/AVRT.

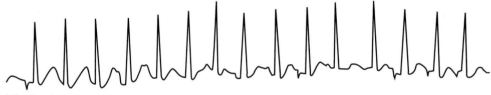

● **Figure 1-20.** Multifocal atrial tachycardia.

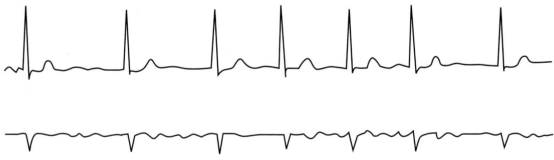

● **Figure 1-21.** Atrial fibrillation.

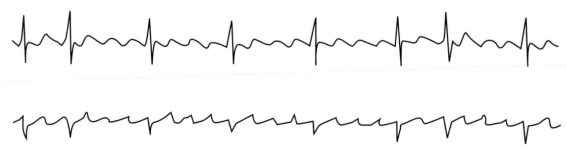

● **Figure 1-22.** Atrial flutter.

pulmonary process. Unifocal atrial tachycardia is often seen in younger patients. Catheter-based radiofrequency ablation is the treatment of choice.

Re-entry Intra-atrial re-entry atrial tachycardia is associated with underlying heart disease or atrial arrhythmia history, such as atrial fibrillation or flutter.

Atrial Fibrillation AF is the chaotic depolarization of the atrium with loss of synchronized mechanical contraction of the atrium during ventricular diastole. AF is associated with multiple conditions, including advanced age, low potassium or magnesium levels, postsurgical state, CHF, hyperthyroidism, and hyperadrenergic states. Because the atrial rate is so elevated at 350 to 600 depolarizations/minute, distinct P waves are not discernible (Fig. 1-21). The ventricular response (QRS complex) is "irregularly irregular" and usually 140 to 160 beats/minute for untreated AF because the AV node can only conduct a fraction of the incoming atrial depolarizations. The clinical consequences of AF include (*a*) increased risk of stroke due to thrombus formation within the fibrillating atrium; and (*b*) hypotension and CHF secondary to a reduced diastolic filling period with sustained rapid ventricular response. Treatment includes decreasing the ventricular rate by further blocking the AV node with beta-blockers, CCBs, or digoxin. Class Ic (propafenone, flecainide) and class III agents (sotalol, amiodarone) can also be used to suppress and terminate AF. If medications are not successful, electrical cardioversion can be applied to restore normal sinus rhythm.

Atrial Flutter Atrial flutter is secondary to a re-entrant circuit usually within the right atrium but can also originate as a re-entrant circuit in other parts of the atrium. The classic ECG pattern is a "sawtooth" P-wave pattern at a rate of 300 beats/minute with a slower ventricular rate that is usually an even multiple of the atrial rate (e.g., atrial flutter with 2:1 block has a ventricular rate of 150 beats/min) (Fig. 1-22). Atrial flutter often degenerates into AF. The treatment of choice for atrial flutter is radiofrequency ablation of the re-entrant circuit. The pharmacologic treatment for atrial flutter is similar to that for AF, and electrical cardioversion can also be applied to restore normal sinus rhythm. The clinical consequences of increased risk for stroke secondary to intra-atrial thrombus formation and CHF are also elevated for prolonged atrial flutter.

Ventricular Arrhythmias

Ventricular arrhythmias originate from ventricular tissue and are classified as VT or VF. VT and VF are the major causes of sudden cardiac death. PVCs are common, benign, and usually asymptomatic. PVCs are the result of ectopic ventricular foci generating an action potential independent of the SA and AV nodal conduction system. PVCs appear as wide QRS depolarizations because the electrical activity travels slowly through myocardium rather than through the normal conduction system. In people with no significant structural heart disease, PVCs do not progress to VT or VF.

Ventricular Tachycardia

VT is a rapid rhythm greater than 100 beats/minute originating in the ventricle and is caused by re-entry, triggered activity, or enhanced automaticity. If three PVCs occur in a row, a diagnosis

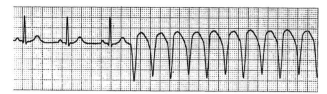

• **Figure 1-23.** Ventricular tachycardia: a wide-complex tachycardia defined as three or more premature ventricular contractions in a row.

of VT is established. VT is subclassified as nonsustained (<30 sec) or sustained (≥30 sec). In VT, the QRS complexes are very broad and occur at a rate of 100 to 200 beats/minute (Fig. 1-23).

VT can also be subclassified by morphology as monomorphic versus polymorphic. All the QRS complexes are the same shape in monomorphic VT because the tachycardia evolves from a single arrhythmogenic focus. The most common cause of monomorphic VT is re-entry in scarred myocardium created after MI. In polymorphic VT, the QRS complexes are different shapes because the tachycardia evolves from several ventricular foci. Polymorphic VT is usually associated with active ischemia rather than with re-entry from myocardial scarring.

Patients with VT usually complain of palpitations, chest fullness, and light-headedness. If VT is sustained, hypotension occurs and loss of consciousness ensues from decreased cardiac output. The treatment of choice for symptomatic VT is electrical cardioversion. Electrical cardioversion produces a transient electrical field over the entire heart to re-establish organized electrical activity and contractile function. Although VT is a life-threatening arrhythmia, degeneration of VT into VF is even more lethal.

Ventricular Fibrillation

VF is the most lethal arrhythmia and is the result of multiple disorganized circulating wave fronts of electrical activity (Fig. 1-24). The most common etiology of VF is ischemia from MI. As a result of the chaotic depolarizations, no coordinated contractile function can occur, and cardiac output suddenly declines. VF presents with sudden loss of consciousness with subsequent sudden cardiac death if electrical defibrillation is not emergently performed.

Wolff-Parkinson-White Syndrome

Wolff-Parkinson-White (WPW) syndrome is a pre-excitation syndrome in which ventricular depolarization occurs by an anomalous conduction pathway before the ventricle is depolarized by the normal AV conduction pathway (Fig. 1-25). Although only half of WPW syndrome cases are symptomatic and present as young adults with either an SVT or AF, the ECG shows a short PR interval and a delta wave. Treatment of choice for WPW syndrome is catheter-based ablation of the accessory pathway.

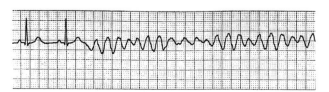

• **Figure 1-24.** Ventricular fibrillation: the most common cause of sudden cardiac death.

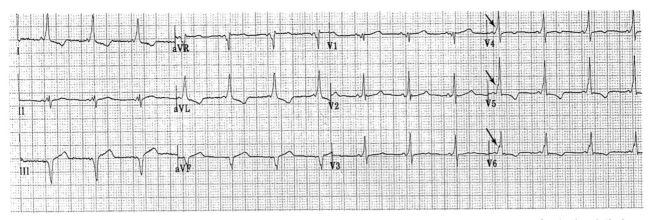

• **Figure 1-25.** Wolff-Parkinson-White syndrome: the ventricle is activated through the AV node as well as via a bypass tract. Conduction via the bypass tract occurs earlier than via the AV node and this earlier activation produces the delta wave (*arrows* in V4–V6) and shortens the PR interval.

Rarely, AF in WPW can induce VF because of rapid ventricular stimulation via the accessory pathway. Therefore, treatment of AF with AV node-blocking agents (CCBs and digoxin) is contraindicated because these agents can precipitate VF by diverting the atrial impulses from the AV node into the accessory pathway. Procainamide is the treatment of choice for AF in the setting of WPW.

Bradyarrhythmias

Bradyarrhythmias are abnormal heart rhythms when the HR is less than 60 beats/minute. Bradyarrhythmias are the result of either decreased impulse formation from the SA node or impaired conduction.

Cardiac Conduction System

Cardiac conduction originates at the SA node, which is a collection of pacemaker cells located in the RA between the superior vena cava and right atrial appendage. In 60% of patients the SA node blood supply is the SA nodal artery from the proximal right coronary artery (RCA). In 40% of patients the SA node blood supply is a branch of the circumflex artery. Although the SA node receives innervation from both the parasympathetic and sympathetic nervous systems, the SA node is predominantly under the influence of the parasympathetic nervous system at rest.

After the spontaneous formation of an electrical signal in the SA node, the impulse is conducted in a delayed fashion to the AV node. This intrinsic delay allows for atrial contraction to be completed before the contraction of the ventricles. In 90% of people, the AV node receives its blood supply from a branch of the RCA (10% from the left anterior descending [LAD] artery). Since the majority of the blood supply to the SA and AV nodes is from the RCA, ischemia of this coronary vessel often causes bradyarrhythmias. The impulse then leaves the AV node and enters the bundle of His. After 1 cm, the bundle of His bifurcates into the right and left bundles. The left bundle bifurcates again into an anterior and posterior fascicle (Fig. 1-26). A common ECG finding is a left or right bundle branch block pattern, which corresponds to a conduction disturbance in the corresponding bundle branch.

SA Node Dysfunction

SA node dysfunction is the result of intrinsic or extrinsic factors. Intrinsic factors are structural changes within the node itself. The most common pathologic finding is replacement of the pacemaker cells with fibrous tissue. Intrinsic causes of SA node dysfunction include connective tissue disorders, infiltrative disease (amyloid), inflammation (myocarditis), chronic ischemia, and idiopathic degeneration.

Extrinsic causes temporarily inhibit SA node automaticity but do not physically modify the node. The most common extrinsic cause is drugs, including beta-blockers, CCBs, digoxin, lithium, and antiarrhythmic drugs. Autonomically mediated syndromes such as carotid SA hypersensitivity, situational (coughing, vomiting), and neurocardiogenic syncope can also cause transient SA node dysfunction. Other extrinsic causes include hypothermia, hypothyroidism, and electrolyte disorders.

Mild SA node dysfunction can result in sinus bradycardia, which is secondary to decreased automaticity of the SA node. Some well-conditioned athletes or older patients have intrinsically high vagal tone and have asymptomatic and benign sinus bradycardia. More severe SA node dysfunction can result in sick sinus syndrome (SSS). In SSS, the automaticity of the sinus node is highly variable, and sinus pauses can be followed by atrial tachyarrhythmias. Treatment usually requires an electronic

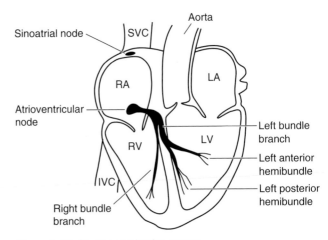

• **Figure 1-26.** Cardiac conduction system.

pacemaker for the bradycardia and antiarrhythmic drug therapy for the tachyarrhythmia.

When SA node activity is suppressed for a prolonged period in severe sinus node dysfunction, pacemaker foci in the AV node or ventricle generate escape rhythms to maintain an adequate heart rate. Junctional escape beats from the AV node are characterized by QRS complexes at a rate of 60 beats/minute and not preceded by P waves since there is no intrinsic atrial activity. Ventricular escape beats are characterized by wide QRS complexes at 30 to 40 beats/minute and also not preceded by P waves. Treatment for extreme intrinsic sinus node dysfunction is implantation of a permanent pacemaker.

Impaired Conduction

Impaired conduction is usually the result of degeneration of the conduction pathway, MI, or drug toxicity.

First-degree AV block is a lengthening of the normal delay between atrial and ventricular depolarization so that the PR interval is greater than 0.2 seconds. The cause of first-degree AV block is similar to the causes of sinus node dysfunction. First-degree AV block usually occurs at the level of the AV node, and most patients remain asymptomatic and require no intervention.

Second-degree AV block is due to intermittent failure of AV conduction so that not every P wave (atrial depolarization) is followed by a QRS complex (ventricular depolarization). Second-degree AV block is further subclassified as Mobitz type I (Wenckebach) or Mobitz type II block. In Mobitz type I block the conduction delay between the atria and ventricles lengthens with each beat until an atrial impulse is not conducted to the ventricle. On an ECG, the PR interval progressively lengthens until a P wave does not generate a QRS depolarization. Mobitz type I block occurs at the level of the AV node and usually does not require treatment. In Mobitz type II block, the PR interval remains constant before the sudden loss of AV conduction manifested by a P wave not followed by a QRS depolarization. Mobitz type II block is more serious and more likely to occur distal to the AV node in the His bundle. Since Mobitz type II block is much more likely to progress to third-degree AV block, the treatment of choice is electronic pacemaker implantation.

Third-degree AV block is complete absence of conduction between the atria and ventricles with no fixed relationship between the P waves and QRS complexes. While the atria depolarize at the intrinsic SA node rate (60–80 beats/min), the ventricles independently depolarize at the ventricular escape rate of 30 to 40 beats/minute. Because third-degree AV block can severely compromise heart rate and cardiac output, emergent pacemaker therapy is necessary.

CASE CONCLUSION

JS is experiencing an AV nodal-dependent SVT precipitated by her hyperthyroidism (low-grade fever, baseline sinus tachycardia, hyperreflexia, and thyroid nodule) and caffeine intake. The termination of the tachycardia by vagal stimulation (cold water stimulus) suggests that the tachycardia involves the AV node. The regular nature of the tachycardia excludes AF, which is usually irregularly irregular. Given her middle age, her diagnosis is most likely AVNRT. After her hyperthyroidism was treated and her caffeine intake was reduced, her tachycardia resolved.

THUMBNAIL: Classification of Antiarrhythmic Mechanisms

Class	General Mechanism	Examples
I	Sodium channel blockage	See subclasses (Ia, Ib, Ic) below
Ia	Decrease phase 0 upstroke rate	Quinidine, procainamide, disopyramide
Ib	Little effect on phase 0 in normal tissue Decreased phase 0 upstroke rate in abnormal tissue Shortens repolarization or little effect	Lidocaine, mexiletine, phenytoin
Ic	Markedly decreases phase 0 upstroke rate Markedly slows conduction	Flecainide, propafenone, encainide, moricizine
II	Beta-blockade	Metoprolol, esmolol, atenolol, propranolol
III	Potassium channel blockers Prolongation of repolarization	Amiodarone, sotalol, ibutilide, dofetilide, bretylium
IV	Calcium channel blockade	Verapamil, diltiazem

☑ KEY POINTS

- AV node-dependent tachycardias (AVNRT and AVRT) usually terminate with administration of an AV node blocking agent (adenosine) or vagal stimulus (carotid sinus massage)

- SVTs are secondary to two basic mechanisms: (1) abnormal impulse formation secondary to abnormal automaticity and (2) abnormal impulse formation secondary to re-entry

- PVCs are common and do not progress to VT or VF in people with no significant heart disease

- Treatment of symptomatic VT or VF is emergent electrical cardioversion

- WPW syndrome is premature ventricular depolarization by an accessory conduction pathway

- Bradyarrhythmias are the result of either sinus node dysfunction or impaired conduction

- First-degree AV block and second-degree Mobitz type I block usually need no further intervention, whereas second-degree Mobitz type II block and third-degree heart block require electronic pacemaker placement

QUESTIONS

1. FD is a 74-year-old man postoperative day 1 from a radical prostatectomy for prostate cancer. After breakfast, he develops palpitations and light-headedness. The surgical intern administers 6 mg IV adenosine, which promptly resolves the tachycardia. The tachycardia recurs 2 hours later and an ECG obtained during the second episode would most likely reveal:

   A. AF
   B. Multifocal atrial tachycardia
   C. Atrial flutter
   D. Sinus tachycardia
   E. AV nodal re-entry tachycardia

2. SH is an 18-year-old woman who complains of palpitations, and her work-up is still pending. She was wondering whether radiofrequency ablation could be the appropriate treatment for her palpitations. Which diagnosis would be the most suitable and straightforward for radiofrequency ablation?

   A. Multifocal atrial tachycardia
   B. AF
   C. Typical atrial flutter

   D. Atypical atrial flutter
   E. Sinus tachycardia

3. A 69-year-old man with a history of two prior MIs presents with recurrent polymorphic VT requiring multiple electrical cardioversions. What would be the next clinical step in his management?

   A. Automatic implantable cardiac defibrillator implantation
   B. IV magnesium replacement
   C. IV antiarrhythmics
   D. Thrombolysis
   E. Emergent cardiac catheterization and possible angioplasty

4. Myocardial infarction of which coronary artery is most likely complicated by severe bradycardia?

   A. Circumflex coronary artery
   B. Obtuse marginal coronary artery
   C. LAD coronary artery
   D. RCA
   E. Ramus intermedius

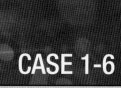

CASE 1-6 Congenital Heart Disease

HPI: JS is a 56-year-old man who presents with the inability to move his right arm and leg for 6 hours. He is otherwise healthy but on review of systems he notes he has been increasingly fatigued and short of breath. An ECG demonstrates RVH, and his chest x-ray reveals RV enlargement and prominent pulmonary arteries. Brain magnetic resonance imaging (MRI) is consistent with an embolic left middle cerebral stroke. Heparin is started and cardiology is consulted for further evaluation.

PE: Vitals: T 37.0°C; HR 70 beats/min; BP 110/60 mm Hg; RR 16 breaths/min. **H/N:** JVP elevated at 12 cm. **Chest:** Clear to auscultation. **Cardiac:** RV lift, accentuated P$_2$, fixed split S$_2$, no significant murmur. **Extremities:** Mild cyanosis. **Neurologic:** Decreased strength and fine motor control of right upper and lower extremities with associated hyperreflexia.

THOUGHT QUESTIONS

- What is the anatomic difference between an atrial septal defect (ASD) and patent foramen ovale (PFO)?
- What pathophysiologic changes occur with left-to-right versus right-to-left shunts?
- What is Eisenmenger syndrome?
- What are the common physical findings and clinical presentations of the common congenital cardiac abnormalities?

BASIC SCIENCE REVIEW AND DISCUSSION

Congenital heart disease is defined as a cardiac abnormality in structure and function present a birth. About 0.8% of live births are complicated by a congenital heart abnormality. Normal cardiovascular embryologic development will be reviewed in the Thumbnail section since congenital abnormalities are usually the result of altered embryonic development of a cardiac structure.

Atrial Septal Defects and Patent Foramen Ovale

Anatomy and Pathology An ASD is an opening within the atrial septum, allowing for flow of blood from the LA to the RA. It is relatively common, representing 6 to 10% of all cardiac anomalies, and is twice as common in females as in males. Although ASDs can occur anywhere along the interatrial septum, the most common is the ostium secundum defect, accounting for 69% of all ASDs. An ostium secundum defect is actually a developmental defect of the septum primum.

A PFO is an open conduit between the superior portion of the septum secundum on the RA side and the septum primum on the LA side. Postnatally, the foramen is normally held shut by overlapping of the two septa and the higher pressure in the LA. However, high RA pressures can cause the two septa to separate, allowing paradoxical embolization from right to left to occur.

Pathophysiology In the setting of a large ASD, a chronic left-to-right shunt imposes a volume overload on the RV and RA, resulting in right-sided chamber hypertrophy and dilatation. The volume overload also causes dilatation of the pulmonary vascular bed and hypertrophy/luminal narrowing of the pulmonary arteries. As a result, 10% of patients with large ASDs can develop severe and irreversible pulmonary HTN secondary to increased pulmonary vascular resistance. With the elevated right-sided pressures, the left-to-right shunting eventually decreases (with a resultant decrease in the murmur) and may even reverse from right to left. The elevation of pulmonary artery pressure to systemic level causing a bidirectional or shunt reversal is known as

Eisenmenger syndrome. Shunt reversal results in systemic hypoxia because deoxygenated blood from the RA mixes with the oxygenated blood in the LA.

Clinical Presentation Most ASDs are asymptomatic and may never be detected if very small. Large left-to-right shunts can result in fatigue and dyspnea. On physical exam, an RV precordial lift may be present due to dilatation of the RV. A widely and fixed split S$_2$ (composed of an aortic component followed by a pulmonary component) is present because the RV volume overload results in prolonged emptying of the RV and a subsequent delay in pulmonic valve closure. The ASD itself does not generate a murmur because there is little pressure gradient across the ASD. However, the increased blood flow through the cardiac chambers can result in two different types of murmurs: (1) a soft systolic murmur at the second intercostal space secondary to increased blood flow across the pulmonic valve; or (2) an early to mid-diastolic murmur secondary to increased blood flow across the tricuspid valve. Chest radiographs demonstrate a cardiac enlargement and RVH. The ECG shows RVH.

Management Elective surgical repair is the preferred treatment for major ASD. If major ASDs are left untreated, CHF can develop, especially in patients older than age 40. If left untreated, CHF is quite common in patients older than age 40 , atrial arrhythmia incidence increases by up to 62% by age 60, and pulmonary HTN can develop in 10% of patients. A percutaneous double umbrella device can also be used to close major ASDs less than 22 mm in diameter with adequate edges around the lumen.

Ventricular Septal Defects

Anatomy and Pathology A VSD is an opening within the interventricular septum, allowing flow of blood from the LV to the RV. VSDs are slightly more common in females than in males. Although VSDs are the most common congenital cardiac anomaly associated with chromosomal abnormalities, 95% of VSDs are not associated with a chromosomal defect.

Although VSDs can occur anywhere along the ventricular septum, the most common type is a defect in the membranous septum, which is beneath the septal leaflet of the tricuspid valve and extends up to the aortic valve.

Pathophysiology Similar to ASDs, VSDs initially result in shunting of blood from a high pressure LV to a lower pressure RV. With right-sided volume overload, narrowing of the pulmonary arteries occurs and pulmonary HTN develops in 10 to 20% of patients (Eisenmenger complex—refer to ASD section for description). LA dilatation, secondary to increased venous return from the lungs, can also cause the foramen ovale to open, creating an additional left-to-right shunt.

Unlike ASDs, there is bidirectional shunting of blood across VSDs with left-to-right shunting during isovolumetric contraction and right-to-left shunting during isovolumetric relaxation. This bidirectional shunting results in LV volume overload, LV hypertrophy, and, eventually, LV systolic dilatation and dysfunction.

Clinical Presentation VSD presentation depends on the size of the VSD and the severity of the left-to-right shunt. A VSD may not be detected in newborns because pulmonary vascular resistance is high at birth, which minimizes the amount of left-to-right shunting. Several weeks after birth, as the pulmonary vascular resistance decreases, the amount of left-to-right shunting and associated signs and symptoms increase. Most VSDs are diagnosed in children when they are referred for a cardiac murmur.

With small VSDs, patients are asymptomatic and present with a high-pitched, lower LSB, holosystolic murmur extending past the S_2 with an associated palpable thrill. As the VSD becomes moderate in size, patients present with tachycardia and mild tachypnea. A mid-diastolic rumble may be present secondary to increase blood flow across the mitral valve, and the precordium is hyperdynamic. When the VSD is large, severe volume overload of the LV and LA occurs, with findings of pulmonary edema (tachypnea, rales) and an S_3.

If secondary pulmonary HTN develops, the holosystolic murmur of the VSD may disappear due to the decline in the pressure gradient between the RV and LV. Pulmonary HTN also causes (*a*) an accentuated pulmonic component of S_2; (*b*) RV lift secondary to RV hypertrophy; and (*c*) an early diastolic decrescendo murmur from pulmonic insufficiency. The increased shunting of deoxygenated blood from the RV to the systemic circulation within the LV (Eisenmenger syndrome) results in cyanosis and systemic hypoxia.

Management Small asymptomatic VSDs require only periodic follow-up and antibiotic prophylaxis for endocarditis because many of them may spontaneously close. As VSDs become larger and patients become symptomatic, diuretics and digoxin are usually administered to alleviate right-heart failure symptoms. Surgical therapy is recommended if there is increasing pulmonary pressure or if the amount of blood flow within the pulmonary circulation exceeds the amount of blood flow with the systemic circulation by a factor of 2 (both determined by cardiac catheterization).

Tetralogy of Fallot

Anatomy and Pathology Tetralogy of Fallot (TOF) is composed of four anatomic features:

1. Pulmonic stenosis
2. RVH
3. VSD
4. Overriding of the aorta (aorta is displaced anteriorly and receives blood from both ventricles)

TOF is the most common cyanotic congenital heart disease in both children and adults and accounts for 4 to 10% of all congenital heart disease. TOF is the result of abnormal anterior and cephalad displacement of the infundibular septum during embryonic development, resulting in unequal division of the conus. This unequal division results in the anterior aortic displacement, VSD, and pulmonic stenosis (which then induces RVH).

Pathophysiology Cyanosis and hypoxemia are present in TOF because deoxygenated blood returning to the RV encounters increased resistance from the pulmonic stenosis. This deoxygenated blood is routed through the VSD and into the aorta. Hypoxemia is induced by situations in which systemic vascular resistance is lowered, systemic venous return is increased, or pulmonic stenosis is worsened. For example, crying or exposure to cold air can precipitate cyanosis because venous return increases and systemic vascular resistance decreases. Severe cases of hypoxemia can induce unconsciousness and convulsions. Compensation for the hypoxemia includes collateral circulation and polycythemia.

Clinical Presentation Cyanosis beginning at 3 to 6 months and a pulmonic stenosis murmur is a classic presentation. Cyanosis often induces clubbing of the nails. An RV precordial lift secondary to RVH is also present. Squatting is a characteristic position for children. In this posture, both the systemic vascular resistance (compression of the abdominal aorta) and systemic venous resistance (from compression of leg veins) increase with a resultant increase in aortic oxygenation.

Management Medical management includes iron supplementation to prevent anemia, antibiotics for endocarditis prophylaxis, and beta-blockers to decrease the degree of infundibular/RV outflow contraction during systole. Definitive treatment is surgical and includes RV outflow tract reconstruction and closure of the VSD.

Transposition of the Great Arteries

Anatomy and Pathology Transposition of the great arteries (TGA) occurs when the origin of the aorta and main pulmonary artery are reversed, with the aorta arising from the RV and the main pulmonary artery arising from the LV. TGA is often associated with VSD, pulmonic stenosis, PDA, and coarctation. It occurs with a 2:1 male-to-female ratio.

Pathophysiology With TGA, there are two separate circulations. The RV acts as the systemic ventricle and recirculates deoxygenated blood back into the systemic circulation. The LV acts as the pulmonic ventricle and recirculates oxygenated blood back to the lungs. Because there is no mixing of the oxygenated LV circuit with the deoxygenated RV circuit, TGA is lethal if not corrected. However, TGA is compatible with life in utero. In the TGA fetus, oxygenated blood from the placenta enters the RA and then passes into either the RV or LA via the PFO. Due to the transposition, LA blood then enters the LV and is pumped into the pulmonary artery (instead of the aorta). However, due to the high pulmonary vascular resistance, the majority of the oxygenated blood in the pulmonary artery flows into the aorta/systemic circulation via the ductus arteriosus instead of into the pulmonary vasculature.

Oxygenated blood that has passed from the RA to the RV is also pumped into the aorta (instead of the pulmonary artery). After birth, the physiologic closure of the ductus arteriosus and the foramen ovale do not permit shunting of oxygenated blood from the right-sided circulation into the deoxygenated left-sided circulation. Without a communication between the two parallel circuits, the infant becomes hypoxic and cyanotic.

Clinical Presentation The most common presentation of TGA is severe cyanosis. Unlike most other congenital cardiac abnormalities, no murmur is appreciated.

Management Medical management includes immediate infusion of prostaglandin E to maintain patency of the ductus arteriosus, which will permit continued mixing of deoxygenated blood in the right-sided circulation with oxygenated blood in the left-sided circulation. Palliative interventional therapy includes balloon atrial septostomy to permit mixing of systemic and pulmonary blood at the atrial level. All patients will eventually need definitive surgical therapy, which includes an atrial baffle procedure (Mustard or Senning procedure) or arterial switch procedure.

THUMBNAIL: Diagrams of Common Congenital Cardiac Abnormalities

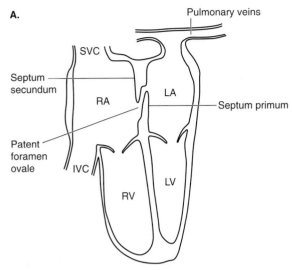

A.

Pulmonary veins

SVC

Septum secundum

RA

LA

Septum primum

Patent foramen ovale

IVC

RV

LV

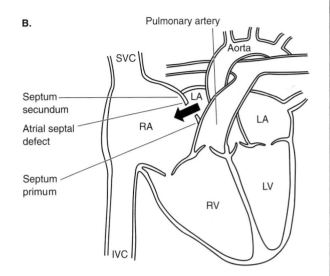

B.

Pulmonary artery

Aorta

SVC

Septum secundum

LA

Atrial septal defect

RA

LA

Septum primum

RV

LV

IVC

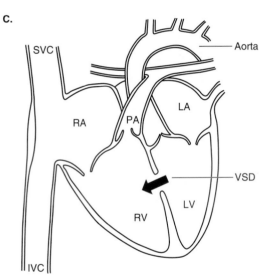

C.

SVC

Aorta

LA

RA

PA

VSD

IVC

RV

LV

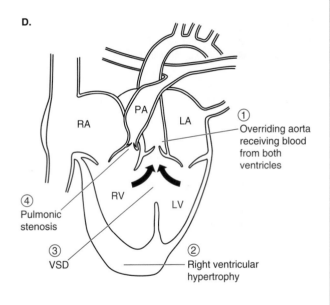

D.

RA

PA

LA

① Overriding aorta receiving blood from both ventricles

④ Pulmonic stenosis

RV

LV

③ VSD

② Right ventricular hypertrophy

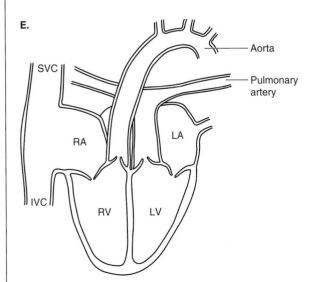

E.

Aorta

SVC

Pulmonary artery

RA

LA

IVC

RV

LV

● **Figure 1-27. A.** Patent foramen ovale (PFO). **B.** Arterial septal defect (ASD). 1. The most common ASD (secundum defect) is secondary to overabsorption of the septum primum or inadequate growth of the septum primum. 2. A large ASD results in a substantial left-to-right shunt with subsequent volume overload of the RA/RV. **C.** Ventricular septal defect (VSD). A large VSD results in a large left-to-right shunt with subsequent volume overload of the RV and pulmonary HTN. **D.** Tetralogy of Fallot (TOF). **E.** Transposition of great vessels (TOGV).

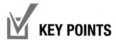

CASE CONCLUSION

A transesophageal echocardiogram demonstrated that JS has a 2.7-cm ASD. His stroke was most likely secondary to a paradoxical embolism that migrated from the lower extremities into the right-sided heart chambers, through the ASD, into the LA and LV, and then to his cerebral circulation. As a result of the chronic left-to-right volume overload, he has developed RV enlargement/hypertrophy (RV lift detected on exam and RV enlargement by CXR and ECG), pulmonary HTN, and reversal of flow via the ASD (Eisenmenger syndrome). His accentuated P_2 on exam is secondary to pulmonary HTN, and the fixed split S_2 is the result of delayed pulmonic valve closure from increased RV flow. Although his initial shunt was left to right, the flow is now right to left secondary to Eisenmenger syndrome, with resultant systemic hypoxia, fatigue, cyanosis, and clubbing. Because the ASD was greater than 22 mm in diameter, he was referred for open heart surgical repair.

KEY POINTS

- PFO/ASD: A PFO or ASD can result in paradoxical embolization (thrombus from the leg can shunt across PFO/ASD into the left heart chambers and cause a stroke if the thrombus lodges within the brain)
- VSD: Eisenmenger complex is defined as pulmonary HTN at the systemic level caused by high pulmonary vascular resistance with reversed or bidirectional shunt through a VSD. Eisenmenger syndrome is identical to Eisenmenger complex, but the shunt is secondary to a congenital defect other than VSD (e.g., ASD or PDA).

- TOF: The tetralogy is pulmonic stenosis, RVH, VSD, and overriding aorta
- TGA: TGA is compatible with life in the fetus due to right-to-left shunting of oxygenated blood at the ductus arteriosus and PFO. After birth, the ductus arteriosus and PFO close, resulting in life-threatening hypoxia.

QUESTIONS

1. A newborn infant is noted to be increasingly cyanotic after birth and an immediate echocardiogram confirms the diagnosis of transposition of the great arteries. Which of the following interventions would be most helpful in reversing the pathophysiologic process?

    A. Supplemental oxygen
    B. Inotropic support with dobutamine
    C. Indomethacin administration
    D. Prostaglandin infusion
    E. Blood transfusion

2. A 6-month-old girl presents with cyanosis and a pulmonic stenosis murmur. Further evaluation of the patient reveals she has TOF. Which of the following interventions would be least helpful in stabilizing her condition until an open surgical correction can be performed?

    A. Antibiotics for endocarditis prophylaxis
    B. Supplemental iron
    C. Supplemental oxygen
    D. Beta-blockers
    E. Hydralazine

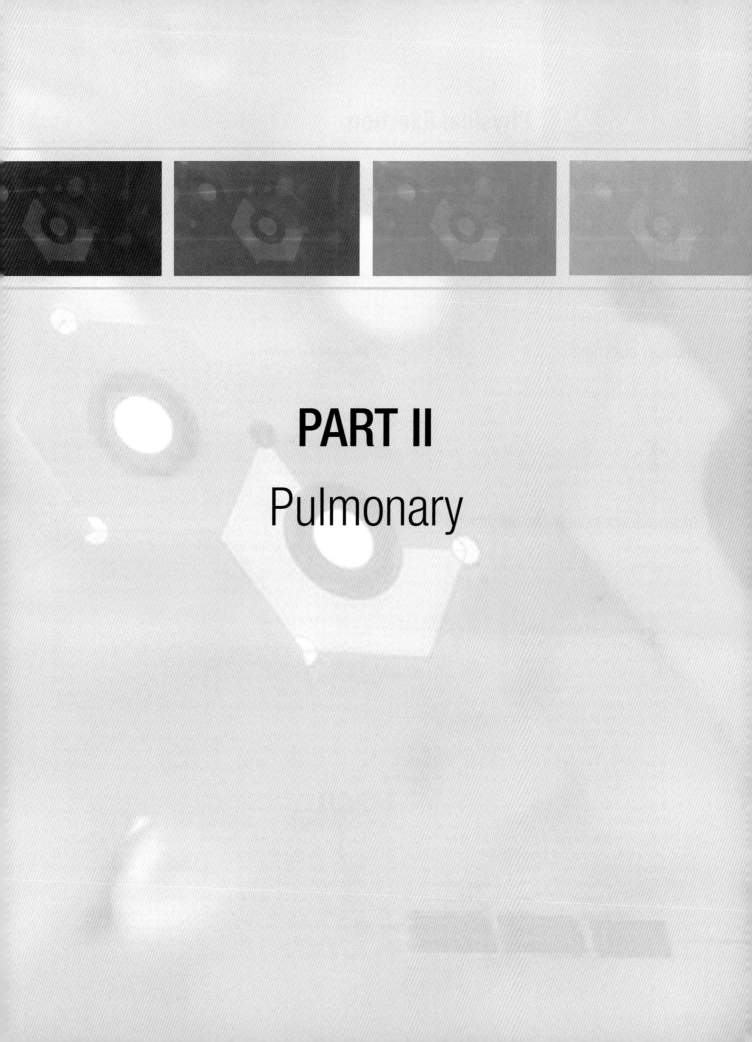

PART II

Pulmonary

CASE 2-1 Physical Exertion

HPI: TS, a 22-year-old college wrestler, is preparing for his upcoming senior season as a heavyweight wrestler. Despite his heavyweight status, TS is in very good shape and likes to run stairs to get ready for the extreme cardiopulmonary demands of wrestling. He runs the 250-step aisle in the stands of his college stadium. It takes TS 2 minutes to run to the top and 3 minutes to walk back down. At maximal workload his total body oxygen consumption increases from about 0.5 liters per minute at rest to about 4.0 liters per minute at maximal exercise workload. To facilitate this increase in oxygen consumption, his cardiac output increases from about 5 liters per minute to 25 liters per minute, and his ventilation increases from 15 liters per minute to 150 liters per minute. As TS arrives at the top the second time, he is breathing at 40 times per minute, his heartbeat is 146 beats per minute, his chest is burning, he feels starved for oxygen, and his muscles begin to fatigue. He is now delivering the maximal amount of oxygen to his muscle tissue, but it is not enough to keep up with the current oxygen consumption rate. He begins to fatigue as anaerobic metabolism creates lactic acid.

THOUGHT QUESTIONS

- Which mechanisms allow oxygen transport from the outside world to enter end-organ tissues that utilize oxygen as fuel?
- Which component of oxygen transport is the rate-limiting factor at maximal workload and oxygen utilization?
- Which respiratory muscles are involved in inspiration and expiration and how does the mechanism of breathing change during exercise?

BASIC SCIENCE REVIEW AND DISCUSSION

Oxygen Transport

There are five major mechanisms of oxygen transport from the outside world to its final destination in end-organ tissues that utilize oxygen for fuel:

1. *Ventilation* is the mechanical process of drawing air into the airways and alveoli via negative pressure created by active expansion of the chest wall.
2. *Alveolar diffusion* is the transfer of oxygen molecules across the alveolar cell membrane, interstitium, and pulmonary capillary membrane into the pulmonary circulation.
3. *Binding* is a function carried out by hemoglobin in red blood cells whereby four oxygen molecules are bound to a hemoglobin moiety.
4. *Circulation* refers to cardiac output that propels oxygenated blood to the peripheral capillary tissue beds.
5. *Peripheral diffusion* occurs in oxygen-utilizing tissues as oxygen molecules are off-loaded from saturated hemoglobin molecules across capillary membranes and interstitial tissue into cells that utilize oxygen.

There is a limit to oxygen utilization and thus a maximum workload achievable before oxygen utilization in peripheral tissues surpasses oxygen delivery. At this point, anaerobic metabolism comes in to play and its byproduct lactic acid begins to accumulate in peripheral tissues. This is referred to as the anaerobic threshold and corresponds with maximal oxygen consumption. Of the five steps of oxygen transport, cardiac output is the rate-limiting factor that determines maximal oxygen consumption in a healthy person.

Mechanisms of Ventilation

The diaphragm is the most important muscle for inspiration. It is attached to the lower portion of the rib cage and—when contracted—pushes the contents of the abdomen downward, which increases the vertical dimension of the thorax. The contraction of the diaphragm also pulls up on the naturally downsloping rib cage that is hinged to the vertebrae in a bucket-handle fashion. Lifting the individual bucket handles acts to increase the anteroposterior dimension of the thorax (Fig. 2-1). The increased volume of the thorax creates a negative intrathoracic pressure that draws air through the airways and into the alveoli. The diaphragm is innervated by the phrenic nerve that originates from the cervical levels C3–C5. The diaphragm is unique in that it acts as both an involuntary and voluntary muscle. During sleep and rest, the diaphragm contracts involuntarily at a rate determined by respiratory centers in the medulla. This process can be overcome voluntarily by conscious breath holding, increased inspiratory excursion, or forceful exhaling.

Also important during inspiration are the external intercostal muscles that connect adjacent ribs. These are oriented in a forward downsloping direction as they connect the top rib with the bottom rib. This contraction acts to lift the rib cage as a whole, increasing the anteroposterior dimension of the thorax. During exercise, the tidal volume can be increased by using accessory muscles of inspiration. These include the scalene muscles that lift the first two ribs and the sternocleidomastoids that elevate the sternum. During maximal exertion, the diaphragm can increase its excursion to 10 cm (usually 1 cm at rest); therefore, the diaphragm is still the most important muscle involved in increasing tidal volume during exercise.

At rest, expiration is a *passive* process whereby the elasticity of lung tissue and the chest wall restore the thoracic dimensions to resting values. During exercise, however, expiration is facilitated by accessory muscles that include the abdominal wall muscles (rectus abdominus, internal and external obliques). Abdominal wall muscles act to compress the contents of the abdomen and thereby push the diaphragm up. The internal intercostal muscles are oriented in the opposite direction from the external intercostals, and therefore when contracted they pull the rib cage downward toward its resting position. The advantage to using accessory muscles of expiration is to shorten expiratory time and thus increase ventilatory rate.

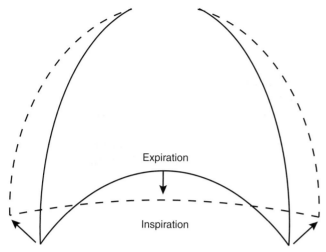

Figure 2-1. Diaphragm depression and rib cage elevation results in increased thoracic volume during inspiration.

CASE CONCLUSION

TS is able to do a total of 10 repetitions up the stairs within 50 minutes. His ventilatory rate and heart rate have changed little since the second repetition, and thus his oxygen consumption has remained fairly constant. However, the workload has exceeded the maximum possible energy produced from aerobic metabolism, and the excess work performed is compensated for by anaerobic metabolism at the level of the muscle. This has resulted in a high concentration of lactate in the muscle beds and a relative acidosis that later results in stiffness and fatigue. However, in the process his overall physical condition has improved due to optimizing the five components of oxygen delivery, especially his ability to increase cardiac output in the setting of high oxygen consumption.

THUMBNAIL: Oxygen Transport and Ventilation

Pathophysiology

The five steps of oxygen transport are ventilation, alveolar diffusion, hemoglobin binding, circulation, and peripheral diffusion.

Circulation (i.e., cardiac output) is the rate-limiting step in oxygen transport.

Inspiration is an active process mediated by respiratory centers in the medulla and pons.

Diaphragm contraction pushes down on the abdomen and pulls up on the rib cage.

Increases the vertical and horizontal dimensions of the thorax.

Creates negative pressure.

Accessory muscles of inspiration include external intercostal, scalene, and sternocleidomastoid muscles.

Expiration is normally a passive process allowed by relaxation of the diaphragm.

Accessory muscles of expiration include the abdominal wall muscles and the internal intercostal muscles.

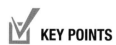

KEY POINTS

- Exercise results in increased oxygen consumption, which requires increased oxygen delivery
- Increased minute ventilation (MV) = (respiratory rate) × (tidal volume)
- Achieved primarily through increased respiratory rate
- Increased cardiac output (CO) = (heart rate) × (stroke volume)
- Achieved primarily through increased heart rate
- Arterial oxygen content (CaO_2 = [oxygen bound to hemoglobin] + [dissolved oxygen] = $[1.36 \times Hgb \times Sa_{O_2}] + [0.003 \times Pa_{O_2}]$)
- Hgb = hemoglobin concentration (13 – 15 mg/dL), Sa_{O_2} = arterial oxygen concentration (98%), Pa_{O_2} = arterial oxygen tension (80 – 100 mm Hg)
- CaO_2 = 20.0 + 0.3 = about 20 mL O_2/dL plasma
- Oxygen delivery = CO × CaO_2
- Achieved primarily through increased CO
- Oxygen delivery increases from about 0.5 L/min to 4 L/min

QUESTIONS

1. Which muscle is *not* used in forceful inspiration?

   A. Diaphragm
   B. Scalenes
   C. Sternocleidomastoids
   D. Internal intercostals
   E. External intercostals

2. Diffusion of gas across the alveolar capillary membrane is *inversely proportional* to which of the following?

   A. Area of the membrane
   B. Difference between partial pressures of the gas on both sides of the membrane
   C. A diffusion constant that is related to the solubility and molecular weight of the gas
   D. Thickness of the membrane
   E. Size of the alveolus

3. Which of the following has the *lowest* pressure in the cardiovascular system?

   A. Pulmonary arteries
   B. Pulmonary veins
   C. Systemic arteries
   D. Systemic veins
   E. Splanchnic vessels

4. Which of the following represents inspired air's partial pressure of oxygen at sea level?

   A. 760 mm Hg
   B. 713 mm Hg
   C. 160 mm Hg
   D. 150 mm Hg
   E. 100 mm Hg

High-Altitude Hypoxia

HPI: When TS graduated from college he no longer had wrestling to stay in shape, so he took up mountain climbing. He and his wife, VS, went on a hike to Mt. Whitney (elevation 14,300 feet) in California with some friends. They left Santa Barbara at sea level on Friday morning and spent the night in the desert at about 1200 feet. The next day they drove to the trailhead at 6000 feet and began backpacking; VS carried a 40-pound pack. By 7:00 P.M. they had hiked eight miles and set up camp at 10,600 feet. VS had difficulty sleeping during the night. Even though they had stopped hiking 2 hours previously, she still felt short of breath and was breathing heavily. TS noticed that throughout the night her breathing pattern was very irregular with periods where she would stop breathing for a number of seconds. The next morning VS felt tired but, despite her fatigue, continued up the trail. After 4 hours they had hiked another three miles and reached 13,100 feet. By that time VS had a horrible headache, body aches, nausea, and she vomited.

THOUGHT QUESTIONS

- What is the primary environmental change at high altitude responsible for VS's illness?
- What is the body's response to this change in the environment?
- Which two main chemoreceptors offer feedback to the respiratory centers?
- What acid-base alteration occurs during high-altitude adaptation?
- How does VS's body compensate for the primary acid-base disturbance?

BASIC SCIENCE REVIEW AND DISCUSSION

Partial Pressure of Oxygen in Inspired Air

Atmospheric pressure (or barometric pressure) is 760 mm Hg at sea level. This pressure decreases at higher altitudes. At 11,000 feet—the height of many peaks in the Rockies, Sierras, and Cascades—the barometric pressure is about 500 mm Hg. Atop Mount Everest (29,000 feet) the barometric pressure is about 250 mm Hg. Water vapor pressure of inspired air is 47 mm Hg and the fractional concentration of oxygen in dry air is 0.21. This results in a partial pressure of inhaled oxygen of $P_{IO_2} = (250 - 47 \text{ mm Hg}) \times 0.21 = 43$ mm Hg, which translates directly to a decreased hemoglobin saturation and lower oxygen delivery capacity. The end result is hypoxemia, or a lower than normal blood oxygen content.

There are five causes of hypoxia (Box 2-1). The A-a gradient is calculated by subtracting the partial pressure of oxygen in the alveoli (PaO2) from the partial pressure in the atmosphere (PAO2). In both hypoventilation and decreased FiO_2 the A-a gradient is normal as both atmospheric and alveolar O_2 concentration are decreased, whereas in ventilation/perfusion (V/Q) mismatch, right-to-left cardiac shunting, and alveolar diffusion defects, the A-a gradient is increased as the PAO2 is normal and only the PaO2 is decreased.

Regulation of Breathing

There are two primary locations for chemoreceptors that offer feedback to the respiratory centers in the medulla and pons. Central chemoreceptors are located in the ventral portion of the medulla and are surrounded by cerebrospinal fluid (CSF). These receptors are stimulated by CO_2 that crosses the blood-brain barrier and are responsible for the minute-to-minute regulation of respiratory rate and volume. Small increases in blood CO_2 tension translate into increases in CSF CO_2 tension and carbonic acid. Receptor stimulation activates the dorsal respiratory group in the medulla, increasing the respiratory rate. Hyperventilation lowers the partial pressure of CO_2 in the alveoli, which facilitates diffusion of CO_2 from the blood into the alveoli.

Peripheral chemoreceptors, which are primarily responsible for hyperventilation during hypoxemia, are located in the carotid bodies at the bifurcation of the common carotid arteries. These chemoreceptors are stimulated by both low oxygen tension (with maximal response at $Pa_{O_2} <70$ mm Hg) and low pH. There are also receptors in the lungs that offer feedback to the respiratory centers, including pulmonary stretch receptors, irritant receptors, and juxtacapillary receptors (J receptors).

High-Altitude Hypoxia and Acid-Base Physiology

As VS gains altitude, she is exposed to a lower partial pressure of oxygen, causing her to become hypoxemic. Stimulation of peripheral baroreceptors causes her to hyperventilate. This facilitates equilibration of alveolar PA_{O_2} and PA_{CO_2} with those of ambient air (i.e., PA_{O_2} increases and PA_{CO_2} decreases). In serum, CO_2 exists in equilibrium with carbonic acid (H_2HCO_3) and bicarbonate (HCO_3^-). Their relationship is described by the Henderson-Hasselbalch equation: $pH = pKA + \log\{[HCO_3^-]/[CO_2]\}$. This equation is depicted graphically by the Davenport diagram (Fig. 2-2). As VS blows off CO_2, her blood becomes alkalotic. This is known as primary respiratory alkalosis. All acid-base disturbances are the result of altering the ratio of $[HCO_3^-] / [CO_2]$, the driving factor in the Henderson-Hasselbalch equation. $[CO_2]$ is regulated primarily by ventilation; therefore, acid-base disorders that stem from a change in $[CO_2]$ are referred to as respiratory acidosis or alkalosis. It is important to understand that O_2 and CO_2 are dissolved gases in serum and that their concentrations $[O_2]$ and $[CO_2]$ are measured by their partial pressures Pa_{O_2} and Pa_{CO_2}. In contrast, HCO_3^- is a dissolved ion in serum and its concentration $[HCO_3^-]$ is measured directly.

$[HCO_3^-]$ is regulated by the kidneys. Primary alterations in $[HCO_3^-]$ occur via metabolic abnormalities and are therefore referred to as metabolic acidosis or alkalosis. Metabolic acidosis is typically caused by an excess of organic or exogenous acids that consume free HCO_3^- (e.g., lactic acid in shock, ketoacids in diabetic ketoacidosis, toxic ingestions such as methanol, paraldehyde, and others). Metabolic alkalosis is less common and usually results from excessive vomiting.

Once a primary acid-base disturbance exists, the buffering action of carbonic acid and its constituents carbon dioxide and

BOX 2-1 Causes of Hypoxia

1. Hypoventilation

2. Decreased FiO2

3. Ventilation/perfusion (V/Q) mismatch

4. Right-to-left cardiac shunting

5. Alveolar diffusion defects

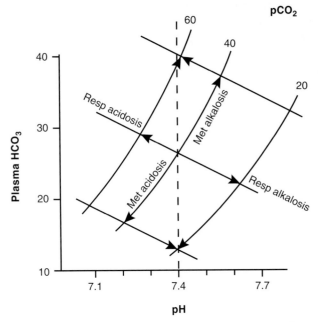

• **Figure 2-2.** Davenport diagram shows how serum pH, [HCO_3^+], and PCO_2 change with the four primary acid-base disturbances (*arrows originating from center*) and how secondary compensation occurs (*secondary arrows* that push the pH back toward 7.4 [*dotted line*]).

bicarbonate will cause a secondary compensation to restore the pH back toward 7.4. It is simple to predict how compensation will occur by considering the ratio [HCO_3^-] / [CO_2] in the Henderson-Hasselbalch equation. For example, in primary respiratory alkalosis, [CO_2] decreases (Pa_{CO_2} decreases) and the pH rises. To restore the pH toward its normal value, [HCO_3^-] must then decrease as well. This does in fact happen as bicarbonate is excreted from the kidneys; however, the process of bicarbonate excretion and complete compensation takes 2 to 3 days. Acetazolamide can be used to help prevent mountain sickness as it hastens the kidneys' bicarbonate diuresis. Another example is metabolic acidosis, in which the primary disturbance is the consumption of bicarbonate by an organic or exogenous acid, resulting in a pH decrease. Again, looking at the ratio [HCO_3^-]/[CO_2], one predicts that to restore a normal pH, [CO_2] must decrease. This is accomplished by increasing minute ventilation, which excretes CO_2 via the lungs. It is important to note that compensation is never complete, meaning that the pH will trend back toward 7.4 but not fully reach it.

CASE CONCLUSION

Once VS became obviously ill, she and TS descended down to 9000 feet and spent the night. At that altitude, the increased partial pressure of inhaled oxygen enabled her to slow her breathing rate and allow her kidneys more time to excrete bicarbonate to compensate for the respiratory alkalosis that had developed. By the next afternoon, VS felt well enough to resume the climb.

THUMBNAIL: High Altitude and Acid-Base

Pathophysiology

Partial pressure of oxygen in inspired air decreases as altitude increases
• Decreased PA_{O_2} results in hypoxemia (decreased PA_{O_2}).
• Hyperventilation is triggered by peripheral chemoreceptors.
• Increased minute ventilation decreases PA_{CO_2}.
• Decreased PA_{CO_2} allows for a relative increase in PA_{O_2}.

Respiratory alkalosis is a result of decreased PA_{CO_2}, decreased serum [CO_2], and increased pH
• Alkalosis and hypoxemia cause symptoms of acute mountain sickness.
• Kidneys compensate by excreting HCO_3^-, which takes 2 to 3 days.

Risk Factors
• Rapid ascent to altitudes greater than 8000 feet.
• Unclear genetic predisposition to acute mountain sickness.

☑ KEY POINTS

■ Central chemoreceptors in the medulla provide the primary regulatory feedback system for normal ventilation
  • Respond to increases in CSF CO_2 levels
■ Peripheral chemoreceptors in the carotid bodies provide secondary feedback to respiratory centers in the medulla and pons
  • Respond to decreased Pa_{O_2}, increased Pa_{CO_2}, and decreased pH
■ Acid-base disorders
  • $[CO_2]$ regulated by lungs and $[HCO_3^-]$ regulated by kidneys
  • pH <7.4 is acidosis

• Pa_{CO_2} >40 is primary respiratory acidosis
• $[HCO_3^-]$ <24 is primary metabolic acidosis
• pH >7.4 is alkalosis
• Pa_{CO_2} <40 is primary respiratory alkalosis
• $[HCO_3^-]$ >24 is primary metabolic alkalosis
■ The ratio $[HCO_3^-]/[CO_2]$ predicts how the body will compensate for the primary disturbance

QUESTIONS

1. Peripheral chemoreceptors are activated by which of the following?
   A. Decrease in pH
   B. Increase in arterial Pa_{O_2}
   C. Decrease in arterial Pa_{CO_2}
   D. Increase in serum bicarbonate
   E. Hyperventilation

2. What is the physiologic advantage to hyperventilating at high altitude?
   A. Increases the partial pressure of oxygen in inspired air
   B. Creates respiratory alkalosis that facilitates oxygen-hemoglobin binding
   C. Decreases alveolar PA_{CO_2} and thereby increase alveolar PA_{O_2}
   D. Opens, or recruits, more alveoli for gas exchange
   E. Compensates for a primary metabolic acidosis

3. A patient presents to the emergency department with decreased mental status and the following arterial blood gas analysis is obtained: pH 7.26, Pa_{O_2} 100 mm Hg, Pa_{CO_2} 26, $[HCO_3^-]$ 12. Which of the following is the primary acid-base disturbance and its accompanying compensatory mechanism?

   A. Respiratory acidosis with a compensatory metabolic alkalosis
   B. Metabolic acidosis with a compensatory respiratory alkalosis
   C. Respiratory alkalosis with a compensatory metabolic acidosis
   D. Metabolic alkalosis with a compensatory respiratory acidosis
   E. None of the above

4. A patient with long-standing chronic obstructive pulmonary disease presents to the emergency department with increased cough and difficulty breathing. The following arterial blood gas analysis is obtained: pH 7.34, Pa_{O_2} 76 mm Hg, Pa_{CO_2} 60, $[HCO_3^-]$ 28. Which of the following is the primary acid-base disturbance and its compensatory mechanism?

   A. Respiratory acidosis with a compensatory metabolic alkalosis
   B. Metabolic acidosis with a compensatory respiratory alkalosis
   C. Respiratory alkalosis with a compensatory metabolic acidosis
   D. Metabolic alkalosis with a compensatory respiratory acidosis
   E. None of the above

Carbon Monoxide Poisoning

HPI: BR lives in the city three blocks down the street from CA, her grandmother. The city was in the grips of the first cold weather spell of winter, and CA had turned on the gas furnace early in the morning. BR came to visit mid-morning and her grandmother complained of a headache and nausea. BR thought that because her grandmother looked pale, she would grocery shop for her while CA stayed home and rested. BR was gone for 2 hours and returned to find her grandmother asleep in bed. BR tried to arouse her but CA wouldn't open her eyes. BR quickly called 911 and the paramedics arrived shortly thereafter. After assessing that CA was breathing spontaneously, they placed her on 100% oxygen and a cardiac monitor. They also established an IV, drew several vials of blood, and administered glucose. As part of the initial blood analysis in the emergency department, one of the vials drawn by the paramedics was sent for a blood gas analysis and carbon monoxide level. The carbon monoxide level returned at 38% (may be as high as 10% in smokers but normal is 0%). BR's grandmother was kept on high-flow oxygen and arrangements were made for more definitive treatment.

THOUGHT QUESTIONS

- When and where is carbon monoxide (CO) poisoning most often seen?
- How is oxygen transported in the blood to peripheral tissues?
- How is carbon dioxide (CO_2) transported from peripheral tissues back to the lungs?
- How does CO interfere with the normal transport of oxygen?
- How does CO affect the oxygen-hemoglobin dissociation curve?
- In which three forms is CO_2 transported from peripheral tissue back to the lungs?

BASIC SCIENCE REVIEW AND DISCUSSION

CO poisoning is most often encountered in building fires, leaking heating systems, and suicide attempts. The most common cause of unconsciousness and death in fires is CO poisoning; therefore, all fire victims should be monitored and treated for CO poisoning. CO poisoning is also common during winter months in large cities in cold climates such as Chicago, New York, or Boston. Poisoning typically affects the elderly, who have little hypoxic reserve. Symptoms are initially vague and include headache, nausea, fatigue, visual disturbances, paresthesias, chest or abdominal pains, and/or diarrhea. Attaching a hose from a car's exhaust into the driver's compartment is a common method of committing suicide. CO is very insidious because it is colorless and odorless, thus making its presence often difficult to detect.

Alveolar Gas Equation

Inspired air has a partial pressure of oxygen of 150 mm Hg, which is calculated based on sea level barometric pressure (760 mm Hg), adjusted for the partial pressure of humidified air (47 mm Hg) and the fractional component of oxygen in air (0.21). The alveolar gas equation is used to calculate the partial pressure of oxygen in the alveoli (PaO2) based on the oxygen partial pressure of inspired gas (PI_{O2}) and the alveolar partial pressure of carbon dioxide (PA_{CO2}): $PA_{O2} = PI_{O2} - (PA_{CO2}/R)$, where PA_{O2} is the actual partial pressure of oxygen in the alveoli, PI_{O2} is the partial pressure of oxygen in inspired air (150 mm Hg), PA_{CO2} is the partial pressure of CO_2 in the alveoli (approximate to PaO2, or 40 mm Hg, which is the partial pressure of CO_2 measured in arterial blood), and R is the ratio of CO_2 produced to O_2 consumed and is approximately 0.8. Therefore, $PA_{O2} = 150 - 40/0.8 = 100$ mm Hg.

Henry's Law

Once oxygen transits the alveolar membrane it dissolves into the blood. Henry's law dictates that the concentration of dissolved gas (C_x) is proportional to its partial pressure (P_x): $C_x = K \times P_x$. For oxygen, 0.003 mL/dL will be dissolved for each mm Hg of P_{O2} (e.g., Ko = 0.003 mL/dL for oxygen), which translates into a blood oxygen concentration of about 0.3 mL/dL given a partial pressure for oxygen of 100 mm Hg in the pulmonary capillaries. The oxygen requirement during exertion is about 15 mL/dL; an alternative means of oxygen transport must therefore exist in order to supply this demand.

Hemoglobin: The Oxygen Carrier

The alternative means of oxygen transport is facilitated by hemoglobin, which is a protein contained within red blood cells. The molecule consists of four globin chains each having an iron-porphyrin moiety that binds oxygen; therefore, four molecules of oxygen can bind to one hemoglobin molecule. The affinity of hemoglobin for oxygen rises as more oxygen-binding sites become filled, which explains the nonlinear shape of the oxygen-hemoglobin dissociation curve (Fig. 2-3). At $P_{O2} >80$ mm Hg, the curve is essentially horizontal, which means oxygen is bound avidly to hemoglobin. Such a condition of high P_{O2} exists in arterial blood where oxygen transport is desired. As the P_{O2} declines, the curve undergoes a sharp descent, which means that oxygen is easily off-loaded. This condition exists in peripheral capillary beds where oxygen delivery to tissues is desired. In addition, there are certain factors that shift the curve to the right, which results in increased dissociation at a given P_{O2}. These factors include increased temperature, H+ concentration, P_{CO2} concentration, and 2,3-DPG concentration. All of these conditions exist in peripheral muscle capillary beds during exertion and thus facilitate in oxygen dissociation and delivery to tissues.

Carbon Dioxide Transport

CO_2 is a normal byproduct of cellular metabolism. It must be transported in the systemic venous system back to the heart, where it is pumped into the pulmonary capillary beds, diffuses across the alveolar-capillary membrane, and is exhaled by the lungs. CO_2 is transported in three forms: dissolved CO_2, carbamino compounds, and bicarbonate. The solubility of CO_2 is 20 times greater than that of oxygen; therefore, a larger proportion of CO_2 is dissolved in blood. Carbamino compounds are formed when CO_2 reversibly binds amine groups on circulating proteins. The

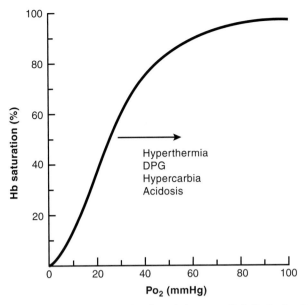

• Figure 2-3. Oxygen-hemoglobin dissociation curve. Note the horizontal shape of the curve above oxygen saturation >90%. Corresponding with PO_2 drops below 70 mm Hg, the oxygen saturation drops rapidly (steep portion of the curve). A shift to the right results in off-loading of oxygen from hemoglobin at higher PO_2.

10% as dissolved CO_2. This is in contrast to oxygen, in which over 98% is transported by hemoglobin.

Pathophysiology of Carbon Monoxide Poisoning

As CO enters the alveoli, it diffuses across the alveolar-capillary membrane similar to oxygen. CO reversibly binds hemoglobin at one of the oxygen-binding sites and converts the molecule into carboxy-hemoglobin (COHb). COHb binds the three remaining sites to oxygen; however, the conformation of the molecule is such that it does not release the bound oxygen. The oxygen saturation of hemoglobin therefore remains essentially the same (and measured oxygen saturation may, in fact, be normal), yet the oxygen cannot be off-loaded in peripheral tissues. For this reason, CO has the effect of shifting the oxygen-hemoglobin dissociation curve to the left. In addition, CO has 240 times the affinity for hemoglobin than for oxygen. Thus, low concentrations of CO can have profound effects on oxygen-transport capabilities.

most abundant of the CO_2-binding proteins is hemoglobin itself, which results in carbamino Hb. Deoxygenated Hb has a higher affinity for CO_2 than does oxygenated Hb, which is referred to as the *Haldane effect*. Bicarbonate is generated from CO_2 in red blood cells by the following reaction:

$$CO_2 + H_2O \xleftarrow{CA} H_2CO_3 \longleftrightarrow H^+ + HCO_3^-$$

The first reaction occurs in the presence of carbonic anhydrase (CA) in red cells, and the second reaction occurs spontaneously. Bicarbonate (HCO_3^-) diffuses out of the cells and is transported in blood plasma. Because H+ cannot freely cross the red cell membrane, chloride shifts into the cells to maintain electric neutrality. This is known as *chloride shift*. In total, 60% of CO_2 is transported as bicarbonate, 30% as carbamino compounds, and

CASE CONCLUSION

CA becomes minimally more responsive during the first 15 minutes in the emergency department with oxygen therapy alone. She is transported immediately to a hyperbaric oxygen chamber where she is placed at three atmospheres and continues to receive 100% oxygen. Because CO binds reversibly to oxygen receptors on the hemoglobin molecule, increasing the concentration of oxygen will reverse binding. Breathing 100% oxygen can achieve this; breathing 100% oxygen at three atmospheres greatly increases the delivered concentration of oxygen, in turn increasing alveolar PAO_2. The binding half-life of CO to hemoglobin is about 240 minutes while breathing room air, 80 minutes while breathing 100% oxygen, and about 20 minutes while breathing 100% oxygen at three atmospheres. After 2 hours in the chamber, CA wakens and answers simple questions.

THUMBNAIL: CO Poisoning and Oxygen Transport

Pathophysiology

CO is an inhaled poison that binds hemoglobin

CO has 240 times the affinity of oxygen

Causes conformational change of hemoglobin
    Remaining sites bind oxygen tightly
        Prevents oxygen off-loading in peripheral tissues
        Results in tissue hypoxemia

Risk Factors

Smoke inhalation, leaking heating systems, car exhaust

✓ KEY POINTS

- Concentration of dissolved arterial oxygen is proportional to the oxygen tension in the alveoli according to Henry's law
- Dissolved oxygen accounts for only about 1.5% of arterial oxygen content
- Hemoglobin is a protein with four binding sites for oxygen
- Carries about 98.5% of oxygen in arterial blood
- Oxygen affinity is high at high oxygen tension (pulmonary capillaries) and low at low oxygen tension (peripheral capillaries)
- Oxygen-hemoglobin dissociation curve has a plateau at high oxygen tension

- Oxygen-hemoglobin dissociation curve is steep at lower oxygen tensions
- Shift to the right of the oxygen-hemoglobin dissociation curve results in off-loading of oxygen from hemoglobin
- Occurs in peripheral tissues as a result of increased temperature, increased P_{CO2}, decreased pH, and increased 2,3-DPG
- CO_2 is transported back to the lungs as bicarbonate, carbamino groups, and dissolved CO_2
- CO_2 is 20 times more soluble than O_2
- Higher percentage of CO_2 is in the dissolved form
- CO_2 diffuses across the alveolar membrane more readily

QUESTIONS

1. Approximately what percentage of oxygen is dissolved in arterial blood plasma?

   A. 1.5%
   B. 10%
   C. 25%
   D. 50%
   E. 80%

2. Compared with carbon dioxide, what is the rate of diffusion of oxygen across the alveolar-capillary membrane?

   A. Higher because of oxygen's smaller molecular weight
   B. Higher because of oxygen's greater solubility
   C. Higher because of oxygen's greater affinity for hemoglobin
   D. Lower because oxygen is less soluble than CO_2
   E. Lower because of oxygen's greater affinity for hemoglobin

3. Which of the following conditions results in a *lower* arterial oxygen tension (mmHg)?

   A. Anemia
   B. Low cardiac output

   C. CO poisoning
   D. High-altitude climbing
   E. All of the above

4. Which of the following is *consistent* with a shift to the right of the oxygen-hemoglobin dissociation curve?

   A. Increased affinity of hemoglobin for oxygen
   B. Decreased P_{50}, or O_2 tension that produces 50% hemoglobin saturation
   C. Facilitated off-loading of oxygen to peripheral tissues
   D. Decreased temperature, increased pH, decreased P_{CO2}, decreased 2,3-DPG
   E. CO poisoning

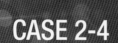

HPI: EZ, a 67-year-old man, presents with dyspnea. He typically experiences shortness of breath on exertion, such as walking up stairs, which has gradually worsened over the past 2 years. For 3 days, EZ has had an increased cough without sputum production and severe dyspnea when walking only a short distance. He has had no fevers or chills. EZ's chest feels tight when he takes a deep breath. He has also noted increased swelling in both feet. He has a history of hypertension, hyperlipidemia, and "asthma"; he takes atenolol and Lipitor. EZ has smoked two packs of cigarettes a day for 50 years.

PE: His vital signs are remarkable for a respiratory rate of 34 and an Sa_{O_2} of 88%. On exam, he is thin, in moderate respiratory distress, and using accessory muscles to breathe. He has distended jugular veins. Despite EZ's overall thin appearance, his chest is large in diameter. His lung sounds are diminished and he has bilateral expiratory wheezes. He has mild peripheral cyanosis obvious around his fingernail beds. EZ also has 1+ peripheral edema.

THOUGHT QUESTIONS

- How is the normal ventilatory cycle affected by obstructive lung disease? How are resting lung volume, vital capacity, and forced expiratory volume affected?
- What is the common characteristic feature of obstructive lung disease and what are the four major obstructive lung diseases?
- What are the pathophysiologic differences between emphysema and chronic bronchitis? How do these contribute to the obstructive pattern of chronic obstructive pulmonary disease (COPD)?
- What is the relationship between lung volume and compliance? How does this affect the work of breathing for someone with COPD?
- In which region of the lung is air trapping in COPD most predominant? How does ventilation, perfusion, and the ratio of ventilation to perfusion (V/Q ratio) differ between the lung base and apex? Why are these differences significant in COPD?

BASIC SCIENCE REVIEW AND DISCUSSION

Lung Volumes and Obstructive Lung Disease

Normal ventilation consists of inspiratory and expiratory phases. Inspiration is an active process of expanding the chest cavity, creating increased negative intrathoracic pressure, and drawing air into the lungs. This is achieved mainly by contraction and downward deflection of the diaphragm, but also through expansion of the thoracic cage by the external intercostal, sternocleidomastoid, and scalene muscles. Exhalation occurs passively because of the inherent elasticity of lung tissue. Obstructive lung disease is characterized either by loss of lung elasticity (e.g., COPD) or increased airway resistance (e.g., asthma). The hallmark of obstructive lung disease is *reduction of expiratory flow rate*. As a result, air trapping occurs, causing an increase in the resting lung volume (i.e., increased functional residual capacity [FRC]) and end-expiratory volume (i.e., increased residual volume [RV]). Total lung capacity (TLC) is also mildly increased (Fig. 2-4). As a result of the disproportionate increase in FRC, the vital capacity (VC = TLC – FRC) is drastically decreased. Forced expiratory volume in 1 second (FEV_1) is decreased as a result of both functional and mechanical obstruction and is therefore a sensitive test for the presence of obstructive lung disease (Table 2-1). Types of obstructive lung disease include chronic COPD, asthma, bronchiectasis, and cystic fibrosis.

Pathophysiology of Chronic Obstructive Pulmonary Disease

Emphysema and chronic bronchitis are the two pathologic entities that comprise COPD. Often, these two entities coexist and patients will exhibit features of both; sometimes patients will exhibit a predominance of one or the other. Emphysema is caused by alveolar wall destruction as a result of excessive protease activity. Inhaled toxins, such as those in cigarette smoke, cause an increase in alveolar macrophages and neutrophils. The present hypothesis is that activated neutrophils release proteases that destroy interstitial elastin and cleave type IV collagen. Alveolar wall destruction leads to loss of pulmonary capillaries and a reduction of oxygen diffusing capacity. It also results in increased pulmonary artery pressure and right heart failure (cor pulmonale). Interstitial elasticity helps maintain patency of terminal and respiratory bronchioles in healthy adults. In emphysema, many of these bronchioles collapse without elasticity of the surrounding interstitium, thus creating obstruction to air outflow.

Chronic bronchitis is characterized by excessive mucus production in the bronchial tree. In response to inhaled toxins and irritants, epithelial goblet cells and subepithelial mucous glands proliferate and the number of ciliated epithelial cells decrease. This results in increased mucus production with chronic cough. Airway obstruction seen with chronic bronchitis is primarily due to bronchiolar inflammation and bronchospasm, both of which are triggered by inhaled irritants or acute respiratory infection. For this reason, systemic corticosteroids, inhaled β2-agonists, and inhaled anticholinergics are helpful in COPD exacerbations.

Pressure-Volume Relationship

Lung expansion is achieved through increasing the volume of the thoracic cage, which results in an increased negative intrapleural pressure. Compliance is a measure of the amount of volume change achieved by a certain amount of negative pressure (i.e., compliance = $\Delta V/\Delta P$). For example, stiff lungs (e.g., interstitial fibrosis) expand less for a given amount of pressure change; therefore, they have a low compliance. As lung volume increases, interstitial elastin becomes taut, and compliance decreases. For this reason, in COPD as FRC increases, lung expansion becomes more difficult because of the lower compliance at higher resting volumes (Fig. 2-5). This leads to increased work of breathing that is characteristic with COPD.

Regional Variation in Ventilation

Intrapleural pressure increases (i.e., it becomes less negative) toward the base of the lung due to the effects of gravity and the

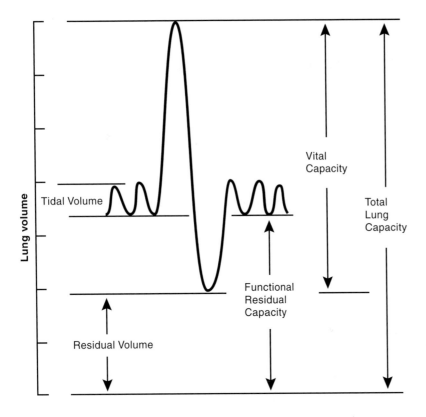

• **Figure 2-4.** Graphical output of spirometer during normal breathing (TV), full inspiration (TLC), and full expiration (RV). Functional residual capacity is the lung volume remaining after passive exhalation.

weight of the lung. For this reason, the alveoli at the base are less distended and thus more compliant. During inhalation, higher compliance at the base results in greater expansion and thus greater ventilation as compared with the apex. However, in COPD, alveolar wall destruction and decreased elasticity of respiratory bronchioles result in alveolar collapse when increased thoracic pressure is created during exhalation. This collapse occurs preferentially at the bases because of their relatively higher compliance than at the apices. Therefore, patients with COPD ventilate the apices more than the bases, which is the opposite of normal physiology.

Regional Variation in Perfusion and Lung Zones

Similar to the regional variation in ventilation, pulmonary capillary perfusion is greater at the lung base compared with the apex. In fact, the difference is even greater than that for ventilation because the pulmonary vascular pressure, which in effect acts like a column of fluid, varies largely from the bottom to the top of the lungs. Alveolar pressure, however, remains constant at atmospheric pressure throughout the lung regions. At the level of the alveolus, capillary flow is exposed to alveolar pressure and thus flow is dependent on relative pressure differences. At the apex where alveolar pressure exceeds pulmonary arterial and venous pressure (zone 1), there is practically no flow (Fig. 2-6). Farther down, in zone 2, pulmonary arterial pressure exceeds alveolar pressure and the capillary flow is proportional to the difference of these two pressures. At the base, in zone 3, pulmonary venous pressure exceeds alveolar pressure and flow is proportional to the difference of pulmonary arterial and venous pressures. Because of the larger decrease in perfusion compared

	Normal	Obstructive	Restrictive
TABLE 2-1 Pulmonary Function Tests in Obstructive versus Restrictive Lung Disease			
VC	4.8 L	3.5	3.5
FRC	3.8 L	6.0	2.2
TLC	6.0 L	8.0	4.5
FEV_1	3.5 L	1.5	3.0
Compliance	0.20 L/cm water	0.35	0.12

VC, vital capacity; *FRC*, functional residual capacity; *TLC*, total lung capacity; *FEV₁*, forced expiratory volume in 1 second

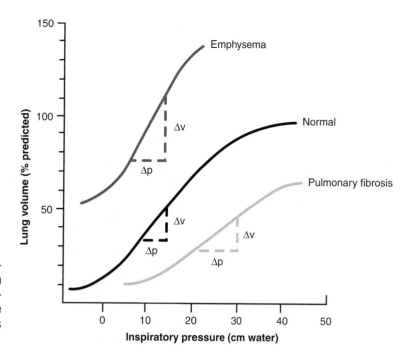

• **Figure 2-5.** Pressure-volume curves for normal, obstructive (emphysema), and restrictive (pulmonary fibrosis) patterns. Note increased compliance ($\Delta V/\Delta P$) in emphysema versus pulmonary fibrosis. In general, compliance (slope of P-V curve) decreases at higher lung volumes as is seen by the flattening of the curves at high volumes.

with ventilation from the base to the apex, the V/Q ratio is larger at the apex. However, this region contributes little to the total pulmonary capillary gas exchange because of its low perfusion.

In COPD, the shift of ventilation from the well-perfused bases to the hypoperfused apices creates a pathologic V/Q mismatch. This impairs overall pulmonary gas exchange and results in hypoxemia. The inability to effectively expire alveolar CO_2 results in CO_2 retention, increased arterial Pa_{CO_2}, and respiratory acidosis. Noninvasive positive-pressure ventilation (NPPV) is a useful technique for treating acute exacerbations of COPD. NPPV consists of a tight-fitting, airtight face mask linked in series to a ventilator. The ventilator provides breaths to the patient at increased inspiratory pressures. This acts to open alveoli that have collapsed due to the increased compliance of the terminal and respiratory bronchioles (Fig. 2-7).

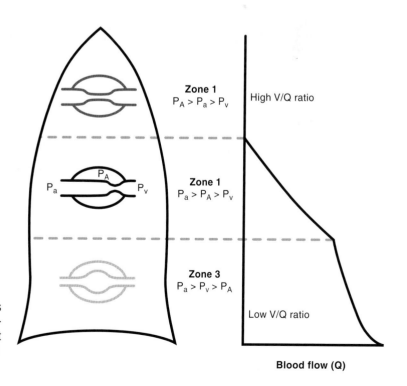

• **Figure 2-6.** Depiction of the three lung zones where P_a is pulmonary arterial pressure, P_v is pulmonary venous pressure, and P_A is alveolar pressure. P_A is constant throughout all zones, whereas P_a and P_v decrease from zone 3 to zone 1 as a result of hydrostatic pressure.

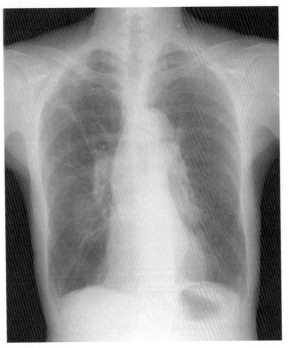

• **Figure 2-7.** Chest x-ray showing characteristics of COPD: hyperinflated lungs, diaphragm flattening, and narrow cardiac silhouette.

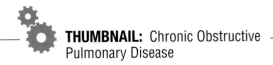

THUMBNAIL: Chronic Obstructive Pulmonary Disease

Pathophysiology

Emphysema
Destruction of alveolar walls and elastin by chronic airway inflammation
Dilated airspaces and increased lung compliance
Cigarette smoke attracts neutrophils and macrophages
Increased protease activity
Respiratory bronchioles affected the most (centrilobular emphysema)
α1-Antitrypsin deficiency results in uncommon hereditary emphysema
Natural defense against proteolytic enzymes
Diffuse involvement of lung tissue (panacinar emphysema)

Chronic bronchitis
Proliferation of mucus glands and goblet cells in bronchi and bronchioles
Destruction of cilia and ability to clear secretions
Increased bronchospasm and airway resistance

Risk Factors
Smoking, air and environmental pollutants, respiratory infection
α1-Antitrypsin deficiency

CASE CONCLUSION

EZ is placed on four liters of oxygen by nasal canula to keep his oxygen saturation above 92%; he is also placed on a cardiac monitor. An IV is obtained and he is given methylprednisolone 125 mg IV and continuous albuterol and ipratropium nebulizers. A chest x-ray shows hyperinflated lungs, flattening of the diaphragm, and narrowing of the cardiac silhouette (Fig. 2-7). He continues to have difficulty breathing and is placed on NPPV via a tight-fitting face mask and a ventilator. An arterial blood gas is obtained prior to NPPV, which shows pH 7.32, P_{O2} 56 mm Hg, P_{CO2} 62 mm Hg. He is admitted to the ICU where he continues to receive oxygen, nebulizers, and NPPV to which he gradually responds.

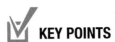

KEY POINTS

■ Reduced expiratory flow rate (FEV1)
■ Patients exhibit features of both emphysema and chronic bronchitis
■ Pulmonary function abnormalities
  • Increased TLC, FRC, RV
  • Decreased VC, FEV_1

■ Ventilation/perfusion mismatch
  • Alveolar collapse during exhalation
  • Inadequate ventilation resulting in hypoxia and hypercapnia

QUESTIONS

1. COPD is characterized by which of the following?

   A. Increased lung compliance
   B. Increased VC
   C. Decreased RV
   D. Decreased physiologic dead space
   E. Decrease in TLC

2. In COPD, air trapping occurs:

   A. more in the upper lobes
   B. more in the lower lobes
   C. centrally greater than peripherally
   D. equally throughout
   E. Cannot be determined

3. Which blood gas result represents compensated respiratory acidosis?

   A. pH 7.30; Pa_{O_2} 85; Pa_{CO2} 30; HCO_3^- 12
   B. pH 7.24; Pa_{O_2} 60; Pa_{CO2} 60; HCO_3^- 26
   C. pH 7.37; Pa_{O_2} 62; Pa_{CO2} 60; HCO_3^- 42
   D. pH 7.48; Pa_{O_2} 70; Pa_{CO2} 30; HCO_3^- 22
   E. pH 7.52; Pa_{O_2} 90; Pa_{CO2} 48; HCO_3^- 48

4. As lung volume increases, lung compliance

   A. increases
   B. decreases
   C. stays the same
   D. first increases, then decreases
   E. cannot be determined

CASE 2-5 Pneumonia

HPI: SS, a 26-year-old woman, smokes a pack of cigarettes daily but is otherwise healthy. She became ill one morning when she developed a sudden shaking chill and spiked a temperature up to 102.4°F. SS noted pain in her right chest when she took a deep breath but had no difficulty breathing. Later that morning she developed a dry cough and the pain increased. SS took acetaminophen for her fever but continued to feel worse. By afternoon, she had not eaten, her fever rose to 103.2°F, and she began to have shaking chills again.

PE: Upon arrival in the emergency department, she looked ill and was mildly dyspneic. Her vital signs included a temperature of 102.8°F, pulse 118, blood pressure 112/74, respiratory rate 32, and oxygen saturation of 92% on room air. On physical exam, she had rhonchi in the right lower lung field with egophony and transmitted upper airway sounds.

THOUGHT QUESTIONS

- How do classical and atypical presentations differ for pneumonia? What are the most common organisms causing each of these syndromes?
- What are some of the most common risk factors for pneumonia?
- Which features of pneumonia result in a worse outcome and subsequently require hospitalization and intravenous antibiotics?
- How are antibiotics selected to treat pneumonia?

BASIC SCIENCE REVIEW AND DISCUSSION

Classical versus Atypical Pneumonia

The classical presentation for pneumonia is the sudden onset of fever, chills, cough with or without purulent sputum, pleuritic chest pain, and dyspnea. This syndrome is most frequently caused by *Streptococcus pneumoniae*; however, *Haemophilus influenzae*, *Moraxella catarrhalis*, *Staphylococcus aureus*, or gram-negative enteric bacteria may also be the culprit. When sputum is available, a diagnosis can be made by Gram stain with an adequate specimen that contains greater then 25 neutrophils and less than 10 squamous cells. Gram stain findings and optimal antibiotic treatment are detailed for each organism in Table 2-2. The chest x-ray in classic pneumonia shows a focal consolidation confined to a particular lobe of the lung that correlates with location of pleuritic chest pain. A consolidation refers to alveolar infiltrates that consist of the bacterial pathogen and exudative inflammatory response, including inflammatory cells, cytokines, and proteinaceous fluid.

Atypical pneumonia usually occurs as a more indolent process that may progress over several days and include more prominent constitutional symptoms, such as a low-grade fever, myalgias, fatigue, arthralgias, headache, sore throat, or skin rash. Pulmonary complaints are often less marked, the cough is usually nonproductive, and pleuritic chest pain is often absent. Atypical pneumonia is most commonly caused by *Mycoplasma pneumoniae*; however, many organisms can possibly cause it, including other bacterial pathogens (e.g., *Chlamydia pneumoniae*, *Legionella*, *Mycobacterium tuberculosis*), viral pathogens (e.g., adenovirus, parainfluenza virus, respiratory syncytial virus), or fungal pathogens (e.g., aspergillosis, coccidiomycosis, histoplasmosis, *Pneumocystis carinii*). The Gram stain in atypical pneumonia contains fewer neutrophils and is less diagnostic. The chest x-ray findings vary but will often show bilateral patchy or interstitial infiltrates.

Risk Factors

As with many infectious diseases, risk factors for pneumonia include the elderly, debilitated, and immunocompromised. More specifically, patients with chronic lung disease, chronic renal failure, diabetes mellitus, and sickle cell disease are more susceptible to pneumonia. Patients who suffer from alcoholism, seizure disorders, or chronic debilitating neurologic disorders are prone to aspiration pneumonia. Immunocompromised patients include those with acquired immunodeficiency syndrome (AIDS) or those taking immunosuppressive medications such as steroids or chemotherapeutic agents. These patients are susceptible to the common bacterial and viral agents but consideration must also be given to opportunistic organisms such as tuberculosis, fungal agents (e.g., *Candida*, *Pneumocystis carinii*), or parasites.

Admission Criteria

The decision to admit a patient with pneumonia for IV antibiotics is multifactorial and based largely on clinical experience; however, there are several clinical features that portend a poor outcome and usually warrant admission. These include patients older than age 70 or those with significant comorbidity, such as renal, heart, or lung disease. Patients who have failed outpatient antibiotic therapy or who cannot tolerate oral medication must also be admitted. Patients with evidence of respiratory failure or sepsis should definitely be admitted. This is evident by persistent tachypnea greater than 30 breaths/minute, tachycardia greater than 120/minute, hypotension less than 90 mm Hg, hypoxia less than 90%, or changes in mental status. Patients with an empyema or large parapneumonic effusion also should be admitted.

Treatment

The selection of antibiotics is based on the suspected agent and on whether the pneumonia was acquired in the community, in the hospital, or in some other chronic care facility. Community-acquired pneumonia in young, healthy adults usually is caused by one of the atypical organisms, such as *Mycoplasma*, *Chlamydia*, or a virus. Smokers are more likely to harbor one of the typical bacterial pathogens, such as *S. pneumoniae*, *H. influenzae*, and *M. catarrhalis*. Macrolide antibiotics (e.g., azithromycin, clarithromycin) provide good coverage against the typical and atypical organisms and are therefore the first-line agents against community-acquired pneumonia. Of course, if a sputum sample can be obtained and a Gram stain performed in a timely fashion, then a specific organism may be identified and the antibiotic tailored (see Table 2-2). Commonly used second-line agents

TABLE 2-2 Gram Stain Findings and Antibiotic Treatment for Common Bacterial Pathogens

Organism	Gram Stain Findings	First-Line Antibiotics
Streptococcus pneumoniae	Gram-positive cocci in pairs	Penicillin
Mycoplasma pneumoniae	Does not stain; diagnosis with positive cold-agglutinin serology	Erythromycin
Haemophilus influenzae	Gram-negative coccobacillus	Trimethoprim-sulfamethoxazole, ampicillin
Staphylococcus aureus	Gram-positive cocci in clusters	Nafcillin
Legionella pneumophila	Rare gram-negative rods, numerous neutrophils; diagnosis with positive urine *Legionella* antigen	Erythromycin
Escherichia coli, Klebsiella pneumoniae, Pseudomonas pneumoniae	Gram-negative rods	Aminoglycosides, third-generation cephalosporin
Chlamydia pneumoniae	Giemsa stain shows cytoplasmic organisms within epithelial cells	Erythromycin

include a fluoroquinolone (e.g., levofloxacin), second-generation cephalosporin (e.g., cefuroxime), amoxicillin/clavulanate (e.g., Augmentin), or doxycycline.

Patients with community-acquired pneumonia who have significant comorbidities and require hospitalization should be covered more broadly for gram-negative pathogens. Therefore, in addition to a macrolide or fluoroquinolone, a third-generation cephalosporin (e.g., ceftriaxone, cefotaxime) should be administered intravenously. For hospital-acquired pneumonia, antibiotic coverage needs to be expanded to cover resistant strains of *Streptococcus* and *Staphylococcus*, *Pseudomonas*, gram-negative organisms, and anaerobes.

Imipenem and meropenem as single agents provide good coverage for these organisms in addition to the typical bacterial pathogens. Despite their broad coverage, these drugs should not be used as first-line agents to avoid drug resistance. A good choice is a third-generation cephalosporin with antipseudomonal activity (e.g., cefepime, ceftazidime) plus an aminoglycoside (e.g., tobramycin, gentamicin), which also possesses antipseudomonal activity. Antipseudomonal penicillins (e.g., ticarcillin, piperacillin) are also good options. Again, sputum and blood cultures are important in hospital-acquired pneumonia in order to specify the organism, identify drug sensitivities, and tailor antibiotic therapy.

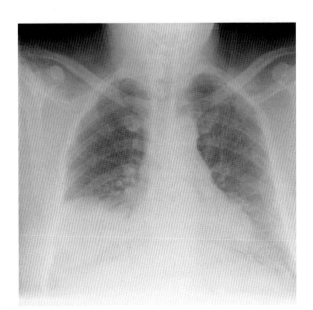
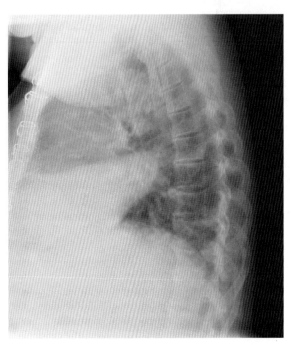

• **Figure 2-8.** Chest x-ray showing a right middle lobe pneumonia. Note that the right heart border and right diaphragm are obscured on the posteroanterior view (**A**) and the wedge-shaped infiltrate on the lateral view (**B**) corresponds to the right middle lobe.

CASE CONCLUSION

SS has the typical symptoms for classic bacterial pneumonia. A chest x-ray showed a consolidation in the right middle lobe (Fig. 2-8). Given that she is a young, healthy smoker, the most likely pathogens are *S. pneumoniae*, *H. influenzae*, and *M. catarrhalis*. If she were treated as an outpatient, azithromycin would be a reasonable choice of antibiotics. However, because SS does not look well, is not tolerating fluids, and her oxygen saturation is in the low 90s, she is admitted for antibiotic treatment and IV rehydration. In the emergency department, she is able to provide a deep sputum sample, which is sent to the laboratory for Gram stain and culture. The Gram stain shows abundant neutrophils with gram-positive cocci in pairs. A diagnosis of pneumococcal pneumonia is made and SS is given IV penicillin G. Her fever breaks that evening and she feels better the next day. She is discharged home on the third day in good condition.

THUMBNAIL: Pneumonia

Pathophysiology

Classic Pneumonia
Rapid onset of symptoms
High fever, rigors, cough, pleuritic chest pain
Physical exam reveals tachycardia, tachypnea, hypoxia, focal rhonchi, egophony, transmitted breath sounds
Chest x-ray shows focal consolidation
Most common pathogens are *S. pneumoniae*, *H. influenzae*, *M. catarrhalis*

Atypical Pneumonia
Symptom onset more gradual or indolent
Low-grade fevers, myalgias and arthralgias, fatigue, headache, rash
Physical exam may reveal low-grade fever, tachycardia or mild hypoxia, diffuse rales
Chest x-ray shows diffuse interstitial infiltrates
Most common pathogens are *Mycoplasma pneumoniae*, *C. pneumoniae*, or a virus

Risk Factors
Mucociliary dysfunction
Smoking, chronic asthma or bronchitis, cystic fibrosis, bronchiectasis
Comorbid disease
Heart disease, renal failure, chronic lung disease, diabetes mellitus
Immunocompromised
Cancer, AIDS, chemotherapeutic agents, chronic steroid use

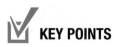

KEY POINTS

- Identification of specific organism is important in tailoring therapy
- Empiric treatment is based on several factors
- Community acquired, healthy adult
- Macrolide, fluoroquinolone, second-generation cephalosporin, amoxicillin/clavulanate, doxycycline
- Community acquired, but ill and requiring hospitalization
- Third-generation cephalosporin PLUS macrolide, fluoroquinolone, second-generation cephalosporin, amoxicillin/clavulanate, doxycycline
- Hospital acquired
- Requires double coverage for *Pseudomonas*
- Antipseudomonal penicillin (e.g., ticarcillin, piperacillin) or antipseudomonal cephalosporin (e.g., cefepime, ceftazidime) PLUS an aminoglycoside (e.g., gentamicin, tobramycin)

QUESTIONS

1. A 26-year-old healthy male smoker presents with sudden-onset shaking chills, fever to 103.0°F, cough, and left-sided pleuritic chest pain. A chest x-ray shows focal consolidation in the left lower lobe. Which organism is *least likely* to be causative?

   A. *S. pneumoniae*
   B. *H. influenzae*
   C. *M. catarrhalis*
   D. *Mycoplasma pneumoniae*
   E. *S. aureus*

2. An outbreak of illness occurs in a large apartment complex, characterized by low-grade fevers, cough, malaise, and diarrhea. In one patient, a Gram stain of induced sputum reveals

several gram-negative rods and many neutrophils. What is the antibiotic of choice for this illness?

A. Penicillin G
B. Ciprofloxacin
C. Erythromycin
D. Gentamicin
E. Cefaclor

3. A 22-year-old college student presents with 2 weeks of low-grade fevers, dry cough, malaise, myalgias, headache, and decreased appetite. A chest x-ray shows diffuse, interstitial, patchy infiltrates. What is the first-line antibiotic for this illness?

A. Azithromycin
B. Doxycycline
C. Ceftriaxone
D. Amoxicillin/clavulanate
E. Levofloxacin

4. A 36-year-old man with AIDS presents to the emergency department with 10 days of a dry, nonproductive cough, intermittent fevers, malaise, and decreased appetite. Over the past 2 days he has developed difficulty breathing and severe dyspnea on exertion. His vital signs are significant for mild tachypnea and an oxygen saturation of 88% on room air. He has oral thrush and his pulmonary exam reveals bilateral fine rales. A chest x-ray shows bilateral perihilar interstitial opacities. What is the first-line antibiotic agent for this condition?

A. Penicillin G
B. Trimethoprim/sulfamethoxazole
C. Azithromycin
D. Doxycycline
E. Rifampin

CASE 2-6 Tuberculosis

HPI: RJ, a 58-year-old man, emigrated to the United States from India 20 years ago. He never experienced health problems until 2 months ago when he began feeling ill. He has had chronic intermittent fevers, mostly at night and associated with drenching sweats. He has had a nagging cough with small amounts of blood-streaked sputum, a decreased appetite, and a 20-pound weight loss over the past 2 months. RJ has not recently traveled out of the country and has had no contacts with persons who were ill. He does not recall if he has ever had a skin test for tuberculosis or if he was ever immunized against tuberculosis in India.

THOUGHT QUESTIONS

- Which organism is responsible for tuberculosis (TB) and what distinguishes it from other bacteria?
- What is the mode of transmission and the host's immunologic reaction to the bacterium?
- What is the difference between primary and secondary TB?
- What is the role of purified protein derivative (PPD) in the diagnosis of TB?
- How is TB treated?

BASIC SCIENCE REVIEW AND DISCUSSION

Pathophysiology and Transmission

TB is caused by the bacterium *Mycobacterium tuberculosis*, which is one of many types of mycobacteria, including *M. leprae* and *M. avium*. *Mycobacteria* are distinguished from other bacteria by their cell wall, which is acid-fast. Its cell wall has a high lipid content such that once it is stained it cannot be decolorized by acid alcohol. *M. tuberculosis* contains highly immunogenic proteins in its cell wall that activate cell-mediated immunity and account for the pathogenesis of the disease.

M. tuberculosis is contracted via respiratory droplets from a person with active TB. Desiccated bacilli can remain airborne for long periods of time. Once the bacilli are inhaled into the lungs, they are phagocytized by macrophages and carried to regional lymph nodes. This initial infection—or primary TB—usually occurs in the lower lobes of the lung where ventilation is highest. Macrophages release chemotactic factors that initiate a cell-mediated immunologic response. Lymphocytes and monocytes migrate to the focus of infection and create a granuloma, that is, an island of inflammatory tissue that contains macrophages with phagocytized bacteria and histiocytes. These lesions typically remain self-contained and heal, forming a ring of calcification that can be seen on chest x-ray. The bacteria, however, remain viable and latent within this granuloma.

Primary Tuberculosis

In most infected hosts, primary TB is asymptomatic. In patients who are immunocompromised or in those who suffer from malnutrition and famine, the primary infection has a greater chance of spreading outside the initial site of infection. This is referred to as *disseminated tuberculosis* and can manifest in many ways, including miliary tuberculosis, which is characterized by numerous small lesions distributed throughout the lungs and simultaneous hematogenous spread with seeding of other organs. Extrapulmonary sites of infection include infected pleural effusions, pericarditis, lymph nodes (e.g., scrofula), bones and large joints (e.g., Pott disease is cavitary lesion and destruction of vertebral body), kidneys, liver, adrenal glands, chorioretinitis and uveitis, and meningitis.

Secondary Tuberculosis

TB usually manifests clinically as reactivation pulmonary disease many years after the initial infection. Typically, there is no inciting event, although reactivation occurs with a higher prevalence in the elderly, debilitated, undernourished, and immunocompromised. Reactivation TB tends to occur in the apical regions of the lung because of the higher V/Q ratio and the fact that *M. tuberculosis* flourishes in areas of higher oxygen tension. Reactivation TB can manifest as a focal lobar consolidation resembling other bacterial pneumonias. Classically, areas of focal inflammation result in caseating granulomas that appear nodular on a chest x-ray. These lesions may become necrotic and form cavitary lesions that can erode into bronchi. Erosion of lesions into blood vessels results in hemoptysis, which is a common feature of TB.

The diagnosis of pulmonary TB is made by sputum microscopic examination and culture. Under the microscope, *M. tuberculosis* appears as a slender, curved rod that is resistant to acid alcohol staining (i.e., acid-fast). *M. tuberculosis* is a slow-growing, aerobic microbe that can take 4 to 8 weeks for growth to occur on a classic culture medium; there are more selective media that facilitate growth in 1 to 2 weeks. Common clinical practice is to keep a patient in isolation if active TB is suspected until three sputum samples are negative on three separate days. The likelihood of identifying organisms by microscopy is related to the degree of disease. One third of patients who ultimately have positive culture results will have negative microscopic smears even after multiple specimens. Therefore, patients with active TB will be missed; however, these are patients with a lower burden of bacteria in the respiratory airways and who are less contagious.

Purified Protein Derivative

Tuberculin PPD is a substance formed from a number of proteins associated with *M. tuberculosis* and is used to identify persons with active TB or prior exposure. The PPD is placed subdermally on the forearm, and a positive reaction will occur in 48 to 72 hours as a raised, discoid, erythematous patch. In patients with prior exposure to TB, memory T cells will be activated by the introduction of the PPD proteins, resulting in proliferation and infiltration into the tissues surrounding the injection. This is the result of a cell-mediated hypersensitivity reaction. A positive result depends on the diameter of the lesion; however, there are different thresholds for a positive result based on the patient being tested and their pretest likelihood of disease

TABLE 2-3 Interpretation of PPD Results

Result	Negative/Positive Interpretation
<5 mm	Negative, except in HIV patients
5–10 mm	Positive in those likely infected (e.g., household contacts, known exposure, healthcare worker)
10–15 mm	Positive in those at elevated risk (e.g., homeless, endemic area)
>15 mm	Positive for general population

HIV, human immunodeficiency virus

TABLE 2-4 Drugs Used to Treat Tuberculosis and Common Toxicities

Drug	Condition
Isoniazid	Hepatitis, peripheral neuropathy
Rifampin	Hepatitis, flu-like illness
Streptomycin	Hearing loss, renal impairment
Pyrazinamide	Hepatitis, hyperuricemia
Ethambutol	Optic neuritis

(Table 2-3). For immunocompromised patients (e.g., AIDS) any reaction is considered positive. For patients with a high likelihood of being infected (e.g., family member of someone with TB, healthcare worker), 5 mm or greater is considered positive. For persons who are at higher risk for TB (e.g., homeless, from an endemic region, institutionalized), 10 mm or greater is considered positive. For those with a low risk for TB, 15 mm or greater is considered positive.

Treatment for TB is difficult because of drug resistance, the required duration of treatment and compliance, and the cost of the drugs. A number of drugs are available for the treatment of TB, with varying toxicities (Table 2-4). When treatment is initiated, typically three agents are used simultaneously until culture sensitivities are obtained. This is done because of the prevalence of resistance. Resistant strains are typically found in populations from endemic regions of the world (e.g., Haiti, Africa, Southeast Asia) where the only available drug for treatment has been isoniazid. As a result, organisms resistant to isoniazid are very common in these regions. Multidrug resistance is becoming more common in the United States as well, where in New York City up to 25% of *M. tuberculosis* is resistant to both isoniazid and rifampin. Therefore, in addition to these two agents, usually pyrazinamide or ethambutol is added to the initial treatment regimen.

CASE CONCLUSION

RJ is admitted to the hospital to an isolation room. His chest x-ray shows a right upper lobe infiltrate that is concerning for secondary TB. He is started on isoniazid, rifampin, and pyrazinamide. A PPD was placed on admission, and by 48 hours a discoid lesion about 20 mm in diameter had formed at the injection site. On the second day, RJ was able to produce sputum that showed several slender, curved organisms in clumps that were acid-fast. Several days after treatment he began to feel better and his cough decreased. After 14 days of isolation, antibiotic therapy, and several sputum samples that showed no organisms, he was discharged from the hospital with a 6-month course of oral isoniazid and rifampin. The culture results came back subsequently showing *M. tuberculosis* sensitive to both isoniazid and rifampin.

THUMBNAIL: Tuberculosis

Pathophysiology

Primary Infection
Mycobacterium has a cell wall that is rich in lipids and is acid-fast.
Proteins in cell walls are highly antigenic.
Inhaled bacilli are phagocytized by macrophages and carried to regional lymph nodes.
Macrophages initiate an inflammatory response by releasing chemotactic factors.
Cell-mediated hypersensitivity results with influx of lymphocytes and monocytes.
Primary granuloma is formed around initial site of infection that consists of macrophages, histiocytes, and lymphocytes.

(Continued)

THUMBNAIL: Tuberculosis *(Continued)*

Latent Phase
Majority of primary infections are asymptomatic
Granuloma self-contained, heals, and forms calcified granuloma that is evident on chest x-ray.
Calcified granuloma "dormant" but contains viable *Mycobacteria.*
PPD test becomes positive several weeks after primary infection and remains so during the latent phase.

Secondary (Reactivation) TB
Disease manifests years later as a result of age, comorbid disease, or immunocompromised state.
Reactivation occurs typically in apices and upper poles of lower lobes where the V/Q ratio is high.
Spread of *Mycobacteria* outside the original granuloma results in formation of caseating granulomas that can necrotize and become cavitary granulomas.
Cavitary granulomas erode into bronchioles and generate sputum with *M. tuberculosis.*
Cavitary granulomas can also erode into blood vessels, causing hemoptysis.

Disseminated TB
More common in immunocompromised persons and in children.
Result of hematogenous spread of *Mycobacteria* and seeding in various organs of the body.

Risk Factors
Endemic regions of the world: Southeast Asia, Africa, India, Latin America
Overcrowded living conditions, homeless, inner-city urban dwellers, jailed or institutionalized

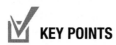

KEY POINTS

- Presenting symptoms of reactivation TB include chronic cough, hemoptysis, intermittent fevers, night sweats, weight loss
- Chest x-ray may show any variety of infiltrate although classically shows granulomatous or cavitary lesions in the upper lobes
- Patients with pulmonary infiltrates suspicious for TB must be kept in isolation until three sputum samples are negative for acid-fast organisms
- Positive PPD suggests prior infection with *M. tuberculosis* but does not necessarily imply active TB
- Any reaction in immunocompromised persons is positive

- For individuals at high risk, 5 mm is positive
- For individuals with several risk factors, 10 mm is positive
- For individuals at low risk, 15 mm is positive
- Initial treatment of active TB consists of a three-drug regimen
- Duration of treatment is at least 6 months due to large number of inactive organisms and poor drug penetration into caseating granulomas and cavitary lesions
- Treatment of asymptomatic patient with positive PPD and normal chest x-ray is typically rifampin for 6 months

QUESTIONS

1. Which of the following is *true* regarding primary TB?

    A. Usually progresses to fulminant disease
    B. Imparts transient immunity to host
    C. Invokes β cell-mediated humoral immunity
    D. Characterized by granuloma formation
    E. Results in contagious host

2. Which of the following is *false* regarding secondary TB?

    A. Typically occurs in the lung apices
    B. Characterized by fevers, chills, night sweats, and weight loss
    C. PPD is usually negative during active disease
    D. Caseating granuloma can necrotize into adjacent bronchi
    E. Risk factors include elderly, debilitated, immunocompromised

3. An 18-year-old Hispanic woman lives with her father who was recently diagnosed with active TB based on symptoms of fevers, cough, weight loss, a chest x-ray showing a cavitary lesion, and a sputum sample with acid-fast bacilli. What size PPD skin reaction would be considered positive and mandate treatment for this woman?

    A. Any reaction
    B. 5 mm
    C. 10 mm
    D. 15 mm
    E. 20 mm

4. What is the *most common* side effect of drug therapy for TB?

    A. Hepatitis
    B. Peripheral neuropathy
    C. Thrombocytopenia
    D. Hyperuricemia
    E. Renal failure

CASE 2-7   Lung Cancer

HPI: HF, a 52-year-old man, is a 30-year smoker and was doing well until about 2 months ago when he began feeling fatigued, general malaise, developed a chronic nonproductive cough, and lost his appetite. HF assumed he had a viral illness and wasn't worried until yesterday when he noticed some blood in his sputum. Today he coughed up about a teaspoon of blood and decided to go see his doctor. He reports that he has lost 25 pounds over the past 6 weeks.

PE: HF's vital signs are unremarkable but he looks pallid and thinner than normal. His chest exam reveals decreased breath sounds over the superior left lung field.

THOUGHT QUESTIONS

- What are the four types of primary lung cancer?
- What is the incidence of metastatic lung cancer compared with primary lung cancer, and which primary cancers metastasize most often to the lung?
- Which paraneoplastic syndromes are often associated with lung cancer?
- Which lung cancers are amenable to surgical resection?
- What are the two most common types of benign pulmonary tumors?

BASIC SCIENCE REVIEW AND DISCUSSION

Types of Lung Cancer

There are four major types of primary lung cancer (Table 2-5) based on their cell type. Squamous cell carcinoma is the most common. It tends to be located centrally, and histologically is characterized by keratin formation and intracellular bridges. Adenocarcinoma consists of malignant glandular cells that produce mucin. Adenocarcinoma is located peripherally and, unlike the other types of cancer, appears to have no link to smoking. Large cell carcinoma is also peripheral and consists of poorly differentiated cells; it is likely an undifferentiated form of adenocarcinoma. Small cell carcinoma is a central tumor that behaves differently from other bronchogenic cancers. It consists of many cells about twice the size of lymphocytes that multiply rapidly, making it highly invasive. Metastasis has usually occurred by the time of diagnosis. Alternatively, metastatic spread to the lung from a primary site outside the lung is actually more common than bronchogenic carcinoma itself. Common sites of the primary tumor include breast, ovary, kidney, thyroid, pancreas, testicles, and bone.

Clinical Findings

Patients with lung cancer usually present with a history of weight loss, fatigue, cough, hemoptysis, chest pain, and dyspnea. Patients with adenocarcinoma present with increased sputum production. Pancoast syndrome refers to an apical tumor that compresses the sympathetic cervical chain and leads to Horner syndrome (ptosis, myosis, and anhydrosis). Superior lobe tumors can also lead to superior vena cava (SVC) syndrome as a result of compression of the SVC. These patients have swelling of the face and upper extremities because of venous engorgement. Many bronchogenic cancers are diagnosed because of a pneumonia that is refractory to antibiotic therapy. Tumors commonly cause bronchial obstruction and a postobstructive pneumonia.

Patients with refractory pneumonia should undergo computed tomography (CT) scan or bronchoscopy to search for an obstructive lesion.

There are several paraneoplastic syndromes associated with bronchogenic tumors. Squamous cell carcinoma typically results in hypercalcemia as a result of bone involvement. As the tumor invades bone, osteoclastic activity releases parathyroid hormone (PTH)-like factors that result in the liberation of calcium. Small cell carcinoma is most often associated with paraneoplastic syndromes, including syndrome of inappropriate antidiuretic hormone (SIADH), resulting in water retention and low serum sodium. Small cell carcinomas can also cause Cushing syndrome by means of ectopic adrenocorticotropic hormone (ACTH) production and various neuromuscular disorders by unknown means.

Diagnosis and Work-Up

The approach to diagnosis of a lung mass depends on the location. The easiest way of making a diagnosis is by sputum cytology. However, the sensitivity is relatively low, especially for peripheral lesions. If the lesion is central, the next approach to diagnosis is bronchoscopy. The sensitivity of bronchoscopy for making the diagnosis for central lesions is about 90%. Peripheral lesions often can be approached with percutaneous CT-guided needle biopsy, which has a diagnostic accuracy of about 80%. However, patients with significant risk factors for lung cancer may go directly to open thoracotomy and resection given a single peripheral lesion.

Once a diagnosis of cancer is made, the next step is to determine whether metastasis has occurred. This is best achieved by a CT scan of the chest. Lymph nodes greater than 1.5 cm suggest metastatic spread and, in that case, mediastinoscopy is indicated for lymph node biopsy to confirm the diagnosis. If mediastinal metastasis has occurred, the patient is likely no longer a candidate for surgery. There is no need to look for extrathoracic metastases unless there are specific symptoms (e.g., neurologic deficits, bone pain) or lab abnormalities (e.g., hypercalcemia, liver function abnormalities) that may suggest so. Pulmonary function tests are also part of the preoperative work-up because patients with lung cancer often have concomitant lung disease, such as COPD. A postoperative predicted FEV_1 is calculated based on the current FEV_1 and the planned amount of lung resection. If the reserve function is adequate and there is no evidence of metastasis, then the patient is a surgical candidate. Surgical techniques continue to improve and in recent years there has been success with resection of affected ipsilateral hilar and mediastinal lymph nodes.

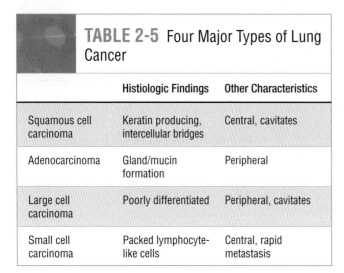

TABLE 2-5 Four Major Types of Lung Cancer

	Histiologic Findings	Other Characteristics
Squamous cell carcinoma	Keratin producing, intercellular bridges	Central, cavitates
Adenocarcinoma	Gland/mucin formation	Peripheral
Large cell carcinoma	Poorly differentiated	Peripheral, cavitates
Small cell carcinoma	Packed lymphocyte-like cells	Central, rapid metastasis

Benign Pulmonary Tumors

Common benign pulmonary tumors include bronchial adenomas and pulmonary hamartomas. Bronchial adenomas are intrabronchial tumors that can cause chronic cough, hemoptysis, and obstructive symptoms. Diagnosis is made by bronchoscopy, and treatment is surgical resection because these tumors have the potential for malignant transformation. About 80% of bronchial adenomas are carcinoids that can be locally invasive and often secrete hormones such as ACTH or ADH. Carcinoids may also metastasize to the liver and cause carcinoid syndrome consisting of cutaneous flushing, bronchoconstriction, and diarrhea. Pulmonary hamartomas are benign, peripheral tumors consisting of smooth muscle and collagen. Their classic appearance on chest x-ray includes small, rounded size with distinct, well-demarcated borders. These typically have central, speckled calcifications known as the "popcorn" pattern. If a nodule on chest x-ray is consistent with these findings, then a repeat x-ray is indicated every 6 months for 2 years to confirm its stability.

CASE CONCLUSION

HF's chest x-ray showed a large mass in the left superior lobe consistent with bronchogenic carcinoma. A chest CT showed diffuse mediastinal adenopathy. Labs showed a calcium of 10.0, which is consistent with early bone metastasis. On the basis of these findings HF is not a candidate for surgery. Over the next several months he received radiotherapy to the left superior lobe and systemic chemotherapy. His condition continued to worsen until he developed pneumonia and sepsis, requiring endotracheal intubation. After discussion with the family and the patient's previous wishes, HF was withdrawn from the ventilator and expired soon after.

THUMBNAIL: Bronchogenic Carcinoma

Pathophysiology

Squamous Cell Carcinoma
Centrally located, consists of keratin and intracellular islands
Often cavitary, locally invasive, bone metastasis (hypercalcemia)

Adenocarcinoma
Peripherally located, glandular cells that produce mucin
No apparent link to smoking

Large Cell Carcinoma
Peripherally located, likely undifferentiated form of adenocarcinoma

Small Cell Carcinoma
Centrally located, islands of numerous lymphocytic-appearing cells
Highly invasive, usually metastatic at time of diagnosis
Often associated with paraneoplastic syndromes due to secretion of hormones such as ADH, ACTH

Risk Factors
Smoking increases risk 13-fold, long-term passive exposure increases risk 1.5-fold
Dose-response relationship such that 40 pack-year smoker has 60-fold risk increase
Asbestos exposure has synergistic effect with smoking increasing risk 200-fold
Other industrial exposures and air pollution

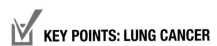

KEY POINTS: LUNG CANCER

- Benign-appearing peripheral nodules on chest x-ray can be followed with repeat chest x-rays at 6-month intervals for 2 years
- In high-risk patients or with suspicious-appearing masses, tissue biopsy required
- Bronchoscopy for central lesions
- CT-guided needle biopsy for peripheral lesions
- Open thoracotomy and wedge resection if suspicion very high
- Anatomic staging determines extent of disease and metastasis
- CT scan of chest defines tumor size, location, and presence of mediastinal lymph node involvement

- Suspicious-appearing lymph nodes require mediastinoscopy for biopsy
- CT scan of abdomen often done to assess for liver or adrenal metastases
- Physiologic staging involves pulmonary function tests
- In general, cancer that is contained within a single lung with minimal hilar and mediastinal lymph node extension is amenable to surgery

QUESTIONS

1. Which of the following will *most likely* present with massive hemoptysis?
   A. Squamous cell carcinoma
   B. Adenocarcinoma
   C. Large cell carcinoma
   D. Small cell carcinoma
   E. Metastatic lung cancer

2. Which of the following manifests as a peripheral lesion and can present as diffuse, multifocal, pneumonia-like infiltrates?
   A. Squamous cell carcinoma
   B. Adenocarcinoma
   C. Large cell carcinoma
   D. Small cell carcinoma
   E. Metastatic lung cancer

3. A 72-year-old smoker develops a left lower lobe pneumonia that is treated with a 5-day course of azithromycin. His symptoms and lobar infiltrate do not improve and he is admitted to the hospital for IV antibiotics. Upon further inquiry, he has also had blood-streaked sputum and lost 25 pounds over the past 2 months. Which of the following is a reasonable next test that will most likely yield a specific diagnosis?
   A. CT scan of thorax
   B. MRI of thorax
   C. Bronchoscopy
   D. Mediastinoscopy
   E. Open biopsy

4. Which finding is *not* known to be associated with bronchogenic carcinoma?
   A. Eyelid drooping
   B. Hoarseness
   C. Facial swelling
   D. Leg swelling
   E. Hematuria

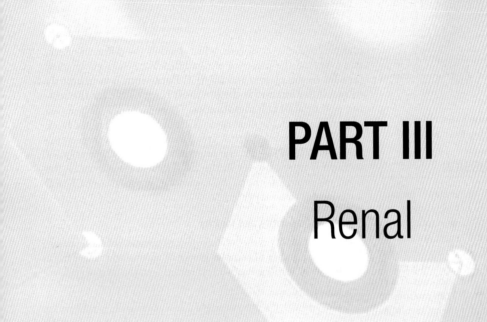

PART III

Renal

HPI: KR is a 70-year-old man who is seen in the doctor's office at a resort in Mexico. He has just returned from a long hike in the noonday sun exploring some Mayan ruins. He didn't drink water during the hike and did not wear a hat. He has no medical problems but is usually sedentary.

PE: Pulse 110; BP 100/60 mm Hg

The patient appears fatigued and flushed. His heart rate is tachycardic and his lungs are clear.

Labs: His chemistry panel is significant for sodium 150 mEq/L, BUN 52 mg/dL, and creatinine 1.3 mEq/L.

THOUGHT QUESTIONS

- What is the distribution of water and electrolytes among the body fluid compartments?
- What are osmolality and tonicity?
- How does the kidney maintain salt and water balance?
- What is the role of thirst in maintaining fluid balance?

BASIC SCIENCE REVIEW AND DISCUSSION

Our bodies are approximately 60% water by weight. The percentage of total body water (TBW) differs between men and women. Men have a higher percent TBW, 60%, due to a greater amount of lean muscle mass. Women have a larger amount of anhydrous adipose tissue, and their TBW comprises approximately 50% of their weight. As we age, lean muscle mass decreases, adipose tissue increases, and our percent TBW decreases. TBW can be broken down into two compartments: the extracellular fluid (ECF) compartment and the intracellular fluid (ICF) compartment. The ECF is composed of the plasma and interstitial fluid (fluid between cells, not in the vasculature).

The ECF is one third of the TBW or 20% of the body weight. The ICF is two thirds of the TBW or 40% of the body weight. The ECF can be further broken down into plasma, which is one fourth of the ECF, and interstitial fluid, which makes up three fourths of the ECF.

To measure the **TBW** one needs a measurable substance, such as tritiated water, that will equilibrate across semipermeable membranes. The formula below allows us to calculate the volume of a fluid compartment if we first know the concentration (C) and the volume (V) we have instilled.

$$C_1 V_1 = C_2 V_2$$
$$mg/L * L = mg/L * x$$
$$x = mg/L * L/mg * L$$

The **ICF** cannot be directly measured because there is no substance that will stay isolated to the intracellular compartment. Mannitol, inulin, and sucrose, all large molecules, will stay distributed in the **ECF** and are good markers of ECF. Evans blue dye is a substance that is largely bound to plasma proteins and is used to measure the **plasma volume.**

The distribution of electrolytes between the intracellular compartment and the extracellular compartment is not the same. The differences in electrolyte composition among the plasma, interstitial fluid, and intracellular compartment are maintained by the electrical potential difference across cell membranes; the semipermeable phospholipid bilayer of cells, which hinders the diffusion of certain ions; and the presence of nondiffusable, negatively charged proteins in the plasma and the ICF. **Potassium is a primarily intracellular ion and is the ion most responsible for the resting potential of cell membranes.** There is a high concentration of protein in both the plasma and ICF but none in interstitial fluid. These nondiffusable proteins create oncotic pressure, preventing fluid from "leaking" into the interstitium. The concentration of **sodium is much higher in the ECF** than in the ICF and is the main determinant of the ECF osmolality and thus ECF and intravascular (plasma) volume.

Osmolality, Osmolarity, and Tonicity

Plasma osmolality is the total solute concentration of a fluid measured as the number of osmoles per kg of plasma and ranges from 285 to 295 mOsm/kg. It can be estimated with the formula below:

$$\text{Osmolality} = 2(Na^+ \, mEq/L) + \frac{\text{glucose mg/dL}}{18} + \frac{\text{BUN mg/dL}}{2.8} = mOsm/kg$$

The contribution of BUN and glucose to plasma osmolality is usually small but may become larger if diabetes or renal failure is present. The term **osmolarity** has units of number of milliosmoles per liter and may also be used when referring to body fluids.

Tonicity is a unitless term that allows us to make comparisons of concentrations between fluids. It describes the hydrostatic force created by osmotically active particles across a semipermeable membrane. A hypertonic fluid has a higher effective osmolar concentration than does plasma. A 0.9% saline solution ("normal saline") is used as plasma replacement fluid because it is approximately isotonic to plasma, having 154 mEq/L of sodium chloride (2 × 154 mEq = 308 mOsm/L). A 0.45% saline solution ("half-normal saline") is hypotonic to plasma, with only 154 mOsm/L of sodium chloride.

Serum osmolality is tightly controlled by antidiuretic hormone (ADH) also known as vasopressin for its vasoconstrictive properties. **ADH** is a nonapeptide synthesized in the supraoptic nucleus of the hypothalamus and released from the posterior pituitary. It is released when the osmoreceptors in the anterolateral hypothalamus are stimulated by increases in serum osmolarity as small as 1%. ADH acts on V_2 luminal receptors in the collecting ducts via the cyclic adenosine monophosphate (cAMP) messenger system. Upon binding ADH, there is an up-regulation of transmembrane water channels, **aquaporins,** which results in an increased reabsorption of water. In the absence of ADH, the distal tubule and

TABLE 3-1 Changes that Occur with Water Loss

Disorder	Osmolarity of Lost Fluid	ECF Volume	ICF Volume	Serum Na⁺
Diarrhea	Iso-osmotic	↓	↔	↔
Sweating	Hypo-osmotic	↓	↓	↑
Diabetes insipidus	Hypo-osmotic	↓	↓	↑
Adrenal insufficiency	Hyper-osmotic	↓	↑	↓

ECF, extracellular fluid; *ICF,* intracellular fluid

collecting ducts are almost impermeable to water, but with ADH, the kidney is able to reabsorb large amounts of water.

Fluid Shifts

Water equilibrates freely across cell membranes to establish an osmotic equilibrium between the ECF and the ICF. Thus, ICF volume varies inversely with the plasma concentration of sodium. The volume of ECF in the intravascular space (i.e., plasma) is a central determinant of blood pressure. Several disorders causing water loss can disrupt plasma volume, leading to dangerously low blood pressures. The effect of fluid loss on ECF volume, ICF volume, and plasma sodium concentration can be determined if we know the osmolarity of the fluid being lost. The average daily loss of water in the urine is approximately 1.5 to 2.0 L and from the feces, 0.1 to 0.2 L. Insensible losses include loss of water from the skin and lungs and account for approximately 0.5 L per day. Table 3-1 catalogues changes that occur with pathologic GI, renal, and insensible water losses.

The effects of ECF volume contraction, decreased cardiac output, tachycardia, and hypotension result in a cascade of events aimed at maintaining blood pressure and perfusion to vital organs. Hypotension is sensed by the cardiac and carotid baroreceptors, which stimulate the sympathetic nervous system and renin-angiotensin-aldosterone hormonal axis. Systemic vasoconstriction due to sympathetic nervous system activation and increased reabsorption of salt and water by the kidney under the influence of aldosterone act to restore normal blood pressure. Under circumstances of hypovolemia, ADH is also secreted in an attempt to increase intravascular volume.

ECF volume can be expanded by the addition of hypertonic or isotonic saline. Hypertonic 3% saline contains 513 mEq/L of sodium chloride and will draw water from the ICF, thereby expanding plasma volume but dehydrating individual cells. Isotonic saline expands the intravascular volume without causing fluid to shift from the cells because the osmolarity of 0.9% saline is similar to the ICF and ECF osmolarity (Table 3-2).

Thirst

What about the role of thirst in preserving intravascular volume? In states of dehydration, a rise of plasma osmolarity of only 2% will stimulate our thirst center, located anterolaterally to the preoptic nucleus of the hypothalamus (near the area that controls the release of ADH). Other stimulants of thirst include decreased blood pressure and a dry mouth.

CASE CONCLUSION

Our weekend warrior went out hiking unprepared. Sweating leads to a loss of hypotonic fluid and volume contraction. As a result, the patient's serum sodium concentration is increased, blood pressure is decreased, and he is tachycardic. Keep in mind that the BUN concentration can also be a useful indication of volume status. Dehydration causes increased reabsorption of urea, resulting in an elevation of the normal BUN-creatinine ratio of 10:1. **A ratio of BUN-creatinine of 20:1 or greater is not unusual in dehydrated patients.**

TABLE 3-2 Changes that Occur with Fluid Gained

Situation	Osmolarity of Fluid Gained	ECF Volume	ICF Volume	Serum Na⁺
3% saline infusion	Hypertonic	↑	↓	↑
0.9% saline infusion	Isotonic	↑	↔	↔
5% dextrose	Hypotonic	↑	↑	↓

ECF, extracellular fluid; *ICF,* intracellular fluid

THUMBNAIL: Renal Physiology—Body Fluids

Compartment	% Total Body Weight	% Total Body Water	Marker	Volume for a 70-kg Person (L)
TBW	60♂ 50♀	100	Tritiated water, deuterium oxide (D_2O)	42
ICF	40	67	TBW-ECF	28
ECF	20	33	Mannitol, inulin, sucrose	14
Plasma	5	8 (1/4 of ECF)	Evans blue dye, radioiodinated serum albumin	3.5
Interstitial	15	25 (3/4 of ECF)	ECF-plasma	10.5

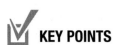

KEY POINTS

- Serum sodium concentration is the main determinant of ECF volume
- Osmolality is the number of particles per kg of water and osmolarity is the number of particles per liter of water
- Tonicity is a measure of the osmotic activity or hydrostatic force exerted by particles in a solution across a semipermeable membrane
- ADH, the main regulator of serum osmolality, is stimulated with small increases in serum osmolality

QUESTIONS

1. A 100-kg man is injected with 250 mL of Evans blue dye with a concentration of 500 mg/mL. After 10 minutes his blood is drawn and the concentration of Evans blue dye is 25 mg/mL. What is his plasma volume?

   A. 1000 mL
   B. 2500 mL
   C. 4000 mL
   D. 5000 mL
   E. 10,000 mL

2. A 24-year-old man presents to your clinic with a history of episodes of diarrhea and crampy abdominal pain for the last 6 years. He comes to your office today after 3 days of severe diarrhea and because he has noticed blood in his stool. Measurement of his blood pressure in the supine position is 100/60 and his heart rate is 90 beats per minute. His upright blood pressure drops to 80/50 and his heart rate increases to 110 beats per minute and he complains of feeling dizzy and nauseous. His serum sodium is 140 mEq/L. What is the most appropriate replacement fluid?

   A. IV 0.9% saline
   B. IV 0.45% saline
   C. IV 5% dextrose
   D. IV 3% saline
   E. Chicken soup

HPI: BB is a 67-year-old woman brought to the emergency department (ED) by her son because of confusion. Her son states that over the past 2 days his mother became increasingly lethargic. When he arrived home from work today his mother was sleeping on the couch and he could not wake her. The son notes that his mother recently started a new medication for hypertension.

PE: BP 130/90 mm Hg; Pulse 80; T 36.6°C; SaO$_2$ 97% at room air.

The patient's heart rate is within normal limits and regular. Her lungs are clear. She is somnolent, responds to voice but quickly returns to sleep and cannot follow commands. There is no facial droop, she resists eye opening, and her pupils are equal and reactive to light. She moves all extremities when stimulated to do so and her reflexes are intact.

Medication: Hydrochlorothiazide

Labs: Sodium (Na$^+$) 120 mEq/L; potassium (K$^+$) 3.0 mEq/L; Cl$^-$ 90 mEq/L; HCO$_3^-$ 26 mEq/L; BUN 32 mg/dL; creatinine (Cr) 1.0 mg/dL.

THOUGHT QUESTIONS

- What is the renal regulation of sodium?
- What are the causes of hypernatremia and hyponatremia?
- Why is this patient so lethargic?

BASIC SCIENCE REVIEW AND DISCUSSION

Sodium is the major cation of the ECF. Normal serum levels range between 135 and 145 mEq/L. The high sodium concentration in the ECF and low concentration intracellularly is an important determinant of the potential difference across cell membranes. The abundance of sodium in the ECF also determines the osmolality of the ECF. The serum osmolality is normally regulated by ADH acting to regulate water reabsorption in the distal nephron. The osmolality may be deranged in disease states as we shall see below.

Sodium Homeostasis

Approximately 99% of filtered sodium is reabsorbed by the end of the nephron (Fig. 3-1). The action of the Na$^+$/K$^+$ ATPase at the basolateral membrane of the tubular cells facilitates sodium movement from lumen to tubular cell to peritubular capillary. The reabsorption of water and chloride (and most other filtered solutes) is closely coupled to the sodium reabsorption throughout the nephron.

Two thirds of the filtered sodium and water is reabsorbed in the proximal convoluted tubule (PCT). When sodium is reabsorbed it creates an osmotic gradient, which facilitates the passive absorption of water, and a negative potential in the tubular lumen, which facilitates the absorption of chloride down its electrical and chemical gradient. Fluid entering the loop of Henle is iso-osmolar with respect to plasma.

Countercurrent Multiplication and Countercurrent Exchange

The primary role of the loop of Henle is to establish a hyperosmolar medullary interstitium that can be used by the collecting tubules to concentrate urine. The loop of Henle establishes this gradient by the mechanism of **countercurrent multiplication.**

The flow of urine through the limbs of the loop run counter to one another. The descending loop of Henle is permeable to water and impermeable to ions. As fluid flows down the descending loop, it becomes increasingly concentrated as water is reabsorbed into the peritubular capillaries. The ascending loop is impermeable to water and actively transports, via an ATPase pump, Na$^+$, 2Cl$^-$, and K$^+$ from the tubular lumen to the medullary interstitium. As the filtrate flows up the ascending loop it becomes more dilute. The active transport of ions into the medulla creates an osmotic gradient that ranges from 300 mOsm/L at the outer medulla to up to 1400 mOsm/L at the tips of the loops of Henle. The gradient is maintained by vasa recta, capillaries that course parallel to the loops of Henle. Because of their ability to perpetuate the high osmotic pressure of the medulla, the vasa recta are termed **countercurrent exchangers.** During their course through the kidney, the plasma within the vasa recta becomes more concentrated as it descends and more dilute as it ascends. The net effect is that the vasa recta are able to perfuse the kidney interstitium without disrupting the steep medullary gradient essential for the production of concentrated urine.

The Concentration of Urine

The collecting tubule becomes permeable to water only under the influence of ADH, which acts on V$_2$ luminal receptors in the collecting ducts. Upon binding ADH, transmembrane water channels, aquaporins, are inserted into the luminal cell surface. Water passively flows through these channels down the osmotic gradient created by countercurrent multiplication and is reabsorbed, resulting in concentration of urine. The concentration of urine varies directly with the plasma concentration of ADH, with urine osmolarity ranging from 50 to 1400 mOsm/L.

Urea is a product of protein metabolism. Approximately 50% of filtered urea is reabsorbed at the PCT. Most nephron segments are relatively impermeable to urea except for the medullary collecting ducts, which, under the influence of ADH, allow urea to diffuse into the medullary interstitium. In this manner, urea contributes to the hyperosmolarity of the medulla and maximal urine concentration.

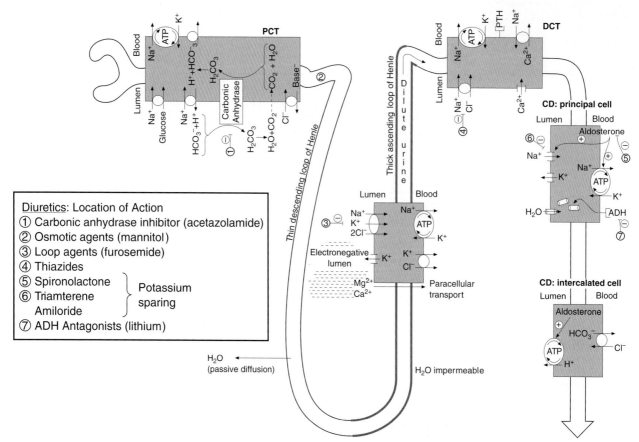

• **Figure 3-1.** The nephron. (Drawing courtesy of Tracie Harris, Class of 2003, University of California, San Francisco, School of Medicine.)

Hypernatremia

Hypernatremia is defined as a serum sodium concentration above 145 mEq/L. There are only two ways to become hypernatremic, either to ingest too much salt or to lose too much water. The latter is far more common. Hypernatremia occurs most commonly in patients with inadequate water intake due to an altered state of consciousness or in elderly patients who are less sensitive to thirst. Insensible water loss via the skin or respiratory tract without replenishment leads to hypernatremia. While diarrhea is usually isotonic, it can lead to hypernatremia when the affected individuals don't replace the water lost. Renal water losses include osmotic diuresis due to diabetes insipidus or hyperglycemia.

Diabetes Insipidus

Diabetes insipidus (DI) is the renal wasting of water due to a lack of or resistance to ADH. Patients with DI present with polyuria, intense thirst, and signs of volume depletion such as hypotension and tachycardia. Patients with DI urinate large volumes of dilute urine, greater than 2 to 3 L/day, that may disrupt sleep or result in enuresis (bedwetting).

Central DI occurs with damage to the hypothalamus or posterior pituitary, leading to impaired ADH secretion. Central DI may be caused by CNS tumors, surgery, intracranial hemorrhage, anoxic injury, infection, or infiltrating disease such as sarcoidosis. Central DI can be primary or idiopathic if no proximate cause is found. Renal insensitivity to ADH leads to the same clinical picture with normal or elevated ADH secretion and is referred to as **nephrogenic DI.** Nephrogenic DI is caused by chronic renal insufficiency, drugs such as **lithium** and **alcohol, hypercalcemia,** and long-standing **hypokalemia.**

The clinical presentation of hypernatremia depends on the rapidity of onset. Acute hypernatremia results in alterations of consciousness, from lethargy to coma, due to cerebral intracellular dehydration. Other neurologic symptoms include weakness, tremor, muscle rigidity, ataxia, and seizures. Hypernatremia that develops over time allows the body, especially the neurons, to produce osmolytes, solutes that allow the cells of the CNS to maintain intracellular volume. This moderates damage to the brain and may not produce any specific pattern of symptoms.

Treatment of hypernatremia includes restoring body water, ADH replacement when indicated, and removing the offending drug. The TBW deficit may be estimated by the following equation:

$$\text{Water deficit} = ((\text{measured serum Na}^+ / \text{normal serum Na}^+) * \text{TBW}) - \text{TBW}$$

where TBW = 0.60 * normal body weight in kg.

The rate of water repletion is determined by how acutely the hypernatremia developed. Chronic onset (greater than 36 hours) allows for the compensatory response by neurons, and care must be taken to correct the hypernatremia slowly. If hypernatremia has occurred over time, rapid correction may result in cerebral edema.

Hyponatremia

Hyponatremia is a serum sodium of less than 130 or 135 mEq/L with a resulting parallel decrease in the osmolality of the serum. This distinguishes true hyponatremia from **pseudohyponatremia,** which is a factitious lowering of the serum sodium concentration due to hyperlipidemia, hyperproteinemia, or hyperglycemia, in which there is increased serum osmolality.

Like hypernatremia, the clinical picture in hyponatremia depends on the rapidity of onset. Mild hyponatremia is usually asymptomatic, but the rapid onset of severe hyponatremia (less than 120 mEq/L) can result in serious morbidity and death due to cerebral edema. Patients commonly present with lethargy, seizures, anorexia, headaches, and muscle cramps.

Patients with hyponatremia can be hypovolemic, euvolemic, or hypervolemic. The serum sodium concentration does not give any information about the patient's volume status. For volume status, we look for clinical signs of dehydration (dry mucous membranes, tachycardia, etc.) or fluid overload (edema).

Disorders that present with hyponatremia and **hypovolemia** include water losses due to diarrhea, excessive sweating with solute-free water replacement, and renal losses due to diuretics, osmotic diuresis, salt-losing nephropathy, and adrenal insufficiency.

Several disorders present with **euvolemia** and hyponatremia. Syndrome of inappropriate antidiuretic hormone secretion (SIADH), deficiencies of glucocorticoid and thyroid hormones, primary polydipsia, and medications that potentiate the effect of ADH all cause euvolemic hyponatremia. The list of drugs that cause a SIADH-like syndrome include nicotine, chlorpropamide, morphine, and carbamazepine. Primary polydipsia or compulsive water drinking usually occurs in psychiatric patients taking psychotropic medications that cause a dry mouth.

SIADH is a diagnosis of exclusion and is usually secondary to ectopic ADH production by tumors (especially non-small cell lung cancer), pulmonary disorders, CNS disorders, or pain. Patients maintain euvolemia in the presence of excess ADH because any increase in TBW leads to sodium excretion to rid the body of the excess water. In addition to elevation of urine sodium concentration, the urine osmolarity will be inappropriately concentrated (i.e., greater than 100 mOsm/L). The hallmarks of SIADH are euvolemia and inappropriately concentrated urine in the presence of hyponatremia.

Disorders that present with **hypervolemia** and hyponatremia include nephrotic syndrome, cirrhosis, CHF, and sepsis with hypotension. In all of these disorders TBW is increased, but water is not retained in the circulation and intravascular hypovolemia is present. Inadequate filling of the arterial circulation leads to inadequate sodium delivery to the renal tubules and increased ADH secretion, culminating in hyponatremia. In addition, diuretics used in the treatment of these disorders also perpetuate hyponatremia.

The treatment of hyponatremia depends on the underlying cause, the volume status of the patient, and the severity of symptoms. Hormonal causes of hyponatremia are treated with hormone replacement. If hyponatremia is drug induced, the offending drug should be discontinued. SIADH, regardless of the cause, usually responds to water restriction.

Emergent treatment of hyponatremia is required if patients have an alteration of consciousness or seizures. The emergent treatment is administration of hypertonic saline (3% NaCl = 513 mEq/L) to replace the sodium deficit to at least 120 mEq/L at a rate not more than 0.5 mEq/L/h. The sodium deficit to be replaced can be calculated as follows:

$$Na^+ \text{ deficit} = TBW * (Na^+ \text{ desired} - Na^+ \text{ measured})$$
$$= 0.60 * \text{wt in kg} * (120 \text{ mEq/L} - Na^+ \text{ measured mEq/L})$$
$$= \text{mEq } Na^+ \text{ deficit}$$

Too rapid correction of hyponatremia may result in **central pontine myelinosis,** a selective demyelination of the pons that can result in quadriparesis and death.

CASE CONCLUSION

The patient has a symptomatic hyponatremia most likely due to diuretic use. She also has hypokalemia. Treatment includes discontinuation of hydrochlorothiazide, restriction of water, repletion of potassium, and infusion of normal saline.

THUMBNAIL: Renal Physiology—Sodium Regulation

	Hypernatremia	Hyponatremia
Etiology	Decreased water intake Increased salt intake Diabetes insipidus Diarrhea Insensible losses	Pseudohyponatremia **Hypovolemic** Renal losses (diuretics) GI losses (diarrhea) Insensible losses Addison disease (adrenal insufficiency) **Euvolemic** SIADH Hypothyroidism Glucocorticoid deficiency Primary polydipsia Medications **Hypervolemic** Nephrotic syndrome CHF Cirrhosis
Symptoms	Impaired consciousness, weakness, tremor, hyperreflexia	Anorexia, headaches, muscle cramps, impaired consciousness, seizure, coma

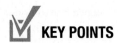

KEY POINTS

■ The reabsorption of sodium occurs throughout the nephron and is coupled to the reabsorption of chloride, amino acids, and glucose.

■ The ascending loop of Henle is the site of active transport of Na^+, K^+, and Cl^- into the medulla of the kidney.

■ The collecting ducts are permeable to water only under the influence of ADH and are responsible for the final concentration of urine.

■ ADH is the hormone primarily responsible for maintaining serum osmolality but is elevated in states of hypovolemia even when the patient is hyponatremic.

■ SIADH results in euvolemic hyponatremia and inappropriate renal sodium wasting.

■ DI is caused by a lack of ADH or a resistance to ADH, resulting in large volumes of dilute urine.

QUESTIONS

1. A 33-year-old, 70-kg woman remains lethargic after surgery for removal of an ovarian cyst. She has no other health problems. She was given 2.5 L of 0.45% saline during her operation and recovery. Her serum sodium is 122 mEq/L. How many milliequivalents of sodium are needed to raise her sodium to 130 mEq/L and how fast should it be replaced?

A. 200 mEq, 10 hours
B. 336 mEq, 16 hours
C. 448 mEq, 40 hours
D. 513 mEq, 20 hours
E. No replacement is needed

2. A 70-year-old man is admitted to the intensive care unit (ICU) after admission via the ED for a subarachnoid hemorrhage. After 12 hours of observation, the astute ICU nurse informs you that the patient's urine output has increased to 400 cc/h. What is his most likely diagnosis?

A. SIADH
B. Diuresis after urinary obstruction

C. Diabetes mellitus
D. Diabetes insipidus
E. Administration of diuretics

3. A 35-year-old woman comes to see you for a checkup required by her new place of employment. She feels well and takes no medication. She complains of a weight gain of 5 pounds over the last year. Her blood pressure is mildly elevated at 130/80 mm Hg. Her serum chemistry profile reveals hyponatremia. Laboratory examination is as follows: Na^+ 125 mEq/L, Cl^- 100 mEq/L, K^+ 4.2 mEq/L, HCO_3^- 24 mEq/L, BUN 9 mEq/L, Cr 0.9 mg/dL, glucose 90 mg/dL. Which of the following is the most likely diagnosis?

A. Hyperthyroidism
B. Diabetes mellitus
C. Hypercholesterolemia
D. Diuretic abuse
E. SIADH

HPI: DK, an 81-year-old man, is brought to the ED by his wife for increasing lethargy at home over the last week. She also reports that he has complained of feeling ill and has had little to eat or drink over the past week.

His past medical history includes hypertension, myocardial infarction, and congestive heart failure. His medical regimen includes metoprolol, furosemide, and lisinopril.

PE: BP 100/60 mm Hg; Pulse 62; T 37°C; SaO_2 97% at room air.

The patient is a thin, frail-appearing man. His oral mucosa is dry. His cardiac rhythm is regular and his lungs are clear to auscultation. He is lethargic but easily aroused and answers questions appropriately.

Labs: Na^+ 148 mEq/L; K^+ 6.1 mEq/L; Cl^- 102 mEq/L; HCO_3^- 20 mEq/L; BUN 60 mg/dL; creatinine 3.4 mg/dL. ECG, see Figure 3-2.

THOUGHT QUESTIONS

- What regulates the serum concentration of potassium?
- How do the kidneys help regulate potassium?
- How does the acid-base balance affect the serum potassium concentration?
- What are the physiologic effects of hyperkalemia and hypokalemia?
- What is the cause of hyperkalemia in this patient?

BASIC SCIENCE DISCUSSION AND REVIEW

Most of the potassium within the body is **intracellular.** The ratio of intracellular to extracellular concentrations determines the resting membrane potential of cell membranes, and alterations in this ratio have profound effects on membrane excitability. Normal serum potassium levels are 3.5 to 5.0 mEq/L. The serum concentration of potassium is regulated by renal excretion and by changes in the distribution of potassium between ECF and ICF compartments. **Aldosterone,** via its action on the kidney, is the main determinant of serum potassium concentration.

Renal Potassium Handling

Approximately 60 to 80% of filtered potassium is passively reabsorbed in the PCT. An additional 25% is actively reabsorbed at the thick ascending loop of Henle by cotransport of Na^+, K^+, and Cl^-. Only 10 to 15% of filtered potassium reaches the distal nephron. Aldosterone determines the final concentration of potassium in the urine. An increased serum concentration of potassium (e.g., by eating lots of bananas) stimulates the production of aldosterone from the zona glomerulosa of the adrenal cortex. Aldosterone stimulates the Na^+/K^+ pump of the principal cells of the cortical collecting tubules, resulting in secretion of potassium. The converse is also true: In potassium depletion (e.g., due to diarrhea), aldosterone production decreases, resulting in decreased potassium secretion. The ability of the kidney to conserve potassium is limited, with an obligatory excretion of 10 mEq/L in the urine even in the presence of hypokalemia.

Transcellular Shifts

The serum concentration of potassium is also regulated by changes in distribution between the ICF and ECF compartments. During acidemic states, hydrogen ions are shifted from the ECF to the ICF in an attempt to maintain a physiologic pH. For every H^+ that enters the cell, a positive ion (K^+) must leave the cell to maintain electroneutrality. If alkalosis is present, potassium is shifted into cells and hydrogen ions are shifted out of cells. **Insulin** and **catecholamines** (epinephrine and norepinephrine) cause increased uptake of potassium by cells, resulting in decreased serum potassium.

Hyperkalemia

Hyperkalemia is defined as a serum potassium greater than 5 mEq/L. The causes of hyperkalemia can be broadly categorized as follows: decreased renal excretion, increased ingestion, redistribution of potassium due to transcellular shifts, pseudohyperkalemia, or hyperkalemia induced by drugs. Decreased renal excretion occurs with poor renal function and aldosterone deficiency due to adrenal disease. Hyperkalemia due to increased potassium intake occurs with oral or parenteral potassium supplementation. A decrease in serum pH causes a transcellular shift of potassium from the ICF to the ECF, as discussed above.

Pseudohyperkalemia is seen if significant hemolysis with release of intracellular potassium occurs during the collection of a blood sample. Leukocytosis or thrombocytosis can also create spurious hyperkalemia by releasing intracellular potassium into the serum collected for testing. Drugs such as angiotensin-converting enzyme inhibitors (ACEIs) and potassium-sparing diuretics can lead to hyperkalemia. ACEIs result in decreased aldosterone production and increased serum potassium. Potassium-sparing diuretics include spironolactone, triamterene, and amiloride. Spironolactone antagonizes the effects of aldosterone in the distal nephron. Triamterene and amiloride act directly on sodium channels in the distal renal tubules causing both sodium and potassium retention.

An increased serum potassium causes a less electronegative resting potential, and cells become more excitable. This causes conduction disorders in cardiac muscle and may result in the electrocardiographic pattern seen in the patient above. ECG changes seen in hyperkalemia include peaked **T waves, widened QRS,** and **prolonged PR,** and may result in cardiac arrest.

The treatment of hyperkalemia includes increasing the movement of potassium into cells with insulin (preceded by glucose administration to avoid hypoglycemia) and β-adrenergic agonists such as inhaled albuterol, and alkalinizing the serum with sodium bicarbonate so as to increase transcellular shifts with H^+.

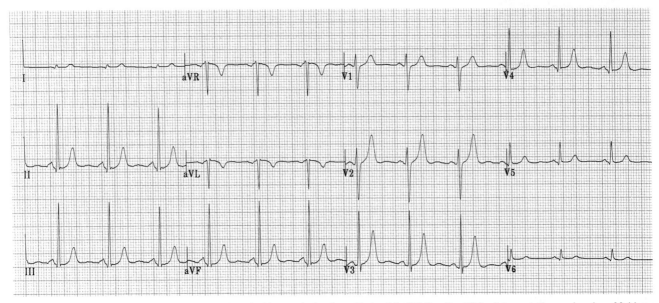

• **Figure 3-2.** ECG with peaked T waves. (Reproduced with permission from Taylor GJ. 150 Practice ECGs: interpretation and review. Malden, MA: Blackwell Science, 2002.)

To protect the heart from dangerous arrhythmias, intravenous calcium is given to antagonize the effects of hyperkalemia on cell membrane potential. Actual removal of potassium can be accomplished through forced diuresis, elimination from the GI tract with an ion exchange resin such as sodium polystyrene sulfonate or hemodialysis.

Hypokalemia

Hypokalemia is defined as a serum potassium of less than 3.5 mEq/L. It may reflect a reduction in total body potassium or it may result from redistribution of potassium in patients with normal or even increased total body potassium. The causes of hypokalemia include dietary deficiency, redistribution with increased entry of potassium into cells, diarrhea, diuretics, aldosterone excess, and hypomagnesemia.

The clinical manifestations of hypokalemia are a result of increased negativity of the resting membrane potential and decreased sensitivity of cell membranes. Skeletal muscles may be weakened, resulting in paresis and rhabdomyolysis. Hypokalemia also causes decreased motility of smooth muscle, leading to decreased intestinal motility and paralytic ileus. ECG changes seen in hypokalemia include decreased T wave amplitude, prolonged QT interval, and a prominent **U wave** (a finding not correlated with the cardiac cycle) and may lead to cardiac arrest.

The cause of hypokalemia should be investigated and treated. Potassium should be replaced according to the severity of the hypokalemia using oral or parenteral potassium.

CASE CONCLUSION

The patient is volume depleted due to poor nutrition and exacerbated by his continuing to take his diuretic. Kidney perfusion is diminished, and substances such as potassium that are normally cleared by the kidney have accumulated. His ability to excrete organic acids is diminished, leading to acidemia and elevated serum K$^+$ as potassium shifts into the ECF. The patient is hospitalized, rehydrated, and treated with sodium bicarbonate, glucose followed by insulin, and inhaled albuterol, which all shift potassium into cells. To prevent potassium uptake from his GI tract, he is given the exchange resin sodium polystyrene sulfonate. His serum potassium and ECG findings normalize over the next few hours and his renal function slowly returns over the next few days.

THUMBNAIL: Renal Physiology—Hyperkalemia vs. Hypokalemia

	Hyperkalemia	*Hypokalemia*
Etiology	Renal failure	Dietary deficiency
	Hypoaldosteronism	Hyperaldosteronism
	Drug induced	Renal losses
	Tubular defects	Diarrhea
	Ingestion	Alkalemia
	Acidemia	
	Insulin deficiency	

(Continued)

THUMBNAIL: Renal Physiology—Hyperkalemia vs. Hypokalemia *(Continued)*

	Hyperkalemia	*Hypokalemia*
Clinical manifestation	Weakness Fatigue Cardiac arrhythmias	Weakness Fatigue Cardiac arrhythmias Hyporeflexia Paralytic ileus
ECG findings	Peaked T waves Decreased P wave amplitude PR lengthening QRS widening	Flattened T waves Prominent U wave ST depression Prolonged QT

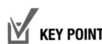

KEY POINTS

- Aldosterone, acting on the cortical collecting ducts, is the main determinant of serum potassium concentration
- A low serum pH shifts potassium from the ICF to the ECF, and a high pH shifts potassium from the ECF to the ICF
- Insulin, catecholamines, and sodium bicarbonate cause potassium to shift from the ECF to the ICF
- Both hyperkalemia and hypokalemia can cause weakness and cardiac arrhythmias, leading to cardiac arrest
- Potassium-sparing diuretics: potassium STAys in = **S**pironolactone, **T**riamterene, **A**miloride

QUESTIONS

1. A patient with known renal failure on hemodialysis presents to the ED in congestive heart failure and is found to have a potassium of 7.0 mEq/L. Which of the following can be used in the ED to treat him prior to initiating dialysis?

   A. Calcium chloride
   B. Insulin
   C. Sodium bicarbonate
   D. Albuterol
   E. All of the above

2. A 60-year-old woman presents to your office with weakness and a heart rate of 38 beats per minute. Her chemistry panel is significant for a potassium of 2.0 mEq/L. Which of the following conditions could be the cause of her hypokalemia?

   A. Hypoaldosteronism
   B. Furosemide

   C. Spironolactone
   D. Metabolic acidosis
   E. Hyperthyroidism

3. A 72-year-old woman was recently started on both triamterene and an ACEI for control of her blood pressure. At her office checkup 2 weeks later, which of the following might be seen on her electrocardiogram?

   A. Peaked T waves
   B. Decreased P wave amplitude
   C. PR lengthening
   D. QRS widening
   E. All of the above

CASE 3-4 | Acid-Base Physiology

HPI: CD, a 47-year-old woman with HIV, was unable to provide a history, as she had been intubated in the ED. Her husband reports that she has been suffering from a cough for the last 2 days. Her HIV is well controlled by antiretroviral therapy and she has never suffered from any opportunistic infections.

PE: T 39°C (rectal); pulse 110; BP 90/40 mm Hg; RR 40; SaO_2 97% on 100% oxygen.

The physical examination is significant for crackles over both lung bases. The patient's extremities are cool and her lower legs have a mottled appearance.

Chest x-ray: Dense infiltrates in the lower lobes bilaterally, cardiac silhouette within normal limits, endotracheal tube present and in proper position.

Labs: A blood gas prior to intubation has the following values: pH 7.27; pCO_2 8 mm Hg; pO_2 50 mm Hg; oxygen saturation 82%; bicarbonate 12 mEq/L. A basic metabolic panel shows the following: Na^+ 130 mEq/L; K^+ 5.5 mEq/L; Cl^- 90 mEq/L; HCO_3^- 14 mEq/L; BUN 37 mg/dL; creatinine 3.0 mg/dL. Her serum lactate is elevated at 8.1 U/L. A complete blood count (CBC) is significant for WBC count 15,000 cells/mL; hemoglobin 10 g/dL; and platelets 113,000 cells/mL.

THOUGHT QUESTIONS

- How do the kidneys regulate acids and bases?
- What is the renal compensation for respiratory and metabolic derangement of serum pH?
- What are the acid-base disorders?
- What is an anion gap?
- What is the acid-base disturbance in our patient?

BASIC SCIENCE REVIEW AND DISCUSSION

The body produces hydrogen ions as a result of the metabolic degradation of glucose, protein, and fatty acids. Under normal circumstances the buffering systems of the blood (bicarbonate and hemoglobin), the exhalation of carbon dioxide (CO_2, a volatile acid), the reabsorption of bicarbonate (HCO_3^-, a base), and excretion of ammonium and phosphoric acid (nonvolatile acids) by the kidney maintain our physiologic pH at approximately 7.4. Blood pH can be determined by blood gas analysis. Normal blood gas values are pH 7.35–7.45, pCO_2 35–45 mm Hg, pO_2 90–100 mm Hg, and a HCO_3^- 20–24 mmol/L. The buffering systems of the blood and the lungs are limited by the amount of buffer in the blood and the ability of patients to increase or decrease their respiratory rate. Thus, the kidney must compensate for acid-base disturbances by either reabsorbing or excreting bicarbonate or excreting protons. The major buffers of the urine include bicarbonate, ammonia, and phosphate. When the blood pH falls below 7.4, the urine becomes more acidic to rid the body of excess acid, and when the blood pH exceeds 7.4, the urine becomes more alkaline.

The reabsorption of bicarbonate occurs primarily at the PCT and ensures there is no loss of bicarbonate from the filtered plasma. This mechanism is highly efficient, and, in general, the kidney reabsorbs all of the filtered bicarbonate. Within renal tubular cells, carbon dioxide is hydrated to form carbonic acid, which is then broken down by the enzyme carbonic anhydrase to hydrogen and bicarbonate [$H_2O + CO_2 \leftrightarrow H_2CO_3 \leftrightarrow H^+ + HCO_3^-$]. The bicarbonate ion is reabsorbed down its electrochemical gradient into the blood. The hydrogen ion is excreted into the tubular lumen by countertransport with sodium (this active transport mechanism allows the hydrogen ion to use energy released when sodium moves down its electrochemical gradient created by the basolateral Na^+/K^+ ATPase). The hydrogen ion derived from bicarbonate combines with the filtered bicarbonate, which is then converted by carbonic anhydrase to water and carbon dioxide, both of which readily diffuse into the renal tubule cell. By this mechanism there is no excretion of either bicarbonate or hydrogen ions but the efficient use of hydrogen ions to conserve bicarbonate. Bicarbonate reabsorption occurs to a great extent (80–90%) at the PCT because carbonic anhydrase is active in the extensive PCT cell brush border.

When hydrogen combines with any buffer other than bicarbonate and is excreted, the body rids itself of excess acid. The kidneys compensate for a sustained acidosis by combining hydrogen ions with ammonia and phosphate. Ammonia (NH_3) is formed from the breakdown of glutamine within renal tubule cells. As a neutral molecule, ammonia can diffuse across the cells of the tubular lumen, where it combines with hydrogen to form a positively charged, hydrophilic ammonium ion (NH_4^+), which is trapped in the urine as it can no longer diffuse across the cell membrane (Fig. 3-3). Up-regulation of ammonia synthesis and subsequent **diffusion trapping** of ammonium ions occurs when blood pH is acidotic for any length of time and is the main mechanism by which the kidney compensates for acidosis. It occurs primarily in the latter segments of the nephron after most of the bicarbonate has been reabsorbed in the PCT. Phosphate, the other major urinary buffer, is largely reabsorbed by the kidney; thus, a limited amount is available to buffer urinary acid.

Disruptions in Acid-Base Homeostasis

Changes in the concentration of the acid-base buffer components cause disturbances in acid-base balance. The acid-base disorders are divided into two categories: metabolic and respiratory. They can be further subdivided into metabolic acidosis, metabolic alkalosis, respiratory acidosis, and respiratory alkalosis.

Metabolic Acidosis

A serum pH of less than 7.35 with normal or low pCO_2 is diagnostic of a metabolic acidosis and is caused by a decrease in blood

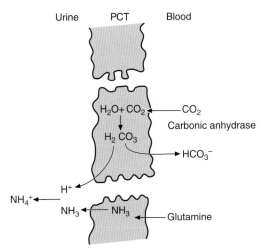

• **Figure 3-3.** Generation of ammonium.

bicarbonate. Hyperventilation is the compensatory response, resulting in hypocapnia. The possible etiologies include loss of bicarbonate through the GI tract or kidneys, an increase in hydrogen ion load from endogenous or exogenous sources, and a decrease in the renal excretion of hydrogen or production of bicarbonate.

An anion gap is important in the diagnosis of the etiology of metabolic acidosis. The anion gap is the mathematical difference between the concentration of the measured major cations and anions in the serum.

$$\text{Anion gap} = Na^+ - (Cl^- + HCO_3^-)$$

Normally, this difference is approximately 12 mEq/L. It is an estimation of the unmeasured anions in the serum such as phosphate, sulfate, and proteins. Although measurable, by convention, potassium, magnesium, and calcium are not included in the formula above. If the anion gap is elevated, it is an indication that an acidic anion (either exogenous or endogenous) is present. The mnemonic **MUD PILERS** summarizes the causes of an elevated anion gap: **m**ethanol, **u**remia, **d**iabetic ketoacidosis, **p**araldehyde, **i**soniazid, **l**actate, **e**thanol, **e**thylene glycol, **r**habdomyolysis, and **s**alicylates.

It is also possible to have an acidosis with no anion gap, also known as a nongap or hyperchloremic acidosis. The etiology is usually a loss of bicarbonate necessitating that sodium be reabsorbed with chloride. Causes of a nongap acidosis are summarized with the mnemonic **HEART CCU: h**ypoaldosteronism, **e**xpansion (volume expansion), **a**limentation (parenteral nutrition), **r**enal tubular acidosis, **t**rots (diarrhea), **c**holestyramine, **c**arbonic anhydrase inhibitors (acetazolamide), **u**reterosigmoidostomy.

Metabolic Alkalosis

Metabolic alkalosis, characterized by a pH greater than 7.45, is caused by an increase in serum bicarbonate. The resultant alkalemia decreases the respiratory rate, causing compensatory hypercapnia. Alkalemia is caused by loss of acid from vomiting or from consumption of alkali (e.g., antacids). Vomiting and/or the use of diuretics leads to hypovolemia, necessitating uptake of sodium. Bicarbonate is absorbed alongside sodium in the place of chloride to maintain electroneutrality. Mineralocorticoid excess leads to a loss of hydrogen ions as aldosterone increases the H+ pump in the distal convoluted tubule. The factors that maintain the disturbance include renal failure with the inability to excrete bicarbonate, decreased availability of chloride and the reabsorption of sodium with bicarbonate to compensate, continuing mineralocorticoid excess, and hypokalemia. In hypokalemia, hydrogen ions shift from the intracellular compartment to the extracellular compartment in exchange for potassium, to maintain electrochemical neutrality. These "excess" hydrogen ions are then excreted into the urine in exchange for the reabsorption of potassium, thereby maintaining the alkalosis.

Compensatory Changes

It is not possible to completely compensate or overcompensate for an acid-base disturbance. The compensatory response to the primary disorder results in only partial correction of the disorder, and the change in pH will reflect the primary disorder. If the pH does not fall within the limits of the primary disorder, one should consider a mixed disorder. The compensatory responses of the various disorders are shown below (see Thumbnail).

CASE CONCLUSION

This patient has an elevated anion gap metabolic acidosis with an anion gap of 26 mEq/L. She is hypoxic due to *Streptococcus pneumoniae* pneumonia, and her cells are metabolizing glucose via anaerobic respiration, producing lactate. She is attempting to compensate for the production of this endogenous acid by increasing her respiratory rate to rid her body of CO_2. She is treated with antibiotics, improves over the course of several days, is successfully extubated, and recovers quickly.

THUMBNAIL: Renal Pathophysiology

Renal compensation for changes in pH

	Primary Disorder	Compensatory Response	Result
Metabolic			
Acidosis	↓ HCO_3^-	↓ pCO_2	↓ pH
Alkalosis	↑ HCO_3^-	↑ pCO_2	↑ pH
Respiratory			
Acute acidosis	↑ pCO_2	(↓) HCO_3^-	↓ pH
Chronic acidosis	↑ pCO_2	↑↑ HCO_3^-	↓ pH
Acute alkalosis	↓ pCO_2	(↑) HCO_3^-	↑ pH
Chronic alkalosis	↓ pCO_2	↓ HCO_3^-	↑ pH

☑ KEY POINTS

- **Carbonic anhydrase** is the enzyme responsible for each step of the following reaction: $H_2O + CO_2 \leftrightarrow H_2CO_3 \leftrightarrow H^+ + HCO_3^-$

- Reabsorption of bicarbonate occurs primarily at the proximal convoluted tubule

- Regulation of bicarbonate reabsorption is how the kidney compensates for acidosis in the short and long term

- Up-regulation of ammonia synthesis and **diffusion trapping** of the ammonium ion (NH_4^+) is the kidney's main compensation for prolonged acidosis

- Anion gap = $Na^+ - (Cl^- + HCO_3^-)$. An anion gap acidosis is present if the gap is greater than the normal gap of 12, indicating the presence of an unmeasured anion.

- A **nongap acidosis** is also known as a **hyperchloremic** acidosis

QUESTIONS

1. A 62-year-old man arrives for his first checkup in 20 years. He is a smoker who received a diagnosis of hypertension many years ago, but did not take medication or return to his primary care physician. On physical examination, his blood pressure is 180/105 mm Hg. He is well-appearing but overweight. His laboratory examination is significant for sodium 138 mEq/L, potassium 5.8 mEq/L, chloride 104 mEq/L, bicarbonate 20 mEq/L, BUN 60 mg/dL, creatinine 2.8 mg/dL, and glucose of 230 mg/dL. What is the most likely cause of his decreased bicarbonate?

   A. Diabetic ketoacidosis
   B. Hypertension
   C. Renal insufficiency
   D. Diarrhea
   E. Chronic obstructive pulmonary disease

2. An elderly homeless woman is found unresponsive in the street, breathing rapidly. A blood gas analysis is performed with these results: pH 7.29, pCO_2 18 mm Hg, pO_2 100 mmHg, O_2 saturation 99%, Na^+ 145 mEq/l, Cl^- 90, HCO_3^- 12. A likely cause of her acidosis is which of the following?

   A. Hypoxia
   B. Diarrhea
   C. Methanol
   D. Vomiting
   E. Chronic obstructive pulmonary disease

3. A young man is brought in by ambulance after attempting suicide. He admits to being severely depressed and trying to end his own life by taking a bottle of aspirin. What abnormalities can we expect to see on his arterial blood gas analysis?

   A. Hypercapnia and hypoxia
   B. Hypocapnia and hypoxia
   C. Hypocapnia and decreased bicarbonate
   D. Hypercapnia and decreased bicarbonate
   E. Hypoxia and increased bicarbonate

4. A teenaged girl visits her primary care physician for her annual checkup. The astute family physician notices several worrisome physical signs, including red puffy eyes, swollen parotid glands, and erosion of her tooth enamel. Her basic metabolic panel is as follows: Na^+ 123 mEq/L, K^+ 2.9 mEq/L, HCO_3^- 32 mEq/L. Which of the following is the likely cause of her metabolic abnormalities?

   A. Hyperventilation
   B. Ingestion of calcium carbonate
   C. Renal failure
   D. Vomiting
   E. Polydipsia

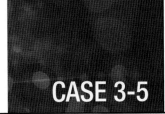

CASE 3-5 Calcium and Phosphate

HPI: LM is a 70-year-old woman with type 2 diabetes and hypertension who presents to the ED complaining of lack of appetite, a dull, constant ache over her entire abdomen, and constipation for the last week. She is recovering from a bout of influenza diagnosed by her primary care physician 2 weeks ago and has not been eating or drinking well since the onset of her illness. She has also had a headache and difficulty concentrating for the last several days. Her diabetes and hypertension are well controlled, and she has continued to take her medications, which include hydrochlorothiazide, lisinopril, glipizide, and metformin.

PE: BP 100/60 mm Hg; HR 60; RR 12/min; T 36.7°C

Her oral mucosa is dry. Her heart rate is bradycardic and regular, and her lungs are clear to auscultation. Her abdomen is protuberant and soft, with few bowel sounds and no tenderness to palpation. She is somnolent, and easily aroused, but falls back to sleep immediately and cannot state where she is.

Labs: Na^+ 139 mEq/L; K^+ 5.5 mEq/L; Cl^+ 98 mEq/L; HCO_3^- 29 mEq/L; BUN 65 mg/dL; Cr 3.4 mg/dL; glucose 200 mg/dL; Ca^{2+} 15 mEq/dL; phos 4.2 mEq/L.

THOUGHT QUESTIONS

- How does the kidney contribute to calcium and phosphate homeostasis?
- How is vitamin D involved in calcium and phosphate regulation?
- What are the causes of and symptoms associated with hypercalcemia and hypocalcemia? Hyperphosphatemia and hypophosphatemia?
- What is the pathophysiology of our patient's condition?

BASIC SCIENCE REVIEW AND DISCUSSION

Homeostasis of both calcium and phosphate can be discussed together because serum levels of both ions are dependent on renal excretion, intestinal absorption, the action of PTH, and regulation of bone metabolism.

Calcium Homeostasis

Calcium is a very important ion in both the physiology and the structure of the body. It is a rapidly fluctuating intracellular messenger, induces microtubule and muscle contraction, enables neurotransmitter release, is an important cofactor in the coagulation cascade, and is a component of the bony skeleton. It is the most abundant electrolyte in the body and most of it is found in the skeleton. The normal serum calcium concentration ranges from 8.5 to 10.0 mg/dL, with approximately 40 to 50% bound to albumin. For every 1 g/dL fall in plasma albumin concentration, there is a 0.8 mg/dL reduction in serum calcium concentration. The active form of calcium is the ionized portion, which accounts for 45 to 50% of serum calcium. The percentage of calcium bound to protein changes with changes in blood pH; binding increases with increased pH.

Ionized calcium is filtered at the glomerulus and approximately 65% is reabsorbed at the proximal tubule and 20% at the thick ascending loop of Henle. **PTH,** the most important regulator of ionized calcium concentration, increases the reabsorption of calcium in the distal convoluted tubule (DCT). Diuretics have a variable effect on calcium excretion, with furosemide increasing calcium excretion and hydrochlorothiazide decreasing calcium

excretion. Opposing PTH and of lesser significance in normal calcium homeostasis is **calcitonin,** released by the parafollicular cells (C cells) of the thyroid, which decreases bone reabsorption of calcium, resulting in decreased serum ionized calcium.

The most important regulator of calcium absorption from the gut is **1,25-(OH) vitamin D** (Fig. 3-4). The precursor to vitamin D, 7-dehydrocholesterol, is converted in the skin in the presence of ultraviolet radiation to cholecalciferol. Cholecalciferol is then hydroxylated in the liver to 25-hydroxycholecalciferol and then further hydroxylated in the kidney to produce the active form 1,25-dihydroxycholecalciferol. PTH directly stimulates 1α-hydroxylase. PTH is synthesized and released from the parathyroid gland in response to a lowered serum ionized calcium level. Vitamin D negatively feeds back on 1α-hydroxylase at the level of the kidney and inhibits the production of PTH, thereby regulating the intestinal absorption of calcium.

Hypercalcemia

Hypercalcemia results from several mechanisms, including increased mobilization of calcium from bone, increased GI absorption, and decreased urinary excretion. Under normal circumstances, PTH increases mobilization of ionized calcium from bone, and in certain malignancies and hyperparathyroidism increased mobilization occurs to an extreme degree, resulting in hypercalcemia. Squamous cell lung cancer produces PTH-related peptide and causes the paraneoplastic syndrome of hypercalcemia. Osteoblastic metastases from breast cancer and osteolytic lesions due to multiple myeloma may also precipitate hypercalcemia, especially in immobile patients. **Primary hyperparathyroidism** usually is due to a single hyperfunctioning adenoma in one of the four parathyroid glands. Long-standing renal insufficiency may lead to chronically elevated levels of PTH and hypercalcemia, termed **secondary hyperparathyroidism.** Secondary hyperparathyroidism may progress until the parathyroid glands autonomously hyperfunction, leading to **tertiary hyperparathyroidism** and hypercalcemia that can only be corrected by parathyroidectomy. Other causes of hypercalcemia include thiazide diuretics and granulomatous diseases. Thiazide diuretics increase the sodium gradient used for the reabsorption of calcium in the DCT and thus elevate serum calcium levels.

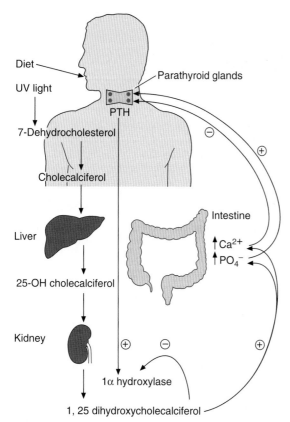

• **Figure 3-4.** Vitamin D metabolism.

2 minutes. Severe hypocalcemia may precipitate **tetany** due to increased neuromuscular excitability including laryngospasm. Treatment of hypocalcemia includes the administration of calcium and vitamin D.

Phosphate Homeostasis

Phosphate is present in various forms in the body. In its ionic form (PO_4^{3-}) it is an important intracellular anion (many essential reactions use the breaking of the high energy phosphate bonds in ATP for energy); in its organic form it is a component of all body tissues, as it forms the backbone of all nucleic acids. Urinary phosphate buffers protons in the urine.

Normal serum phosphorus levels range from 2.5 to 4.5 mg/dL. Serum phosphate concentration is determined by both intestinal absorption and renal excretion, with renal excretion being most important. In the kidney, approximately 90% of the filtered phosphorus is reabsorbed in the proximal tubule. Vitamin D increases absorption of phosphorus in the gut.

Hyperphosphatemia

Hyperphosphatemia is caused by decreased renal excretion, increased cell turnover, acidosis, exogenous administration of phosphorus or vitamin D, and magnesium deficiency. A complete list of etiologies is given below (see Thumbnail). Phosphate inhibits renal hydroxylation of vitamin D; thus, elevated phosphorus levels may lead to hypocalcemia. Hyperphosphatemia in the presence of a normal calcium level may result in metastatic calcification as phosphate complexes with calcium and deposits in the tissues.

The treatment of hyperphosphatemia includes using phosphate binders such as calcium carbonate or calcium acetate, alkalization of the urine with a carbonic anhydrase inhibiting diuretic, or dialysis.

Hypophosphatemia

Hypophosphatemia is due to renal loss, decreased intestinal absorption, or redistribution during various conditions. A complete list of etiologies is given below (see Thumbnail). Clinical manifestations may include anorexia, confusion, paresthesias, and bone pain due to skeletal abnormalities. The treatment is a high phosphate diet and oral or parenteral phosphate.

Granulomatous diseases such as sarcoidosis may cause hypercalcemia because macrophages convert vitamin D precursors to the active form of vitamin D. A complete list of etiologies of hypercalcemia is given below (see Thumbnail).

Symptoms of hypercalcemia include anorexia, nausea, abdominal pain, polydipsia, polyuria, headache, impaired concentration, loss of memory, confusion, hallucinations, and muscle weakness. Hypercalcemia induces a nephrogenic DI that impairs the kidney's ability to concentrate urine, resulting in dehydration. Hypercalcemia may result in nephrocalcinosis and nephrolithiasis. The treatment of hypercalcemia is aimed at hydration with normal saline, forced diuresis with furosemide, and bisphosphonates to bind calcium to bone. Hemodialysis may be necessary.

Hypocalcemia

The causes of hypocalcemia include hypoparathyroidism, decreased calcium mobilization from bone, and reduced absorption of calcium from the gut. Long-standing renal insufficiency may contribute to hypocalcemia due to the lack of nephron mass available to hydroxylate vitamin D. Hypocalcemia may be seen in association with hypomagnesemia because low magnesium levels inhibit PTH release. A complete list of etiologies is given below (see Thumbnail).

Symptoms of hypocalcemia include paresthesias such as perioral or acral (fingertip) tingling and muscle cramps. Classic physical exam signs of hypocalcemia include the **Chvostek sign,** a twitching of the lip brought about by tapping on the facial nerve just anterior to the ear below the zygomatic bone, and the **Trousseau sign,** carpal spasm after the inflation of a blood pressure cuff for

CASE CONCLUSION

The patient has many of the symptoms of hypercalcemia: anorexia, constipation, impaired concentration, and abdominal pain. Symptoms of hypercalcemia are often referred to as **moans (abdominal pain), groans (bone pain), stones (kidney stones), and psychic overtones (mental status changes).** During the patient's illness, her oral fluid intake decreased while she continued to take her thiazide diuretic. Her hypercalcemia was precipitated by dehydration, worsened by renal insufficiency, and exacerbated by immobilization. Her increased serum calcium further impaired her kidney's ability to concentrate urine, worsening her dehydration. Following rehydration and correction of her serum calcium, her serum calcium levels slowly normalized and her kidney function returned.

THUMBNAIL: Renal Pathophysiology—Calcium and Phosphate Abnormalities

	Etiology	Symptom	Sign
Hypercalcemia	Malignancy	Fatigue	Lethargy to coma
	Hyperparathyroidism	Muscle weakness	Seizure
	Primary	Abdominal pain	Dilute urine
	Secondary	Constipation	Metastatic calcification
	Tertiary	Anorexia	Arrhythmia
	Renal disease	Nausea	Paralytic ileus
	Thiazide diuretics	Polydipsia	↓ QT segment
	Hyperthyroidism	Polyuria	
	Vitamin D intoxication	Headache	
	Vitamin A intoxication	Impaired concentration	
	Hypophosphatemia	Loss of memory	
	Immobilization		
	Granulomas		
	Sarcoidosis		
	Milk alkali syndrome		
Hypocalcemia	Hypoparathyroidism	Muscle cramps	Carpal spasm
	Post-thyroidectomy	Tetany	Pedal spasm
	Chronic magnesium deficiency	Paresthesias	Laryngospasm
	Vitamin D deficiency		Arrhythmia
	Pseudohypoparathyroidism		↑ QT segment
	Hyperphosphatemia		
	Pancreatitis		
	Alcohol withdrawal		
Hyperphosphatemia	Renal failure	Symptoms of hypocalcemia	Decreased urine volume
	Hypoparathyroidism	Weakness	Arrhythmias
	Pseudohypo-PTH	Fatigue	Paralytic ileus
	Lysis of cells with chemotherapy	Anorexia	Heart failure
	Hemolytic anemia	Nausea	
	Rhabdomyolysis		
	Acidosis		
	Vitamin D intoxication		
	Magnesium deficiency		
Hypophosphatemia	Hyperparathyroidism	Bone pain	Seizures
	Hypomagnesemia	Weakness	Coma
	Corticosteroids	Anorexia	Reduced glomerular filtration rate
	Malabsorption	Lethargy	Heart failure
	Alcoholism	Confusion	
	Phosphate binders	Paresthesias	
	Vitamin D deficiency		
	Sepsis		
	Salicylate poisoning		
	Alkalosis		
	Glucose/insulin refeeding syndrome		

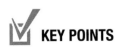 **KEY POINTS**

■ The renal contribution to calcium homeostasis is the production of vitamin D and, via the influence of PTH, the renal excretion of calcium.

■ The primary regulation of serum phosphate levels is via renal excretion of phosphate.

■ Long-standing renal disease results in hypocalcemia and hyperphosphatemia.

QUESTIONS

1. A healthy 27-year-old woman presents to your office for a routine exam and is found to have a serum calcium level of 12 mEq/L and a phosphorus level of 2.2 mEq/L. What is the most likely diagnosis?

   A. Renal insufficiency
   B. Familial hypocalciuric hypercalcemia
   C. Hyperparathyroidism
   D. Pseudohypoparathyroidism
   E. Excessive use of vitamin D

2. A patient of yours has suffered for many years from severe chronic renal insufficiency due to hypertension. His blood pressure is well controlled with a combination of an ACEI and a beta-blocker. Which of the following electrolyte abnormalities is he most likely to have?

   A. Hypercalcemia and hyperphosphatemia
   B. Hypercalcemia and metabolic alkalosis
   C. Hypercalcemia and hypophosphatemia
   D. Hypocalcemia and hyperphosphatemia
   E. Hypercalcemia and metabolic acidosis

3. A very anxious medical student complains of anxiety attacks characterized by tingling of his hands and around his mouth. Which of the following is the pathophysiology of his complaint?

   A. Hypercalcemia
   B. Hypocalcemia
   C. Hyperphosphatemia
   D. Metabolic acidosis
   E. Metabolic alkalosis

CASE 3-6 Hypertension

HPI: DB, a 40-year-old African American man, presents to his primary care provider's office for an annual physical. He has not seen a doctor for some time, and has no complaints, but wants to have his cholesterol checked because his 48-year-old brother just had a heart attack. He jogs and plays basketball to stay in shape but knows he doesn't eat the right foods. Both his father and his mother have hypertension.

PE: BP 154/92 mm Hg; pulse 72

The patient has an athletic build. His fundi are within normal limits. His heart has a regular rate and rhythm with an S_4 present. His lungs are clear to auscultation.

THOUGHT QUESTIONS

- What is essential hypertension (HTN) and what mediates it?
- What are the consequences of HTN on the kidney?
- What is accelerated/malignant HTN?
- What are the causes of renovascular HTN and when should we suspect them?
- How can we best treat this patient?

BASIC SCIENCE REVIEW AND DISCUSSION

Essential HTN is an elevation in BP, without a proximate cause, above an ambiguously defined "normal level." Current guidelines are listed in Table 3-3.

No single value should be considered proof of high BP. BP values should be well established over several visits. The definitions of HTN are changing because it is now apparent that lower BPs significantly reduce cardiovascular morbidity and mortality and are renal protective.

Although the etiology of essential HTN is unclear, there are endocrine, neural, genetic, and environmental factors responsible for the apparent upward resetting of BP homeostatic set points. It is likely that many different, interrelated factors contribute to the development of HTN in susceptible individuals.

The prevalence of essential HTN varies among the population. It is estimated that 10 to 15% of Caucasian adults and up to 30% of African Americans have BPs greater than 140/90 mm Hg. For unclear reasons, African Americans have a more serious form of the disease. The incidence of HTN increases with age. Women have a lower incidence of HTN until menopause, when incidence rapidly approaches that of men. The incidence of **secondary HTN,** attributed to causes such as renal artery stenosis, fibromuscular dysplasia, pheochromocytoma, primary hyperaldosteronism, Cushing disease, and coarctation of the aorta comprises only 2 to 5% of all cases of HTN. It is particularly important to suspect secondary HTN in young adults.

Etiologies of Hypertension

Renin-angiotensin-aldosterone Axis The renin-angiotensin-aldosterone hormonal axis (Fig. 3-5) is an important determinant of BP. **Renin** is an enzyme produced and secreted from the juxtaglomerular cells of the kidney. Its substrate, angiotensinogen, is an α-globulin produced in the liver and cleaved by renin to produce angiotensin I. **Angiotensin I** is cleaved by ACE, found on the surface of endothelial cells—primarily in the lung—to angiotensin II. **Angiotensin II** is a potent vasoconstrictor and stimulates the production of aldosterone from the adrenal cortex. **Aldosterone,** a steroid hormone, is produced in the zona glomerulosa of the adrenal cortex. Its main actions are increased sodium reabsorption, potassium secretion, and hydrogen ion secretion. Aldosterone acts on the principal cells of the cortical collecting duct to increase the permeability of luminal sodium channels and increase the activity of the sodium-potassium pumps in the basolateral membrane, facilitating the uptake of sodium and the secretion of potassium.

Another determinant of BP is **sympathetic tone** mediated by the catecholamines of the adrenal medulla. This is often termed the neural hormonal axis as atrial baroreceptors are activated by a decrease in BP to stimulate the adrenal medulla to release epinephrine and norepinephrine. These vasoactive substances vasoconstrict both arteries and veins, stimulate heart rate and contractility, and increase renin secretion.

A drop in BP results in renal hypoperfusion and increased renin secretion from the cells of the juxtaglomerular apparatus. Decreased BP is also sensed by the cardiac baroreceptors and stimulates epinephrine and norepinephrine release from the adrenal medulla. Renin secretion is further stimulated by epinephrine and norepinephrine. Increased plasma renin results in increased levels of angiotensin I, which is converted to angiotensin II in the lungs. Renin also stimulates the adrenal cortex to produce aldosterone, resulting in increased salt and water reabsorption from the kidney, thereby increasing intravascular volume. The combination of angiotensin II-mediated vasoconstriction and an aldosterone-mediated increase in salt and water reabsorption is the mechanism by which normal BP is maintained. Increased BP and plasma volumes negatively feed back to the kidney to lower renin levels.

Both an overactive renin-angiotensin-aldosterone axis and a tonically active sympathetic nervous system have been postulated to cause HTN, but neither etiology can fully explain the pathogenesis of HTN. Only 15% of patients with essential HTN have elevated renin levels. Increased sympathetic activity has been linked with transient elevations in BP but cannot account for the sustained HTN seen in essential HTN.

Other Etiologies of Hypertension Noninherited factors that increase BP include a high-sodium diet, obesity, and alcohol ingestion. The mechanism for sodium-sensitive HTN is not clear, and only 40 to 60% of hypertensives respond to a reduction in dietary salt. In

TABLE 3-3 Current Guidelines for Assessing Blood Pressure

BP Stage	Systolic (mm Hg)	Diastolic (mm Hg)
Pre-hypertension	120–139	80–89
Mild HTN	140–159	90–99
Moderate HTN	160–179	100–109
Severe HTN	>180	>110

BP, blood pressure; *HTN*, hypertension

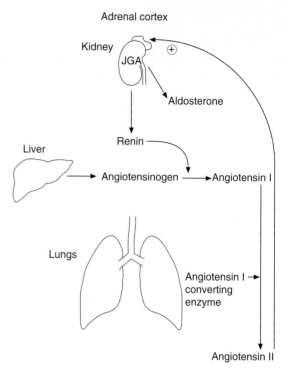

● **Figure 3-5.** The renin-angiotensin-aldosterone axis. *JGA*, juxtaglomerular apparatus.

these patients, sodium restriction and diuretics decrease plasma volume and aid in BP reduction. **Syndrome X** is a triad of insulin resistance, HTN, and hypercholesterolemia found in patients with centripetal obesity. Alcohol is also associated with HTN by an unclear mechanism, and a reduction in BP is seen with the cessation of alcohol consumption.

Renal artery stenosis is one cause of secondary HTN. It is found in older patients with atherosclerotic vascular disease and suggested by an abdominal bruit. It usually causes severe HTN and may present as a rapid rise in BP in a patient with HTN that was previously well controlled. Renal artery stenosis can be bilateral or unilateral and may cause HTN by activation of the renin-angiotensin cascade in response to kidney hypoperfusion. The gold standard for diagnosis is an angiogram.

Fibromuscular dysplasia is another cause of secondary HTN in younger patients. Most commonly the disease affects young women who have dysplasia or hyperplasia of the media of many different vessels. The characteristic appearance of the renal arteries on angiogram is a **"string of beads."** The bead-like appearance is due to areas of arterial wall hyperplasia alternating with normal-appearing segments.

Genetic factors clearly play a role in HTN, although a specific gene (or set of genes) has not been identified. Patients with one or two hypertensive parents are two to three times more likely to develop HTN than are patients with a family history negative for HTN.

Effects on the Kidneys

HTN is a chronic illness that can result in cumulative injury to the kidney if left untreated. The typical course of renal damage is a slow decline in renal function, with sclerosis of the glomerular arteries and arterioles, cortical glomeruli being most affected. Sclerotic glomeruli are thickened and hyalinized, decreasing renal perfusion. Eventually the tubules and supportive stroma atrophy, leading to shrunken and scarred kidneys bilaterally.

An accelerated form of HTN also occurs and leads to acute renal failure. **Malignant HTN,** more correctly referred to as **accelerated HTN,** is associated with diastolic BPs above 130 mm Hg. It often occurs in patients with long-standing HTN who have stopped taking their medications. BPs in this range are an urgent matter and become an emergent matter when associated with renal failure, retinal hemorrhages and exudates, papilledema, encephalopathy, CHF, MI, or aortic dissection. A diagnosis of hypertensive emergency does not depend on the absolute value of the patient's BP but on the rapidity of the rise and the patient's associated symptoms. The renal failure causes glomerular damage and is thus associated with proteinuria and dysmorphic RBCs seen on urinalysis. The histologic lesions are cortical petechial hemorrhages, fibrinoid necrosis of the small vessels, and **"onion skinning"** of the arterioles due to intimal hyperplasia. When seen together, the above findings are termed **malignant nephrosclerosis.**

CASE CONCLUSION

DB had two repeat blood pressures of 146/96 and 158/101 mm Hg. After education about the risks of hypertension, including stroke, renal failure, heart failure, and retinopathy, the patient was started on a thiazide diuretic and a beta-blocker. He was also referred to a nutritionist for counseling and began to eat a low-sodium diet. He remained physically active and his hypertension is well controlled on this regimen.

THUMBNAIL: Renal Pathophysiology—Essential vs. Renovascular Hypertension

	Essential HTN	*vs.*	*Renovascular HTN*
Etiology:	Idiopathic		Renal artery stenosis
Age:	Older than 40 years		Younger than 30 or older than 50 years
Gender:	Males more than females		Female in fibromuscular dysplasia
With medications:	Responds to treatment		Refractory to treatment
Clues:	No atherosclerosis		Atherosclerosis likely
			Accelerated HTN
			Pulmonary edema
			Flank bruit

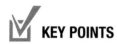

KEY POINTS

- Essential HTN is far more common than secondary HTN
- Accelerated HTN is high BP associated with neural, renal, and cardiovascular compromise
- Secondary causes of HTN include renal artery stenosis, pheochromocytoma, primary hyperaldosteronism, Cushing disease, and coarctation of the aorta
- Good BP control reduces the risk of stroke, heart attack, retinopathy, and kidney damage

QUESTIONS

1. A 67-year-old man with a history of MI, diabetes, and HTN is started on lisinopril. What are the potential complications?

   A. Acute renal failure
   B. Hyperkalemia
   C. Hypotension
   D. Angioedema
   E. All of the above

2. A 29-year-old woman presents to your office for a general checkup. She has not seen a doctor other than to have Pap smears for many years. Her BP is found to be 200/140 mm Hg. On physical exam she has narrowing of her retinal arteries, a carotid bruit, and an S_4. She has no family history of hypertension. Her most likely diagnosis is which of the following?

   A. Hyperaldosteronism
   B. Cushing syndrome
   C. Fibromuscular dysplasia
   D. Pheochromocytoma
   E. Atherosclerotic renal disease

3. A 61-year-old women in otherwise good health has HTN. In your office today her BP is 180/100 mm Hg. Her BP has been well controlled with medication in the past but she refuses to take medication because she feels well. Which of the following is she at risk for?

   A. Renal failure
   B. Retinopathy
   C. Left ventricular failure
   D. Stroke
   E. All of the above

Immunologic Glomerular Injury

HPI: LR is an 8-year-old Asian girl with fever, nausea, oliguria, and dark-colored urine. At about 10 A.M. this morning, the patient began feeling and looking ill. Her mother noticed that she was urinating infrequently and that when she did urinate, it looked like "Coca-Cola." Her mother is also concerned about the swelling around her eyes. The mother states that her daughter is generally a healthy child and has never had similar symptoms. Upon further questioning, she admits her daughter was recently (~2 weeks ago) out of school for a few days with a sore throat, which resolved on its own. LR lives with her mother and older brother. Her father shares custody and sees her on weekends. She attends Stuart Day School and is in the third grade.

PE: The patient is febrile with a temperature of 39.0°C, moderately elevated blood pressure at 117/78 mm Hg, and normal pulse and respirations. She has periorbital edema.

Labs: Serum evaluation reveals a slightly elevated serum BUN and creatinine, depressed C3 concentration, cryoglobulins, and an elevated antistreptolysin O (ASO) titer. Urinalysis and urine cytology reveals mild proteinuria and red cell casts.

THOUGHT QUESTIONS

- Describe the pathophysiology and the associated microscopic and immunofluorescence findings of the glomerular diseases.
- How is the immune system involved in the etiology of glomerular diseases?
- What is the difference between nephritic and nephrotic syndrome?

BASIC SCIENCE REVIEW AND DISCUSSION

There are many glomerular diseases, and the task of keeping them straight is overwhelming. However, there are a few guiding principles that help with organization. There are two ways to approach these diseases, either pathophysiologically or clinically. The pathophysiology of most cases of glomerulonephritis (GN) is immune related, through the formation of antigen-antibody (Ag-Ab) complexes. Nonimmune mechanisms include hereditary defects in the glomerular basement membrane (GBM) and the pathologic processes involved in systemic diseases like amyloidosis and diabetes. Glomerular diseases present with different clinical syndromes including nephritic syndromes, discussed in this case, and nephrotic syndromes, discussed in the subsequent case.

Pathophysiology

Immune-complex GN Ag-Ab complexes can form when antibodies attach themselves to antigens that constitute the normal GBM, as in **Goodpasture syndrome/anti-GBM disease.** As a result, antibodies and complement line up along the GBM, forming linear patterns on immunofluorescence (IF). There are no **circulating** immune complexes to form lumpy deposits.

Alternately, Ag-Ab complexes can form when circulating antigens are bound by circulating antibodies, and then deposit in the glomeruli because of their physical or chemical properties. In this case, antigens are either endogenous, as in **lupus GN,** or exogenous, as in **poststreptococcal GN.** Once these Ag-Ab complexes have deposited in the glomerulus, they activate the alternate complement pathway, causing inflammation and injury to the glomerular filtration apparatus, leading to proteinuria and hematuria. Leukocytes infiltrate and mesangial cells proliferate in an attempt to repair the injury. Immune complexes appear as electron-dense deposits in the **mesangium** (as in **immunoglobulin A [IgA] nephropathy**), between the *endo*thelium and the GBM (**sub***endo***thelial** deposits as in **membranoproliferative GN**), or between the outer surface of the GBM and the podocytes of the glomerular *epi*thelial cells (**sub***epi***thelial** deposits as in **poststreptococcal GN**). The charge and size of the Ag-Ab complexes determine where they get lodged.

Another variant of immune-complex associated GN is **antineutrophil cytoplasmic antibodies (ANCAs)-associated GN. Wegener granulomatosis, Churg-Strauss syndrome,** and **microscopic polyangiitis** are small vessel vasculitides and, as such, impact the glomerular capillary tuft. They are associated with the ANCAs that bind endothelial cells. However, the mechanism of glomerular injury is not simply immune-complex deposition since antibodies are not seen on IF (these are sometimes referred to as "pauci-immune GNs").

Hereditary GN Alport syndrome is a primarily X-linked dominant mutation in the gene encoding part of collagen IV, which composes the GBM. It presents with hematuria and, rarely, nephrotic syndrome. It frequently progresses to renal failure over 20 to 30 years and is associated with nerve deafness and eye problems. **Thin basement membrane disease** (benign familial hematuria) also results from hereditary defects in type IV collagen. However, it presents with asymptomatic hematuria, requires no treatment, and never causes renal failure.

Clinical Syndromes

Clinically, glomerular diseases can be divided into those that present with *nephrotic* syndrome and those that with *nephritic* syndrome. **Nephrotic syndrome** ("o" for proteinuria) is characterized by heavy proteinuria (>3.5 g/d) with resulting hypoalbuminemia and edema, hyperlipidemia, and lipiduria. **Nephritic syndrome** is characterized by hematuria, red cell casts in the urinary sediment, azotemia (increase in serum nitrogenous compounds, including BUN), oliguria, mild to moderate HTN, and only mild edema/proteinuria. Another clinical syndrome, **rapidly progressive (crescentic) GN,** is a final common pathway of rapid progression to renal failure in weeks to months. It is often associated with Goodpasture syndrome, ANCA-associated vasculitides, or systemic lupus erythematosus.

Definitions

Lesions can be described as:

- *Focal:* involves <50% of the glomeruli
- *Diffuse:* involves >50% of the glomeruli
- *Segmental:* involves *part* of the individual glomerular tuft
- *Global:* involves *all* of the individual glomerular tuft
- *Proliferative:* involves an increase in glomerular cell number (either WBCs or local proliferation of glomerular cells)
- *Crescentic:* half-moon–shaped collection of cells in the Bowman space

- *Membranous:* expansion of the GBM by immune deposits
- *Sclerotic:* increase in extracellular material
- *Fibrotic:* deposition of type I and II collagen; consequence of healing inflammation

Immune-complex deposits can be described as:

- *Subendothelial:* between the *endo*thelium and the GBM
- *Mesangial:* in the mesangium
- *Subepithelial:* between the GBM and the podocytes of the glomerular *epi*thelium

CASE CONCLUSION

After arriving at a clinical diagnosis of poststreptococcal GN, you admit the child to the hospital. Treatment includes antibiotics to eliminate any remaining streptococci, bed rest, diuretics and antihypertensives to control blood pressure, and careful monitoring and correcting of fluid and electrolyte abnormalities. You reassure the patient's parents that she has an excellent prognosis, with 95% recovery, and recommend regular follow-up appointments for 1 year to ensure that the hematuria resolves.

THUMBNAIL: Renal Pathophysiology—Nephritic Syndromes

Disease	Most Common Clinical Presentation and Findings	Pathogenesis	Pathology
Postinfectious GN	Acute nephritis • 2 weeks postpharyngitis/impetigo • Children; self-resolving • Group A β-hemolytic strep (elevated ASO titers)	Trapped Ag-Ab complexes	LM: diffuse proliferation IF: IgG + C3, granular EM: **subepithelial humps**
IgA nephropathy (Berger disease) and Henoch-Schönlein purpura	Hematuria • Associated w/upper respiratory or GI infection	Unknown	LM: focal/mesangial proliferation IF: IgA, (+/− IgG, IgM, C3) EM: mesangial deposits
Goodpasture syndrome/anti-GBM GN	**Rapidly progressive GN** • Young men • Goodpasture if also with pulmonary hemorrhage	Abs against fixed Ags in GBM	LM: crescents IF: IgG + C3, linear along GBM EM: widening of BM
ANCA-associated GN (pauci-immune GN)	**Rapidly progressive GN** • Wegener granulomatosis, Churg-Strauss syndrome, microscopic polyangiitis • Systemic involvement common	Unknown	LM: crescents IF: **No Ig** EM: No deposits
Alport syndrome	Hematuria • Most cases **X-linked** dominant • <20 years old • Associated w/deafness and eye disorders	Structural defect in type IV collagen leads to leaky GBM	EM: **GBM splitting**
Thin basement membrane disease (benign familial hematuria)	Hematuria • Asymptomatic • Familial	Defect in type IV collagen	EM: diffusely thin GBM

LM, light microscopy; *IM*, immunofluorescence; *EM*, electron microscopy; *BM*, basement membrane

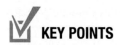

KEY POINTS

- **Nephritic syndrome** is characterized by hematuria, red cell casts, azotemia, oliguria, and HTN
- Nephritic syndromes result from defects in the GBM caused by:

1. Immune responses initiated by deposition of circulating Ag-Ab complexes or Ab attack of GBM components
2. Hereditary defects in components of the GBM

QUESTIONS

1. A 6-year-old boy presents with a gross hematuria and no other symptoms 2 days after a sore throat. A kidney biopsy reveals mesangial proliferation on light microscopy and IgA deposits on immunofluorescence. What is his likely diagnosis?

    A. Poststreptococcal GN
    B. Henoch-Schönlein purpura
    C. Alport syndrome
    D. Benign familial hematuria
    E. IgA nephropathy

2. A 24-year-old man presents with hemoptysis and hematuria. A renal biopsy reveals crescents on light microscopy and linear IgG on immunofluorescence. What is the inciting event in the pathophysiology of the implicated disease?

    A. Circulating endogenous antigens are trapped by circulating antibodies and lodge along the GBM in a linear pattern.
    B. There is an autosomal dominant mutation in a component of type IV collagen in the GBM and lung endothelium.
    C. Exogenous circulating antigens bind to local stationary antibodies as they pass through the glomerulus and lung endothelium.
    D. Autoimmune antibodies bind to normal components of the lung and kidney endothelium.
    E. The pathophysiology is unknown.

3. A 45-year-old woman with a history of adult-onset asthma presents with microscopic hematuria, HTN, and acute renal failure as evidenced by significantly increased BUN and creatinine. Her renal biopsy reveals eosinophil infiltration in the mesangium but no evidence of Ag-Ab complex deposition on light microscopy or immunofluorescence. Serum evaluation is ANA negative but ANCA positive. What is her likely diagnosis?

    A. Wegener granulomatosis
    B. Churg-Strauss
    C. Amyloidosis
    D. Minimal change disease
    E. Thin basement membrane disease

4. A 17-year-old boy with deafness and near-blind vision is referred to a research nephrologist by his primary care doctor, who is concerned about the microscopic hematuria discovered during a routine physical exam. His father was also deaf but was adopted, so no other family history is available. This nephrologist has easy access to electron microscopy and finds splitting of a thick GBM. What is the likely diagnosis?

    A. Goodpasture syndrome
    B. Alport syndrome
    C. Berger syndrome (IgA nephropathy)
    D. Type IV lupus GN
    E. Type I membranoproliferative GN

CASE 3-8 | Glomerular Filtration Apparatus

HPI: L.M. is a 6-year-old Asian boy with sudden-onset lower extremity edema. Over the past 4 days, the patient's father noticed significant and worsening swelling that began in the patient's feet and seems to be moving up his legs. The father reports his son is urinating infrequently, but there is no gross blood in the urine. The patient recently recovered from an upper respiratory infection 2 weeks ago. The patient lives with his parents and younger sister, attends the local public school, and is in the first grade.

PE: The patient is afebrile and his vital signs are normal. There is no periorbital edema; however, he has pitting edema to his knees.

Labs: Urinalysis and urine cytology reveal significant proteinuria (albumin only), with no red cells or casts. Serum evaluation reveals a serum BUN and creatinine at the upper limits of normal.

THOUGHT QUESTIONS

- Proteinuria represents a failure of the glomerular filtration apparatus. Describe the elements of the glomerular filtration apparatus.
- What is the difference between the nephritic and nephrotic syndromes?
- What are the nephrotic syndromes? Describe the general pathophysiology and the associated microscopic and IF findings.

BASIC SCIENCE REVIEW AND DISCUSSION

Glomerular Filtration Apparatus

The glomerular filtration apparatus (Fig. 3-6) is composed of three layers: the **endothelium** of the glomerular capillary, the **basement membrane,** and the Bowman capsule (BC) **epithelium.** The capillary endothelium is fenestrated with 50- to 100-nm fenestrations, providing a *size* barrier to filtration. The basement membrane is thicker than most, is secreted by the BC epithelium, consists of collagen, glycoproteins, and mucopolysaccharides, and is negatively charged, thus providing a *charge* barrier to filtration. Finally, the BC epithelial cells, "podocytes," have foot processes that embrace the capillary basement membrane (BM). These processes are coated with and bridged by a negatively charged glycocalyx, providing another mechanical and charge barrier to filtration. The end result is that size, electrical charge, and molecular configuration determine the permeability of the filter to macromolecules. Molecules smaller than molecular weight (MW) 65,000 can pass (e.g., free hemoglobin), but molecules larger than MW 68,000 are blocked (e.g., albumin). Negatively charged molecules (e.g., albumin) are blocked by the filter's strong electronegativity. Molecules that are trapped on the epithelial side of the basement membrane are phagocytosed by podocytes, and those trapped on the endothelial side are phagocytosed by mesangial cells.

Nephrotic Syndrome

Nephrotic syndrome is characterized by excretion of protein in the urine greater than 3.5 g/day, which leads to **hypoalbuminemia.** This decrease in oncotic pressure in the vasculature leads to fluid extravasation into the surrounding tissues, leading to **edema.** The drop in oncotic pressure also leads to increased hepatic production of lipids and **hyperlipidemia.** This, in turn, leads to **hyperlipiduria** or **oval fat bodies** (grape-like clusters) in the urine, seen as **maltese crosses** when the urinary sediment is examined under polarized light microscopy (LM). This is in contrast to nephritic syndrome, which is characterized by hematuria, red cell casts in the urinary sediment, azotemia, oliguria, mild to moderate HTN, and only mild edema and proteinuria.

Nephrotic syndrome results from deposition of immune complexes, as a complication of a systemic illness, or idiopathically (i.e., with unknown pathophysiology). The most common nephrotic syndrome in adults is **membranous nephropathy.** It is characterized by BM thickening forming a "**spike and dome**" pattern between subepithelial immune complex deposits. IF reveals granular IgG and C3 lining capillary loops. It is usually secondary to other diseases such as systemic lupus erythematosus or hepatitis B, or drugs such as gold and penicillamine.

The most common nephrotic syndrome in children ages 2 to 6 years is **minimal change disease** (aka lipoid nephrosis). It is characterized by the effacement of foot processes of podocytes. Electron microscopy (EM) is required for definitive diagnosis since there are no unusual findings on LM (thus "*minimal change*"). Edema is the usual presenting symptom. Other symptoms such as renal failure and HTN are less common, particularly in children. As with other nephrotic syndromes, laboratory studies reveal severe proteinuria (in this case, selective for albumin) with rare hematuria, and an elevation of the total cholesterol and triglycerides. Fortunately, more than 90% of children respond dramatically to steroid treatment (e.g., prednisone).

Like minimal change disease, **focal segmental glomerulosclerosis (FSGS)** is characterized by effacement of foot processes on EM but normal findings on LM and no immunoglobulin deposition on IF. In FSGS, there is sclerosis in a proportion of the glomeruli (thus, it is *focal*) and each affected glomeruli is only partly sclerosed (thus, it is *segmental*). FSGS often is associated with HIV infection, heroin abuse, sickle cell disease, and morbid obesity. It is grouped with the nephrotic syndromes because of significant proteinuria, although it does present with microscopic hematuria as well. Treatment is with steroids. Unlike minimal change disease, FSGS has a poor prognosis, with 50% progressing to end-stage renal disease (ESRD) in 5 to 10 years.

Nephrotic Glomerular Diseases Secondary to Systemic Disorders

Amyloidosis is a systemic disease characterized by deposits of one of many types of insoluble fibrous proteins (e.g., monoclonal

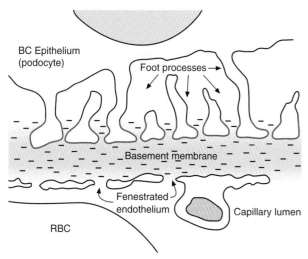

BC Epithelium
(podocyte)

Foot processes →

Basement membrane

Fenestrated
endothelium

Capillary lumen

RBC

• **Figure 3-6.** Glomerular filtration apparatus. *BC*, Bowman capsule; *RBC*, red blood cell

Ig light chains) in multiple organ systems. These deposits stain positive with **Congo red** and show **apple green birefringence** under polarized light, and lead to nephrotic syndrome and ultimately renal failure when they deposit in the glomerulus.

Diabetes is a systemic disease with macrovascular and microvascular impact. The afferent and efferent arterioles lose their ability to regulate GFR as they undergo **hyaline arteriosclerosis.** The basement membrane of the smaller glomerular capillaries becomes thickened as a result of hyperfiltration that occurs in diabetic nephropathy. There is diffuse or nodular (**Kimmelstiel-Wilson nodules**) glomerulosclerosis, which slowly progresses to renal failure.

Systemic lupus erythematosus may present with nephrotic syndrome, nephritic syndrome, or a combination. The World Health Organization (WHO) has developed a classification schema to represent the five patterns seen on biopsy. The important point is that **WHO IV (diffuse proliferative)** has the worst prognosis, and **wire-loop** lesions are seen on IF.

CASE CONCLUSION

Based on the findings of edema and albuminuria in the absence of hematuria or systemic disease, minimal change disease tops the differential diagnosis list for this 6 year old. LM's parents will be reassured by the likelihood that LM will improve quickly with a long-term course of prednisone.

THUMBNAIL: Renal Pathophysiology—Nephrotic Syndromes

Disease	Clinical Presentation and Associated Findings	Pathogenesis	Pathology
Minimal change disease (lipoid nephrosis)	Nephrotic syndrome • **Leading cause in children** • Albumin selectively secreted • Idiopathic; also associated w/allergy, Hodgkin's • Responds well to steroids	Unknown	LM: normal IF: negative/normal EM: **fusion of podocytes;** no deposits
Membranous nephropathy	Nephrotic syndrome • **Leading cause in adults** • Sudden lower extremity edema • Associated w/hepatitis B, malignancy, gold therapy, lupus GN type V	In situ Ag-Ab complex formation	LM: thickened GBM with **"spike and dome"** pattern IF: IgG + C3, granular, along capillary loops EM: **subepithelial** deposits
Focal segmental glomerulosclerosis	Nephrotic syndrome +/− hematuria • Associated w/heroin, HIV, obesity, sickle cell disease • 50% to ESRD	Unknown	LM: focal segmental sclerosis IF: IgM + C3 in sclerotic parts EM: fusion of podocytes
Diabetic nephropathy	Nephrotic syndrome • Associated w/retinopathy, type IV RTA • 10-20 years after onset of diabetes	Unknown	LM: nodular (**Kimmelstiel-Wilson nodules**) or diffuse sclerosis; hyaline arteriosclerosis of afferent and efferent arterioles IF: No Ig EM: No deposits
Amyloidosis	Nephrotic syndrome • >60 y.o. • Associated w/multiple myeloma, etc.	Deposition of light chains	LM: **Congo red** staining mesangial deposits; **apple green birefringence** w/polarized light

THUMBNAIL: Renal Pathophysiology—Diseases with Nephritic and Nephrotic Elements

Disease	Clinical Presentation and Associated Findings	Pathogenesis	Pathology
Lupus GN	• Five WHO patterns, each with proliferation in different parts of the glomerulus and with different degrees of nephrotic and nephritic syndromes • **ANA and anti-dsDNA** associated	Trapped Ag-Ab complexes	LM: crescents; **"wire loop" appearance in type IV** IF: IgG, IgM + C3, granular EM: subepithelial, subendothelial, mesangial deposits (anywhere)
Membranoproliferative GN	Type I: Nephrotic • Recent upper respiratory infection • < 30 y.o		IF: IgG, IgM + C3/C1/C4 granular EM: splitting of GBM; **"train track"** appearance
	Type II: hematuria, CRF		LM: mesangial proliferation IF: C3 only EM: dense subendothelial deposits

C3, complement; y.o., years old; RTA, renal tubular acidosis; ANA, antinuclear antibody; dsDNA, double-stranded DNA; CRF, chronic renal failure

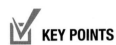 **KEY POINTS**

■ **Nephrotic syndrome** is characterized by proteinuria, hypoalbuminemia, edema, hyperlipidemia, and lipiduria

■ **Nephritic syndrome** is characterized by hematuria, red cell casts, azotemia, oliguria, and HTN

QUESTIONS

1. A 45-year-old male, homeless HIV+ IV drug user comes to the ED for gross hematuria and peripheral edema. A urinalysis with cytology reveals significant proteinuria and oval fat bodies, but few red cells and no casts. Serum analysis reveals hypoalbuminemia. ED doctors diagnose a nephrotic syndrome. This patient has a disease that requires electron microscopy for definitive diagnosis. Which one of the following is his likely diagnosis?

A. Membranous glomerulonephritis
B. FSGS
C. Lupus glomerulonephritis
D. Diabetic nephropathy
E. Minimal change disease

2. A 52-year-old woman is being treated by her primary care doctor for a chronic illness. At this year's annual checkup, her BUN and creatinine are significantly elevated and she has 3+ proteinuria on urine dipstick. A renal biopsy reveals + Congo red staining and apple green birefringence under polarized light. Which chronic disease does this patient have?

A. Lesch-Nyhan syndrome (a syndrome of hyperuricemia)
B. Diabetes mellitus, type 2
C. Diabetes insipidus
D. Systemic lupus erythematosus
E. Amyloidosis

CASE 3-9 | Acute Renal Failure

HPI: MM is a 77-year-old Latina sent to the ED after being seen at her local clinic for a regular follow-up appointment. On routine laboratory tests, her BUN and creatinine were significantly increased above her baseline creatinine of 1.1 and her physician was concerned. She is remarkably healthy for her age. Osteoarthritis and hypertension are her only medical problems. Her medications include metoprolol, benazepril, furosemide, and occasional ibuprofen for arthritis pain. Upon further questioning, she reveals that she has been more active lately. She joined a quilting group and has begun gardening again. Her arthritis has been "acting up," and she has been taking significantly more ibuprofen, up to 2400 mg per day.

PE: Her physical exam is significant for moderate pitting bilateral ankle edema.

Labs: Electrolytes: Na$^+$ 142; K$^+$ 4.1; Cl$^-$ 101; Bicarb 16; BUN 60; Cr 3.2. Urine dipstick shows negative leukocyte esterase, negative nitrates, a slightly elevated specific gravity, and no protein, ketones, or glucose. Urine microscopy is pending.

THOUGHT QUESTIONS

- Define acute renal failure (ARF).
- What are the three broad categories of ARF?
- How does a urinalysis help distinguish between causes of ARF?

BASIC SCIENCE REVIEW AND DISCUSSION

ARF is a syndrome characterized by a **decline in glomerular filtration rate (GFR)** over hours to days (as measured clinically by an increasing creatinine), azotemia, and disturbances in fluid and electrolyte balance. **Azotemia** is an excess of BUN or other nitrogenous compounds in the blood. ARF is initially characterized by nonspecific symptoms like malaise but becomes more seriously symptomatic when BUN exceeds 100 mg/dL. Signs and symptoms include **oliguria,** cardiovascular complications (pericardial effusions, arrhythmias), neurologic abnormalities (asterixis, confusion, seizures), GI complications (nausea, vomiting, abdominal pain), electrolyte abnormalities (including an anion gap metabolic acidosis), or bleeding secondary to uremic platelet dysfunction. Fortunately, most ARF is reversible. Although ARF often presents with similar symptoms, it is distinguished from chronic renal failure in which the decline in GFR occurs over months to years.

Broadly speaking, ARF can result from problems arising in the kidney itself (*renal* causes ~50%), from inadequate blood flow to the kidney (*prerenal* causes ~45%), or from obstruction downstream from the kidney (*postrenal* causes ~5%).

Prerenal Failure

In prerenal failure, the kidneys themselves function more or less normally and the problem lies in the inability of the circulatory system to deliver the proper perfusion to the kidney to produce a normal GFR. This occurs with **hypovolemic** states (hemorrhage, dehydration), impairment of renal **autoregulation** (as seen with cyclooxygenase inhibitors, like NSAIDs and aspirin, or ACE inhibitors), or **low effective plasma flow** states. Low effective plasma flow states include low cardiac output states (arrhythmias, valvular disease, CHF), systemic vasodilation (sepsis, antihypertensives), or congestion (cirrhosis with ascites → hepatorenal syndrome). Once the underlying deficit is corrected, the kidneys usually recover rapidly.

Intrinsic Renal Failure

In intrinsic renal failure, the renal parenchyma is itself malfunctioning. The malfunction may be glomerular, vascular, tubular, or interstitial. *Glomerular* causes include glomerular diseases and the thrombotic microangiopathies such as hemolytic-uremic syndrome (HUS), thrombotic thrombocytopenic purpura (TTP), and disseminated intravascular coagulation (DIC). *Macrovascular* causes include narrowing of the renal arteries and arterioles by atherosclerosis, vasculitis, scleroderma, or malignant hypertension.

Acute *interstitial* nephritis (AIN) and acute *tubular* necrosis (ATN) comprise 90% of intrinsic renal ARF. The pathophysiology of AIN is acute hypersensitivity (allergic), infection, or infiltration. **Allergic AIN** is most commonly a reaction to drugs, especially antibiotics or NSAIDs, with onset approximately 2 weeks after exposure. ARF occurs in about 50% of those with AIN and may be accompanied by fever, eosinophilia, rash, and urinary abnormalities such as hematuria and **eosinophils** in the urine. **ATN** may be ischemic or nephrotoxic. **Ischemic ATN** occurs when prerenal conditions of poor perfusion persist so long that renal tubule cells begin dying. **Nephrotoxic ATN** occurs when exogenous (drugs, radiocontrast) or endogenous (myoglobin, hemoglobin) toxins damage the renal tubules. In either case, the necrotic tubular cells slough off, forming **muddy brown casts** in the urine.

In an oliguric patient (<500 cc/24 hours), measuring urine electrolytes can help distinguish between prerenal and intrinsic renal failure. In prerenal failure, the urine sodium concentration should be tiny (<10 mg/dL), as the kidneys avidly retain sodium and water. The fractional excretion of sodium (**FE$_{Na+}$**) compares the clearance of sodium with that of creatinine. An FE$_{Na+}$ less than 1% suggests prerenal failure, while an FE$_{Na+}$ 1% or greater suggests intrinsic renal failure, as the kidneys have lost their ability to reabsorb sodium.

$$FE_{Na+} \ [\%] = \frac{U_{Na+}/P_{Na+} \times 100}{U_{Cr}/P_{Cr}}$$

In addition, BUN is reabsorbed by normally functioning tubules far in excess of creatinine, which is not reabsorbed. Therefore, a BUN:Cr ratio greater than 20:1 indicates properly functioning tubules and prerenal failure.

Postrenal Failure

Severe urinary tract obstruction is the hallmark of postrenal failure. In men, the most common cause of postrenal failure is prostate enlargement from benign prostatic hyperplasia or prostate cancer.

Other causes include obstruction by bladder or cervical cancer, kidney stones (lodged in the urinary tract such that flow from both kidneys is obstructed), phimosis (nonretractable foreskin), and a neurogenic bladder.

CASE CONCLUSION

MM's urinalysis and electrolytes shows hyaline casts, an FE_{Na+} less than 1%, and a U_{Na+} of 6 mg/dL, which suggest prerenal failure. MM was dehydrated (secondary to furosemide and decreased intake of fluids with increased activity), and her ACEI inhibitor and NSAID compromised her kidney's ability to autoregulate to conserve GFR.

ACEI inhibitors decrease the production of angiotensin II (AII), a potent constrictor of the efferent arteriole. AII also induces the synthesis of local prostaglandins (PGs), powerful dilators of the afferent arteriole. Both constricting the efferent arteriole and dilating the afferent arteriole are mechanisms for preserving renal blood flow in times of hypovolemia. NSAIDs and aspirin inhibit cyclooxygenase, the enzyme that helps convert arachidonic acid into PGs. With neither AII nor PGs, the glomerulus has lost both sources of protection from hypoperfusion. Consequently, GFR drops and BUN and creatinine climb as the kidney can no longer clear substances from the blood. If this situation persists, the renal parenchyma itself becomes ischemic and dies (i.e., ATN). The other category to consider is allergic AIN, also associated with NSAID use, suggested by eosinophils in the urine or a convincing clinical presentation with fever and rash, less likely in this case.

Treatment for this patient involves discontinuing nephrotoxic drugs, appropriate volume regulation (diuretics, water restriction, IV fluids, as needed), and monitoring and correcting electrolyte abnormalities, including by emergent dialysis if needed.

THUMBNAIL: Renal Pathophysiology—Causes of Acute Renal Failure

Prerenal	Intrinsic Renal	Postrenal
Hypovolemia	ATN	Obstruction
• Hemorrhage	• Ischemic (end point	• Bilateral ureteric
• Dehydration	of prerenal ARF)	• Prostatic hyperplasia
• Burns	• Nephrotoxic	• Urethral stricture
• GI losses	• Exogenous (radiocontrast,	• Stones
• "Third space" sequestration	chemotherapy)	• Phimosis
(pancreatitis, burns, hypoalbuminemia)	• Endogenous (rhabdomyolysis,	Neurogenic bladder
Low effective renal plasma flow	hemolysis)	
• Low cardiac output states	Interstitial nephritis	
• Increased systemic vasodilation	• Allergic (drugs: especially	
(sepsis, antihypertensives)	antibiotics, NSAIDs)	
• Cirrhosis with ascites	• Infection (pyelonephritis)	
Impaired renal autoregulation	• Infiltration (sarcoidosis,	
• Cyclooxygenase inhibitors (NSAIDs, aspirin)	leukemia, lymphoma)	
• ACE inhibitors	Diseases of the glomeruli	
• Renal vasoconstriction	• Glomerulonephritis	
(epinephrine, norepinephrine)	• Nephritic	
Renovascular obstruction	• Nephrotic	
Renal artery stenosis	• Thrombotic microangiopathy	
	• HUS	
	• TTP	
	• DIC	
	Macrovascular diseases	
	• Artery (atherosclerosis, vasculitis,	
	malignant HTN, scleroderma)	
	• Vein (thrombosis, compression)	
	Acute renal transplant rejection	
FE_{Na+} <1%	FE_{Na+} >1%	
U_{Na+} <10 mg/dL	U_{Na+} >20 mg/dL	
Plasma BUN:Cr >20	Plasma BUN:Cr < 10–15	

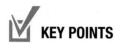

KEY POINTS

- ARF may be divided into prerenal, intrinsic renal, and postrenal causes
- The urinalysis and urine electrolytes provide clues to diagnosis:
  - **Leukocyte esterase:** released by granulocytes; evidence of pyuria
  - **Nitrites:** nitrates are converted to nitrites by gram-negative rods; indicates bacteriuria
  - **Ketones:** indicate metabolic acidosis (diabetic ketoacidosis, starvation)
  - **Lipid:**   Oval fat bodies   Nephrotic syndrome

                   Maltese crosses (polarized light)
  - **Casts:**   Red cell casts   GN

                   White cell casts   Interstitial nephritis

                   Muddy brown casts   ATN
  - **Cells:**   Red cells   GN, tumors, trauma, urinary tract infection

                   Dysmorphic red cells (acanthocytes)   GN

                   White cells   Cystitis (lower urinary tract infection)

QUESTIONS

1. A 62-year-old woman is admitted to the hospital for ARF and a 24-hour urine collection is obtained. Urine volume is 600 cc/day. U_{Na+} is 5 mg/dL, U_{Cr} is 25 mg/dL, P_{Na+} is 140 mg/dL, and P_{Cr} is 3.5 mg/dL. What is the FE_{Na+}?

   A. <1%, suggesting prerenal failure
   B. >2%, suggesting intrinsic renal failure
   C. 1.5%, of limited use in this nonoliguric patient
   D. <1%, of limited use in this nonoliguric patient
   E. 1.2%, making diagnosis difficult but prerenal unlikely

2. A 75-year-old man is referred to the ED after being seen in the clinic with an elevated BUN and creatinine on routine exam.

The patient is not ill-appearing and has stable vital signs. A pelvic ultrasound from several years ago shows two normal-appearing kidneys. What is the most likely cause of renal failure in this patient?

   A. Kidney stone lodged in the right ureter → postrenal failure
   B. Diabetes mellitus → renal insufficiency
   C. Benign prostatic hypertrophy → postrenal failure
   D. Sepsis → prerenal failure
   E. Goodpasture syndrome → intrinsic renal failure

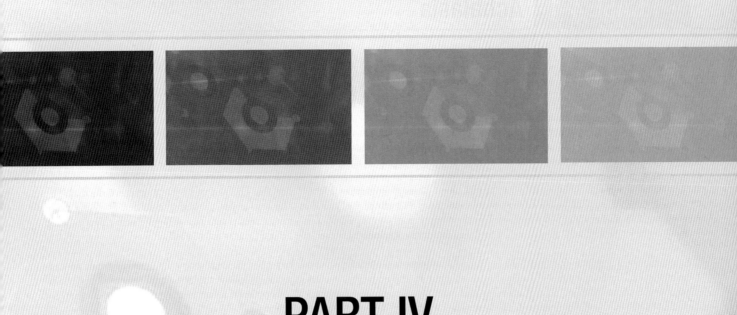

PART IV

Gastrointestinal

HPI: JS a 45-year-old man who complains about his inability to eat. He reports that over the past 12 months he has had difficulty swallowing. JS has lost approximately 40 pounds over the past 8 months. He reports that it "feels like food is getting stuck in my throat." During the first few months of this problem, JS was able to drink increasing amounts of liquids to "push it (the food bolus) through" into his stomach. He was able to eat soups to get nutritious benefit but now he is unable to swallow soup. Over the past few weeks JS has noted that when he leans forward he regurgitates small bits of partially digested and foul-smelling food. Coworkers have always joked about his "bad breath" (halitosis). JS denies any pain associated with swallowing (eating or drinking); he does not vomit. He notes no blood in his regurgitated foods. JS's past medical history is notable for scleroderma, pneumonia treated with antibiotics, and hypertension treated with atenolol.

PE: JS is 5'8" tall and weighs 189 pounds. His blood pressure measures 138/90 mm Hg. The rest of his vital signs are normal. The physical exam is notable for JS's skin—there is sclerosis and atrophy of the skin over his fingers, arms and shoulder. The lung exam reveals crackles bilaterally at both bases. His abdominal exam is normal; his extremity exam is significant for the skin changes listed above; otherwise, there is no cyanosis, clubbing, or edema. Peripheral pulses are intact; fingers move easily.

Labs: Albumin 2.0 (3.5–5.5 g/dL). To work up his symptoms further, you order an upper GI endoscopy. The study reveals no cancerous lesions, large amount of food in dilated esophagus, and no peristalsis. The specialists follow this abnormal result with manometry, which shows increased basal pressure and inability of the lower esophageal sphincter to relax. Finally, JS undergoes a barium swallow (BS) with telling results: dilated esophagus with "bird's beak" and distal stenosis.

THOUGHT QUESTIONS

- What is the *most likely* diagnosis for this patient?
- What is the relevant anatomy and microanatomy?
- How does normal swallowing proceed; what are the functions of the lower esophageal sphincter?
- What are the proposed etiologic agents and how is JS's past medical history linked to his new complaint?
- Which other diseases may present with the complaint of dysphagia? Is all painless dysphagia achalasia?

BASIC SCIENCE REVIEW AND DISCUSSION

The most likely diagnosis for JS is **achalasia.** The combination of progressive painless dysphagia associated with a history of scleroderma and abnormal lab data and imaging studies ensures the diagnosis. The muscular tube of the esophagus is bordered by two rings of muscle: the **upper esophageal sphincter (UES)** and **lower esophageal sphincter (LES).** These act as opening and closing doors that allow food to travel through while protecting the lining of the esophagus. The UES and LES work in conjunction with the peristaltic smooth muscle of the body of the esophagus. If these are synchronous, food reaches the stomach; if not, major problems result.

Anatomy of the Esophagus

The physiology of swallowing is complicated and framed by examining the form and function of the esophagus. Like other components of the GI tract, the esophageal wall is composed of the mucosa, submucosa, muscularis propria, and adventitia. The **mucosa** (or inner lining of the esophagus) is composed of stratified squamous epithelial cells. Beneath it lies the **lamina propria** (mostly connective tissue) and **muscularis mucosa** (thin layer of longitudinal muscle). The next layer is the **submucosa,** which consists of a layer of blood vessels, inflammatory cells, lymphoid follicles, and nerve fibers, including the **Meissner plexus.** Following the submucosa is the **muscularis propria,** which includes the inner circular layer and outer longitudinal layer of smooth muscle. The **myenteric (Auerbach) plexus**—believed to be dysfunctional in achalasia—is located in this layer. Of note, the upper third, or approximately 6 to 8 cm, of the esophagus includes a layer of striated muscle.

Physiology of Swallowing

The bolus of food or drink in the oropharynx sets off a chain reaction beginning with relaxation of the UES followed by waves of coordinated peristalsis that propels the bolus to the lower esophagus; with its relaxation, the bolus enters the stomach. Extrinsic and intrinsic innervation, smooth muscle properties (response to distension), and humoral properties are all involved in the coordination of this event. The LES must open at the correct moment to allow the bolus of food to enter the stomach and close to prevent reflux of the acidic gastric contents that are under positive pressure relative to the esophagus.

Pathophysiology of Achalasia

Because the LES does not relax in achalasia, JS suffers from dysphagia. Many patients find that drinking large quantities of liquids immediately after consuming food can overcome the abnormalities of achalasia. Abnormalities verified by manometry include the lack of peristalsis, incomplete relaxation of the LES with swallowing, and increased resting tone of the LES. Some hormones and other chemical agents (gastrin, acetylcholine, histamine, prostaglandin $F_{2\alpha}$) can increase the resting tone of the LES, leading to progressive dilation. The wall of the esophagus may thicken secondary to hypertrophy of the muscularis or later become thinner after marked dilatation and stretching of the fibers. The ganglia of the myenteric plexus are absent in the body of the esophagus; in the LES these may be absent or present and dysfunctional. The pathophysiology of these abnormalities is poorly understood; however, it appears that the ganglion cells that normally secrete vasointestinal peptide are destroyed or are absent from the myenteric plexus. One theory purports that a virus infects the dorsal vagus motor nucleus; another theory links LES dysfunction to increased sensitivity to gastrin. Less commonly, achalasia can result from an identifiable cause such as advanced scleroderma.

Secondary achalasia can arise from infection with *Trypanosoma cruzi*, resulting in Chagas disease. Chagas disease causes widespread destruction of myenteric plexus in many portions of the GI tract, resulting in progressive dilation. Other causes of secondary achalasia may result from sarcoidosis, amyloidosis, and paraneoplastic syndromes or even diabetic autonomic neuropathy.

Achalasia Patients with this rare (1:100,000) disorder may suffer from a collagen vascular disease such as **scleroderma or calcinosis, Raynaud phenomenon, esophageal disease, sclerodactyly, telangiectasia (CREST) syndrome.** Achalasia can lead to malnutrition, aspiration secondary to nearby gastric contents, or subsequent aspiration pneumonia. These patients also experience an increased incidence of abscess, bronchiectasis, pulmonary fibrosis, candidal esophagitis, lower esophageal diverticula, and esophageal ulceration. The most worrisome are those patients who develop esophageal squamous cell carcinoma (5%).

CASE CONCLUSION

JS questions the association between the scleroderma and achalasia. He wants to know more about the disease, as well as treatment options. You explain that in patients with scleroderma, the muscularis layer progressively atrophies and is slowly replaced by collagen. As the disease progresses, the fibrosed esophageal wall leads to atony and dilatation, associated with the "bird's beak" finding on imaging. Late scleroderma achalasia may be complicated by gastroesophageal reflux disease (GERD) as the LES becomes atrophic.

Treatment options for primary achalasia are both medical and surgical. Medical options are CCBs, nitrates, or botulinum toxin injection via endoscopy to relax the LES. The surgical options include balloon dilation, fundoplication, or cardiomyotomy, which is an incision in the LES muscle. JS chose conservative medical management.

THUMBNAIL: Achalasia

Epidemiology: Men > women, middle-aged, incidence 1:100,000

Pathogenesis: Decreased numbers of ganglion cells in the body of the esophagus with decreased/normal nonfunctioning ganglion in the LES

Impaired inhibitory innervations of the myenteric (Auerbach) plexus

No peristalsis, poor relaxation of the LES, increased resting tone of the LES; progressive dilatation of esophagus "bird's beak" sign on BS, malnutrition

Uncertain etiology

Secondary causes: Chagas disease, collagen vascular disease (especially scleroderma and CREST syndrome), diabetes with autonomic neuropathy, paraneoplastic syndrome, sarcoidosis, amyloidosis, invasion of nerve ganglion by a virus (polio)

Imaging: Upper GI/BS—"bird's beak" (stenosis) with dilatation

Sequelae: Aspiration pneumonia, esophageal diverticula, esophageal ulceration, candidal esophagitis, pulmonary fibrosis, bronchiectasis, abscess, 5% risk of squamous cell carcinoma

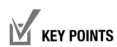

KEY POINTS

- Presents with progressive, painless dysphagia, regurgitation of foods, halitosis
- Often diagnosed in middle-aged males
- Differential diagnosis: primary achalasia with no other comorbidity, cancer etiology often unknown
- Secondary achalasia is often associated with scleroderma and CREST syndrome dermatomyositis, Chagas disease, diabetes mellitus, paraneoplastic syndromes, amyloidosis, and sarcoidosis

QUESTIONS

1. Which of the following is *less likely* to occur with achalasia based on the abnormality of the LES?

   A. Scleroderma
   B. GERD
   C. *Helicobacter pylori* dyspepsia
   D. Hiatal hernia
   E. Mallory-Weiss tears

2. Hirschsprung disease and achalasia both have which of the following in common?

   A. Increased risk of GI cancers (e.g., squamous cell cancer of the esophagus)
   B. Congenital loss of bowel function
   C. Absence of ganglion cells
   D. Increased incidence of collagen vascular disease
   E. Inability to pass stool normally

3. Which of the following is *not* a sequela of achalasia?

   A. Collagen vascular disease
   B. Pulmonary fibrosis
   C. Esophageal diverticula
   D. Aspiration pneumonia
   E. Squamous cell esophageal cancer

4. Which of the following is *not* a component of CREST syndrome?

   A. Esophageal dysmotility
   B. Raynaud disease
   C. Congenital megacolon
   D. Calcinosis
   E. Telangiectasia

CASE 4-2 Peptic Ulcer Disease

HPI: GS, a 40-year-old male, complains of an intermittent gnawing, aching, and burning pain in his abdomen. He characterizes his pain eloquently while pointing to his epigastrium. Although GS is uncertain, he reports that the pain worsens at night and occasionally after meals—usually 2 or 3 hours afterward. His wife takes Tums (calcium carbonate) on a regular basis (to prevent osteoporosis). GS has symptomatic relief using two to three of these tablets. He denies deep or "penetrating" pain to his back or left side and does not report weight loss, nausea, or vomiting. GS also denies hematemesis or melena. His past medical history is significant for chronic headaches, stress type for which he takes ibuprofen, approximately 3 to 4 days a week.

PE: GS is 5'6" tall, his blood pressure measures 112/59, and his pulse is 76. In general, he is in no acute distress; his cardiovascular and pulmonary exams are unremarkable. Abdominally, GS has normal bowel sounds, mild epigastric pain, no guarding or rebound; his rectal exam is significant for normal tone but positive for microscopic blood (heme +).

Labs: WBC 8.5 ($4.5-11 \times 10^3$ per µL); hemoglobin (Hgb) 12 (12−16 g/dL); Hct 35 (35−45%); platelets (Plt) 215 ($159-450 \times 10^3$ per µL); mean corpuscular volume (MCV) 77 (80−100).

To complete his workup, GS undergoes an upper GI series that reveals a gastric ulcer with gastric folds radiating to the base of the ulcer as well as a thick radiolucent edematous collar around a smooth-appearing crater. Following the upper GI series, an endoscopy is ordered, which also shows abnormalities. On gross inspection, the endoscopic exam reveals an oval, sharply punched-out defect in the antrum near the lesser curvature, with no active bleeding or clotted blood. The pathology report describes penetration into the mucosa and muscularis mucosa and partially into the muscularis propria. Additionally, there are no features of malignancy. Biopsy of characteristic areas are stained with silver and reveal many gram-negative S-shaped rods along the gastric epithelial cells. A urease breath test is positive.

THOUGHT QUESTIONS

- What is the *most likely* diagnosis for this patient?
- What are the risk factors for GS's illness?
- Which bacterial agent is commonly associated with this illness?
- How can this agent be identified and eradicated?
- How would you describe the pathogenesis of this illness?
- What are the major sequelae of this illness?
- What is *acute gastric ulceration*?

BASIC SCIENCE REVIEW AND DISCUSSION

GS has **peptic ulcer disease (PUD)**—a disruption in the mucosa of the stomach or duodenum that extends through the muscularis at varying depths. PUD is a chronic disease, characterized by periods of relapse and appears to occur in the presence of increased acid and **pepsin.** Almost exclusively, ulcers are solitary and present in the duodenum or the stomach and are exceedingly rare in other parts of the GI tract. Patients who suffer from PUD have characteristic symptoms: The ulcer pain is often characterized as gnawing, burning, or aching with worsening symptoms at night and vary in relation to meals dependent on the location of the ulcer (duodenum vs. gastric). If a patient describes a penetrating pain or referral to the back, chest, or right upper quadrant, as well as nausea and vomiting, this suggests a perforation of the stomach or duodenal wall. Weight loss—always a red flag for its

association with cancer—should alert the clinician to a possible malignancy.

Epidemiology and Risk Factors

PUD is a common illness seen more often in men than in women (duodenal 3:1 and gastric 3:2 in favor of men) and often diagnosed in middle age. PUD is not associated with genetics or race and can be frustrating to a patient because it often has no obvious precipitating factor, heals spontaneously, and later recurs. However, PUD is associated with *Helicobacter pylori*, alcoholic cirrhosis, chronic obstructive pulmonary disease (COPD), chronic renal failure (CRF), and hyperparathyroidism. Additional risk factors include cigarette smoking, chronic nonsteroidal anti-inflammatory drug (NSAID) use, chronic corticosteroid use, and psychological stress.

Duodenal and gastric ulcerations often can be differentiated based on the history of the illness. More common in incidence, duodenal ulcers often have decreased pain coincident with a meal; the pain recurs 1 to 3 hours following the meal. The theory is that the increased pH of the food bolus soothes the ulcer as it exits the stomach at the pylorus. These patients often complain that they are awakened at night from the gnawing pain. Duodenal ulcers are frequently associated with increased acid, increased parietal cell mass, and impaired mucosal barrier. Gastric ulcers, on the other hand, are less common and are associated with burning upon eating and relieved with antacids. These are more common in the setting of a defective mucosal barrier secondary to *H. pylori* infection, bile reflux, alcoholic cirrhosis, and COPD. Gastric ulceration is associated with an increased risk of gastric cancer; duodenal ulcer is not.

Anatomy and Histology

Most patients with PUD have a single ulcer, but up to 20% have two or more ulcers; most ulcers are in the first part and anterior location of the duodenum. Stomach ulcers are often in the antrum region along the lesser curvature but can occur anywhere in the stomach. Other less-common locations include within Barrett mucosa, at the margin of a gastroenterostomy site, near a Meckel diverticulum with ectopic gastric mucosa, or in patients who suffer from Zollinger-Ellison syndrome. On visual inspection—often during endoscopic exam—the ulcers are small (6 mm in diameter) but can be up to 4 to 6 cm in diameter and appear to be "punched out" of the epithelial lining. The depth of the ulcer varies from shallow (through only the mucosa) to penetration (through the gastric or duodenal wall).

On microscopic exam, the margins are often level with the mucosa or slightly elevated, but a clear drop off from the nearby epithelial lining is apparent. The nearby gastric mucosa is almost always hyperemic, likely secondary to concurrent gastritis. Histologically, there are three common considerations: active necrosis, inflammation, and healing. The active ulcer has several characteristics that are seen on biopsy specimens: fibrinoid debris at the margins and base of the ulcer, neutrophilic infiltration, granulation tissue with a proliferation of monocytes, and a fibrinous or collagenous layer resting on scar. In addition to the characteristics of the ulcer itself, there are typically signs of chronic gastritis, as well as *Helicobacter pylori* infection. One may wonder how to distinguish between gastritis and peptic ulcer disease. It should be noted that chronic gastritis is usually absent in cases of **acute erosive gastritis** or in acute ulceration secondary to stress but is consistently present in patients with PUD.

Pathophysiology of PUD

Despite much interest in PUD, little is known about the pathogenesis; in simple terms, the mucosal defense is outmatched by the damaging forces. However, the presence of gastric acid and pepsin are necessary for ulcer formation. The specifics are not entirely clear but the association with acid is obvious by examining the situation in patients suffering from **Zollinger-Ellison syndrome.** This disease is most commonly caused by a pancreatic tumor that secretes **gastrin,** leading to markedly increased acid levels and peptic ulcerations. Several broader theories exist regarding the specific cause of ulcers: increased basal acid secretion or increased parietal cell mass. Other theories point to increased sensitivity or limited inhibition of regulatory mechanisms controlling acid secretion or rapid stomach emptying leading to increased exposure to acid.

In addition, the bacterium *H. pylori* is known to produce urease that produces ammonia as well as a protease that breaks down proteins important to the function of the mucus barrier. *H. pylori* and its association with PUD is well described, accompanying nearly 100% of duodenal and many gastric ulcers. Another theory purports an impaired mucosal defense (i.e., those patients with normal acid and pepsin and void of *H. pylori*). Unfortunately, no clear defects in the mucosal barrier, bicarbonate, or blood flow can be elucidated clearly.

Some of the risk factors associated with PUD have clearer links to a weakened mucosal defense or possibly a stronger offense. NSAID use inhibits prostaglandin synthesis—an important factor of the mucus barrier. Smoking slows healing of existing ulcers, is thought to suppress prostaglandin synthesis, and favors more frequent recurrence. In GS, elimination of the smoking could have a beneficial effect on his illness. Corticosteroids and increased psychological stress have been clearly shown to increase ulcer formation.

Acute Gastric Ulceration

Acute gastric ulceration occurs following severe stress and often encompasses multiple ulcers in all portions of the stomach. Typically, this is thought of as an extension of severe acute gastritis. Acute gastric ulceration is common in the ICU and often occurs in patients with the following risk factors: shock, sepsis, burns (result in Curling ulcers), trauma, and conditions with increased intracranial pressure (Cushing ulcers). Several common processes can occur in one or several of these conditions: impaired oxygenation of the tissue, vagal stimulation resulting in increased acid productions, or systemic acidosis. Commonly, patients who are acutely ill requiring intensive care are prescribed a proton pump inhibitor or H_2 blocker as prophylaxis. However, the only treatment is to correct the underlying condition.

CASE CONCLUSION

GS is diagnosed with PUD and begins treatment with bismuth, tetracycline, metronidazole, and a proton pump inhibitor for varying times. The treatment is effective and GS asks about the potential sequelae of PUD with a gastric ulcer. Complications can be serious but, fortunately, are uncommon. The most common complication is bleeding, which can occur in up to one third of all patients with PUD. With this patient, it is likely the source of his microcytic anemia. Another serious complication is perforation, which can occur in approximately 5% of patients with PUD; this complication is the cause of death in two thirds of patients with PUD. Additionally, obstruction from scarring can occur, typically in duodenal ulcers with vomiting and crampy abdominal pain.

THUMBNAIL: Gastrointestinal Pathophysiology—Duodenal versus Gastric Ulcer

	Duodenal	Gastric
Location	Duodenum, first portion Often the anterior wall	Between the body and antrum, along the lesser curvature
Association with *H. pylori*	Yes, 90–100% of cases	Yes, 70%
Associations	COPD, alcoholic cirrhosis, CRF, hyperparathyroidism	Bile reflux, smoking, COPD, alcoholic cirrhosis
Frequency	Up to 80% of PUD	Up to 20% of PUD
Pathogenesis	Excess acid production, increased parietal cell mass, decreased bicarbonate in the mucus barrier (*H. pylori*)	Defective mucosal barrier secondary to *H. pylori*, reduced prostaglandin secondary to ischemia
Male:female ratio	3:1	1.5–2:1
Complications	Recurrence, hematemesis, melena, perforation into pancreas	Recurrence, hematemesis, melena, perforation (air under diaphragm)
Associated with cancer	No	Yes, −1 to 4%
Symptoms that may differentiate	Pain 1 to 3 hours after eating Pain relieved by food, antacids	Pain aggravated with meals Pain relieved by antacids

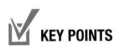

KEY POINTS

- Presents with chronic, intermittent epigastric pain
- Often diagnosed in young adults or middle-aged men with alcoholic cirrhosis, COPD, CRF, hyperparathyroidism, NSAID use, in smokers, in those infected with *H. pylori*, with corticosteroid use, under psychological stress
- Etiology determined by history and physical exam, endoscopy, biopsy results, urease breath test

- Differentiate from acute gastric ulceration by nearby gastric tissue (unremarkable margins); comorbid conditions such as shock, sepsis, burns, trauma; increased intracranial pressure, location (throughout the stomach), and number (often >2)

QUESTIONS

1. A common treatment for PUD is the H_2 blocker cimetidine, which has several side effects including tremor, confusion, inhibition of the cytochrome P_{450} system, and which of the following?

    A. Stevens-Johnson syndrome
    B. Agranulocytosis
    C. Gynecomastia
    D. Microcytic anemia
    E. Depression

2. Aspirin and other NSAIDs *most likely* promote ulcer formation by which of the following pathogenic mechanisms?

    A. Ischemia
    B. Suppression of mucosal prostaglandin
    C. Increased acid production via stimulation of parietal cell mass
    D. Increasing parietal cell mass
    E. Increasing gastric emptying

3. Gastric ulcers *increase the risk* of which of the following cancers?

    A. Liver
    B. Pancreatic
    C. Duodenal
    D. Esophageal
    E. Gastric

4. A patient with a known history of PUD presents with acute abdominal pain. The kidney, ureter and bladder x-ray reveals free air under the diaphragm. What is the next best step in management?

    A. Barium swallow
    B. Outpatient management with proton pump inhibitor
    C. Outpatient management with H_2 blockade
    D. Emergency surgery
    E. Admission with serial abdominal exams

CASE 4-3 Malabsorption Syndromes

HPI: TV, a 43-year-old female, complains of years of diarrhea and belly pain. She has had diarrhea with abdominal pain and bloating for as long as she can remember. TV says that her stomach always sticks out, she has flatus and bulky greasy stools, which, upon query, are described as always floating in the toilet. TV also reports decreased appetite secondary to the abdominal pain and notes chronic fatigue and itchy red skin.

PE: HEIGHT- 5'4"; WEIGHT- 95 pounds; normal VITAL SIGNS (VS); GENERAL- (Gen) thin; HEENT- head, eyes, ears, nose, throat, temporal wasting; SKIN- erythema, excoriation of abdomen and legs; ABDOMEN- positive bowel sounds, soft, nontender, distended, no rebound, no guarding; EXTREMITIES- 2+ pitting edema to the knees.

Labs: WBC 6.5 $(4.5-11 \times 10^3$ per µL); Hgb 9 $(12-16$ g/dL); Hct 26 $(35-45\%)$; Plt 243 $(159-450 \times 10^3$ per µL); bilirubin (tot) 0.2 $(0.2-1.0$ mg/dL); bilirubin (dir) 0.1 $(0-0.2$ mg/dL); aspartate aminotransferase (AST)/SGOT 12 $(7-40$ U/L); alanine aminotransferase/serum glutamic pyruvic transaminase (ALT/SGPT) 23 $(7-40$ U/L); alkaline phosphatase (alk phos) 100 $(70-230$ U/L); amylase 34 $(25-125$ U/L); lipase 65 $(10-140$ U/L); albumin 2.0 $(3.5-5.5$ g/dL).

TV undergoes several diagnostic exams to better elucidate the source of her symptoms. A 72-hour stool sample analysis is performed that reveals elevated fecal fat content without other abnormalities. A D-xylose test reveals decreased uptake of sugar. A tissue sample of the small intestine is obtained that shows marked atrophy and blunting of villi, increased numbers of intraepithelial lymphocytes and other immune cells (plasma cells, macrophages), but normal mucosal thickness.

THOUGHT QUESTIONS

- What is the *most likely* diagnosis for this patient?
- What are the necessary physiologic steps to digestion of nutrients?
- What key components of the history and lab results lead to this diagnosis?
- What are the common and rare sequelae of this disorder?
- What is the etiology?

BASIC SCIENCE REVIEW AND DISCUSSION

TV has **malabsorption** (decreased absorption of nutrients) secondary to **celiac sprue.** Malabsorption is a general term that refers to the decreased absorption of proteins, carbohydrates, fats, electrolytes, water, vitamins, and minerals. Simply, it results from a disturbance in one or more of the following components: (*a*) intraluminal digestion; (*b*) terminal digestion (i.e., brush border of intestine); or (*c*) transepithelial transport. In some cases of malabsorption there is a single, identifiable cause that can be identified at biopsy (e.g., parasitic infection); however, the clinical picture is often similar and in some cases of malabsorption the etiologies may be multiple. In the United States, the most frequent causes of malabsorption are **Crohn** disease, **pancreatic insufficiency** (e.g., chronic pancreatitis), **bile salt deficiency** (e.g., cirrhosis, cholestasis), and celiac sprue. Table 4-1 outlines some of the less common causes of malabsorption.

Celiac Sprue

TV suffers from chronic celiac sprue, an autoimmune disorder with a prevalence of 1:3000 whites (nonexistent in native Africans, Japanese, Chinese) that is theorized to begin in childhood with introduction of wheat **gluten.** Antibodies are developed against a component of gluten—**gliadin**—that lead to immunologic destruction of the villi in the small intestine (atrophy) as well as hyperplasia of the intestinal crypts. There is a hereditary component

to celiac sprue with clusters in families with **DQw2 histocompatibility** antigen, which is linked to **B8. DR3** also increases an individual's risk. In addition to a familial component, there may be an important environmental factor, as a protein from **adenovirus** 12 cross-reacts with gliadin antibodies. The immune response in the small intestinal mucosa leads to the congregation of B lymphocytes and other immune cells. In the long term, celiac sprue is associated with an increase incidence of T-cell lymphomas and GI and breast carcinomas.

Physiology of Digestion

The physiology of digestion of nutrients is salient to a discussion of the causes of TV's malabsorption and ensuing symptoms. One of the digestive tract's objectives is to cleave foodstuffs into assimilable forms that can cross the gut epithelium to be used for energy metabolism (fat, carbohydrates, proteins) or other metabolic processes (electrolytes, minerals, water). This process begins in the mouth and ends in the colon. In the mouth, the salivary glands produce **amylase** that begins the process of digesting starch. Amylase hydrolyzes α **1,4 bonds** resulting in maltose, maltotriose, and α-limit dextrins. This process continues with the aid of pancreatic amylase that encounters food in the duodenal lumen, which results in more maltose, maltotriose, and oligosaccharides. Digestion of starches by **disaccharidases** concludes at the brush border of the small intestine producing glucose, galactose, and fructose, which are all monosaccharides and capable of transepithelial transport. Protein digestion begins in the stomach with **pepsin,** after the chief cell-secreted pepsinogen is cleaved by a pH of < 2.

As part of its exocrine function the pancreas secretes **zymogens** such as trypsinogen. In this case, **trypsin,** which is hydrolyzed from its precursor trypsinogen by **enterokinase** (enteropeptidase) along the brush border of the small intestine, breaks down peptides into smaller polypeptides and amino acids. **Bile salts** and pancreatic enzymes couple to break down fats into absorbable fatty acids. Bile salts, an integral part of bile secreted by hepatocytes,

TABLE 4-1 Malabsorption—Uncommon Etiologies

Cause	Differentiating Factors
Whipple disease	Malabsorption, joint pain, CNS complaints, abnormal pigmentation, lymphadenopathy; bacteria in intestinal biopsy Predominantly in white males, age 30–40 Response to antibiotics (ceftriaxone and streptomycin)
Bacterial overgrowth syndrome	Small bowel with large numbers of anaerobic and aerobic Organisms; seen in patients with (*a*) intestinal stasis; (*b*) hypochlorhydria or achlorhydria; (*c*) immune deficiencies or impaired mucosal immunity; biopsy—mucosa normal, jejunal aspiration with increased number of bacteria is diagnostic, response to antibiotics
Disaccharidase deficiency	Two types of lactase deficiency—acquired is far greater than congenital; common in African Americans; causes osmotic diarrhea; increased hydrogen on exhaled gas chromatography; inherited—revealed after first feeding—abdominal distension with explosive watery diarrhea; biopsy normal
Abetalipoproteinemia	Autosomal recessive inborn error of metabolism in which infant cannot synthesize apolipoprotein B; no assembly of fatty acid and cholesterol into chylomicrons; biopsy reveals lipid vacuolation, no absorption of essential fatty acids or any chylomicrons, very low-density lipoprotein (VLDL) or low-density lipoprotein (LDL); burr cells on hematology smear; vitamin E deficiency

emulsify larger fat globules into smaller, uniformly distributed particles by lowering the surface tension. The fat particles are then cleaved by pancreatic enzymes such as **phospholipase A, lipase,** and **colipase** into absorbable fatty acids. The fatty acids undergo transepithelial transport and are converted to triglycerides, which, with the addition of cholesterol, are converted into chylomicrons for lymphatic transport.

Malabsorption

The broad consequences of malabsorption include obvious findings such as pain and diarrhea but also endocrine disorders, skin abnormalities, and nervous system changes that may lead to diagnosis and illustrate the importance of nutrients. **Diarrhea,** distension, and pain stem from the inability of the gut to absorb nutrients with increased intestinal secretions; this creates an **osmotic diarrhea.** The endocrine consequences result from decreased absorption of calcium and vitamin D, leading to **osteopenia** and **tetany.** Additionally, individuals may suffer from **amenorrhea, impotence,** and **infertility** secondary to generalized malnutrition and **hyperparathyroidism** from calcium and vitamin D deficiencies. Patients with malabsorption may suffer from **anemia** from low levels of iron, folate, and B12 and also increased bleeding with **purpura** and **petechiae** secondary to vitamin K deficiency. B12 and vitamin A deficiency result in peripheral **neuropathy.** Vitamin A deficiency coupled with zinc, essential fatty acids, and niacin can lead to **dermatitis.** TV had pitting edema because of her low protein state and hypoalbuminemia.

CASE CONCLUSION

TV started a diet without oats, barley, rye, and so on, and had resolution of symptoms and signs of her illness. Her follow-up biopsy results were negative. TV's case illustrates the hallmarks of the illness that can be diagnosed correctly only after the following three criterion are met: The patient has sprue with clinical documentation of malabsorption (fecal fat/pentose tests), tissue diagnosis with characteristic findings, and improvement in symptoms and mucosal histology on gluten withdrawal of the diet.

THUMBNAIL: Gastrointestinal Pathophysiology—Malabsorption

Epidemiology: Infancy to adulthood, fifth decade; incidence approximately 1:2000–3000

Pathogenesis: Poor intraluminal digestion secondary to defective hydrolysis or solubilization (e.g., pancreatic insufficiency, bacterial overgrowth)
Mucosal cell abnormality (enzyme deficiency, Vitamin B12 malabsorption due to pernicious anemia, abetalipoproteinemia)
Reduction in intestinal surface area (celiac sprue, Whipple disease, Crohn disease, lymphoma-associated enteritis)
Infection (parasite)
Lymphatic obstruction (lymphoma)
Drug induced (cholestyramine)
Unexplained (endocrine disorders: diabetes mellitus, hypothyroid/hyperthyroid, hypoparathyroid, hypoadrenocorticism)

(Continued)

THUMBNAIL: Gastrointestinal Pathophysiology—Malabsorption *(Continued)*

Sequelae by System and Deficiency in Parentheses

Gastrointestinal: Diarrhea, pain, increased flatus, stool bulk
Mucositis (vitamin A, E)

Blood: Anemia (iron, pyridoxine, folate, B12); increased bleeding (K)

Musculoskeletal: Osteopenia (calcium, vitamin D); tetany (Ca^{++}, Mg$^+$, vitamin D)

Endocrine: Infertility, impotence, amenorrhea (malnutrition); hyperparathyroidism (vitamin D, Ca^{++})

Skin: Petechiae, purpura (vitamin K); edema (protein); dermatitis (niacin, vitamin A, zinc, fatty acids)

Nervous system: Neuropathy (B12)

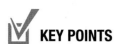

KEY POINTS

- Malabsorption is characterized by increased fecal fat, with malnutrition and vitamin/mineral deficiencies
- Presents with diarrhea, weight loss, bloating, increased flatus, pain
- Failure to thrive in infants
- Contributing genetic factors are 90 to 95% of patients with DQw2 histocompatibility antigen; HLA B8, DR3
- Often diagnosed in infants, those exposed to adenovirus 12, adults up to age 50 years
- Increased incidence with T-cell lymphoma of small bowel, GI and breast carcinoma
- Determine etiology with tissue biopsy, fecal fat test, absorption of sugars (D-xylose test)

QUESTIONS

1. Fat-soluble vitamins can be poorly absorbed in a case of malabsorption. Of the following, which deficiency is *correctly matched* to the fat-soluble vitamin?

   A. Vitamin A—arthralgia
   B. Vitamin D—hypercalcemia, anorexia
   C. Vitamin E—dermatitis
   D. Vitamin K—elevated PT, aPTT resulting in abnormal bleeding
   E. Folic acid—macrocytic, megaloblastic anemia

2. A patient tells you she has been suffering from chronic celiac sprue. She reports bulky stools, with distension, flatus, fatigue, and bleeding from her gums. She has red spots on her abdomen, arms, and legs. She has not adhered to her diet for some time. What is the most important *immediate* step to take?

   A. A shot of vitamin K
   B. You should have a long discussion with her about the importance of her adherence to her diet and participation in her own healthcare
   C. Small intestinal biopsy
   D. Screen other family members for sprue
   E. Test stool for fecal fat

HPI: HW, a 55-year-old male, complains of weakness, lack of appetite, and increasing abdominal girth for a long period of time. He reports that he is a scotch drinker and has been since he was a young man. HW consumes about one bottle each day. He also notes that he has been losing weight even though his pants are too tight. On questioning, HW states that his stools are black and sticky, his urine is tea-colored, and he is impotent.

PE: HW is 5' 7" tall and weighs 139 pounds. HR 100; T 36.8°C; BP 110/75. Gen: appears thin with muscle wasting. HEENT: scleral icterus, yellow under tongue. His skin displays a mild jaundice, he has no chest hair, enlarged breast tissue, palmar erythema, caput medusae, and spider nevi on abdominal wall. The abdomen is positive for bowel sounds, soft, nontender, markedly distended with fluid wave present, no rebound, no guarding, liver edge enlarged with irregular, nodular consistency, and nontender splenomegaly. The rectal exam is significant for guaiac-positive stool. There is testicular atrophy. The extremities display 2+ pitting edema, and there is mild asterixis of HW's hands.

Labs: WBC 6.5 ($4.5-11 \times 10^3$ per µL); Hgb 9 ($12-16$ g/dL); Hct 26 ($35-45\%$); MCV 105 ($80-100$); Plt 110 ($159-450 \times 10^3$ per µL); prothrombin time (PT) elevated; bilirubin (tot) 4.5 ($0.2-1.0$ mg/dL); bilirubin (dir) 2.2 ($0-0.2$ mg/dL); AST/SGOT 230 ($7-40$ U/L); ALT/SGPT 120 ($7-40$ U/L); alk phos 450 ($70-230$ U/L); amylase 34 ($25-125$ U/L); lipase 65 ($10-140$ U/L); albumin 2.0 ($3.5-5.5$g/dL).

You order a CT-guided biopsy of the liver and test for acute hepatitis. The hepatitis panel is negative but the biopsy reveals regenerating nodules of parenchyma with fibrotic changes, including perivenular and sinusoidal fibrosis. The nodules represent a micronodular and macronodular pattern. Individual hepatocytes are swollen and some are necrotic with significant neutrophilic infiltrate.

THOUGHT QUESTIONS

- What is the *most likely* diagnosis for this patient?
- What are the key components of the history, physical exam, and lab results that lead to this diagnosis?
- What is the architecture of the liver; how does the liver follow the dictum "form follows function"?
- How does the liver respond to injury?
- What is the pathophysiology of this disorder?
- What are the common and rare sequelae of this disorder?

BASIC SCIENCE REVIEW AND DISCUSSION

Liver Architecture, Physiology, and Injury

Unlike the majority of the GI tract, the liver is responsible for the processing of nutrients (e.g., amino acids, cholesterol, vitamins), phagocytosis of material in the splanchnic circulation, synthesis of protein, biotransformation of circulating metabolites, and detoxification and excretion of pollutants and wastes. How the liver is essential in so many vital processes is inherent in its architecture.

Liver Microanatomy and Physiology

The hexagonal lobule is the fundamental unit of liver architecture; it revolves around the terminal hepatic venule with portal triads located at three of the six angles. Each **portal triad** consists of the **portal vein** ($60-70\%$ of liver flow), the **hepatic artery** ($30-40\%$ of flow), and the outgoing **common bile duct.** Incoming blood is processed by hepatocytes via sinusoids that eventually drain into the central hepatic vein and continues to the inferior vena cava. The sinusoids are lined by endothelial cells that demarcate an extra sinusoidal space called the **"space of Disse";** this area is important in the pathophysiology of cirrhosis. Between the hepatocytes are the bile ducts that drain bile toward the common bile duct.

In relation to the architecture of the liver exists the metabolic organization in which the parenchyma is subdivided into three zones. **Zone I,** the periportal, receives the greatest amount of nutrients, toxins, and oxygen. **Zone III** is closest to the terminal venule and receives the least amount of nutrients, metabolites, toxins, and oxygen. **Zone II** is intermediate. There is a gradient of enzyme activity, and injury may exist in a zonal distribution.

Liver Injury Liver damage—regardless of the etiologic agent—is classified by five separate stages of injury. **Necrosis** of the liver is characterized by a cellular response of necrosis. In ischemic necrosis, the coagulative pattern dominates with mummified necrotic cells. When the insulting agent is immune related or a toxin, the cells undergo apoptosis with pyknotic cells with intensely eosinophilic **councilman bodies.** Necrotic changes are also described according to the extent and the areas involved: focal, such as with viral damage; zonal, which can be centrilobular (zone III), secondary to toxins or drugs; massive, such as in response to drug toxicity or extensive viral injury.

Other types of injury less severe than necrosis include **degeneration,** wherein hepatocytes have **ballooning degeneration** and cells become edematous. **Inflammation** is marked by a large influx of inflammatory cells, often lymphocytes or macrophages, and is called hepatitis regardless of the etiology. When directly assaulted with a toxin or inflammation, the liver responds with deposition of collagen, or **fibrosis,** which can lead to cirrhosis. Finally, **regeneration** is characterized by proliferation of hepatocytes from the remaining intact structural framework of the cords.

Pathophysiology and Biochemistry of Alcohol-Related Liver Disease

Alcohol abuse and related **alcoholic liver disease** are a staggering global problems; approximately 33% of Americans have had an adverse health outcome related to alcohol abuse. However, not all patients are affected equally by their consumption of alcohol.

Of course, the duration and amount of alcohol consumed is a risk factor, but gender, nutritional factors, and genetics also play a considerable role in who suffers most from liver damage. Only 10 to 15% of alcoholics develop cirrhosis. Chronic alcohol consumption results in liver disease in three classifications: **fatty liver disease, alcoholic hepatitis,** and **alcoholic cirrhosis. Hepatic steatosis** (fatty liver) may become evident with mild liver transaminase, bilirubin, and alkaline phosphatase elevations; this stage usually is not symptomatic, however. **Alcoholic hepatitis,** in contrast, and often after a period of binge drinking, presents acutely with malaise, anorexia, abdominal pain, weight loss, and abnormal lab values. In many patients, with cessation of alcohol use the symptoms remit and the liver heals. But even after cessation of alcohol use, a small portion of the population progresses to cirrhosis. Alcoholic cirrhosis can result in symptoms and physical manifestations such as portal HTN, ascites, splenomegaly, hepatic encephalopathy, and liver failure. These conditions are discussed later.

Alcohol is converted to **acetaldehyde** and **nicotine adenine dinucleotide, reduced form (NADH)** by alcohol dehydrogenase. Acetaldehyde interferes with normal hepatocytes secretion of protein by cellular swelling, termed fatty change. Acetaldehyde also disrupts microtubule formation in the hepatocytes and stimulates **Ito** cells in the space of Disse to transform into fibroblast-like cells and secrete collagen. This represents a final pathway to permanent liver damage and distortion of the architecture. Alcohol metabolism also results in elevated levels of NADH. **NADH** reverses the NAD$^+$ (nicotine adenine dinucleotide, oxidized form)/NADH ratio, which favors the production of lactic acid and triglycerides shunting normal substrates from catabolism to lipid synthesis. There is increased peripheral catabolism of fat and impaired assembly of lipoproteins. **NAD$^+$** is converted to acetate and NADH by aldehyde dehydrogenase. Acetate transforms into **acetyl-CoA,** which leads to ketogenesis.

The cytochrome P$_{450}$ system is induced with increased alcohol use, therefore metabolizing other drugs and metabolites at a faster rate. Finally, alcohol induces an immunologic attack on hepatic neoantigens, altering hepatic proteins.

History of Alcoholic Liver Disease Alcoholic **fatty liver** is the histologic description of the liver even after a moderate amount of alcohol is consumed. Lipid droplets form in hepatocytes; with continued alcohol use all hepatocytes contain large lipid vacuoles. Following this completely reversible stage, alcoholic hepatitis forms. **Alcoholic hepatitis** causes several, sometimes permanent, changes. Liver cell necrosis occurs with ballooning of the centrilobular regions. Additionally, **Mallory bodies** are formed that are hepatocytes with eosinophilic cytoplasmic inclusions. Recognizing an alteration, neutrophils and macrophages surround these abnormal cells, leading to an inflammatory reaction. Finally, sinusoidal and perivenular fibrosis is observed in **alcoholic hepatitis.**

Irreversible **alcoholic cirrhosis** evolves slowly as the liver shrinks and becomes more nodular in appearance. Collagen is formed in response to continued injury connecting portions of the parenchyma. The fibrous septae initially connect the central portions to the portal regions and finally from central to central and portal to portal. Micronodules are the first to form (<3mm), and eventually some enlarge into macronodules, resulting in a mixed picture.

Pathophysiology of Cirrhosis HW suffers from alcoholic cirrhosis secondary to his years of alcohol abuse. The other major causes of cirrhosis include chronic hepatitis, biliary disease, and iron overload, as well as the rarer diseases—Wilson disease and α_1 antitrypsin deficiency. **Cirrhosis** means three distinct things histologically: diffuse fibrosis, an alteration in the parenchymal architecture secondary to fibrosis, and parenchymal nodules regenerated by small foci of hepatocytes. These nodules are termed **micronodular (<3 mm) or macronodular (>3 mm).** Cirrhosis begins predominantly with micronodules but, as it progresses, it leads to a mixed histologic picture. The fibrous liver results from relentless diffuse parenchymal injury of different etiologies—in HW's case, the etiology is alcohol. The fibrosis is irreversible. The nodularity reflects the balance between fibrosis and hepatocyte regeneration. Finally, with the fibrosis comes reorganization of the vascular connections.

In a normal liver, collagen is dispersed to provide a framework for the hepatocytes to perform their vital function; in patients who suffer from cirrhosis, collagen types I and III are dispersed throughout all parts of the lobule. This leads to vascular disruption that impairs blood flow and diffusion of nutrients and solutes through the metabolic zones. Collagen is deposited in the **space of Disse,** impairing the movement of proteins such as clotting factors, albumin, and lipoproteins. Chronic inflammation, inflammatory mediators (TNF-α, TNF-β, and IL-1), Kupffer cell mediators, toxin effects, and disruption of the extracellular matrix are all proposed initiators of the Ito cell transformation. The Ito cell abandons its tasks and transforms into a collagen-forming cell, resulting in widespread fibrosis. These histologic changes result in anatomic and physical changes, many of which are present in HW.

The increased resistance of portal blood flow, **portal HTN,** is a direct result of the abnormal vascular channels secondary to cirrhosis. This portal HTN results in ascites, formation of portosystemic shunts, congestive splenomegaly, and hepatic encephalopathy. The key to the **ascites** in a cirrhotic patient lies in the starling forces. As described above, the abnormal vascular channels increase the pressure in the sinusoids (sinusoidal HTN). Additionally, cirrhotic patients have low levels of albumin because of the aforementioned decrease in synthetic function. With the abnormal starling forces the lymphatic channels initially pick up the extra fluid but are soon overwhelmed; the fluid percolates from the liver capsule to the peritoneal cavity. Also, secondary hyperaldosteronism with salt and water retention contributes to ascites. In addition to ascites, the increased portal pressure is shared by all vascular beds that have systemic and portal circulation. Increased pressure causes dilation of the veins in the vasculature of the rectum, the cardioesophageal junction, the retroperitoneum, and the falciform ligament leading to **hemorrhoids, varices,** and periumbilical and abdominal wall *caput medusae,* respectively. The esophageal varices can lead to life-threatening hematemesis in the cirrhotic alcoholic who retches or vomits as a result of drinking. Additionally, the spleen can enlarge secondary to vascular congestion and result in various hematologic manifestations.

Pathophysiology and Sequelae of Liver Failure Regardless of the etiology, when over 80% of liver parenchyma ceases functioning, **liver failure** ensues with severe clinical implications. Indeed, mortality from liver failure is 75 to 90%. HW possesses many of the classic physical and laboratory findings of liver disease. The cause of failure is often grouped according to one of three main categories: **chronic liver disease** (e.g., chronic hepatitis, cirrhosis, inherited); **ultrastructural lesions** (e.g., tetracycline toxicity, Reye syndrome); and rapid **parenchymal necrosis** (e.g., viral hepatitis, acetaminophen toxicity). Specific problems elucidate the importance of the functioning liver. For instance, HW has jaundice, elevated transaminases and bilirubin reflecting ongoing liver cell necrosis, and altered bilirubin metabolism. He has small testicles, increased breast tissue, and telangiectasias on his skin and red palms—all related to elevated estrogen levels. In addition to poor hepatic clearance of hormones, HW has poor synthetic function. This includes clotting factors, which leads to increased bleeding. He also is at great risk for a GI bleed from ruptured esophageal varices.

HW also has sour, pungent breath secondary to sulfur-containing mercaptans that are encephalopathic. **Hepatic encephalopathy** results from shunting the blood around the liver and severe loss of parenchymal cell function. Hepatic encephalopathy often

presents with a range of altered consciousness. Common behaviors include confusion, stupor, and coma. These behaviors are often accompanied by hyperreflexia and limb rigidity and asterixis, or "liver flap." When HW stretched his arms and dorsiflexed his hands, asterixis was observed; that is, his hands rapidly extend and flex. Patients with severe liver failure also suffer from **hepatorenal syndrome,** which is renal failure in the setting of liver failure with no other obvious source. Patients have elevated BUN and creatinine (which resolves if the liver failure is reversed) and decreased urine output. The pathophysiology is not entirely clear, but decreased renal blood flow is suspected as the cause.

CASE CONCLUSION

HW is now in liver failure, is admitted to the hospital, given supportive measures, and improves slightly. However, while on the liver transplant list he expires secondary to a massive GI bleed.

THUMBNAIL: GI Pathophysiology—Clinical Implications of Hepatic Failure

Clinical/Laboratory Outcome	Pathophysiology
Elevated AST/ALT	Parenchyma cell death
Jaundice	Altered bilirubin metabolism; conjugated hyperbilirubinemia
Ascites	Decreased albumin (decreased oncotic pressure), increased hepatic lymph formation, secondary hyperaldosteronism
Hypoalbuminemia	Decreased synthetic function of liver
Coagulopathy	Decreased synthetic function of liver, clotting factors (2, 5, 7, 9, 10); could lead to DIC poor clearance of activated factors
Fetor hepaticus (breath of the dead)	Mercaptan formation in GI tract
Gynecomastia/testicular atrophy/ palmar erythema telangiectasia/	Hyperestrogenism (poor liver clearance of estrogen)
Hepatic encephalopathy	Bypass of liver circulation, severe hepatocyte dysfunction
Hepatorenal syndrome	Elevated BUN, creatinine, decreased urine output; pathophysiology theorized to decreased renal blood flow

KEY POINTS—ALCOHOLIC CIRRHOSIS

- Risk factors include amount and duration of alcohol use/abuse, male gender, genetics
- Fatty liver disease; fatty change
- Alcoholic hepatitis, which is inflammatory hepatitis with inflammatory infiltrate
- Irreversible cirrhosis with collagen deposition

- Presents with elevated transaminases, physical findings
- Acetaldehyde, which interferes with hepatocyte production of protein; microtubule dysfunction; stimulates collage synthesis by Ito cells; results in immunologic injury secondary to inflammatory infiltrate
- NADH, which favors production of lactic acid and triglycerides
- Sequelae: liver failure (above) psychosocial distress (alcoholism)

QUESTIONS

1. A 55-year-old male patient presents to the clinic complaining of RUQ pain, fever, and yellow skin. He has tender hepatomegaly on exam, and you suspect alcoholic hepatitis. Which of the following liver function abnormalities will confirm your diagnosis?

   A. Elevated AST > elevated ALT, total bilirubin elevated, direct bilirubin normal
   B. Normal AST, elevated ALT, total bilirubin normal, direct bilirubin normal
   C. Elevated AST, normal ALT, total bilirubin elevated, direct bilirubin elevated
   D. Normal AST, normal ALT, total bilirubin elevated, direct bilirubin normal
   E. Elevated AST > elevated ALT, total bilirubin elevated, direct bilirubin elevated

2. A 40-year-old male suffering from alcoholic liver disease visits your office. He questions you regarding the pathophysiology of his many ailments. Which of the following is the appropriate mechanism for the clinical entity?

   A. Melenic stools with poor clearance of clotting factors
   B. Hematemesis (i.e., poor production of clotting factors)
   C. Spider angiomas; secondary to dysfunctional metabolism of hormones
   D. Hemorrhoids with decreased intravenous pressure
   E. Hypogonadism—poor production of testosterone

CASE 4-5 Jaundice

HPI: BG, a 4-day-old Caucasian girl, is brought in for a yellowish hue in her eyes and skin. Her mother, RG, noted the yellow color the day after discharge from the hospital (third day of life) and states that it has worsened. RG reports that BG is feeding well, breast-feeding approximately 12 times a day. The infant is otherwise healthy, with normal bowel movements and urination. No fevers are reported.

PE: BG's vital signs are normal and her development is good. The infant does not appear to be in any distress. HEENT exam shows no cataracts, positive scleral icterus, and a yellow hue of the sublingual mucosa. The baby's skin has an apparent yellow hue. Bowel sounds are positive. The abdomen is soft, nontender, with no masses, no hepatosplenomegaly. The stool is of normal color.

Labs: WBC 4 ($4.5-11 \times 10^3$ per µL); Hgb 16 ($12-16$ g/dL); Hct 45 ($35-45$%); Plt 243 ($159-450 \times 10^3$ per µL); bilirubin (tot) 3.5 ($0.2-1.0$ mg/dL); bilirubin (dir) 0.8 ($0-0.2$ mg/dL); AST/SGOT 12 ($7-40$ U/L); ALT/SGPT 23 ($7-40$ U/L); alk phos 100 ($70-230$ U/L); infant and mother's blood type both B+.

THOUGHT QUESTIONS

- What is the *most likely* diagnosis for this infant?
- How is bilirubin metabolized?
- What is the significance of conjugated and unconjugated hyperbilirubinemia?
- What are the key components of the history and lab results that lead to this diagnosis?
- What are the common and rare etiologies of this disorder?
- What is the pathophysiology of jaundice and cholestasis?

BASIC SCIENCE REVIEW AND DISCUSSION

Physiology of Bile and Bilirubin Formation

The patient with yellow skin and mucous membranes suffers from clinical **jaundice,** that is, the retention of bilirubin. BG has physiologic jaundice of the newborn. Neonates can have an **unconjugated hyperbilirubinemia** secondary to decreased hepatic enzyme activity, as well as other reasons, which are discussed below. To understand why BG appears yellow, it is necessary to discuss the physiology of bilirubin. **Bile** consists of **bilirubin, bile acids, cholesterol,** and **phospholipids** and is secreted by hepatocytes. It has two purposes: emulsification of fats for digestion and elimination of wastes. Bile salts are amphipathic (i.e., hydrophilic and hydrophobic areas) and can therefore serve to solubilize lipids into micelles for absorption. Bile also acts to eliminate cholesterol, bilirubin, and other wastes that are insoluble in water. The removal of these wastes and bilirubin is complex and has many steps in which disruption may occur, leading to jaundice or **cholestasis.** With cholestasis, there is retention of solutes in addition to bilirubin.

Yellow-colored bilirubin is the end product of heme and hemoprotein (e.g., P_{450} cytochrome) breakdown. At the end of their lifespan (120 days), immature erythroid cells or red blood cells are taken up by reticuloendothelial cells in the spleen, marrow, or liver and reduced to heme. **Heme** is broken down into **biliverdin** by heme oxygenase and to **bilirubin** by biliverdin reductase. Bilirubin is insoluble in aqueous solutions so it is bound by albumin and transported to the liver where it must undergo several critical steps. It must be taken up by the liver, bound by intracellular proteins (**ligandin**), and transported to the endoplasmic reticulum. In the endoplasmic reticulum, the bilirubin is conjugated by **uridine diphosphate (UDP)-bilirubin glucuronosyltransferase** (**UGT**), resulting in a bilirubin-glucuronic acid conjugate. This water-soluble, nontoxic, conjugated bilirubin is actively secreted into bile ducts and the small intestine. In the small intestine, most of the bilirubin glucuronides are deconjugated by bacterial **β-glucuronidases** into colorless **urobilinogens.** Approximately 20% of the urobilinogens made are reabsorbed via enterohepatic circulation and returned to the liver for reconjugation. Urobilinogen is water soluble, and small amounts may be excreted in the urine; however, most urobilinogen is oxidized to urobilins in the colon, which gives stool its characteristic color.

In addition to bilirubin, the liver secretes a substantial amount of **bile acids** into the bile canaliculi. Bile acids (taurine, cholic, and chenodeoxycholic acid) are lost in the feces but are matched by de novo synthesis from cholesterol so that balance is maintained. The enterohepatic circulation allows a large pool of bile acids to be available for digestion and excretion (Fig. 4-1).

Pathophysiology of Jaundice and Cholestasis

BG has increased levels of bilirubin in her blood as demonstrated by the lab values and physical exam. Bilirubin is deposited in the skin and mucous membranes, resulting in jaundice; a level of at least 2.0 mg/dL is necessary for clinical jaundice. **Cholestasis** results from bile secretory failure, which leads to an accumulation of cholesterol bile salts and bilirubin. Severely elevated cholesterol and bile acids can manifest as xanthomas and pruritus, respectively. This discussion is limited to pathologic situations that result in jaundice *without* cholestasis.

Jaundice can be classified as **unconjugated** or **conjugated** depending on the pathophysiologic process. **Unconjugated hyperbilirubinemia** occurs when less than 20% of the bilirubin is conjugated and is circulating in the plasma attached to albumin. Unconjugated bilirubin is insoluble and as such cannot be excreted in the urine. In infants, unconjugated hyperbilirubinemia can be disastrous because the blood–brain barrier is immature, allowing for deposition of bilirubin in the brain, leading to **kernicterus.** Unconjugated hyperbilirubinemia can result from excess production of bilirubin; examples include hemolytic anemia, pernicious anemia, thalassemia, and resorption of a large volume of blood from internal hemorrhage. Additionally, unconjugated hyperbilirubinemia can be caused by decreased hepatic uptake caused by drug interference (e.g., rifampin) with membrane carrier systems. Finally, impaired hepatocyte bilirubin conjugation secondary to hepatocellular disease

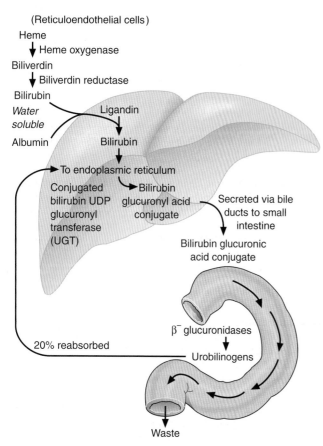

● **Figure 4-1.** Metabolism of bilirubin.

(e.g., hepatitis, cirrhosis), immature hepatocytes (physiologic jaundice) or inherited deficiencies (discussed below) can all lead to unconjugated hyperbilirubinemia.

A **conjugated hyperbilirubinemia** results when more than 50% of the bilirubin is conjugated. Conjugated bilirubin is water soluble and nontoxic and may result in bilirubinuria and clay-colored stools (no urobilin). The causes follow the physiologic pathway of bilirubin excretion. Decreased hepatic excretion or obstruction of bile flow after conjugation can result from intrahepatic bile duct disease (e.g., primary biliary cirrhosis, primary sclerosing cholangitis, graft–versus-host disease) or extrahepatic bile duct disease (e.g., gallstone, obstructive cancer, flukes). Other causes of decreased excretion include hepatocyte disease (e.g., hepatitis, total parenteral nutrition) and medication effects (e.g., oral contraceptives) leading to a conjugated type of jaundice.

Microanatomy of Jaundice

Increased levels of yellow bile pigment in hepatocytes appear wispy with bile pigment and "foamy degeneration"; bile canaliculi are full of bile. Occasionally, these ducts burst and Kupffer cells phagocytose the bile remnants, which are easily observed. In cases of obstruction of the bile tree (intrahepatic or extrahepatic), the pressure leads to swelling ducts and ductal proliferation. Prolonged obstructive cholestasis leads to destruction of the parenchyma, causing "bile lakes" of cellular debris and pigment.

Pathophysiology of Hereditary Hyperbilirubinemias

Just as adult hyperbilirubinemias are classified according to the conjugation status of the bilirubin, so are the causes of jaundice in neonates, infants, and children. Severe hereditary disease must be differentiated from asymptomatic and benign disease as well as physiologic jaundice. The most common cause of unconjugated jaundice in a neonate is secondary immaturity of the activity of hepatocyte bilirubin UGT, termed **physiologic jaundice of the newborn.** The enzyme typically reaches normal activity within 2 weeks of life. Of note, infants who are breast-fed are more likely to have physiologic jaundice of the newborn secondary to β-glucuronidases in the breast milk.

There are five main causes of unconjugated hyperbilirubinemia in neonates and infants. The first is physiologic jaundice of the newborn, which is what BG has (discussed below). **Hemolytic disease of the newborn** caused by blood group (ABO) incompatibility between mother and child results in jaundice and kernicterus from unconjugated hyperbilirubinemia. In this disease, increased production of heme overwhelms the hepatocyte ability to conjugate the substrate. **Crigler-Najjar syndrome type I** is a rare and lethal cause of severe unconjugated jaundice in which there is *no* bilirubin UGT. Without that enzyme, a severe unconjugated hyperbilirubinemia exists leading to deposition in the neonatal brain, resulting in an often fatal kernicterus. This disorder is inherited in an autosomal recessive fashion. **Crigler-Najjar syndrome type II** is a less severe, nonfatal form with a mild decrease in UGT that is inherited in a autosomal dominant pattern with variable penetrance. **Gilbert syndrome** is also inherited in the dominant pattern and is related to decreased levels of UGT; however, it is common and benign and patients with this disorder present with mild fluctuating levels of unconjugated bilirubin.

There are also several causes of **conjugated hereditary hyperbilirubinemia. Dubin-Johnson syndrome** results from the autosomal recessive inheritance of a defective transport in the canalicular membrane of the bile duct. As a consequence, excretion of conjugated bilirubin is impossible. Fortunately, these patients have a normal life expectancy because the conjugated bilirubin is nontoxic to a neonate. Of note, pathologic exam reveals a black liver that distinguishes it from Rotor syndrome. In **Rotor syndrome,** patients have an asymptomatic conjugated hyperbilirubinemia *without* liver discoloration. Rotor syndrome is also inherited in an autosomal recessive fashion.

☑ CASE CONCLUSION

BG has physiologic jaundice of the newborn. She is at a higher risk for several reasons. UGT has decreased activity until about 2 weeks of life. Also, neonates have an increased bilirubin load secondary to increased red cell mass and a relatively short half-life of those cells. Additionally, neonates have decreased intestinal bacterial flora with rare conversion of conjugated bilirubin to urobilinogen. Coupled with an increased enterohepatic circulation, neonates less than 2 weeks old are at risk for physiologic jaundice of the newborn. Like most neonates with physiologic jaundice, BG's was not present on the first day, peaked on the fifth, and resolved without complication on day 14.

THUMBNAIL: Liver Physiology and Pathophysiology—Hyperbilirubinemia

Bilirubin Metabolism	Derangement leads to...	Examples
Heme degradation	Unconjugated hyperbilirubinemia	Hemolytic anemia, resorption of hematoma or large GI bleed, ineffective erythropoiesis (thalassemia, pernicious anemia)
Reduced hepatic uptake (rifampin)	Unconjugated hyperbilirubinemia	Drug interference with carrier Gilbert (rare; usually conjugated)
Decreased bilirubin uptake at level of hepatocyte	Unconjugated hyperbilirubinemia	Physiologic jaundice of newborn, Crigler-Najjar, Gilbert, hepatocyte disease (hepatitis, cirrhosis)
Limited intrahepatic excretion of bilirubin	Conjugated hyperbilirubinemia	Dubin-Johnson, Rotor, hepatocyte disease (hepatitis, cirrhosis), intrahepatic bile disease (biliary cirrhosis, sclerosing cholangitis, transplant)
Limited extrahepatic excretion of bilirubin	Conjugated hyperbilirubinemia	Gallstones, obstructive cancer, fluke

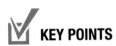 **KEY POINTS**

Unconjugated Hyperbilirubinemia

Crigler-Najjar type I
- Defect/genetics: No bilirubin UGT; autosomal recessive
- Life expectancy: Fatal at 18 months kernicterus/jaundice; seizures
- Pathology: Cholestasis

Crigler-Najjar type II
- Defect/genetics: Decreased bilirubin UGT; autosomal dominant, variable penetrance
- Life expectancy: Normal, occasional; mild kernicterus
- Pathology: Usually normal

Gilbert
- Defect/genetics: Decreased bilirubin UGT; autosomal dominant, heterogeneous
- Life expectancy: Normal, asymptomatic
- Pathology: Normal

Conjugated Hyperbilirubinemia

Dubin-Johnson
- Defect/genetics: Defective canalicular membrane; decreased excretion of bilirubin; autosomal recessive
- Life expectancy: Normal; chronic jaundice
- Pathology: Black liver

Rotor
- Defect/genetics: Altered biliary; excretion; unknown
- Life expectancy: Normal
- Pathology: Normal

QUESTIONS

1. A 3-week-old neonate presents with a seizure and on physical exam you note jaundice. You order the appropriate laboratory tests and diagnose the neonate with Crigler-Najjar, type I. You remember that this is an unconjugated hyperbilirubinemia. Which of the following are *both* conjugated types and syndromes of hyperbilirubinemia?

   A. Dubin-Johnson and Gilbert
   B. Gilbert and hemolytic disease
   C. Crigler-Najjar and physiologic jaundice
   D. Rotor and Dubin-Johnson
   E. Dubin-Johnson and Crigler-Najjar

2. A 45-year-old male presents with jaundice. You order laboratory tests that reveal a total bilirubin of 4.5 and a direct bilirubin of 1.2. You appropriately diagnose an unconjugated disorder. Which of the following pathophysiologic steps is *correctly* matched with the type of hyperbilirubinemia?

   A. Decreased excretion of bilirubin glucuronides; unconjugated
   B. Decreased bile flow; unconjugated
   C. Excess production of bilirubin; conjugated
   D. Decreased hepatic uptake; conjugated
   E. Hemolysis of red blood cells; unconjugated

3. Which of the following represents appropriately matched hereditary hyperbilirubinemia?

   A. Gilbert; decreased hepatic uptake of bilirubin
   B. Crigler-Najjar, type I; absent UDP-bilirubin glucuronosyltransferase
   C. Rotor; black pigmented liver
   D. Dubin-Johnson; autosomal dominant
   E. Rotor; canalicular transport deficiency

CASE 4-6 Acute Cholecystitis

HPI: SP, a 43-year-old Native American female, presents to the ED complaining of right upper quadrant pain. The pain began approximately 8 hours ago and became worse after a meal (within 30 minutes) at a fast-food restaurant. SP reports that the pain "shoots up" to the right shoulder and back (points to her scapula). She took acetaminophen without relief; following that she experienced three episodes of nausea and vomiting. SP remembers one other episode of this pain that resolved with over-the-counter (OTC) pain remedies and a bland diet. She has lost 30 pounds over the past month and this was the first fastfood or fatty food she has eaten in 2 months. SP believes that what she's now experiencing may be a reaction to this food. She has not taken her temperature but has felt a bit warm.

SP has a history of type 2 diabetes mellitus, Crohn disease, and hypercholesterolemia for which she is treated with Glucophage and clofibrate. She is also taking oral contraceptive pills (OCPs) to prevent conception.

PE: SP is 5'4" tall, weighs 254 pounds, and is obese. Her temperature is elevated at 38.6°C; her other vital signs are normal. She has no scleral icterus or jaundice of her skin or under her tongue. Her abdominal exam reveals epigastric and right upper quadrant tenderness, voluntary guarding, and rapid inspiratory arrest with deep palpation of the right upper quadrant.

Labs: WBC 17 (4.5–11 × 10³ per μL); diff-neutrophil 88% (57–67%); seg 60% (54–62%); bands 18% (3–5%); Hgb 13 (12–16 g/dL); Hct 36 (35–45%); Plt 322 (159–450 × 10³ per μL); bilirubin (tot) 1.0 (0.2–1.0 mg/dL); bilirubin (dir) 0.2 (0–0.2 mg/dL); AST/SGOT 25 (7–40 U/L); ALT/SGPT 34 (7–40 U/L); gamma-glutamyltransferase (GGT) 102 (8–40 U/L); alk phos 455 (70–230 U/L); amylase 90 (25–125 U/L); lipase 56 (10–140 U/L); erythrocyte sedimentation rate (ESR) 56 (<20 mm/hr); RUQ ultrasound reveals thickened gallbladder wall with sludging and several gallstones, one of which appears at the junction of the cystic duct.

THOUGHT QUESTION

- What is the *most likely* diagnosis for this patient?
- Which key laboratory results led to this diagnosis?
- What is the relevant anatomy, that is, the liver, gallbladder, ducts, adjacent organs, and so on?
- How is a cholesterol gallstone formed?
- How is a pigment gallstone formed?

BASIC SCIENCE REVIEW AND DISCUSSION

The most likely diagnosis is **acute cholecystitis,** which is an acute inflammation of the gallbladder. The symptoms of RUQ pain with referred pain, nausea, and emesis following a meal with high fat content along with the patient's risk factors place her at greater risk of acute cholecystitis. The physical exam, laboratory, and ultrasound findings confirm the diagnosis. To better understand this patient's condition, the physiology and pathophysiology of the gallbladder and the sequelae that can result from having gallstones are discussed below.

Anatomy and Physiology of the Gallbladder

The gallbladder is inferior to and flush against the liver typically at the anatomic division of the right and left lobes. In preparation for digesting fatty meals, 500 to 1000 cc of **bile** is secreted each day by the liver (exocrine secretion); in between meals, bile is stored in the gallbladder (approximately 50 cc capacity) and concentrated by active absorption of electrolytes and passive water (H_2O) movement. Bile is a fluid that is composed of **bile salts, phospholipids, cholesterol,** and **bilirubin.** Bile facilitates the emulsification, digestion, and absorption of fatty acids and cholesterol, minerals, and the fat-soluble **vitamins A, D, E,** and **K.** Hepatocytes secrete the bile through the right and left hepatic ducts that meet to form the (common) hepatic duct.

The hepatic duct joins with the cystic duct, which leaves the gallbladder at the **spiral valves of Heister** to form the common bile duct. The common bile duct courses to the duodenum through the head of the pancreas and releases bile into the duodenum via the **ampulla of Vater.**

Formation of Gallstones

In the gallbladder, cholesterol is solubilized by water-soluble **bile salts** and insoluble **lecithin.** When there is an excess of cholesterol such that the detergent capacity of bile salts and lecithin are overwhelmed, cholesterol stones can form. More specifically, there are three conditions that must occur for cholesterol stones to form. Bile salts and lecithin must be confronted with too much cholesterol. Along with this state of "supersaturation" there must be stasis in order for the cholesterol crystals to have time to aggregate (form) into stones. Stasis occurs in pregnancy or in rapid weight loss; the latter is what affects SP. The third criterion is that nucleation of the cholesterol monohydrate must be chemically favorable. Other promoters of stone formation include biliary sludge, mucins, and calcium salts.

Pigment stones are formed by complex mixtures of insoluble calcium salts. Although patients may not possess any identifiable risk factors, details from a patient's past medical history may indicate that the stones are likely pigmented. For instance, the presence of high levels of unconjugated bilirubin secondary to hemolysis can predispose to pigmented stones. Additionally, the risk of pigmented stones increases with infection of the biliary tract by *Escherichia coli* or *Ascaris lumbricoides*. Of note, pigmented stones are often (50–75%) radiopaque.

Cholelithiasis There are two types of stones: **cholesterol** and **pigment gallstones.** In the United States, approximately 80% of stones are cholesterol gallstones that contain more than 50% of crystalline cholesterol monohydrate. Cholesterol stones are more common in patients with a positive family history and those from Native American, Mexican American, Northern European, and North and South American populations. Additional risk factors including hyperlipidemia, obesity, recent rapid weight loss, gender, pregnancy, and medications such as OCPs and clofibrate are associated with excess estrogen and increased secretion of biliary cholesterol and thus cholesterol stones. Risk factors associated with the less common pigment gallstones include Asian ancestry, rural living, chronic hemolytic syndromes, and biliary infection and also patients with ileal diseases such as Crohn disease or cystic fibrosis with concomitant pancreatic insufficiency. Patients with gallstones are deemed to have **cholelithiasis.**

Choledocholithiasis If a patient also presents with jaundice and elevated direct bilirubin with the clinical and laboratory picture described above, the obstruction is likely in the common bile duct (and is mild). This is termed **choledocholithiasis.** These patients may present with acholic (no bile, pale) stools or biliuria (bile in urine). Also of note, these patients may present with fluctuating jaundice, differentiating it from jaundice of intrahepatic origin. Finally, increases in amylase and lipase indicate involvement of the pancreas where the distal common bile duct courses

through the pancreas. Commonly termed **gallstone pancreatitis,** these patients suffer mid-epigastric with RUQ pain.

Acute Cholecystitis In acute cholecystitis, the stone often becomes impacted in the gallbladder neck where it narrows or in Hartman pouch, which is a nearby outpouching. Pain is often intense and occurs when the gallbladder contracts in response to **cholecystokinin** that is released by the I cells of the duodenum and jejunum after a fatty meal. In SP, this is the most likely scenario, with elevated **alkaline phosphatase** and **GGT** (both specific to duct cells) and mild or absent transaminitis **(AST/ALT). Hyperbilirubinemia,** if present, is typically very mild. As is the case with our patient, fever and **leukocytosis** indicate infection of the gallbladder.

With the stone impacted, the gallbladder becomes more distended, inflamed, and edematous. Blockage is followed by chemical irritation and inflammation of the gallbladder wall. Enzymes produce lysolecithin, which is toxic to the mucosa. If hyperbilirubinemia is present, it is commonly due to the inflamed and edematous gallbladder that obstructs the adjacent common hepatic duct. When infection is present, the most common organisms include *E. coli, Enterobacteriaceae, Clostridium welchii* or *perfringens,* or *Bacteroides.*

CASE CONCLUSION

The diagnosis of acute cholecystitis with the stone location most likely in the gallbladder neck is made based on history and includes risk factors, physical exam, and laboratory and imaging data. All patients with acute cholecystitis should be admitted to the hospital, administered IV fluids, and treated with antibiotics. Approximately two in three cases of acute cholecystitis will resolve spontaneously; therefore, expectant management is ideal in patients with many medical issues. Serious consideration of a surgical solution should be entertained for any patient who deteriorates during the hospital stay to avoid the complications of acute cholecystitis, such as perforation, empyema, or ascending **cholangitis.** However, many patients choose to have an early or interval cholecystectomy. SP chose an interval laparoscopic cholecystectomy, which proceeded without complications.

THUMBNAIL: Cholesterol versus Pigment Gallstones

	Cholesterol	Pigment
Composition	Cholesterol monohydrate	Insoluble calcium salts
Pathogenesis	Cholesterol supersaturation nucleation; time to allow formation (stasis)	Presence of (abnormal) calcium salt, bilirubin calcium salts, infection
Frequency	>80%	Up to 20%
High-risk groups (ethnicity)	Northern European, Native American, North and South American, Mexican American, African American	Asian, rural
High-risk comorbidity	Estrogen (female gender, oral contraceptive, pregnancy), obesity, gallbladder stasis, hyperlipidemia, inborn errors of bile acid metabolism	Chronic hemolytic syndrome, biliary infection, ileal disease, Crohn disease, cystic fibrosis
Appearance on x-ray	10–20% radiopaque	50–75% radiopaque

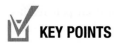

KEY POINTS

- Patients present with RUQ pain, fever
- Often diagnosed in obese women around age 40 years, with high levels of estrogen due to pregnancy or OCPs
- Persons at high risk include those of African American, Native American, and Mexican American heritage; other risk factors include diabetes, chronic extravascular hemolysis
- Cholelithiasis is differentiated by biliary colic, risk factors
- Acute cholecystitis is associated with fever; elevated white blood cells, alkaline phosphatase, GGT; transaminases (AST/ALT) and bilirubin with normal to mild elevation

- Signs of cholecystitis include fever; elevated WBCs; jaundice; elevated direct bilirubin, alkaline phosphatase, GGT; transaminases (AST/ALT) mildly elevated or normal
- Pancreatitis presents with elevated amylase, lipase; pain may be in mid-epigastrium

QUESTIONS

1. A patient presents to the ED with acute RUQ pain, fever, nausea, and vomiting after consuming a meal with high fat content. You suspect acute cholecystitis and consider the pathophysiology of the illness. Which of the following is the *inciting event* of cholecystitis?

   A. Obstruction
   B. Increased production of cholesterol stones
   C. Bacterial infection with gram-negative gut flora
   D. Enzyme degradation of the mucosal wall
   E. Schistosomes

2. Which of the following is deemed the most efficacious antibiotic to use against bacterial organisms that are *most likely* causing acute cholecystitis?

   A. Tetracycline
   B. Azithromycin
   C. Piperacillin-tazobactam or ampicillin-sulbactam or ticarcillin-clavulanate
   D. Trimethoprim-sulfamethoxazole
   E. Third-generation cephalosporin plus metronidazole or clindamycin

3. A patient with a history of acute cholecystitis presents with abdominal pain, nausea, and vomiting. On exam you note distension and absent bowel sounds. The *most likely* diagnosis is

   A. Acute cholecystitis
   B. Choledocholithiasis
   C. Ascending cholangitis
   D. Gallstone ileus
   E. Cystic fibrosis

4. Which of the following is *not* included in the layers of the gallbladder?

   A. Mucosal lining (single layer of columnar epithelial cells)
   B. Muscularis mucosa
   C. Peritoneal covering (except where the gallbladder is directly adjacent to the liver)
   D. Subserosal fat
   E. Fibromuscular layer

CASE 4-7 Appendicitis

HPI: EZ, a 22-year-old male, complains of 1-day history of sharp abdominal pain. He first noted the pain around his belly button, but now is pointing to the right lower quadrant (RLQ). EZ also complains of nausea and vomiting (N/V), which began after his pain; he also notes fever and chills and has no appetite. Otherwise he is healthy.

PE: EZ is 5' 7" tall and weighs 145 pounds. Vital signs: T 38.3°C; HR 102 beats/min; BP 129/66 mm Hg; RR 18 breaths/min. Gen: discomfort, diaphoretic. EZ's abdomen has positive bowel sounds but is hypoactive and soft, with marked tenderness in the RLQ at McBurney point. There is distension, positive rebound, and involuntary guarding.

Labs: WBC 12.5 ($4.5-11 \times 10^3$ per μL); diff-neutrophil 88% (57−67%); seg 60% (54−62%); bands 18% (3−5%); Hgb 14 (12−16 g/dL); Hct 44 (35−45%); Plt 243 ($159-450 \times 10^3$ per μL).

An x-ray and a CT of the abdomen are ordered. The kidneys, ureters, bladder (KUB) radiograph reveals a normal gas pattern with no free or intraperitoneal air. The CT reveals fat stranding and an oval appendicolith.

THOUGHT QUESTIONS

- What is the *most likely* diagnosis for this patient?
- Which key components of the history and lab results lead to this diagnosis?
- What are the common and/or rare sequelae of this disorder?
- What is the etiology of this disorder?
- What is the differential diagnosis of abdominal pain?

BASIC SCIENCE REVIEW AND DISCUSSION

From the history, physical exam, laboratory, and imaging findings it is clear that EZ has **appendicitis,** which is often diagnosed in adolescents and young adults who were previously well. Classically, but not always, the presentation is as follows: peri-umbilical pain followed by RLQ pain at McBurney point (between the umbilicus and the anterior superior iliac spine), then nausea and vomiting. Tenderness and possibly rebound and guarding (indications of peritoneal irritation) are elicited during a physical exam. Next, a low-grade fever followed by an elevation in the WBC count is observed. This sequence does not apply to patients who are pregnant, have a retrocecal appendix, or have a malrotated gut. In pregnant patients, the pain may be in the right lower, middle, or upper quadrant, whereas in those patients with a retrocecal appendix the pain may be in the flank. In those with a malrotated gut, the pain would be in the RUQ. Additionally, the presentation may differ in the very young and the very old.

Pathophysiology of Acute Appendicitis

Appendicitis is associated with obstruction of the appendix in over 50% of the cases. Often the obstruction is caused by lymphoid hyperplasia, a fecalith, or, less commonly, a tumor, gallstone, or even worms. The obstruction leads to increased pressure secondary to continual secretion of mucinous fluid (physiologic), which results in the collapse of the lymphatics and veins; this collapse leads to ischemia. Afterward, secondary bacterial invasion occurs, in which secretion of an exudate results in more edema and inflammation. With ischemia and invasion, gangrene results secondary to venous thrombosis. The bowel wall may rupture secondary to ulceration, bacterial infection, and ischemia.

Morphology of Appendicitis

Initially in appendicitis there is a neutrophilic invasion of the mucosa and submucosa. The neutrophils secrete an exudate that is apparent on the serosa as it grossly changes from pink and normal to granular and red. As the neutrophilic invasion expands to include the muscularis the gross appearance is a fibrinous purulent serosal reaction. As bacterial invasion ensues, an abscess can form followed by ulceration and necrosis. Finally—in the final step prior to rupture—gangrene sets in with a green or green-black appearance. Major sequelae of appendicitis in addition to rupture include peritonitis, pylephlebitis with thrombosis of the portal vein, liver abscess, peri-appendiceal abscess, or bacteremia.

Differential Diagnosis of Acute Abdominal Pain

There are several causes of acute abdominal pain that can often be diagnosed based on history, physical exam, laboratory tests, and imaging studies. Epigastric pain from a **perforated ulcer** classically presents as severe epigastric pain with rapid progression to the entire abdomen in conjunction with the history of an ulcer. The pain is often accompanied by signs of peritoneal irritation (e.g., rebound and guarding). Free air is observed on radiograph. **PUD** is more common in men than in women and is associated with *Helicobacter pylori* infection as well as COPD, chronic NSAID use, and tobacco and alcohol use/abuse.

Biliary tract disease presents in middle-aged female patients (age 35–55) with RUQ crampiness. History of multiparity, obesity, and OCP use are risk factors. On laboratory and imaging evaluation, patients have elevated GGT and alkaline phosphatase levels and stones in the gallbladder, as well as ductal dilation. With an elevated WBC count and fever, patients may have cholecystitis or cholangitis. Acute epigastric pain with radiation toward the back accompanied by nausea, vomiting, and low-grade fever in a patient with a history of alcohol abuse is often diagnosed as **pancreatitis.** On physical exam the pain seems out of proportion to the findings and only in the most severe cases does the examiner find rebound or guarding because the organ is in the retroperitoneum.

Kidney stones or ureteral colic (**nephrolithiasis**) often afflicts men in their 30s with risk factors that can lead to stone formation, such as family history, gout, *Proteus* genitourinary tract infection, cystinuria, or renal tubular acidosis. Upon presentation, these patients are writhing in bed with an acute onset of flank pain that radiates toward the groin. Ureteral colic is often associated with nausea and vomiting and patients have costovertebral angle tenderness (CVAT), a benign abdominal exam, and hematuria. Spiral CT or intravenous pyelography is the mainstay of diagnosis. Patients of any age—infants to adults—may have periumbilical pain with vomiting and a tender, distended abdomen with hyperactive bowel sounds, leading to the diagnosis of intestinal **obstruction.** Abdominal films are a good way to diagnose; obstruction is more common in at-risk patients (those with cancer, adhesions, hernias, abscess, intussusception, or volvulus).

Patients with **diverticulitis** complain of left lower quadrant (LLQ) pain and changing stool consistency. They may have fever, LLQ tenderness without rebound, heme-positive stool,

or even a palpable mass. Risk factors include age greater than 50 years and high-fat, low-fiber Western diet. The diagnosis is made by CT.

Additional causes of lower abdominal pain in women patients include **pelvic inflammatory disease** (PID) and **ovarian torsion.** PID occurs in young, often sexually active women. They present with lower abdominal pain, fever, elevated WBC count, cervical motion, and adnexal and uterine tenderness on bimanual exam. These patients are diagnosed on a clinical basis only. Young women with adnexal masses who present with an acute onset of severe unilateral pain may have had torsion of an ovary. In torsion, the size of the mass allows the ovary to twist, cutting off the vascular supply. Emergent ultrasound can indicate presence of a mass, as well as absence of blood flow.

CASE CONCLUSION

EZ is admitted to the hospital for surgical management of the appendicitis. He undergoes an uncomplicated laparoscopic appendectomy and stays in the hospital for 3 days. EZ is released when his pain is controlled and he is tolerating a regular diet.

THUMBNAIL: Differential Diagnosis of Acute Abdominal Pain

Diagnosis	Epidemiology/Etiology	Presentation/Physical Exam	Studies
PUD	Male, age 50s, bacteria, COPD, NSAID, alcohol (EtOH) abuse, tobacco use	Epigastric pain, often relieved by food/antacids, diffuse abdominal pain; when perforates, peritoneal irritation	Endoscopy, urease breath test
Biliary colic	Female, obese, age 40s, OCPs, multiparous	RUQ pain, radiates to scapula, Murphy sign, fever in cholecystitis	Alk phos, WBC elevated, ultrasound
Pancreatitis	Male, EtOH abuse, gallstones, hyperlipidemia, history of endoscopic retrograde cholangiopancreatography (ERCP), hypercalcemia	Acute onset, epigastric, N/V, radiates toward back, pain out of proportion of PE, fever, no rebound guarding (retroperitoneal)	Amylase, lipase, CT, ultrasound
Appendicitis	Young adults; appendix, obstruction, ischemia, infection, perforation	Epigastric/peri-umbilical then RLQ pain, fever, anorexia, RLQ tenderness, rebound guarding	WBC elevated, CT
Ureteral colic	Male, age 30s, gout, family history, *Proteus* infection, stone in ureter	Acute flank pain, radiates to groin, CVAT, abdomen is benign	CT, IV pyelogram
Obstruction	Infants to adults, history of surgery (adhesions), cancer, volvulus, intussusception	Crampy, diffuse abdominal pain, vomiting, hyperactive bowel sounds, distension, tenderness, peritoneal signs if strangulated	Abdominal radiograph
Diverticulitis	Males, elderly, low-fiber diet, colonic diverticula	LLQ pain, N/V, stool abnormalities, fever, rectal bleeding, no rebound tenderness	WBC elevated, CT
PID	Females, sexually active, high-risk behavior	Low abdominal pain, N/V, fever, uterine and adnexal tenderness, cervical motion tenderness, cervical discharge	Clinical exam
Ovarian torsion	Females, adnexal mass twists; stops blood supply	Acute onset, unilateral low abdominal pain, N/V, tenderness	Ultrasound with vascular evaluation

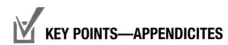

KEY POINTS—APPENDICITES

- Presents with pain, cramping, inability to pass flatus/stool, nausea, vomiting, abdominal distension, hyperactive bowel sounds with rushes, rectal bleeding (currant jelly stool); infarction

- Usually seen in young adults and adolescents; however, persons of any age can be affected; slightly more common in males than in females

- Classic peri-umbilical pain followed by RLQ pain

- Progresses from quadrant pain, then nausea and vomiting; after which patients have fever and leukocytes

- Obstruction followed by increased intraluminal pressure; collapsed lymph drainage and veins leads to bacterial invasion, pus, and ulceration; compromised arterial blood supply leading to gangrenous necrosis; rupture

- Caused by luminal obstruction secondary to (*a*) lymphoid hyperplasia, (*b*) fecaliths, (*c*) foreign body, (*d*) tumor, (*e*) gallstone, and (*f*) worms

- KUB x-ray and CT revealing oval, calcified appendicolith and gas filled appendix with air-fluid levels are pathognomonic; other evidence include nearby gas-fluid levels or evidence of inflammation; fat streaking or obliteration of the right peritoneal fat line

- Perforation, liver or peri-appendiceal abscess, peritonitis, pylephlebitis with thrombosis of portal vein, bacteremia

QUESTIONS

1. A 23-year-old woman presents to the ED. She complains of 3 to 4 days of low abdominal pain, fever, nausea, and vomiting. She has normal bowel movements. The patient reports a history of an ectopic pregnancy, several sexual partners, as well as a chlamydial infection 3 months ago. Her last menstrual period was 9 days ago. Her exam is notable for cervical motion tenderness and RLQ abdominal pain. Which of the following is the likely diagnosis?

   A. Right ectopic pregnancy
   B. PID
   C. Gastroenteritis
   D. Renal calculi
   E. Crohn disease

2. In which of the following is the pathogenesis of acute appendicitis and diverticulitis similar?

   A. Lymphoid hyperplasia
   B. Increased bulk of stool
   C. Western diet
   D. Primary bacterial invasion
   E. Obstruction by a fecalith

CASE 4-8 Inflammatory Bowel Disease

HPI: LC, a 23-year-old woman, presents with 9 months of low abdominal pain and intermittent diarrhea. The pain has intensified over the past few months and is greater on the right side. She characterizes it as crampy and constant; nothing worsens or relieves the pain. LC's bowel movements have become looser but do not contain any mucus or blood. She also notes weight loss, malaise, fatigue, and intermittent fevers.

PE: LC is 5' 8" tall and weighs 115 pounds. She has normal vital signs and is afebrile. She is thin and appears ill. Her abdomen has positive bowel sounds, is soft, nontender, and slightly distended, with no rebound, no guarding, and a slight RLQ fullness. Her rectum has normal tone, guaiac (+).

Labs: WBC 15 (4.5−11 × 10³ per μL); Hgb 11 (12−16 g/dL); Hct 32 (35−45%); Plt 243 (159−450 × 10³ per μL); bilirubin (tot) 0.2 (0.2−1.0 mg/dL); bilirubin (dir) 0.1 (0.0−0.2 mg/dL); AST/SGOT 12 (7−40 U/L); ALT/SGPT 23 (7−40 U/L); alk phos 100 (70−230 U/L); amylase 34 (25−125 U/L); lipase 5 (10−140 U/L); albumin 2.7 (3.5−5.5g/dL); ESR 60 (<20 mm/hr).

LC undergoes several diagnostic exams to better elucidate the source of her symptoms. An abdominal radiograph reveals dilated loops of small bowel with air-fluid levels and moderate air in the colon. Next, she undergoes a barium enema, which is significant for a normal colon and a stricture noted in the distal ileum with proximal dilation. Finally, endoscopy is performed that is diagnostic. The findings include a granular mucosal surface with nodules and areas of friability, as well as erosions and aphthous ulcers. A serpigos linear ulceration is observed with sharply demarcated areas of normal mucosa. Mucosal biopsy of the affected areas reveals transmural involvement with noncaseating granulomas and significant inflammatory infiltrate.

THOUGHT QUESTIONS

- What is the *most likely* diagnosis for this patient?
- Which key components of the history, physical exam, lab, and study results led to and confirm this diagnosis?
- How do you differentiate between the two main causes of this disorder?
- What are the common and rare sequelae of this disorder?
- What are the proposed etiologies of these disorders?

BASIC SCIENCE REVIEW AND DISCUSSION

LC has a chronic relapsing disorder broadly termed **inflammatory bowel disease** (IBD) and, specifically, **Crohn** disease. There are two types of IBD: Crohn disease and **ulcerative colitis (UC).** Each possesses a unique presentation, sequelae, and gross and histologic findings; however, they share in common an elusive etiologic process that results in a final common pathway of inflammatory damage. IBD runs in families, as there is a tenfold increase in first-degree relatives as well as concordance in twin studies. Normally, the physiologic state of the intestine is one of balance between immune activation and down-regulation. It is unclear what tips the scales in favor of activation in cases of Crohn disease and UC; many theories exist but none adequately explain the pathogenesis. Proposed infectious etiologies are ambiguous at best with culprits including viruses, bacteria, atypical bacteria, and even food antigens, but the data are unclear. Another theory stems from the observation of increased mucosal permeability and abnormal mucosal glycoproteins in patients with IBD; other theories point to psychological associations. The most plausible theory stems from altered immune system functioning. Possible causes include abnormal proliferation of cytokines, abnormal antigen-presenting cells (APCs) or lymphocytes, or antiepithelial antibodies. Regardless of the exact mechanism, the immune system is activated and mucosal injury occurs.

Pathophysiology of Crohn Disease

LC suffers from **Crohn disease**—a chronic inflammatory condition affecting mostly young women in their late teens and 20s (a second peak incidence occurs among women in their 50s and 60s). Crohn disease affects all layers of the tract wall (i.e., **transmural**), most commonly in the small bowel and colon (40%), the terminal ileum alone (30%), or the colon alone (20%), but it can affect any place in the alimentary tract. Patients present with chronic colicky pain often in the area where the disease is first active. LC's pain is in the LRQ, which is the area where the stricture was discovered. Another hallmark of Crohn disease is the discontinuous nature of the lesions, or "skip" areas (**skip lesions**) that are sharply contrasted with areas of normal mucosa. Several hallmarks help differentiate Crohn disease from UC. Initially, the shallow ulcerations resemble canker sores. As these lesions grow, the ulcerations coalesce into linear lesions, contrasted with nearby normal mucosa; the classic description is a **"cobblestone"** appearance. These linear lesions are at danger of becoming fistulae into any nearby structures (e.g., bowel, skin, bladder, vagina). On gross inspection, the mucosal wall is noted to be rubbery, thick, and erythematous secondary to edema, inflammatory infiltration, fibrosis, and hypertrophy of the muscularis propria. This results in a narrowed lumen seen as a **"string sign"** on barium enema. Histologically, there is mucosal ulceration and inflammation characterized by neutrophils that invade the crypts and result in crypt abscesses. The destructive process continues with crypt atrophy. As in our patient, the inflammation and ulcerative destruction occurs through all layers; hence, the pathognomonic, **transmural** involvement. Finally, Crohn disease is commonly accompanied by noncaseating granulomas.

The course of Crohn disease is of relapsing and remitting symptoms, occasionally worsened by physical or psychological stress. **Microcytic anemia** is common with nearly perpetual loss of RBCs. Other associations and sequelae help describe the disease, direct treatment, and differentiate Crohn disease from UC. As discussed earlier, strictures can complicate affected regions often in the small intestine, as can fistulas to the bowel or other organs. If the small bowel has significant disease, the patient can suffer from malabsorption, protein loss, and various vitamin deficiencies (e.g., B12). Additionally, Crohn sufferers can have a multitude of extra-intestinal manifestations, including arthritis, ankylosing spondylitis, erythema nodosum, clubbing of the nails, perihepatic cholangitis, or uveitis. There is a five- to sixfold increased risk of GI cancers in patients with long-standing Crohn disease.

Pathophysiology of Ulcerative Colitis

UC is also a chronic ulceroinflammatory condition of unknown etiology affecting only the colon. UC is rare but has a slightly higher incidence than Crohn disease. In the United States, whites and females are more often affected than their counterparts and the onset of disease often occurs in the 20s. Patients complain of crampy pain, rectal bleeding, tenesmus, and chronic diarrhea with blood and mucus. UC affects only the colon and the diseased tissues extend only into the submucosa; the anus is not involved. The disease begins at the rectum and extends proximally, leaving behind a friable red mucosa. Characteristically, the diseased mucosa progresses to ulcerations with pseudopolyps that progress histologically into **crypt abscesses** with eventual atrophy. In only the most severe cases does the illness progress past the submucosa into the muscularis propria; in these severe cases there is a higher risk of toxic megacolon (complete cessation of bowel function). Histologically, there is mucosal damage and ulceration in affected areas with a mononuclear infiltrate in the propria with neutrophils and mast cells. As in Crohn disease, there is an increased incidence of adenocarcinoma of the colon, which is proportional to the duration of the illness. Dysplasia can arise in different sites, increasing a patient's risk of adenocarcinoma by almost 30 times. Clearly, surveillance is important. Common associations include sclerosing pericholangitis and ankylosing spondylitis (with HLA B-27).

CASE CONCLUSION

LC was treated with immunosuppressive medications and her symptoms improved greatly. She also noted the importance of limiting her psychological stressors because her number of exacerbations appeared to be related to the stress level of her job and personal life. LC's anemia and hypoalbuminemia also improved with immunosuppressive therapy. She has not had any extra-intestinal manifestations of her illness.

THUMBNAIL: Inflammatory Bowel Disease—Ulcerative Colitis versus Crohn Disease

	Ulcerative Colitis	*Crohn Disease*
Location	Begins at rectum, extends to colon commonly; rarely affects the anus	Small intestine, colon commonly, but any part of alimentary tract
Depth	Mucosa, submucosa	Transmural
Gross	Diffuse ulceration, pseudopolyps, no strictures, thin wall, dilated lumen	Skip lesions with strictures, thick or thin wall (thick in small bowel), cobblestone appearance
Histology	Crypt atrophy and abscess, many pseudopolyps, mild lymphocytes and polymorphonuclear cells (PMNs)	Deep linear ulcers, noncaseating granulomas, marked inflammatory infiltrate (lymphocytes, PMNs), fistulas
Sequelae	Increased risk for adenocarcinoma (30–35 years after diagnosis), sclerosing pericholangitis, toxic megacolon	Increased risk for GI malignancy (not as high as in UC) extra-intestinal manifestations (polyarthritis, uveitis, clubbing of the nails, ankylosing spondylitis), strictures, fistulas, malabsorption, protein-losing enteropathy, fat-soluble vitamin deficiency

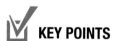

KEY POINTS

Ulcerative Colitis

- Presents with relapsing attack of bloody diarrhea, tenesmus, mucus in stool, pain
- Labs: may have no abnormalities, rarely microcytic anemia
- Etiology: ultimately idiopathic, several theories exist: infections, genetics, intestinal mucosal structural abnormalities, abnormal immunoreactivity
- Treatment: immunosuppression, surgery

Crohn Disease

- Presents with intermittent colicky abdominal pain, diarrhea, fever
- Labs: fat and vitamin malabsorption (low albumin, deficiency of fat-soluble vitamins A, D, E, and K), abnormal liver function tests (cholangitis), elevated creatinine (strictures obstructing the ureters) and electrolytes
- Etiology: ultimately idiopathic, several theories exist: infections, genetics, intestinal mucosal structural abnormalities, abnormal immunoreactivity
- Treatment: immunosuppression, surgery

QUESTIONS

1. A 28-year-old female presents with an 8-month history of bloody diarrhea, intermittent crampy abdominal pain, persistent spasms of the bowel, and stringy mucus in her stools. You suspect IBD, with the likely diagnosis of UC. Which of the following will allow you to differentiate it from Crohn disease?

   A. Areas of affected and unaffected mucosa, "skip" lesions
   B. Transmural involvement on biopsy
   C. Involvement of the small bowel
   D. Pseudopolyps
   E. Fistula formation

2. A 33-year-old white female presents with colicky RLQ abdominal pain, diarrhea, and rectal bleeding for more than 10 years. You perform the appropriate work-up. Her biopsy reveals colon and small bowel involvement with characteristic transmural skip lesions, a cobblestone appearance, and a narrow lumen in the distal small bowel. She presents 3 months later with electrolyte abnormalities and low albumin and complains of tingling and numbness in her hands and feet.

   Which of the following laboratory abnormalities would you expect to see?

   A. Decreased hemoglobin and hematocrit, macrocytosis
   B. Low albumin
   C. Decreased hemoglobin and hematocrit and microcytosis
   D. Abnormal clotting profile
   E. Decreased bone mineral density

3. A 55-year-old white female with a 30-year history of UC returns for a follow-up visit. She recently recovered from an acute exacerbation for which she was hospitalized and given immunosuppressive therapy, to which she responded. She knows about her increased risk for adenocarcinoma of the colon. Which of the following is *more common* in patients who suffer from UC?

   A. Fistula formation
   B. Aphthous ulcers
   C. Toxic megacolon
   D. Granulomas
   E. Malabsorption

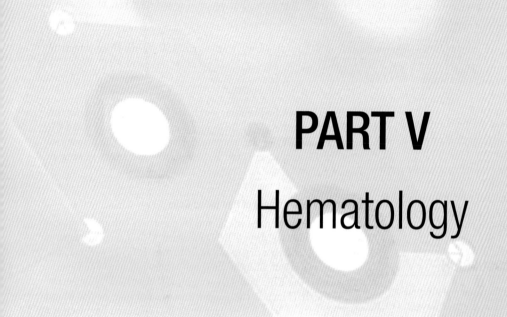

PART V

Hematology

HPI: RC, a 25-year-old woman, comes to your office complaining of increasing fatigue and occasional heart palpitations for the last several weeks. She occasionally feels short of breath while having the palpitations, but denies any fever, chills, or weight loss during this time. She does not have a history of asthma or any cardiac problems. She has never had symptoms like this before.

PMH: Seasonal allergies. Last menstrual period was 1 week prior. Her periods are moderately heavy, lasting 5 to 7 days, cycling regularly every 30 days. She is not taking any medications.

PE: T 36.2°C; HR 72 beats/min; BP 125/72 mmHg

Her conjunctiva look pale, and she has a soft systolic murmur heard best at the left second intercostal space. The rest of the exam is unremarkable.

Labs: Hgb 10 g/dL (low); Hct 30% (low); MCV 76 fL (low); serum iron 40 µg/dL (low); transferrin 450 µg/dL (high); ferritin 8 µg/dL (low).

THOUGHT QUESTIONS

- What is the general structure and function of red blood cells in the human body?
- What is anemia and what are the general mechanisms for its development?
- How are the different types of anemia usefully classified?
- What is the pathophysiology of iron deficiency anemia, how does it present, and how is it treated?

BASIC SCIENCE REVIEW AND DISCUSSION

Red blood cells (RBCs or erythrocytes) are discoid-shaped cells, roughly 8 µm in diameter, that function to transfer oxygen (O_2) from the lungs to other tissues and carry carbon dioxide (CO_2) from those tissues back to the lungs. The plasma membrane of a mature erythrocyte is made up of many transmembrane proteins that regulate the unique properties of deformability, tensile strength, and cell shape. An RBC must repeatedly deform through 2- to 3-µm capillaries during its 120-day lifespan and it must withstand the shear stresses of the circulation. The flattened shape of the erythrocyte maximizes surface area, allowing for faster diffusion and absorption of O_2 and CO_2.

Hemoglobin

During erythropoiesis or RBC maturation, RBCs lose all cellular organelles and function anaerobically to preserve O_2 that is meant for other cells. The cytoplasm is filled with millions of oxygen-carrying proteins called **hemoglobin (Hgb)**. Each Hgb molecule has tetramer of globin subunits and each subunit has a heme group with a central iron atom, which binds O_2 directly. Iron, therefore, plays an essential role in heme (and subsequently RBC) production.

Each of the four heme groups can carry an O_2 molecule; Hgb can carry a maximum of four O_2 molecules. When Hgb is saturated with O_2, it has a bright red color; as it loses O_2 (deoxyhemoglobin), it becomes bluish (cyanosis). Hgb's affinity for O_2 increases as successive molecules of O_2 bind. More molecules bind as the O_2 partial pressure increases until the maximum amount that can be bound is reached (100% saturation). As this limit is approached, very little additional binding occurs and the curve levels out, having a sigmoidal or S shape. The affinity of Hgb for O_2 is also affected by several other factors as seen in Figure 5-1.

Laboratory Assessment of Red Blood Cells

In the lab, Hgb can be measured in a certain volume of blood and functions as a "direct" RBC measure. Other direct measures include the **mean corpuscular volume** (MCV), which is the average volume of an individual cell, and a red blood cell count (also called the RBC count). A commonly reported measure, the **hematocrit** (Hct), is the proportion, by volume, of the blood that consists of RBCs. The Hct is easily measured by placing a sample of blood in a tube and centrifuging down the red cell mass. The Hct is the proportion of the total length of the tube made up of RBCs. This can also be calculated by multiplying the red cell count by the MCV.

Various RBC disorders, such as anemia, can be identified by changes in RBC size or shape. This qualitative analysis of RBCs is done by microscopically examining a **peripheral blood smear**.

Anemia

Anemia occurs when there is a decrease in red cell mass and is usually defined by an Hgb less than 12 g/dL in women and less than 14 g/dL in men. There are three general mechanisms for the development of anemia. The first is **decreased production** of RBCs (hypoproductive anemia), which can result from nutritional deficiencies (iron, vitamin B12, or folate), low levels of erythropoietin (such as in CRF), bone marrow failure (aplastic anemia), or replacement of normal marrow by malignant cells (leukemias or metastatic bone disease). Another cause of anemia is **increased destruction** of circulating erythrocytes, as seen in hemolytic anemias, spherocytosis, and sickle cell disease. Finally, **blood loss** can be the cause of anemia. In the latter two mechanisms, a normal bone marrow compensates with an increase in RBC production, or erythropoiesis (hyperproductive anemia).

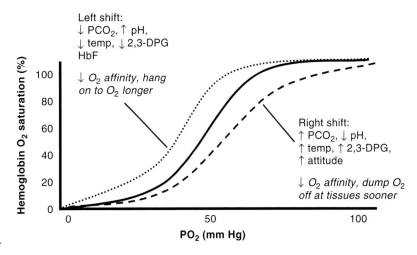

Left shift:
↓ PCO₂, ↑ pH,
↓ temp, ↓ 2,3-DPG
HbF

↓ O₂ affinity, hang
on to O₂ longer

Right shift:
↑ PCO₂, ↓ pH,
↑ temp, ↑ 2,3-DPG,
↑ attitude

↓ O₂ affinity, dump O₂
off at tissues sooner

• **Figure 5-1.** Hemoglobin-oxygen dissociation curve.

To determine whether a patient has a hypoproductive or hyperproductive anemia, one can measure the number of reticulocytes (immature blood cells) in the peripheral blood. An increased number of reticulocytes indicates hyperproduction of RBCs, while a normal or decreased number of reticulocytes means the bone marrow is not able to compensate. A useful classification of anemia is one based on the MCV (see Thumbnail, below).

Iron Deficiency Anemia

RC is diagnosed with anemia since her Hgb is less than normal. Her MCV of 76 fL indicates a microcytic anemia. Iron deficiency anemia, a microcytic type, is the most common form of anemia. Hence, when evaluating someone for a microcytic anemia, it is important to order iron studies. While the largest compartment of iron is found in Hgb (two thirds total body iron), it is also found in a storage compound, ferritin, located in almost every tissue of the body. **Ferritin** synthesis is controlled by the amount of iron in the body. **Transferrin,** a transport molecule, binds much of the iron in the serum and is also an important indicator of iron status. Unbound serum iron, transferrin, and ferritin are all important iron studies. In iron-deficient states, serum iron is low and ferritin is low (not much iron to store), while transferrin is high (the body is mobilizing any stored iron because it is deficient). Our patient's lab values fit these parameters of iron deficiency. A peripheral smear would likely reveal small **hypochromic** (pale) erythrocytes.

Iron deficiency can be caused by **increased requirements** of iron, as seen in growing children and pregnant women; **decreased iron absorption,** sometimes seen in patients after GI surgery; and, most commonly, **iron loss.** For premenopausal woman, menstrual blood loss is the most common cause. For men and postmenopausal women, blood loss from the GI tract is usually the cause.

Iron-deficient patients have the typical indications of anemia, including dizziness, fatigue, heart palpitations, shortness of breath with activity, and skin/mucous membrane pallor. Other complaints or findings related more specifically to the low iron state include headache, paresthesias, glossitis (red, swollen, smooth tongue), stomatitis (inflammation of the oral mucosa), angular cheilitis (fissures at the mouth angle), and koilonychia (spooning of the nails). Standard treatment for iron deficiency anemia is oral iron, usually ferrous sulfate. Up to 20% of patients have significant side effects such as nausea, abdominal pain, constipation, or diarrhea; therefore, the supplements are often given with meals. Steps to stop or decrease any bleeding are advisable. Intramuscular (IM) or IV administration of iron is used in extreme cases or when severe malabsorption impairs iron absorption.

Anemia of Chronic Disease

Anemia of chronic disease (ACD), the second most common type of anemia, is found in patients with chronic inflammatory, infectious, or neoplastic disorders. Systemic lupus erythematosus, rheumatoid arthritis, Crohn disease, osteomyelitis, tuberculosis, lymphoma, and solid tumors are all examples. ACD can appear as microcytic or normocytic. Impaired iron metabolism is a key feature of its etiology, namely impaired iron mobilization. Iron studies can distinguish it from iron deficiency. Hallmark findings of ACD are low serum iron despite normal to high ferritin (storage) levels. Treatment is directed at the underlying disease.

CASE CONCLUSION

The patient is treated with oral iron supplements given three times a day with meals. Because the likely source of her iron deficiency anemia is her heavy periods (menorrhagia), she is also begun on OCPs to decrease the monthly blood loss. Within 6 weeks, her Hgb has increased to 13.5 g/dL. She continues on iron supplementation once per day thereafter.

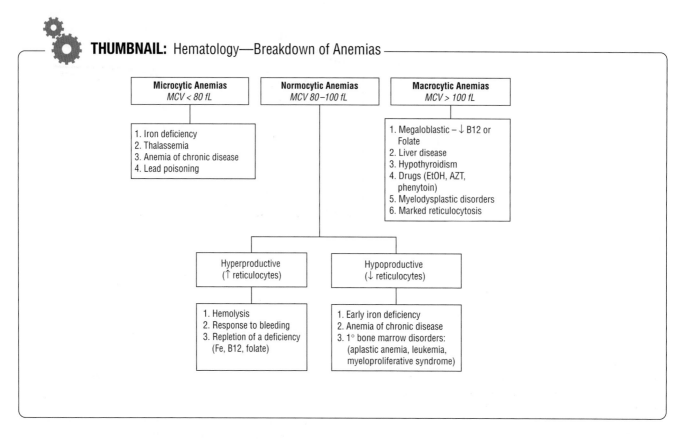

THUMBNAIL: Hematology—Breakdown of Anemias

| Microcytic Anemias
MCV < 80 fL | Normocytic Anemias
MCV 80–100 fL | Macrocytic Anemias
MCV > 100 fL |

Microcytic Anemias:
1. Iron deficiency
2. Thalassemia
3. Anemia of chronic disease
4. Lead poisoning

Macrocytic Anemias:
1. Megaloblastic – ↓ B12 or Folate
2. Liver disease
3. Hypothyroidism
4. Drugs (EtOH, AZT, phenytoin)
5. Myelodysplastic disorders
6. Marked reticulocytosis

Hyperproductive (↑ reticulocytes):
1. Hemolysis
2. Response to bleeding
3. Repletion of a deficiency (Fe, B12, folate)

Hypoproductive (↓ reticulocytes):
1. Early iron deficiency
2. Anemia of chronic disease
3. 1° bone marrow disorders: (aplastic anemia, leukemia, myeloproliferative syndrome)

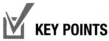

KEY POINTS

- RBCs contain Hgb molecules, each with four O_2-binding iron groups
- Hemoglobin-oxygen dissociation follows a sigmoidal curve
- Three general mechanisms for anemia: ↓ production, ↑ destruction, blood loss
- Iron deficiency is the most common type of anemia

- Iron deficiency lab values: ↑ transferrin, ↓ serum iron, ↓ ferritin, ↓ MCV (microcytic), small hypochromic cells on peripheral smear
- Blood loss is the most common cause of iron deficiency
- Anemia of chronic disease: ↓ transferrin, ↓ serum iron, ↑ or normal ferritin

QUESTIONS

1. A 78-year-old man comes to your office for a routine checkup. His medical history is significant for mild hypertension and hypercholesterolemia, for which he has been taking prescription medications for the last several years. He denies any alcohol or tobacco use, and describes his diet as "healthy." On physical exam you find an elderly, mildly cachectic ("wasted") man with pale conjunctiva. Lab tests reveal an Hct and iron studies consistent with iron deficiency anemia. His last Hct (1 year prior) was normal. What would you do next?

   A. A trial of iron and recheck Hct at next physical exam
   B. Repeat labs since the patient is asymptomatic
   C. Work up for occult GI bleed
   D. Bone marrow biopsy
   E. Hgb electrophoresis

2. A 58-year-old woman with a long history of iron deficiency anemia now presents with progressive dysphagia (difficulty swallowing), primarily with solid foods. On exam she has a swollen, painful, smooth-appearing tongue (glossitis) and spooning of her nails (koilonychia). Endoscopy reveals she has a large esophageal web, which has been obstructing food passage. Her most likely diagnosis is:

   A. Fanconi anemia
   B. Lead poisoning
   C. Esophageal cancer
   D. Plummer-Vinson syndrome
   E. Porphyria

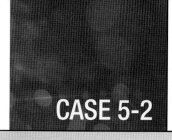

CASE 5-2 Macrocytic Anemia

HPI: PT, a 75-year-old man, comes to your clinic for a routine physical exam. His medical history is significant for mild hypertension, coronary artery disease, degenerative lumbar disc disease, and glaucoma. He denies alcohol or tobacco use and describes his diet as "good." (He cooks often with his wife and eats a variety of foods.)

PE: The patient is slightly overweight and has pale conjunctiva. There is a loss of vibratory sense in the bilateral upper and lower distal extremities and loss of proprioception bilaterally in the toes. These findings are new since last year's exam.

Labs: Hgb 11 g/dL, MCV 111 fL, peripheral blood smear: megaloblasts and hypersegmented neutrophils noted.

THOUGHT QUESTIONS

- What are the causes of macrocytic anemia?
- Why are folate and vitamin B12 important in the human diet?
- How are the clinical manifestations of folate and vitamin B12 deficiency similar? How are they different?
- What can you determine from a Shilling test?

BASIC SCIENCE REVIEW AND DISCUSSION

DNA synthesis is dependent on a derivative of folic acid, called tetrahydrofolate (H4 folate). The enzyme, **dihydrofolate reductase,** is responsible for converting folic acid to H4 folate (remember that the antibiotic trimethoprim and the chemotherapeutic agent methotrexate inhibit this enzyme).

The "folate" contained in dietary supplements is folic acid, but the "folate" in the unsupplemented human diet is a methylated H4 folate. The methyl group is transferred to homocysteine via a reaction that requires vitamin B12 as a coenzyme. This reaction yields methionine and the utilizable H4 folate.

The tissues with the highest turnover of cells (such as the hematopoietic system) have the highest requirement for folate and therefore rely heavily on dietary intake of both folate and vitamin B12. Deficiencies in either compound can result in a macrocytic anemia.

Folate Deficiency

Folate is found in all tissues of the body, and most of the excess storage occurs in the liver. Stores are limited; serum levels fall after 3 weeks of insufficient intake and anemia begins to occur after 4 to 5 months. Folate is found naturally in many fruits and vegetables (e.g., in asparagus, broccoli, spinach, bananas, melons), and in the United States grains and cereals are often supplemented. Folate is absorbed in the proximal jejunum and sometimes in the ileum after surgical resection of the jejunum.

Causes of folate deficiency include increased requirements (such as during pregnancy or after renal dialysis), decreased intake (often in alcoholics or in those who have poor diets), and decreased absorption (in patients with celiac sprue or regional enteritis or in those who have undergone extensive resection of their small intestine).

Clinical manifestations are those of a slowly developing anemia. Patients often do not have symptoms of anemia until their hemoglobin is very low. Other symptoms include glossitis (painful tongue) and mucositis (mouth sores) because mucosal cells also have high turnover. Folate deficiency in pregnant women can result in **neural tube defects** in the fetus; therefore, it is important to have sufficient folate prior to the onset of pregnancy.

Vitamin B12 Deficiency

Vitamin B12 (a derivative of **cobalamin**) is found only in foods of animal origin (meat, eggs, and dairy products). Similar to folate, vitamin B12 can also be found in cereals and grains due to supplementation. Unlike folate, the human body has plentiful stores of vitamin B12; deficiency only manifests itself after years of deficit. Absorption of vitamin B12 requires several steps. In the stomach, vitamin B12 is released from food and binds to transport proteins, which protect it from the acidic environment. In the duodenum, vitamin B12 is released from the protein complex and is bound by **intrinsic factor** (IF). IF is synthesized by parietal cells located in the stomach. The vitamin B12-IF complex is finally absorbed in the **distal ileum.**

Causes of vitamin B12 deficiency include increased requirements (occasionally in pregnancy), decreased intake (usually in strict vegetarians who exclude dairy products from their diet), and decreased absorption. Malabsorption of vitamin B12 can occur for several reasons. The most common cause of B12 deficiency is **pernicious anemia,** with a prevalence of 1% in the U.S. adult population. This is an autoimmune disease in which antibodies destroy gastric parietal cells, resulting in little or no IF production. Patients with stomach resection or distal ileum resection or disease (Crohn, Whipple) also have absorption difficulty. Infestation with the fish tapeworm *Diphyllobothrium latum* is a rare cause in the United States.

Clinical manifestations of vitamin B12 deficiency, like folate, are of a slowly developing anemia. Unique to vitamin B12 are **neurologic abnormalities,** which generally begin with paresthesias, loss of vibratory sense, and loss of proprioception (joint position sense). Findings can progress to gait ataxia, motor weakness, and altered mental state including dementia, depression, and even psychosis. Patients may present with neurologic deficits and no finding of anemia.

Lab Tests

Folate can be measured in the serum or in the red blood cells. RBC levels correlate better with long-term tissue levels. Vitamin B12 levels are usually measured in the serum. Both folate and vitamin B12 deficiencies are "hypoproductive" and have a low reticulocyte count. **Macrocytosis** means a high MCV (>100 fL). On the peripheral smear, RBCs with large immature nuclei (called megaloblasts) can be seen. (Remember, normal RBCs do not have nuclei). Anemias secondary to folate and vitamin B12

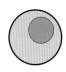

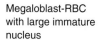

Megaloblast-RBC
with large immature
nucleus

Hypersegmented
neutrophil

• **Figure 5-2.** Peripheral blood smear findings in folate and vitamin B12 deficiencies.

deficiencies are sometimes called **"megaloblastic anemias."** One diagnostic finding on the smear is **hypersegmented neutrophils** with five or more lobes (Fig. 5-2).

The **Shilling test** is a nuclear medicine study specific for detecting vitamin B12 deficiency and its cause. The first step is to give radiolabeled vitamin B12 orally and unlabeled vitamin B12 by IM injection (the latter to saturate body stores). A 24-hour urine collection is then measured for radiolabeled vitamin B12 excretion. A less than normal excretion suggests that vitamin B12 is being malabsorbed. If this is the case, step 2 is performed. This is similar to step 1 with the addition of IF given with the oral radiolabeled vitamin B12. If urinary excretion improves (meaning absorption improved), pernicious anemia is diagnosed. If excretion remains low, other causes of malabsorption are considered.

Treatment

Folate deficiency is treated with oral supplements. Vitamin B12 is best given by IM injection, usually done monthly. It is important **not** to give folate to a patient with vitamin B12 deficiency. This may improve the anemia but can actually worsen the neurologic problems. Early diagnosis of vitamin B12 deficiency is extremely important, as chronic neurologic deficits (e.g., >1 year) are often irreversible despite treatment. Vitamin B12 levels should be checked in every patient with a suspected macrocytic anemia, even if folate levels are low.

Other Causes of Macrocytic Anemias

Liver disease can cause macrocytosis due to altered cholesterol metabolism, which results in RBC membrane changes. Patients with **myelodysplastic syndromes** can have a macrocytic anemia, as well as abnormal WBC and platelet formation. **Drugs** (such as alcohol, phenytoin, or zidovudine [AZT]) can cause macrocytosis, through interference with folate metabolism. **Hypothyroidism** is an additional cause; the mechanism is unknown.

CASE CONCLUSION

Additional labs: serum folate 7 ng/mL (normal 6–20); serum vitamin B12, 97 pg/mL (normal 140–800). The patient was sent for a Shilling test, which revealed normal vitamin B12 absorption with the addition of IF. The diagnosis of pernicious anemia was made. The patient was started on daily IM injections of cyanocobalamin (vitamin B12) for 1 week, then weekly injections for 1 month, and monthly injections for the remainder of his life. At 2 months, the patient had a normal hemoglobin count and improvement in his neurologic exam.

THUMBNAIL: Comparison of Folate and Vitamin B12 Deficiencies

	Folate	Vitamin B12
Biology	Involved directly in DNA synthesis (H4 folate) Limited tissue stores	Involved in reaction that converts natural dietary folate to an H4 folate **Plentiful tissue stores**
Clinical manifestations	Anemia symptoms, **neural tube defects** (in developing **fetus**)	Anemia symptoms, **neurologic deficits** (decreased vibratory and proprioceptive sense, ataxia, altered mental status)
Causes	• ↑ requirements (pregnancy, dialysis) • ↓ intake (alcoholism, poor diet) • ↓ absorption (jejunum—celiac sprue, regional enteritis)	• ↑ requirements (pregnancy) • ↓ intake (strict vegetarians) • ↓ absorption (gastric parietal cells produce **IF** needed for transport to the distal ileum) Pernicious anemia—parietal cells/IF Crohn, Whipple disease—ileum
Lab findings	Low serum or RBC folate level; macrocytic anemia, low reticulocyte count, megaloblasts, hypersegmented neutrophils	Low serum vitamin B12 level; macrocytic anemia, low reticulocyte count, megaloblasts, hypersegmented neutrophils, **possible abnormal Shilling test**
Treatment	**Daily oral** folate supplement	**Monthly IM** vitamin B12 (cyanocobalamin) injection

H4 folate = tetrahydrofolate

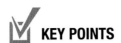

KEY POINTS

■ Folate and vitamin B12 deficiency are both common causes of macrocytic anemia

■ Pernicious anemia (autoantibodies induce atrophy of parietal cells/↓IF) is the most common cause of vitamin B12 deficiency

■ It is important not to give folate to a patient with vitamin B12 deficiency. This may worsen neurologic deficits, which may become irreversible.

■ Liver disease, myelodysplastic syndromes, drugs (alcohol), and hypothyroidism can all cause macrocytic anemias

QUESTIONS

1. A patient is referred to you for a Shilling test. Yesterday, an injection of nonradiolabeled B12 and an oral dose of radiolabeled B12 was administered. A 24-hour urine collection reveals abnormally low excretion of vitamin B12 today. What do you do next?

   A. Call the referring physician and suggest that this patient likely has a decreased dietary intake of B12 as the cause for his anemia.

   B. Call the referring physician and suggest that this patient likely has autoantibodies to his gastric cells as the cause for his anemia.

   C. Repeat the test and give radiolabeled B12 by injection and nonlabeled B12 orally.

   D. Repeat the test and give oral IF with the radiolabeled B12.

   E. Treat the patient with both B12 and folate.

2. An elderly woman is admitted to the hospital for pneumonia. On her admission labs it is noted that her Hgb is 9 g/dL and MCV is 106 fL. A serum folate level is ordered and is 2 ng/mL (normal 6–20). What do you do next to treat her anemia?

   A. Do nothing; her anemia will resolve with resolution of her pneumonia.

   B. Begin an oral folate supplement and continue with treatment of her pneumonia.

   C. Check a serum vitamin B12 level before treating her anemia.

   D. Do not check iron studies before treating her anemia. You already have a diagnosis.

   E. Supplement her diet with iron.

CASE 5-3 Thalassemia

HPI: NT is an 8-month-old boy of Italian parents who are recent immigrants from Sardinia. The baby has been crying frequently and often refuses to eat. He has not been febrile and has not had any symptoms of vomiting, diarrhea, or constipation. Upon questioning, the mother discloses she has had mild anemia since she was a child. The father has no known medical problems, and the patient has no siblings. The patient's birth was full term and uneventful.

PE: This pale baby has a slightly enlarged spleen and appears small for his age. The rest of the exam is unremarkable.

Labs: Hgb 5 g/dL (normal 10–13), the MCV is low. Peripheral blood smear reveals pale microcytic cells with variations in size and shape; a target cell is seen. Hgb electrophoresis reveals elevated Hgb F and Hgb A$_2$ and no Hgb A.

THOUGHT QUESTIONS

- What is the structure of hemoglobin?
- What is the pathophysiology of thalassemia?
- How do the syndromes of α- and β-thalassemia compare?

BASIC SCIENCE REVIEW AND DISCUSSION

In general, the Hgb tetramer found in RBCs is made up of two α-globin and two non-α-globin subunits. Normal adult hemoglobin (or Hgb A) is made up of two α-globin subunits and two β-globin subunits. A less abundant adult hemoglobin, Hgb A$_2$, is composed of two α-globin and two δ-globin chains and fetal hemoglobin, Hgb F, is composed of two α-globin and two γ-globin chains. The α and β genes are expressed on different chromosomes, although their production in normal adults is balanced. A group of genetic disorders that lead to *quantitative* abnormalities of Hgb subunit production are called **thalassemias,** which are causes of varying severities of anemia.

β-Thalassemia

β-Thalassemia is due to absent or diminished expression of β-globin genes. There is normally one β-chain gene located on each chromosome 11, for a total of two gene copies. With little or no β-chains to pair with, the α-chains (produced in normal amounts) remain unpaired, precipitate, and cause premature RBC destruction. Excess α-chains also precipitate in the bone marrow. The varying degree of disease severity depends on the number of abnormal genes inherited.

β-**Thalassemia major** (also known as "Cooley's anemia" or plain "thalassemia major") occurs when a person is homozygous for (or has inherited two copies of) the faulty β-gene. The disease becomes apparent approximately 6 months after birth when Hgb F production declines. At this time, a severe microcytic, hypochromic anemia begins, requiring lifelong transfusions. Lack of oxygen delivery to the tissues sends signals to the bone marrow to increase production of erythrocytes. The bone marrow is teeming with abnormal erythrocyte production, a process called "ineffective erythropoiesis." With time, the marrow cavities (skull bones, facial bones, and ribs) expand, leading to the classic facial or skull bone distortions in an untreated patient due to excessive extramedullary hematopoiesis. Erythrocytes that do enter the circulation are identified as abnormal by the reticuloendothelial system (spleen and liver) and are taken up by these organs with ensuing enormous hepatosplenomegaly. Life expectancy in these patients is approximately 30 to 40 years.

A much milder syndrome, β-**thalassemia minor,** caused by the inheritance of only one faulty β gene (heterozygosity), is characterized by mild anemia (or no anemia), microcytosis, hypochromia, target cells, and basophilic stippling. This can often be mistaken as iron deficiency anemia, but it is important to avoid unnecessary iron therapy in these patients (see Treatment, below). There is generally no effect on the lifespan of β-thalassemia minor patients. An intermediate form of β-thalassemia, appropriately named β-thalassemia intermedia, is caused by inheritance of β genes with reduced (not absent) synthesis of β-globin. β-Thalassemia is most prevalent where malaria is endemic (especially in Mediterranean populations). It is proposed that thalassemia and/or the gene abnormalities that cause it provide a protective mechanism against the parasitic infection and has been naturally selected for in these areas.

α-Thalassemia

There are two α-chain genes located on each chromosome 16, for a total of four gene copies. Deletion of one or more α-globin genes is the usual cause of α-thalassemia. In these syndromes, excess β-chains can form β-4 tetramers (Hgb H), which, similar to unpaired α-chains, precipitate in the RBC. **Hydrops fetalis** is due to loss of all four α genes and results in γ-4 tetramers called **Hgb Barts.** These infants are often stillborn due to CHF. Three missing genes results in **Hgb H disease,** characterized by acute hemolysis when a patient is exposed to oxidant-forming medications or infections. Oxidative reactions increase the precipitation of Hgb H and subsequent damage to RBCs. Two missing α genes (and two normal α genes) cause α-**thalassemia trait,** characterized by mild or no anemia and mild microcytosis. This should be distinguished from iron deficiency anemia to avoid unnecessary iron therapy.

Individuals with one missing α gene are phenotypically normal (silent carriers) but can pass the gene to offspring. α-Thalassemia gene frequencies are highest among southern Chinese, Southeast Asians, and Pacific Island populations. African and Mediterranean descendants also have increased gene frequencies.

Lab Tests

Iron studies can rule out the much more common microcytic anemia, iron deficiency. Hgb Barts (γ-4) can be quantified in umbilical cord blood and correlates with the amount of α-globin deficiency. β-Thalassemia can be detected by electrophoresis. Hgb A$_2$ and Hgb F are elevated since the excess α-chains can pair with δ- and γ-chains, respectively.

Genetic Counseling

The inheritance of thalassemia is **autosomal recessive** and follows mendelian principles. Afflicted individuals and couples from endemic areas should seek counseling to determine the risk of passing thalassemia genes to their offspring.

Treatment

No therapy is indicated for mild forms of thalassemia (β-thalassemia minor, α-thalassemia trait, and α silent carrier). These patients should avoid iron therapy, which can cause toxic iron buildup (hemosiderosis) that can damage the heart, liver, and pancreas (in these patients the body has a sufficient iron supply and is being signaled to absorb excess iron due to the perceived anemia). β-Thalassemia major and Hgb H disease require frequent transfusion therapy and iron chelation therapy to rid the body of excess iron. Bone marrow transplant has been successful in some β-thalassemia major patients.

CASE CONCLUSION

NT was diagnosed with β-thalassemia major. Both his parents are carriers of the β-thalassemia gene (which is why his mother had anemia and the father did not—both common presentations.) NT will continue regular blood transfusions and begin iron chelation therapy at around age 5, but will likely continue to have growth retardation and delayed sexual development. Unfortunately, it is unlikely he will make it past the fifth decade of his life.

THUMBNAIL: Thalassemia

β-Thalassemia	α-Thalassemia
1 β-chain gene = 2 inherited copies	2 α-chain genes = 4 inherited copies
Caused by absent or diminished expression of β-globin genes	Caused by deletion of one or more of the α-globin genes
2 main syndromes: β°/β°—β-thalassemia major (chronic anemia, splenomegaly, bone distortions, hemosiderosis, ↑ Hgb F) β/β°—β-thalassemia minor (mild or no microcytic anemia)	4 main syndromes: 4 missing genes—hydrops fetalis (incompatible with life) 3 missing genes—Hgb H disease (acute hemolysis 2° to oxidative insult) 2 missing genes—α-thalassemia trait (mild or no microcytic anemia) 1 missing gene—α-thalassemia silent carrier (asymptomatic)

β, normal allele; β°, mutant allele

KEY POINTS

- Thalassemia is a heterogeneous group of genetic disorders that lead to *quantitative* abnormalities of Hgb subunit production
- β-Thalassemia is more common than α-thalassemia (especially in Mediterranean origins)
- Avoid iron therapy in thalassemia patients, which can cause toxic iron buildup

---

QUESTIONS

1. An African American couple would like to have children. Both individuals are silent carriers of α-thalassemia (- α/α α). You are asked to provide them with genetic counseling. What percent of offspring would you predict to also be silent carriers?

   A. 0%
   B. 25%
   C. 50%
   D. 67%
   E. 100%

2. If the frequency of the β-thalassemia major disease is 1/1600, what is the probability that a person in the general population (asymptomatic and no family history) is heterozygous for a mutant β-thalassemia allele?

   A. 1/1600
   B. 1/800
   C. 1/40
   D. 1/20
   E. 2/3

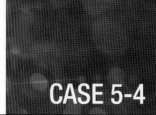

CASE 5-4 Transfusion Reaction

HPI: A 61-year-old man with CAD and HTN underwent a coronary artery bypass graft (CABG) procedure. Before the operation the surgeon ordered four units of packed RBCs to be cross-matched to the patient's type A, Rh negative blood. The patient required three units during the surgery. The patient had an uneventful recovery until the fifth postoperative day, at which time his Hgb dropped from 15 to 8 g/dL. The patient appeared jaundiced and spiked a temperature of 39.1°C; his urine appeared "tea-colored." As part of a work-up for a suspected hemolytic anemia, a direct Coombs test was ordered.

THOUGHT QUESTIONS

- What are blood groups and why are they important in transfusion medicine?
- What is an indirect Coombs test, and what other tests are used to match transfusion products?
- What are some common transfusion reactions?

BASIC SCIENCE REVIEW AND DISCUSSION

Blood Groups

The major **blood types, A, B, O,** and **AB,** are based on the presence or absence of carbohydrate antigens on the RBC surface. Type A blood has the "A" antigen, type B blood has "B" antigen, type AB has both antigens, and individuals with type O blood have neither of these antigens. Individuals have "naturally" occurring antibodies in their serum (stimulated by the environment) directed against the AB antigen(s) that are not found on their red cells. For example, a person who has type B blood has anti-A in her plasma. These antibodies are usually IgM, which react at room temperature, bind complement, but do not cross the placenta. IgG forms of anti-A and anti-B are produced when individuals are exposed to red cells by pregnancy or transfusion.

The presence of the AB antigens on the surface of the red cell and the presence of AB antibodies in the plasma dictates what blood products can be safely transfused. Red cell products must be transfused only to recipients who lack the corresponding AB antibody in their plasma. Plasma products containing AB antibodies must be transfused only to recipients who lack the corresponding antigen on their red cell membranes. Since group O individuals lack any A or B antigens on their red cells, they are considered **universal blood donors.** Group AB individuals are **universal plasma donors,** as they lack AB antibodies.

Another type of blood grouping is the **Rh** system. Of the numerous antigens in the Rh system, the D antigen is the most important. Rh-positive blood denotes the presence of the D antigen on the red cells of an individual's blood. The D antigen is strongly immunogenic, and anti-D (anti-Rh) antibodies are the leading cause of **hemolytic disease of the newborn.** When an Rh-negative pregnant woman carries an Rh-positive fetus, small amounts of D-positive red cells can enter her circulation. Her body can then produce anti-D IgG antibodies. If she becomes pregnant in the future with an Rh-positive fetus, the antibodies can cross the placenta and attack the red cells of the fetus. Rh-negative pregnant women are given a small amount of Rh immunoglobulin (anti-D), RhoGAM, which prevents their own formation of anti-D antibodies.

More than 600 red cell antigens are known, but only a small amount are considered clinically significant (capable of stimulating IgG antibodies) and may cause hemolytic transfusion reactions. Some examples are Kell, Duffy, or Kidd antigens.

Blood Testing

When a patient requires a blood transfusion, there are several tests that are done to find a compatible match in the blood bank. First, the patient's red cells are tested for the presence of A, B, and D antigens (blood typing). Next, an antibody screen (also known as an **indirect Coombs test**) is performed by mixing a patient's serum with reagent red cells with known antigens (Fig. 5-3). If the patient has serum antibodies directed against any of the red cell antigens, the specimen will agglutinate (clump) after antiglobulin is added. Another test is the **direct Coombs test,** during which the patient's RBCs are mixed directly with antiglobulin (Fig. 5-4). Patients with delayed hemolytic transfusion reactions or with autoimmune hemolytic anemias have red cells coated with antibodies that agglutinate, yielding a positive reaction.

Transfusion Reactions

Reactions to blood transfusions do occur and can even result in death. Reactions can be acute (immediate) or delayed, occurring days or weeks after transfusion. **Febrile nonhemolytic transfusion reactions (FNHTRs)** are one of the most common acute transfusion events. The patient often experiences chills, rigors, and a temperature increase of 1°C or more during or after the transfusion. This reaction is due to pyrogenic cytokines (IL-6 or TNF) that are stimulated in the recipient by leukocytes in the transfused product or that have already been produced in the transfusion product during storage. Most patients are pretreated with an antipyretic (e.g., acetaminophen) to avoid this reaction.

A **hemolytic transfusion reaction,** a less common but more serious transfusion reaction, also causes fever. These reactions can be acute or delayed. Acute hemolytic transfusion reactions occur most commonly when ABO incompatible blood is transfused. The most common cause is human error in matching identification of the patient and appropriate blood product! Antibodies in the patient's serum react with antigens on the transfused cells and complement-mediated **intravascular hemolysis** occurs. Along with fever, patients may have chills, chest pain, hypotension, and diffuse bleeding. Renal failure, shock, and DIC can follow. This is an extremely serious reaction, as death occurs in 10 to 40% of cases. Delayed reactions occur when a person is sensitized during a previous transfusion but has undetectable antibodies on pretransfusion testing. Several days to weeks after the second transfusion, the patient produces more antibodies, which coat the surface of the transfused cells. Presenting symptoms are fever, anemia, and jaundice due to **extravascular hemolysis** as the

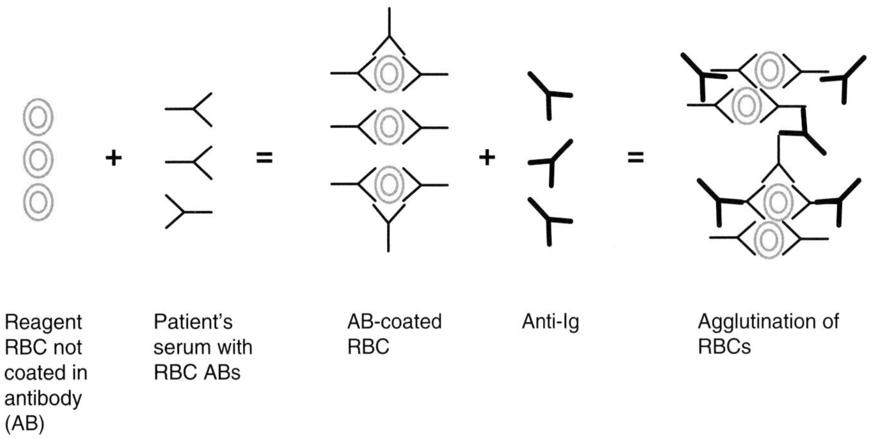

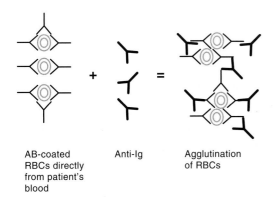

• **Figure 5-3.** Indirect Coombs test.

Reagent
RBC not
coated in
antibody
(AB)

Patient's
serum with
RBC ABs

AB-coated
RBC

Anti-Ig

Agglutination of
RBCs

AB-coated
RBCs directly
from patient's
blood

Anti-Ig

Agglutination
of RBCs

• **Figure 5-4.** Direct Coombs test.

antibody-coated RBCs are removed in the spleen. A direct Coombs test is often positive. These reactions may go undetected due to their delayed nature. Treatment includes a procedure, called *elution*, that removes antibodies from the surface of the red cells.

Another common reaction is an **allergic transfusion reaction,** occurring in 1 to 3% of all transfusion recipients. These are mediated by preformed IgE in the recipient to some transfused allergen. Hives and pruritus are common, but reactions can progress to bronchospasm, hypotension, and anaphylaxis. Treatment is with antihistamines, which are often given to all patients before a transfusion to prevent this event.

CASE CONCLUSION

The direct Coombs test was positive. According to the patient's records, he had been transfused two units of RBCs the previous year for his first CABG procedure. A formal investigation of a suspected transfusion reaction was performed. There was no evidence of clerical or laboratory error. The pretest direct Coombs test of the transfused blood was negative. As a part of the patient's treatment, an elution was performed and the antibodies were then identified in the laboratory as JKb, a Kidd antigen. It was determined that the patient underwent a delayed hemolytic transfusion reaction. He was sensitized to the Kidd antigen during the previous transfusion, but his antibody titer was too low to be detected on pretransfusion testing. The patient was given further supportive care and was discharged from the hospital on day 9. It was noted in his records that all future transfusion products be screened for this antigen and avoided.

THUMBNAIL: ABO Blood Group Antigens, Antibodies, and Compatibility

Group	ABO Antigens of Red Cells	Compatibility of Red Cells	Antibodies in Plasma	Compatibility of Plasma
O	None	Transfuse to all patients (*universal donor*)	Anti-A Anti-B	O patients only
A	A	A and AB only	Anti-B	A or O
B	B	B and AB only	Anti-A	B or O
AB	A and B	AB only	None	Transfuse to all patients (*universal donor*)

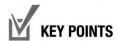

KEY POINTS

- ABO blood types are based on red cell antigens. Patients receiving blood products from another person must have a compatible blood type.

- An antibody screen (also known as an indirect Coombs test) is performed by mixing a patient's serum with reagent red cells with known antigens to determine which RBC antibodies are present in the patient's serum

- A direct Coombs test detects the presence of preformed antibody-coated RBCs in the patient's blood and can be positive in autoimmune hemolysis and delayed transfusion reaction

- Hemolytic disease of the newborn occurs when Rh-negative mothers are sensitized by Rh-positive babies. If pregnant with a subsequent Rh-positive child, Anti-D (Rh) antibodies can cross the placenta and attack the newborn's RBCs. RhoGAM is given early to prevent this occurrence.

- Acute hemolytic transfusion reaction is caused by direct ABO incompatibility. Delayed hemolytic transfusion reactions can be caused by antibody sensitization during pregnancy or prior transfusions.

- Allergic transfusion reactions, mediated by IgE, can cause hives and, in severe cases, shock and anaphylaxis

QUESTIONS

1. Which of the following correctly describes how a direct Coombs test is performed?

   A. The patient's serum is mixed with test RBCs and agglutination is measured.

   B. The patient's serum is mixed with mouse RBCs and agglutination is measured.

   C. The patient's RBCs are mixed with anti-human immunoglobulin/complement mouse antibodies and agglutination is measured.

   D. The patient's RBCs are mixed with anti-mouse immunoglobulin/complement human antibodies and agglutination is measured.

2. Which of the following statements is correct regarding Rh immunoglobulin (RhoGAM)?

   A. It prevents the production of anti-D antibodies.

   B. It is given to all Rh-positive pregnant women at the time of delivery.

   C. It blocks IgM antibodies from crossing the placenta.

   D. It can trigger hemolytic disease of the newborn in some patients.

CASE 5-5 Coagulation Cascade

HPI: HK is an 18-month-old boy who presents with a painful left knee. His father relates that the child had large bruises following the immunizations at 15 months. He also states that someone in his wife's family, possibly the wife's father, had a similar history of "easy bruising" as a child.

PMH: Increased bleeding postcircumcision.

PE: Warm, tender, and swollen left knee with decreased muscle size in left quadriceps in comparison to right quadriceps. Remainder of physical exam is normal.

Labs: Plt (normal) 330,000/dL; PTT (high) 80 seconds; PT (normal) 12 seconds.

THOUGHT QUESTIONS

- What diagnostic considerations are most likely based on the patient's presentation and bleeding times?
- What is the inheritance pattern and variable expression of this disorder?
- How should this patient be treated and managed to prevent recurrent episodes?
- What infectious organisms are possible complications of treatment?

BASIC SCIENCE REVIEW AND DISCUSSION

Patients with coagulation disorders may present with one of two general symptom profiles. Patients who have a **platelet disorder** present with **mucosal bleeding** (e.g., gums, nosebleeds), **ecchymoses**, as well as **purpural and petechial rashes**. Those with **deficient clotting factors** present more commonly with **hemarthroses, bleeding into soft tissue or muscle, or increased bleeding after trauma or surgery** (Table 5-1).

Coagulation Cascade

For proper blood coagulation to occur, soluble plasma fibrinogen must be converted to fibrin. A deficiency in fibrin or more commonly an inability to convert fibrinogen to fibrin prevents normal fibrin function. Therefore, the primary platelet plug is not encapsulated and will not form a stable hemostatic clot. The process of activating fibrin requires a functional coagulation cascade. Each factor, except factor XIII, is a **serine protease**, which activates the following reaction in the cascade. The activated form of the factor is represented with a lowercase *a*. In the classic view, the intrinsic and extrinsic pathways converge in the common pathway (Fig. 5-5).

Modeling the extrinsic and intrinsic pathways allows the use of prothrombin time (PT), partial thromboplastin time (PTT), and thrombin time (TT) in diagnosing coagulation disorders; however, in vivo the model is not accurate. The modified view is currently most representative of the clotting pathway within the human body.

The modified pathway links the extrinsic and intrinsic through VIIa's activation of IX. This allows two means of activating X. This is necessary due to an in vivo inhibitor of VIIa and tissue factor—tissue factor pathway inhibitor (TFPI). Increased thrombin is then dependent on IXa activating X. This explains the bleeding seen in patients with hemophilia A despite a normal PT. This model also accounts for the bleeding seen in a small number of patients deficient in factor XI (Fig. 5-6).

Hemophilia

A diagnosis of moderate or severe **hemophilia** is the most likely consideration in this case due to the patient's labs (increased PTT with normal [nl] PT and nl platelet count), the clinical presentation (bleeding postcircumcision and recurrent joint bleeds with increased activity), and the described inheritance pattern (**X-linked recessive**). Hemophilia A is five times more common than hemophilia B; however, both are inherited in the same pattern.

Hemophilia A is the most common form of a factor deficiency. While the majority of patients inherit the disease, 33% of cases result from random mutation of the *FVIII* gene on the long arm of the X chromosome. Variable amounts of viable protein are produced in affected individuals, which are grouped as mild, moderate, or severe. Mild hemophiliacs (5–20% coagulation factor activity compared with normal expression) present with bleeding posttrauma. Moderate hemophiliacs (1–5%) bleed posttrauma, and occasionally spontaneously. Severe hemophiliacs (<1%) present with frequent spontaneous bleeding episodes and are likely to develop joint deformities, which can be crippling if not properly treated. While it is unusual for females to develop the disease due to its pattern of inheritance, carrier females may present with bleeding following severe trauma. Most carriers express 50 to 70% normal FVIII levels.

Treatment of hemophilia A or B is determined by the level of factor that is functionally produced by the patient. Patients are advised on limiting physical activity and contact sports. Families are also routinely screened to determine if the mother is a carrier and if future children should be tested during pregnancy. Severe hemophiliacs require a prophylactic regimen of FVIII transfusions to prevent spontaneous bleeding, yet mild hemophiliacs require replacement therapy only for surgeries or following trauma. Mild hemophiliacs may also show benefit with **deamino-8-D-arginine vasopressin (DDAVP)** (desmopressin) treatment. DDAVP causes a transient rise in FVIII levels by triggering its release from endothelial cells. Currently, FVIII replacement therapy uses recombinant FVIII and immunopurified FVIII, which has greatly reduced the degree of infectious diseases spread by blood products. During the 1980s, over 50% of hemophiliacs contracted **HIV** through blood transfusions. Prior to the surge in HIV among hemophiliacs, the incidence of hepatitis C was on the rise as well. Both of these have caused AIDS, chronic hepatitis, and cirrhosis to be among the leading causes of death among severe hemophiliacs.

TABLE 5-1 Comparison of Bleeding Disorders

Patient Presentation	Category	Most Common Diagnoses
Spontaneous mucosal bleeding; nonpalpable purpuric rash and ecchymoses	Platelet disorder	Qualitative platelet disorder—*von Willebrand disease, Bernard-Soulier syndrome, Glanzmann thrombasthenia, storage pool diseases* Reduced platelet count—*thrombocytopenias*
Hemarthrosis with muscle and joint involvement, spontaneous or post minor trauma; prolonged bleeding following surgery	Clotting factor deficiency	*Hemophilia A* (factor VIII deficiency), *hemophilia B* (factor IX deficiency)

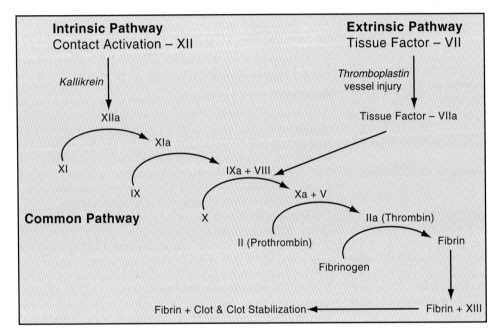

Figure 5-5. Coagulation cascade.

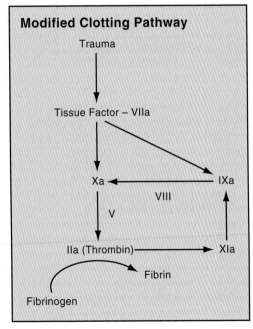

Figure 5-6. Modified clotting pathway.

CASE CONCLUSION

HK was admitted to the hematology day clinic and transfused with recombinant FVIII to 30% correction. The hemarthroses of the left knee were treated symptomatically with elevation and ice. Additional labs showed a 0% production of FVIII protein, and HK was diagnosed with severe hemophilia A. A follow-up visit was scheduled to discuss prophylactic treatment and to screen.

HK's mother and sisters undergo genetic testing by restriction fragment length polymorphism (RFLP) analysis to determine their carrier status.

THUMBNAIL: Hematology—Lab Tests of Coagulation

PT and **PTT** are common laboratory measures of a patient's intrinsic and extrinsic clotting pathways. PT may be expressed as international normalized ratio (INR), which is the ratio of a patient's PT over the normal PT. **TT** is a third, less commonly used, measure of the coagulation cascade.

Laboratory Value	Potential Deficiency	Most Common Diagnoses
TT nl 14–16 seconds	Fibrinogen—deficient or abnormal Inhibition of thrombin	*DIC* Heparin therapy
PT nl 10–14 seconds, a measure of extrinsic pathway function	Deficiency or abnormality in one or multiple of factors II, V, **VII**, X, and fibrinogen	*Liver disease* *warfarin therapy* DIC
PTT nl 30–40 seconds, a measure of intrinsic pathway function	Deficiency or abnormality in one or multiple of factors II, V, **VIII**, **IX**, X, XII, and fibrinogen	*Hemophilia A* (VIII) *Hemophilia B* (Christmas disease, IX) *Heparin therapy* Warfarin therapy DIC

Factor XIII is not assessed by either PT or PTT. For this reason, a patient with nl PT and PTT yet recurrent bleeding episodes is suspect for a factor XIII deficiency.

Factor XII and, in most cases, **factor XI**, deficiencies show increased PTT but no increased bleeding clinically.

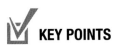

KEY POINTS

- The most common factor deficiency leading to increased bleeding is hemophilia A, FVIII
- Both *FVIII* and *FIX* genes are located on the long arm of the X chromosome with an X-linked recessive inheritance pattern
- PT and PTT provide an in vitro assessment of the factors involved in the extrinsic and intrinsic pathways, respectively
- Platelet disorders present clinically as mucosal bleeding, ecchymoses, and purpural and petechial rashes
- Clotting factor deficiencies present clinically as hemarthroses, bleeding into soft tissue or muscle, and bleeding posttrauma or after surgery

QUESTIONS

1. Elective surgery is scheduled for a 14-year-old boy with no history of bleeding problems. During routine labs an elevated PTT is found and determined to be a deficiency in FXII. The patient's PT, platelet count, and all other labs are normal. The family consults you to determine if the surgery should be performed. The most appropriate action is which of the following?

   A. Cancel the surgery and determine if replacement therapy is needed.
   B. Reassure the family and proceed as planned.
   C. Perform the surgery only after infusing purified FXII.
   D. Cancel the surgery and reorder labs including PTT, PT, and TT.
   E. Perform the surgery after vitamin K supplements and fibrinogen IV are given.

2. Which of the following regarding FVIII deficiency is true?

   A. PT is prolonged.
   B. Vitamin K administration is adequate treatment to prevent bleeding.

   C. It is less common than FIX deficiency.
   D. Girls are affected more commonly than boys.
   E. Severe hemophiliacs should be placed on prophylactic therapy despite the risk of HIV transmission.

3. A 22-year-old man is brought to the ED following a gang fight. Two deep lacerations are observed in the LRQ of his abdomen. The lacerations are bleeding profusely despite applied pressure for 20 minutes. Diffuse swelling, erythema, and rubor are noted in his right ankle and left knee. The patient is unresponsive. An astute medical student notices a medical alert bracelet among the pile of the patient's belongings. It indicates the patient has mild hemophilia A. The expected labs and treatment plan are which of the following?

   A. Normal PT, prolonged PTT; treatment with recombinant FVIII
   B. Normal PT, prolonged PTT; treatment with recombinant FIX
   C. Prolonged PT, normal PTT; treatment with recombinant FVIII

D. Prolonged PT, normal PTT; treatment with recombinant FIX

E. Prolonged PT, prolonged PTT; treatment with recombinant FVIII

4. A 4-year-old boy presents with recurrent bleeding into soft tissue and muscle. Some rib fractures are noted in the child's chart. At the prior visits, PT, PTT, and TT were tested. All normal results were reported consistently, except for a transient period as an infant during which PT and PTT were slightly elevated. During this visit the father is concerned since the child's bruising has continued. The physician identifies symmetric bruising along the child's midaxillary line. X-ray of the ribs indicates new rib fractures overlaid on healing fractures. His PT, PTT, and TT are currently normal. The next step in working this child's case up is which of the following?

A. Reorder PT, PTT, and TT.

B. Order a von Willebrand factor count including multimers and ristocetin.

C. Check the platelet count.

D. Check vitamin K levels.

E. Contact Child Protective Services and the team's social worker on call.

CASE 5-6 Cells of Innate Immunity

HPI: AA is a 68-year-old African American man who presents with 3 weeks of gradually worsening **fatigue, epistaxis,** and **nonhealing oral lesions.** He noticed increasing **dyspnea on exertion** with his daily 1-mile walks and now can, at most, walk around the house. His epistaxis has occurred daily and is now becoming increasingly difficult to stop. He also notes **increased bruising** to minor trauma. He developed multiple oral ulcers 1 week ago, which have not improved since. Prior to this, he had had an upper respiratory infection after visiting his granddaughter, who was sick with a fever and rash. His past medical history is significant for a recent history of **hepatitis with negative serologies,** and thus presumed to be due to alcohol, although he denies heavy alcohol use. His family history is significant for **sickle cell anemia,** although he has never had symptoms suggestive of this disease nor has he been evaluated for it. He worked for a **petroleum** company for 40 years and is now retired.

PE: T 37.6°C; HR **109** beats/min; BP 135/65 mm Hg; RR **36** breaths/min; SaO$_2$ 99% at room air.

The patient is a thin, ill-appearing man in mild respiratory distress during exertion. His physical exam is significant for **scleral pallor,** dried blood in his nares, **mucosal petechiae,** multiple buccal and labial **aphthous ulcers,** and **diffuse ecchymoses** on his upper and lower extremities with no evidence of bone tenderness. His cardiovascular and abdominal exams are benign; he has no organomegaly.

Labs: WBC 3500/μL, absolute neutrophil count 358/μL, monocytes 1%, lymphocyte 25%, Hct 26%, MCV 105 fL, Plt 85,000/μL. *Peripheral blood smear* revealed **large RBCs, few platelets and granulocytes,** with **rare hyperlobulated neutrophils.** *Bone marrow biopsy* produced a **pale and dilute aspirate,** which microscopically appeared **fatty** with **less than 20% cellularity,** consisting of a few red cells, lymphocytes, and scant megakaryocytes. Blood cultures were negative for bacteria.

THOUGHT QUESTIONS

- What are the basic functions of WBCs?
- What are the causes of pancytopenia? How are these diagnosed?
- What are the clinical features of pancytopenia? How is pancytopenia treated?

BASIC SCIENCE REVIEW AND DISCUSSION

The leukocytes of the **innate immune system** rely on the non-specific recognition of **pathogen-associated molecular patterns (PAMPs),** molecular structures commonly expressed by many microorganisms in order to carry out their multiple functions. This recognition activates various mechanisms of pathogen elimination, including phagocytosis, cell killing, and recruitment of other leukocytes that have their own roles in amplifying, refining, or suppressing the immune response (Table 5-2).

Pancytopenia is defined as a decrease in circulating mature blood cells, leading to the characteristic *leukopenia, anemia,* and *thrombocytopenia.* In the simplest terms, it results from some insult leading to a dynamic abnormality in blood cell production, distribution, usage, and survival. Such abnormalities may occur in two compartments, either within the bone marrow or in peripheral circulation. An insult may cause enough damage to hematopoietic stem cells that their numbers no longer adequately support the body's requirements. In **aplastic anemia,** pancytopenia is accompanied by a marked reduction of all hematopoietic precursors in the bone marrow. Alternatively, damage may result in cytogenetic abnormalities that simply *impair* cell proliferation and differentiation, and thus prevent adequate replenishment of circulating blood cells, as found in **myelodysplastic syndromes (MDSs).** Abnormal bone marrow cell replacement may also occur with **myelophthisic diseases,** wherein fibroblasts are stimulated to lay down collagenous material in the bone marrow, thereby crowding out normal hematopoietic cells and causing abnormal

release of immature cells. Three possible categories of bone marrow histopathology can result, as shown in Table 5-3.

The main clinical features of pancytopenia are those associated with anemia, thrombocytopenia, and neutropenia. Physical exam findings include petechiae, ecchymoses, retinal hemorrhage, and skin and mucosal pallor. Pelvic and rectal exams may reveal cervical bleeding or blood in the stool. Hepatosplenomegaly may also be present as a sign of extramedullary hematopoiesis when the bone marrow is unable to meet the body's requirements. Often, the etiology of pancytopenia is suggested by history. In **aplastic anemia,** in which pancytopenia arises from the destruction of hematopoietic precursors, a blood smear reveals *normal-appearing cells but in markedly reduced numbers,* with evidence of compensatory RBC production. In **MDS** in which there is abnormal cell proliferation and differentiation, a blood smear would reveal a distinct population of large RBCs along with *abnormal-appearing and hypofunctioning platelets and neutrophils.* Other causes of pancytopenia with cellular bone marrow must be ruled out, such as severe malnutrition, B12 or folate deficiency, drug reaction, and infection wherein aplasia is transient or reversible. In **myelophthisic disease,** the peripheral smear reveals cell morphologies consistent with **disturbances in the blood-bone marrow barrier** where mature and immature WBCs, RBCs, and platelets are abnormally released into circulation. Circulating red cells are nucleated or **teardrop-shaped;** WBCs include myeloid precursors; platelets are elevated and giant in size.

Bone marrow studies provide definitive diagnosis. In aplastic anemia, bone marrow destruction results in a dilute, fatty, and grossly pale aspirate that is **hypocellular with less than 20% cellularity.** In MDS, the bone marrow is normal or hypercellular with **dysplastic morphologies,** including RBCs with **ringed sideroblasts,** hypogranulated and hyposegmented myeloblasts, and poorly nucleated megakaryocytes. Lastly, myelophthisic disease is characterized by a "dry tap," wherein no aspirate can be produced. The presence of granulomas suggests an infectious etiology. Treatable causes such as tuberculosis and fungus must be ruled out.

TABLE 5-2 Review of White Blood Cells of the Innate Immune System

Cell Type	Characteristics and Functions
Neutrophils (PMNs)	• **Primary phagocyte of the innate immune system;** recognizes PAMPs; have no class II MHC proteins for antigen presentation • Can better recognize and phagocytose pathogens opsonized with immunoglobulin and complement component C3b via Fc surface receptors
Eosinophils	• **Parasite recognition**—leukocyte with *red-staining cytoplasmic granules* that recognize and *attack large extracellular pathogens* (e.g., parasites) • Recognize parasites opsonized with IgE via the Fcε receptor, which activates degranulation of vesicles containing lytic enzymes • **Parasite killing**—lytic enzymes, including *major basic protein*, are released extracellularly to attack pathogen membranes; may also cause local tissue damage • **Immediate hypersensitivity reactions** (e.g., asthma)—eosinophil granules contain *histaminase,* which degrades histamine, a mediator of allergic reactions • Recruited and activated by T$_H$2 **helper cells** via cytokines **IL-4** and **IL-5**
Basophils and mast cells	• **Basophils,** leukocytes with *blue-staining cytoplasmic granules* • **Mast cells** are functionally similar to basophils but *reside in tissue*, e.g., skin, mucosa, and have *receptors with bound IgE* that recognize certain allergens • **Immediate hypersensitivity reaction**—releases histamine (which increases vascular permeability, smooth muscle contraction, and glandular secretion), adenosine (activates masts cells, inhibits platelet aggregation), SRS-A, ECF-A, etc. • Both have **Fcε receptor,** which binds IgE-opsonized allergens → induces degranulation of cells, which initiates inflammatory reaction • Massive degranulation can lead to severe reaction such as **anaphylaxis** • Late-phase response involves recruitment of other leukocytes
Macrophages/monocytes	• Monocytes are circulating leukocytes, while macrophages are monocytes that have migrated to an extravascular site like lymph nodes, spleen, bone marrow, etc. • **Phagocytosis** of bacteria, viruses, and other *small* foreign particles via Fc receptors that recognize immunoglobulins opsonizing foreign antigen; eliminates tumor cells • **Antigen presentation**—ingested foreign particles are processed and fragments are bound to class II MHC on macrophages for antigen presentation to T cells, activating the adaptive immune response • **Cytokine production**—released **IL-1, IL-6, IL-10,** and **TNF-α** mediate several aspects of the inflammatory reaction
Dendritic cell or Langerhans cells *(when associated with skin or mucosa)*	• Lymphoid/myeloid-derived cells important in both innate and adaptive immunity • **Innate immunity**—recognize bacterial PAMPs, which bind dendritic cell TLR → up-regulate class II MHC and coreceptor expression → enhance antigen presentation and cytokine production → promote adaptive immune response • **Antigen presentation**—most important function; has both class I and II MHC • **Cytokine production**—produces **IFN-α** in response to viral infections → *activates NK cells* to kill virally infected cells; *recruits T and B cells*
NK cells	• **Nonimmune cytotoxic killing**—recognize reduced expression of class I MHC and stress-induced protein expression on the cell surface of virally infected cells, cancer cells, as well as foreign cells; *does not require prior exposure to target* • Kills via **perforins** and **granzymes,** inducing *apoptosis* of targeted cell

PMN, polymorphonuclear cell; *PAMP,* pathogen-associated molecular patterns; *Fc,* constant fragment of antibody; *IL,* interleukin; *SRS-A,* slow-reacting substance of anaphylaxis; *ECF-A,* eosinophil chemotactic factor of anaphylaxis; *TNF,* tumor necrosis factor; *MHC,* major histocompatibility complex; *TLR,* toll-like receptor; *IFN,* interferon; *NK,* natural killer; *APC,* antigen-presenting cell

CASE CONCLUSION

AA is diagnosed with a pancytopenia with apparent hypocellular bone marrow suggestive of bone marrow failure. He is thus treated with supportive care, prophylactic antibiotics, fluids, packed RBCs, and platelet transfusions. This is followed up with GM-CSF therapy to support bone marrow regrowth.

TABLE 5-3 Causes of Pancytopenia by Bone Marrow Histopathology

Hypocellular Bone Marrow	Cellular Bone Marrow	Bone Marrow Fibrosis
Acquired aplastic anemia: • Idiopathic (>80% of cases) • Toxic exposure—radiation, chemotherapy, benzene (in petroleum) • Drugs—chloramphenicol, carbamazepine, cimetidine • Viruses—EBV, non-A/B/C hepatitis, CMV, B19 *Inherited aplastic anemia:* • Fanconi anemia *Immune diseases:* • Transfusion—GVHD • PNH *Pregnancy*	*Myelodysplastic syndromes* • Radiation, benzene • Late toxicity of chemotherapy/radiation therapy *Substrate deficiencies:* • Megaloblastic anemia • Anorexia nervosa, starvation *Other bone marrow diseases:* • Chronic leukemia/lymphoma • Metastatic bony infiltration usage: *Overwhelming infection* *Sequestration:* hypersplenism *Nonspecific toxicity:* alcohol *Immune disease:* PNH, SLE	*Primary myelofibrosis* • Myelofibrosis with myeloid metaplasia *Secondary myelofibrosis* (myelophthisis) • Mycobacterial infection • Fungal infection • HIV • Sarcoidosis • Radiation therapy • Gaucher disease • Chronic leukemia/lymphoma

EBV, Epstein-Barr virus; CMV, cytomegalovirus; B19, parvovirus B19; GVHD, graft-versus-host disease; PNH, paroxysmal nocturnal hemoglobinuria; SLE, systemic lupus erythematosus; HIV, human immunodeficiency virus

THUMBNAIL: Hematology—Pancytopenia

	Aplastic Anemia	Myelodysplastic Syndrome	Myelophthisic Anemias
Pathophysiology	*Destruction* of bone marrow stem cells, causing insufficient production of circulating blood cells	*Damage* to stem cells causing *abnormal* proliferation and differentiation → release of hypofunctioning blood cells	Bone marrow fibrosis → replacement of normal cells and disturbance of blood-bone marrow barrier → release of premature and abnormally shaped cells
Etiology	Idiopathic (80%) Viruses Environmental exposures Chemotherapy/radiation Drugs Congenital disease Autoimmune disease Pregnancy	Environmental exposures Chemotherapy/radiation *Rule out:* Nutritional deficiencies Overwhelming infection Hypersplenism Myeloproliferative disease	Primary hematologic disease Metastatic tumor in bone marrow Infection Infiltrative disease Radiation therapy
Epidemiology	Biphasic age distribution: young and elderly	Elderly, mean age 68 years Male > female	Adults >50 years old
History	Abrupt or insidious onset of bleeding, bruising → fatigue, palpitations → frequent mucosal infection	Insidious onset of anemia signs and symptoms (S/Sx) → thrombocytopenia → neutropenia	Insidious onset of anemia S/Sx → thrombocytopenia → neutropenia Abdominal fullness
Physical exam	Petechiae, ecchymoses, bleeding, heme+ stool Pallor, ↑RR, ↑HR Signs of infection (mucosa)	Pallor, tachycardia, tachypnea Signs of bleeding, diathesis Signs of infection	Massive splenomegaly Signs of anemia, thrombocytopenia Signs of infection

Laboratory findings	Pancytopenia
	<20% bone marrow cellularity
	Severe aplastic anemia
	includes 2 of 3 criteria:
	  1. ANC <500/μL
	  2. Platelets <20,000/μL
	  3. Reticulocytes <1%
		Pancytopenia
		Normal or hypercellular bone marrow
		Morphologically and functionally abnormal blood cells with elevated blasts in blood and bone marrow
			Pancytopenia
			Teardrop-shaped RBCs
			Leukoerythroblastic blood
			↑WBC, RBC blasts
			Giant abnormal platelets

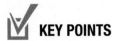 **KEY POINTS**

- WBCs provide basic functions of immune defense through phago-cytosis, cell killing, and leukocyte recruitment for the amplification, refinement, and even suppression of the immune response

- Pancytopenia is the combined presence of *leukopenia, anemia,* and *thrombocytopenia* that results from an insult causing a dynamic abnormality in blood cell production, distribution, usage, and survival

- Most etiologies of pancytopenia can be diagnosed by peripheral blood smear and bone marrow biopsy, which will reveal a hypocel-lular bone marrow, a normal or hypercellular bone marrow, or bone marrow fibrosis

QUESTIONS

1. What is the least likely etiology of AA's pancytopenia from the history?

   A. Parvovirus B19 infection

   B. Posthepatitis aplasia

   C. Benzene exposure during his years working in a petroleum plant

   D. Fanconi anemia

   E. Undiagnosed sickle cell trait with new overlying cyto-megalovirus infection compromising already compro-mised hematopoietic capacity

2. PR is a 59-year-old woman who presents with respiratory dis-tress and is eventually diagnosed with *Streptococcus* pneumo-nia. Her recent medical history includes recent initiation of the antiseizure drug carbamazepine after a recent stroke. She has a long history of alcohol abuse and is noted by her case-worker to have poor appetite and food intake. Her exam is significant for rhonchi in the right upper lobe. Her labs reveal a pancytopenia with hypersegmented neutrophils. Subse-quent bone marrow biopsy reveals a normal-appearing cellu-lar bone marrow. What is the least likely cause of her pancytopenia?

   A. Drug reaction

   B. Vitamin B12 deficiency

   C. Parvovirus B19 infection

   D. Alcohol toxicity

   E. Pernicious anemia

HPI: A 68-year-old man is admitted to the hospital for pneumonia.

PMH: Significant for diabetes mellitus, cardiovascular disease, and severe aortic stenosis.

PE: The patient has significant scleral icterus (yellow sclera) and appreciable jaundice.

Labs: Hgb 10 g/dL; Hct 30%; MCV 85 fL; reticulocytes 6% (nl 0.5–1.5%); total bilirubin 2.5 mg/dL (normal 0.2–1.0)

A direct Coombs test was done.

THOUGHT QUESTIONS

- What are the signs and symptoms of hemolytic anemia?
- What are schistocytes and in what type of anemia are they found?
- What underlying diseases are associated with autoimmune hemolytic anemias?
- Why does glucose-6-phosphate dehydrogenase (G6PD) deficiency lead to hemolysis?

BASIC SCIENCE REVIEW AND DISCUSSION

In general, hemolytic anemias are **normocytic** (normal MCV) and **hyperproductive** (increased reticulocytes). Symptoms and signs of hemolytic anemia include those of anemia (headache, fatigue, shortness of breath, heart palpitations) and those of hemolysis: **jaundice, scleral icterus** (yellow skin and eyes, respectively), and a high incidence of gallstones (all due to increased bilirubin). Laboratory findings of hemolysis include an **increased serum LDH** (released from RBC during hemolysis), **increased serum bilirubin** (a breakdown product of hemoglobin), and **decreased free plasma haptoglobin** (a hemoglobin-binding protein that gets quickly cleared when bound).

Microangiopathic Hemolytic Anemia

Microangiopathic hemolytic anemia (MAHA) is an acquired anemia in which erythrocytes undergo lysis in the circulation. This intravascular red cell fragmentation is caused by **mechanical damage** to the RBC membrane. The damage can be caused by either shear stress force, such as when RBCs pass through damaged (e.g., in aortic stenosis) or faulty prosthetic cardiac valves, or when RBCs come into contact with abnormal vascular endothelial surfaces, such as in patients with aortic aneurysms, TTP, malignant HTN, vasculitis, and DIC. Patients present with typical signs of a hemolytic anemia and features of their underlying cardiac or vascular disease. The hallmark of MAHA is the presence of **schistocytes** (cells with two or more membrane projections or pointy ends) and RBC fragments on the peripheral blood smear caused by the direct damage of the RBC membrane. Treatment is targeted at correcting the underlying disease, such as resection of the aortic aneurysm or replacement of a damaged cardiac valve. While the hemolysis continues, patients should be supported with iron and folate so that the bone marrow can continue to be hyperproductive. In extreme cases, red cell transfusions may be necessary.

Autoimmune Hemolytic Anemia

Autoimmune hemolytic anemia (AIHA) is an acquired anemia caused by the presence of circulating autoantibodies that bind to RBCs and cause their premature destruction. The complement system plays a role in the lysis of targeted RBCs. The majority of AIHA cases (80–90%) are mediated by **warm-reacting autoantibodies** (antibodies that bind to red cells at 37°C). **IgG** antibodies and/or complement bind to the red cell membrane and target it for macrophage phagocytosis. Part of the red cell membrane is internalized by the macrophage, and when the red cell is released, it reseals and forms a sphere (due to lost surface area). These rigid **spherocytes** get trapped in the spleen and are prematurely removed by phagocytosis (extravascular hemolysis). A smaller portion of AIHA cases are mediated by **cold-reacting autoantibodies** (antibodies that bind to red cells at <37°C). These antibodies are typically **IgM** and they activate and bind complement optimally at 20° to 25°C. They can also directly agglutinate red cells at temperatures from 0° to 5°C. The formation of spherocytes and extravascular hemolysis occur as described above.

AIHAs can occur in otherwise healthy individuals or in patients with underlying diseases. Warm-reacting antibodies are associated with lymphoproliferative malignancies (lymphoma, chronic lymphocytic leukemia), and rheumatic disorders (SLE). Cold-reacting antibodies can be associated with infectious mononucleosis and *Mycoplasma pneumoniae* infections. The clinical manifestation of AIHA can be rapid in onset or insidious, developing over months. The symptoms are that of anemia (headache, dizziness, shortness of breath) and jaundice. Individuals with cold-reacting antibodies experience cold-induced acrocyanosis (blue fingers, toes) because of cold-mediated vasoocclusion at these peripheral sites, where the body temperature is lower.

Common laboratory test findings are those for general hemolysis and the presence of spherocytes on the blood smear. A more definitive test for AIHA is a **positive direct Coombs test** in which the patient's red cells are reacted with specific reagents to determine the presence of immunoglobulin or complement bound to the red cells. In warm antibody autoimmune hemolysis, one would expect the presence of any of the following: (*a*) IgG alone; (*b*) IgG plus complement components (C3 and C4); or (*c*) C3 or C4 alone. In cold antibody disease the direct Coombs test is positive only for the presence of C3 or C4 because IgM falls off during the washing procedures. The initial treatment for AIHA is systemic **steroids** (e.g., prednisone), although only two thirds of patients respond. Additional treatment includes **splenectomy.** Occasionally cytotoxic drugs or plasmapheresis is used. The most effective treatment for cold-reacting antibody disease is to keep the patient warm, which sometimes requires the patient moving to locations with warm weather year round.

G6PD Deficiency

G6PD is an enzyme in the pentose phosphate pathway. G6PD deficiency is a **sex-linked** genetic disorder that causes episodic hemolysis in response to infection, to exposure to oxidant drugs (sulfas, quinine), or to eating fava beans. Infection, certain drugs, and fava beans cause the formation of free radicals that can oxidize glutathione and complex it with hemoglobin. This results in oxidized hemoglobin, which precipitates inside red cells as

Heinz bodies. Normal cells protect themselves against oxidant damage by reducing glutathione with reduced nicotinamide adenine dinucleotide phosphate (NADPH). Individuals deficient in the enzyme G6PD are unable to regenerate NADPH. Red cells with Heinz bodies are identified as abnormal and undergo premature phagocytosis. Sometimes **bite cells** are seen on a peripheral blood smear. Eleven percent of African American males have a mutant form of the enzyme, and enzyme activity is reduced to 5 to 15% of normal. A Mediterranean variant causes a more severe disease, as individuals have less than 1% normal enzyme activity. Individuals with G6PD deficiency are instructed to avoid drugs known to precipitate hemolysis (the list is very long), and they are supported with transfusions through episodes of hemolysis.

CASE CONCLUSION

The patient's direct Coombs test came back negative. Review of the peripheral blood smear showed schistocytes and RBC fragments. The patient's findings are consistent with microangiopathic hemolytic anemia. (If the direct Coombs test was positive and blood smear showed spherocytes, one might suspect an autoimmune hemolytic anemia.) Severe aortic stenosis can cause shear stress on RBC membranes while they pass over the calcified valve. Treatment for the anemia is surgical replacement of the diseased valve. In the meantime, the patient was started on folate and iron supplements to maintain his active reticulocytosis. There was not an indication for transfusion at this time, but the patient will be monitored regularly.

THUMBNAIL: Comparison of Select Hemolytic Anemias

	Microangiopathic Hemolytic Anemia	Autoimmune Hemolytic Anemia		G6PD Deficiency
		Warm-Reacting	Cold-Reacting	
Etiology	Mechanical damage → RBC fragmentation • Aortic stenosis • Aortic aneurysm • Prosthetic cardiac valves • TTP • Malignant HTN • DIC • Vasculitis	IgG +/− Complement binds RBC → partial phagocytosis → RBC reseals → spherocyte → trapped/lysed in spleen • Idiopathic • Lymphoproliferative disease • Rheumatic disease	IgM autoantibody agglutinates RBCs (at low temp) and binds complement → phagocytosis → spherocyte → lysed in spleen • Idiopathic • Lymphoproliferative disease • Mononucleosis infection • Mycoplasma infection	Free oxygen radicals → oxidizes Hgb → Hgb precipitates (Heinz body) → phagocytosis/lysis of RBCs • Oxidant drugs • Infection Fava beans
Clinical picture	Underlying cardiac or valvular disease	Previously healthy or underlying disease	Acrocyanosis	• Sex-linked genetics • ↑ in African Americans • Episodic hemolysis
Laboratory	• Schistocytes ☾ • RBC fragments	• Spherocytes ● • (+) Direct Coombs • IgG +/− C3/C4 or C alone	• Spherocytes ● • (+) Direct Coombs • C3, C4 only	• Bite cells ☽ • ↓ G6PD enzyme activity
Treatment	• Treat primary disease • Folate/iron supplement	• Steroids • Splenectomy • Cytotoxic drugs • Plasmapheresis	• Warmth • Steroids • Splenectomy	• Avoid precipitating drugs • Red cell transfusion during severe episodes

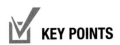

KEY POINTS

- Hemolytic anemias are normocytic and hyperproductive
- Specific signs of hemolysis include jaundice and scleral icterus
- Laboratory findings include an increased serum LDH, increased serum bilirubin, and decreased free plasma haptoglobin

QUESTIONS

1. An African American college student is planning a trip to South America. A week prior to departure he begins a course of anti-malarial pills (Mefloquine) that you have given him while working at the university travel clinic. Several days later he begins feeling ill and comes back to see you. His labs are as follows: Hgb 10 g/dL, Hct 30%, MCV 87 fL, and reticulocytes are 8%. The peripheral smear shows bite cells. His blood is direct Coombs negative. What is the pathophysiology of his illness?

   A. IgG autoantibodies bind RBCs and cause partial phagocytosis by macrophages.
   B. IgM-drug complexes bind RBCs and cause complement-mediated lysis.
   C. Mechanical vascular damage causes RBC fragmentation.
   D. Cold-mediated vasoocclusion of peripheral veins.
   E. Oxidized Hgb precipitates in the RBC and causes phagocytosis by macrophages.

2. A 33-year-old woman presents to the ED with a fever and appears confused. She is alert and oriented only to person. Her exam is unremarkable except for some moderate scleral icterus. Laboratory results: Hgb 9 g/dL, Hct 27%, MCV 88 fL, reticulocytes 5%, Plt 50,000, total bilirubin 2.2 mg/dL, and creatinine 2.4 mg/dL. What do you expect to see on the peripheral blood smear?

   A. Bite cells
   B. Schistocytes
   C. Target cells
   D. Spherocytes
   E. Hypersegmented PMNs

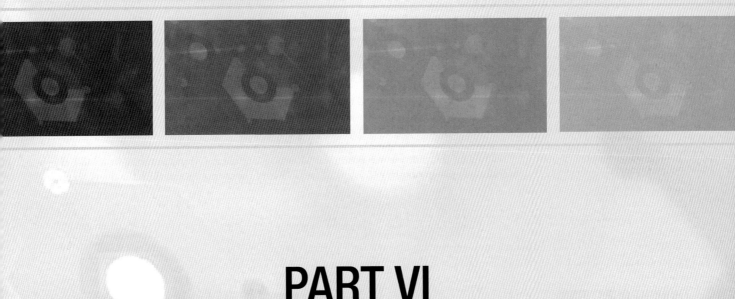

PART VI

Oncology

HPI: TL, a 59-year-old woman, presents with 5 days of **fever and night sweats.** She also noted 20 lb of **unexplained weight loss** in the last 3 months from her previous weight of 150 lb. She has also had an intermittent cough with mild wheezing when lying on her right side. She has had no sick contacts nor symptoms suggesting infection. She had a negative PPD 1 year ago and has no risk factors for tuberculosis exposure.

PMH: Hashimoto thyroiditis during her 20s; now hypothyroid and taking L-thyroxine. No history of smoking or drinking.

PE: T 38.6°C; BP 135/75 mm Hg; HR 85 beats/min; RR 20 breaths/min; SaO$_2$ 98%.

The patient is thin and ill-appearing. Her exam is significant for **positional wheezing** audible anteriorly in the right middle chest when lying on the right side and **nontender lymphadenopathy** consisting of two 2.5-cm rubbery nodules in the left axillary and right inguinal regions.

Labs: CBC and other routine labs are normal.

Chest x-ray reveals a 3-cm **mediastinal mass** protruding into the right pleural cavity.

THOUGHT QUESTIONS

- What are the neoplasms of lymphoid origin and how do they arise?
- What are the histologic subtypes of these neoplasms and what are their characteristics?
- What are the clinical manifestations of lymphoid neoplasms?
- How are lymphoid neoplasms diagnosed, staged, graded, and treated?

BASIC SCIENCE DISCUSSION AND REVIEW

Lymphomas are solid tumors of lymphoid origin that arise from the malignant transformation of a lymphoid cell leading to its clonal proliferation. They are related to leukemias and are different only in that they do not arise in the bone marrow and are not characterized first by their presence in circulation. Figures 6-1 and 6-2 are diagrams of B-cell and T-cell differentiation and the leukemias and lymphomas associated with different stages of maturation.

Hodgkin disease (HD) is a lymphoma characterized by the presence of **Reed-Sternberg cells** (or "owl's eye cells"), which are the true neoplastic components of the tumor. These cells are thought to secrete cytokines and thereby recruit reactive infiltrates, which make up the bulk of the tumor. All other lymphomas are categorized as **non-Hodgkin lymphomas** (Table 6-1).

HD presents as singular nontender lymphadenopathy (LAD) along the **central axis** of the body with contiguous spread to other nodal groups. In contrast, non-Hodgkin lymphomas present at multiple sites in peripheral nodal groups with noncontiguous spread. Both diseases may present with **"B symptoms,"** namely

fever, night sweats, and weight loss, associated with cytokine release of lymphocytes.

Diagnosis of lymphoma is established by exam of a tissue biopsy. For non-Hodgkin lymphoma, prognosis depends on *grade*. Cells are either *mature* or *immature, B cell* or *T cell* in origin. Growth patterns either adhere to the normal *follicular* structure or grow in *diffuse* sheets. In general, the more mature the malignant cells, the less aggressive and slower growing the neoplasm, and vice versa. Paradoxically, more mature cells of low-grade lymphomas disseminate earlier and wider as normal lymphocytes do, while less mature, high-grade lymphomas disseminate later, often presenting as a localized mass. Untreated, low-grade lymphomas can develop into high-grade lymphomas.

HD is classified by histologic subtype (Table 6-2). Prognosis for HD is most dependent on *stage* (size and nodal involvement) and is poorer among those with "B symptoms" (Table 6-3). Generally, localized disease is treated with **radiation therapy.** More disseminated disease is treated with **chemotherapy.** HD has among the most successful rates of cure.

Multiple myeloma and **Waldenström macroglobulinemia** are both neoplasms of *immunoglobulin-secreting B lymphocytes* (Table 6-4). They occur among older adults (mean age 60 years) and present with anemia and serum hyperviscosity (blurry vision, priapism, headaches, altered mental status, and peripheral blood smear showing **Rouleaux formation** of red blood cells) due to massive overproduction of immunoglobulin proteins. These diseases can be distinguished by identifying monoclonal immunoglobulin via serum protein electrophoresis **(SPEP)** and **Bence-Jones proteins** consisting of κ and λ light chains by urine protein electrophoresis **(UPEP),** by the radiographic presence or absence of lytic bone lesions, and by bone marrow exam. They are both incurable and have a mean survival of 3 to 4 years.

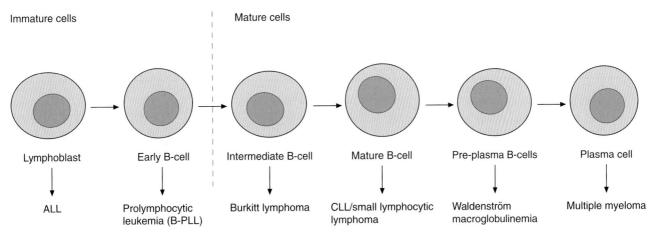

• **Figure 6-1.** B-cell differentiation and malignant transformation into lymphomas and leukemias.

CASE CONCLUSION

Biopsies of the left axillary and right inguinal nodes reveal follicular lymphoma. Given that the patient presented with fever, night sweats, and weight loss, she was thought to have more advanced disease, and combination chemotherapy was initiated with chlorambucil, vincristine, and prednisone. She achieved complete remission but relapsed 2 years later, presenting with repeated B symptoms and LAD. She was found to have histologic transformation of follicular lymphoma to diffuse large B-cell lymphoma. She is now undergoing aggressive chemotherapy for her relapse.

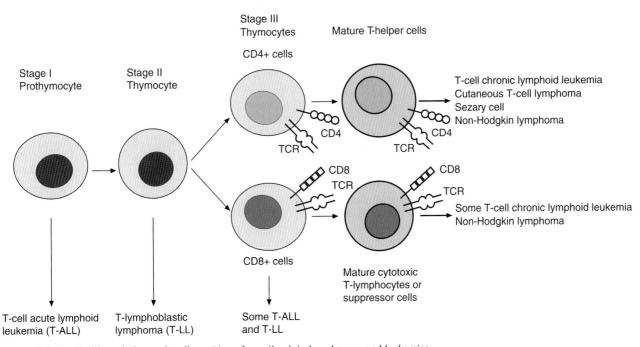

• **Figure 6-2.** T-cell differentiation and malignant transformation into lymphomas and leukemias.

TABLE 6-1 Common Non-Hodgkin Lymphoma Subtypes

Common Adult Subtypes	
Follicular lymphoma[a]	**Germinal center B-cell lymphoma** (*mature and follicular*) *Most common form of NHL*, age >40 years; indolent course **t(14,18)** linking proto-oncogene, *bcl-2*, to Ig-heavy chain locus → **bcl-2** prevents apoptosis of lymphocyte
Small lymphocytic lymphoma	**Solid tumor counterpart to chronic lymphoid leukemia,** *mature B cells in diffuse pattern* are slow growing and migratory; indolent course; age 50–60 years Asymptomatic LAD, bone marrow/organ involvement; evolves into CLL
Diffuse large B-cell lymphoma[a]	Aggressive tumor, **usually *intermediate- or high-grade cells, diffuse pattern*** 20% of NHL; mean age = 60 years old; associated with immunodeficiency Presents with localized solid tumor then later dissemination; rapidly fatal
Mycosis fungoides	Cutaneous T-cell lymphoma infiltrating dermal/epidermal junction Mid-50s; common in males, blacks; indolent progressive course; incurable
Sézary syndrome	**Cutaneous T-cell lymphoma infiltrating skin and peripheral circulation** Sézary cells have "cerebriform" nuclei; median survival 8–9 years
Adult T-cell leukemia/lymphoma	**T-cell neoplasm of HTLV-1 infected patients** → skin lesions, LAD, HSM, lymphocytosis, hypercalcemia, CD4+ "flower cells" in blood; rapidly progressive, fatal within 1 year
Common Childhood/Adolescent Subtypes	
Lymphoblastic lymphoma	**Solid tumor counterpart to *immature* B-cell acute lymphoblastic leukemia** Leukocytosis LAD, HSM, bone marrow failure, CNS/skin infiltration
Burkitt lymphoma[a]	**Peripheral B-cell lymphoma/leukemia** of *mature* B lymphocytes, *diffuse* pattern, *high grade* → most rapidly proliferating of any cancer ***Endemic in Africa and South America, associated with HIV*** ***EBV infection is thought to mediate malignant transformation*** Peripheral LAD, intra-abdominal mass, CNS infiltration **"Starry sky"** appearance of lymphoid tissue

[a]*Most tested lymphomas on USMLE Step 1.*
NHL, non-Hodgkin lymphoma; *LAD,* lymphadenopathy; *CLL,* chronic lymphocytic leukemia; *HTLV-1,* human T-cell leukemia virus; *HSM,* hepatosplenomegaly; *EBV,* Epstein-Barr virus

TABLE 6-2 Rye Classification System for Hodgkin Disease Histologic Subtypes

Subtypes	Epidemiology	Pathology	Prognosis
Lymphocyte predominant	Least common	*Mostly* lymphocytes, L+H cells, rare RS cells	Best
Nodular sclerosing	Most common, esp. in women	Nodular fibrosis with lymphocytes, lacunar cells, eosinophils, histiocytes, RS cells	Intermediate
Mixed cellularity	Older and HIV+ patients	No nodular fibrosis, irregular scarring, necrosis, *many* RS cells	Intermediate
Lymphocyte depleted	Rare; common in HIV+ patients	*Few* lymphocytes, RS cells, more atypical cells	Worst

L+H, lymphohistiocytic ("popcorn cells"); *RS,* Reed-Sternberg

TABLE 6-3 Ann Arbor Staging System for Hodgkin Disease

Stage 1	*Single* lymph node region or single extralymphatic organ involvement
Stage 2	Involvement of two or more lymphoid tissues on the *same side of the diaphragm*
Stage 3	Involvement of lymph node regions on *both sides of the diaphragm*
Stage 4	*Disseminated involvement* of organs, tissues, bone marrow, lymph nodes
Category A:	Patients are **A**symptomatic
Category B:	"**B** symptoms"—fever, night sweats, and weight loss >10% original body weight

TABLE 6-4 Plasma Cell Disorders/Monoclonal Gammopathies

	Multiple Myeloma	Waldenström Macroglobulinemia
Pathophysiology	**Monoclonal IgG and κ or λ light chain-secreting B-lymphocyte neoplasm**—bone marrow infiltration	**IgM-secreting plasma cell neoplasm**—variant of diffuse small lymphocytic lymphoma—no bony infiltration
Clinical presentation	Anemia, hyperviscosity syndrome, **bone pain,** bone fractures, recurrent infection, renal failure, proteinuria	Anemia, hyperviscosity syndrome, **no bone pain,** HSM, LAD, peripheral neuropathy, proteinuria

Diagnosis
  SPEP
  X-ray
	SPEP, UPEP, PBS, x-ray
	Monoclonal **IgG** spike
	Lytic bone lesions diffusely
		SPEP, UPEP, PBS, x-ray
		Monoclonal **IgM** spike
		No lytic bone lesions

HSM, hepatosplenomegaly; *LAD,* lymphadenopathy; *SPEP,* serum protein electrophoresis; *UPEP,* urine protein electrophoresis; *PBS,* peripheral blood smear

THUMBNAIL: Non-Hodgkin Lymphoma vs. Hodgkin Lymphoma

	Non-Hodgkin Lymphoma	*Hodgkin Disease*
Epidemiology	**75%** of all lymphomas Mean age of onset = 42 years Risk factors: ionizing radiation exposure, viral infection (EBV, HTLV-1), autoimmune disease, immunosuppression	**25%** of all lymphomas **Bimodal distribution:** 20s and >50s Men > Women Increased in HIV+ with more aggressive disease
Pathophysiology	Varied translocations affect cellular proliferation of lymphoid cells	Malignant Reed-Sternberg cells recruit inflammatory cells
Clinical presentation	Nontender enlargement of **multiple nodes** in **peripheral nodal groups** with **noncontiguous spread** to other nodes; extranodal lymphoid tissue involvement; generalized pruritus; B symptoms	Nontender enlargement of a **single node or nodal group** with **contiguous spread** to adjacent nodes along the **central axis;** mediastinal or abdominal LAD; generalized pruritus; B symptoms; clinical anergy
Diagnosis	Lymph node/tissue biopsy; histologic exam	**Reed-Sternberg cells** on lymph node biopsy
Staging/grading	Prognosis **depends on grade:** follicular vs. diffuse; small vs. large; B cell vs. T cell vs. mixed	Prognosis **depends on stage** (spread and pattern of nodal involvement): Ann Arbor stage 1–4, category A/B
Common histologic subtypes	Follicular lymphoma Diffuse large B-cell lymphoma Burkitt lymphoma	Lymphocyte predominant Nodular sclerosing Mixed cellularity Lymphocyte depleted
Therapy	Radiation therapy, chemotherapy, immunotherapy, autologous, allogeneic stem cell transplantation	Radiation therapy for stages I and II Combination chemotherapy for stages III and IV

☑ KEY POINTS

■ Lymphomas are solid tumors of lymphoid origin; HD is defined by the presence of Reed-Sternberg cells, while all other lymphomas are designated as non-Hodgkin lymphomas

■ HD manifests with central axis LAD with contiguous spread to other lymph nodes, while non-Hodgkin lymphoma manifests as a peripheral LAD with noncontiguous spread

■ Plasma cell neoplasms hypersecrete monoclonal IgM, IgG, or immunoglobulin light chains (κ or λ) and produce disease related to serum hyperviscosity

QUESTIONS

1. A 62-year-old man presents with anemia, bone pain, and blurry vision. Which lymphoma does he most likely have, what would be the most useful diagnostic test or procedure one would order, and what would be the characteristic finding?

   A. Waldenström macroglobulinemia, serum protein electrophoresis, IgM spike
   B. Multiple myeloma, serum protein electrophoresis, IgG spike
   C. Follicular lymphoma, lymph node biopsy, small-cleaved cells in follicular pattern
   D. HD, lymph node biopsy, lymphocyte-predominant morphology
   E. Burkitt lymphoma, lymph node biopsy, mature B lymphocytes in diffuse pattern

2. A 40-year-old woman presents with isolated cervical LAD with no fever, night sweats, or weight loss. A lymph node biopsy is performed and histopathology reveals small lymphocytes and rare Reed-Sternberg cells. Staging is done with MRI and she is found to have disease limited to one cervical nodal group. How would one classify her disease and what would be her prognosis?

   A. Follicular lymphoma with a prognosis of 5 to 10 years without treatment and 50 to 75% response to chemotherapy and radiation with complete remission
   B. HD stage IA with 85 to 95% 5-year survival and high potential for cure

   C. HD stage IIA with 85 to 95% 5-year survival and high potential for cure
   D. HD stage IB with poorer prognosis than stage IA
   E. Diffuse large B-cell lymphoma, which is rapidly fatal without treatment but highly responsive to chemotherapy

3. A 55-year-old HIV+ man with a CD4 count of 180 and viral load of 25,000 on highly active retroviral therapy presents with 4 days of fever and night sweats and 4 weeks of nonproductive cough. He has a history of a positive PPD with negative chest x-ray. On exam, he has multiple enlarged cervical, axillary, and inguinal lymph nodes, which he had noted to be slowly growing over the last several months. Subsequent chest and abdominal x-rays reveal a mediastinal mass and a single pulmonary nodule and abdominal mass. A repeat PPD is done and is found to be negative. Which of the following is the least likely explanation for his presentation?

   A. HD with anergy due to T-cell dysfunction associated with the lymphoma
   B. Diffuse large B-cell lymphoma with mediastinal involvement causing nonproductive cough
   C. Multiple myeloma causing T-cell dysfunction and recrudescence of tuberculosis
   D. Burkitt lymphoma with several rapidly growing lymph nodes and anergy caused by advanced AIDS
   E. All answers above can explain his presentation

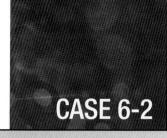

CASE 6-2 Epidermal Carcinomas

HPI: A 63-year-old man comes to your primary care clinic for a refill of his allergy medication. You notice a **lesion on his nose** and question him about it. He recalls the lesion has been present for about 5 years and seems to be **gradually enlarging.** It is intermittently **itchy** and occasionally **bleeds** and scabs if he scratches vigorously. The patient adds that he worked as a **lifeguard** for 15 years and has always enjoyed swimming at the beach. With the exception of mild seasonal allergies, he is otherwise in good health.

PE: The patient is a **light-skinned** man. He has a 3 × 4 cm erythematous papule on the left side of his nose. It has a **pearly, translucent appearance** with visible telangiectatic vessels. The center is **ulcerated** and covered with a crust. He has no other lesions on his skin. The remainder of his exam is within normal limits.

THOUGHT QUESTIONS

- What is the differential diagnosis of this lesion?
- What are major risk factors for malignancy?
- How do basal cell carcinoma and squamous cell carcinoma differ?
- What type of treatment do you recommend? Does this patient need to be seen in follow-up?

BASIC SCIENCE REVIEW AND DISCUSSION: PREMALIGNANT AND MALIGNANT EPIDERMAL TUMORS

Nonmelanoma Skin Cancers

Nonmelanoma skin cancers are divided into two categories: basal cell carcinoma and cutaneous squamous cell carcinoma. Despite the fact that there are over a million cases of nonmelanoma skin cancers diagnosed each year, only 2000 patients die from the disease annually. This low mortality rate is primarily due to the low rate of metastasis in either of these malignancies. However, it is important that physicians be able to recognize and treat these epithelial malignancies because they may progress to metastasis if neglected over the years.

Basal Cell Carcinoma

Basal cell carcinoma (BCC) is the **most common type of skin cancer.** In the United States alone, there are between 750,000 and 950,000 cases diagnosed annually; 85% of cases involve head and neck structures, especially the nose. The risk of developing BCC is directly proportional to cumulative ultraviolet (UV) exposure and inversely proportional to degree of skin pigmentation. Other risk factors include sites of chronic inflammation or injury, such as with scars or burns.

Technically, the name basal cell carcinoma is a misnomer, as the cells more closely resemble follicular cells than basal layer cells. Nevertheless, BCC cells do appear histologically "basaloid," with palisading nuclei. BCC **grows slowly,** approximately 1 to 2 cm per year. Thus, the morbidity of BCC is largely due to local damage caused by relentless growth with invasion of adjacent structures. Nonetheless, there is almost no risk of metastasis. The extremely rare event of metastasis has occurred only in large, long-standing lesions that have been neglected for decades.

The classic presentation of BCC is as a **pink-pearly white papule** with prominent telangiectatic vessels. However, the morphology of individual cases is diverse enough that BCC is often confused with actinic keratosis, squamous cell carcinoma, melanoma, chronic inflammation, or psoriasis. Definitive diagnosis is made by biopsy. Primary treatment is by Mohs surgical excision, a technique that involves removal of the lesion followed by immediate inspection of frozen pathology sections and reexcision if positive margins are found. Reconstructive surgery is often required after removal of large lesions. Close follow-up is also necessary because BCC has a high rate of recurrence, and the larger the tumor the more likely it is to recur. Lesions greater than 2 cm have a recurrence rate of 25% even after full surgical treatment of the primary lesion.

Actinic Keratoses

Actinic keratoses are dysplastic **precursors of squamous cell carcinoma.** Also known as solar keratoses, these lesions are extremely common; as many as 50% of fair-skinned adults develop actinic keratosis. This dysplasia is caused by prolonged exposure to the sunlight with a resultant buildup of keratin. Some lesions produce so much keratin that a **"cutaneous horn"** develops. While most lesions may regress or remain stable over a lifetime, the risk of malignant transformation is sufficient to warrant the removal of these potential precursor lesions. Removal can be accomplished in the same manner as for a common wart: by gentle curettage or by freezing.

Cutaneous Squamous Cell Carcinoma

Cutaneous squamous cell carcinoma (SCC) is the second most common type of skin cancer and occurs primarily in the elderly. The underlying cause of SCC is DNA mutagenicity. Accordingly, factors that predispose or cause epithelial damage have been found to be risk factors. These include fair skin, **excessive sunlight UV rays,** industrial carcinogens, chronic ulcers, old burn scars, and ionizing radiation. Early-onset SCC is observed in xeroderma pigmentosum, which arises from a defect in DNA repair mechanisms of the skin. In addition, immunosuppressed individuals (such as organ transplant recipients) are also at increased risk for developing SCC.

Clinically, preinvasive carcinoma in situ (also known as **Bowen disease**) appears as sharply defined, red scaling plaques. More advanced invasive lesions are nodular with evidence of hyperkeratosis and ulceration. Note that SCC can occur anywhere on the skin, including even the lip, mouth, and genitalia. On microscopic inspection, there is full-thickness atypia of the epidermis, with sheets of squamous epithelium and central foci of keratinization ("**keratin pearls**").

SCCs are usually recognized early while they are still easily treatable with Mohs excision. The incidence of metastasis is greater than that for BCC, but it is still low. Indeed, the risk of metastasis is lower if the malignancy occurs de novo than if the cancer arises from a precursor lesion. If metastasis does occur, however, mortality is high (5-year survival rate of 35%).

CASE CONCLUSION

Punch biopsy demonstrated irregular clusters of darkly staining basaloid cells with peripheral palisading nuclei. A diagnosis of infiltrative BCC was made. The patient successfully underwent Mohs surgical excision of the lesion, followed by reconstructive surgery. He was scheduled for regular follow-up visits every 6 months. Three years later, a recurrent lesion was noticed at the site of the initial lesion. The patient underwent repeat excision of the entire lesion. Postoperative radiation therapy was delivered to the surgical site. The patient has been disease-free since then.

THUMBNAIL: Basal Cell Carcinoma and Squamous Cell Cancer

Name	Epidemiology	Appearance	Risk Factors	Prognosis
Basal cell carcinoma	Most common skin tumor	Morphology: pearly, translucent nodule with telangiectasias Histology: "basaloid" cells with palisading nuclei	UV light, fair skin, age, chronic skin inflammation	High recurrence rate, almost never metastasizes
Squamous cell carcinoma	Second most common skin malignancy	Morphology: red, scaly plaque Histology: sheets of epithelial cells, "keratin pearls"	UV light, fair skin, age, actinic keratosis, Bowen disease, chronic skin inflammation, xeroderma pigmentosum	Rarely metastasizes

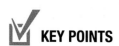

KEY POINTS

- BCC is the most common skin cancer; SCC is the 2nd most common skin cancer
- Both BCC and SCC have low overall mortality rates
- Definitive diagnosis of skin cancer is by biopsy, and treatment is by surgical excision

QUESTIONS

1. Both SCC and BCC share many of the same risk factors. Which of the following is a major risk factor for SCC but not for BCC?

   A. Excessive sunlight exposure
   B. Actinic keratosis
   C. Chronic decubitus ulcer
   D. Tanning salons
   E. Dysplastic nevus

2. JR is a 38-year-old recipient of a kidney transplant. She has been on immunosuppressive medication for 6 years to ensure that her body does not reject the transplant. She now comes to you with a suspicious skin lesion on her left forearm and you are concerned about malignancy. What histologic feature on her biopsy would confirm your suspicions of SCC?

   A. Palisading nuclei
   B. Acanthosis
   C. Keratin pearls
   D. Basaloid cells
   E. Follicular cells

3. It is important to know where to look for skin malignancies in order to diagnose them. Among the following sites, where is BCC most likely to be located?

   A. Ears
   B. Hands and feet
   C. Chest
   D. Genitalia
   E. Shoulders

HPI: KE is a 51-year-old man who presents to the ED after his wife saw him "have a seizure." After breakfast he collapsed to the ground for 4 to 5 minutes with outreached extremities experiencing jerky movements. He does not have a known seizure disorder. During the episode he was incontinent of urine and bit his tongue. He was disoriented to place and date for 20 to 30 minutes after the movements ceased. Past medical history is significant only for hypertension, for which he takes a low dose of hydrochlorothiazide. He does not smoke, and he drinks an occasional beer on holidays. His family history is significant for coronary artery disease, and both of his parents died in their 70s from MIs. On review of systems (ROS), it was noted that in the last 2 months he had been experiencing some new early morning headaches that were not relieved with OTC analgesics. He said he generally felt more "clumsy" than usual.

PE: Overweight man sitting comfortably on gurney. Head and neck: pupils equally round and reactive to light and accommodation (PERRLA), extraocular movements intact (EOMI), conjunctiva clear. No lymphadenopathy. Neuro: cranial nerves (CN) II-XII intact. Motor: 4/5 on L upper/lower extremities; 5/5 on R; deep tendon reflexes (DTRs): decreased on the L bicep and knee jerk; negative Babinski test bilaterally. Sensory: intact to light touch. Gait: wide-based gait. Difficulty standing on heel/toe on L side. A head CT was ordered.

THOUGHT QUESTIONS

- What are the most common types of brain tumors in adults? In children?
- Are "benign" brain tumors really benign?
- What is glioblastoma multiforme?

BASIC SCIENCE REVIEW AND DISCUSSION

It is estimated that 17,000 malignant tumors of the brain or spinal cord were diagnosed in 2002 in the United States. Approximately 13,100 will die from these malignant tumors. Cancer of the CNS accounts for approximately 1.4% of all human cancers and 2.4% of all cancer-related deaths, with men slightly more affected than women in a 3:2 ratio. CNS tumors are mostly intracranial; tumors of the spinal cord are much less frequent. Unlike other solid tumors in the body, primary malignant CNS tumors rarely metastasize.

In **adults,** the majority of intracranial tumors are **supratentorial** (occurring in the cerebral hemispheres). **Metastatic tumors are the most commonly occurring tumors of the brain,** followed by astrocytomas (including glioblastoma) and meningiomas. In **children,** the majority of intracranial tumors are **infratentorial** (occurring in the cerebellum/brainstem), with **medulloblastoma** occurring most frequently. CNS tumors are about equal to acute lymphocytic leukemia (ALL) as the most commonly occurring childhood cancer.

Brain tumors can be benign or malignant. Benign tumors have clear borders, do not invade adjacent brain tissue, and rarely reoccur after removal. Yet benign tumors can still result in devastating clinical consequences due to mass effect and compression of important brain structures.

Glioblastoma Multiforme

Glioblastoma multiforme (GBM) is the most common and most malignant adult primary intracranial brain tumor. It is also known as the WHO grade IV astrocytoma. The peak incidence is age 45 to 70 years. The clinical history of patients with GBM is usually short (<3 months) and is consistent with the presence of a fast-growing diffuse brain lesion. Patients frequently present with headache, nausea, vomiting, and/or cognitive impairment. Patients can develop slowly progressing neurologic deficits such as motor weakness or visual changes. Seizures are not uncommon. It is widely accepted that several different genetic alterations may lead to the formation of glioblastoma. In approximately 40% of GBMs, the epidermal growth factor receptor (EGFR) is truncated, causing it to be continually turned on, leading to uncontrolled cell growth. Histologically, GBMs are composed of poorly differentiated, often pleomorphic, astrocytic cells with marked nuclear atypia and brisk mitotic activity. Necrosis is an essential diagnostic feature, and prominent microvascular proliferation is common. A hallmark finding is a **pseudopalisade** arrangement of cells around an area of necrosis. Imaging studies are also essential to making the diagnosis of GBM. On CT, GBMs appear as irregularly shaped hypodense lesions with a peripheral ring-like zone of contrast enhancement and surrounding edema. MRI is also useful. Unfortunately, the prognosis for patients with GBM is poor; survival is often less than 18 months after diagnosis. Treatment is primarily focused on palliation. Surgery is performed to debulk the tumor mass followed by radiation and/or chemotherapy to control remaining tumor cells.

CASE CONCLUSION

The head CT revealed a large, irregularly shaped intracranial mass spanning the right parietal region. A large area of edema surrounded the lesion and much of the parenchyma was compressed. A presumptive diagnosis of GBM was made. The patient was scheduled for surgery with the neurosurgeon, who removed a large portion of the mass. The pathology report commented on pseudopalisading glial cells around necrotic areas of tissue, confirming the diagnosis. The patient was scheduled to meet with both a medical and radiation oncologist for further follow-up.

THUMBNAIL: Nervous System Tumors

Tumor Type	Who Likely Gets It	Significant Features
Astrocytoma grade IV: GBM	Age 45–70 years Men > women	Most common adult primary intracranial tumor; neural tube origin; in cerebral hemispheres; hemorrhagic necrosis with pseudo-palisading cells; highly malignant
Meningioma	Middle-aged women	Second most common adult primary intracranial tumor; originates in arachnoid cells; external to brain; neural crest origin; psammoma bodies on histology; benign, slow growing
Medulloblastoma	Children	Most common childhood intracranial tumor; in cerebellum; neural tube origin; highly malignant
Neuroblastoma	Children	Related to neuroblastoma of adrenals; in cerebral hemispheres; N-*myc* oncogene amplification; neural crest origin
Retinoblastoma	Young children	Retinal tumor; sporadic (unilateral) or familial (bilateral) forms; linked to Rb (tumor suppressor gene) inactivation on both chromosome copies; neural tube origin
Schwannoma (acoustic neuroma)	Middle age to later life	Involves CN XIII; benign, often resectable; neural crest origin; presents with hearing loss, ataxic gait
Craniopharyngioma	Children	Most common supratentorial brain tumor in children; ectodermal origin (Rathke pouch); enlarged sella turcica causing pituitary abnormalities, papilledema, and bitemporal hemianopsia (tunnel vision)
Ependymoma	Children	Line ventricles, often 4th ventricle; obstructed CSF, hydrocephalus; rosette histology
Metastatic	Anyone	Most common brain tumor; usually from lung, breast, GI, melanoma, kidney, thyroid primaries

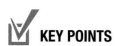

KEY POINTS

- In adults, brain tumors are often supratentorial (cerebral hemispheres). Metastatic brain tumors are more common than astrocytomas (glioblastomas), which are more common than meningiomas.

- In children, brain tumors often are intratentorial (cerebellum); medulloblastoma is the most common type

- Benign brain tumors can have devastating clinical consequences due to mass effect

- GBM (grade IV astrocytoma) is the most common adult primary brain tumor; characterized by necrosis, pseudopalisading arrangement of cells, and a poor prognosis

QUESTIONS

1. A patient is found to have bilateral acoustic neuromas. What hereditary syndrome do you suspect?

   A. von Hippel–Lindau disease
   B. Neurofibromatosis type 1 (von Recklinghausen disease)
   C. Neurofibromatosis type 2
   D. Li-Fraumeni syndrome
   E. Multiple endocrine neoplasia type I
   F. Multiple endocrine neoplasia type III

2. A 63-year-old man comes to your office after suffering from 2 months of new headaches, which do not resolve with OTC analgesics. A CT of the brain shows multiple enhancing lesions in both cerebral hemispheres. What is your preliminary diagnosis?

   A. GBM
   B. Pilocytic astrocytoma
   C. Meningioma
   D. Medulloblastoma
   E. Metastasis

HPI: DC is a 55-year-old woman who presents with a **breast lump.** She had noted the lump 2 weeks ago in the shower and describes it as **painless.** She noted no bloody or green **discharge** from her nipples, no **nipple retractions, skin changes, breast dimpling** or **enlargement,** axillary **masses,** or **bone pain.** She has no **family history** of breast or ovarian cancer. She has no significant past medical history and no previous screening mammographies, and takes no medication. She has **never been pregnant.**

PE: The patient is a thin woman in no acute distress. She is afebrile with normal vital signs. She has no gross **breast asymmetry,** dimpling, skin changes, or retractions. She has a 2-cm firm, **nontender, and immobile breast nodule** at the **upper outer quadrant** of her left breast. She has no palpable **axillary lymph nodes** and no expressible nipple discharge.

THOUGHT QUESTIONS

- How are tumors categorized histologically?
- What is the difference between benign and malignant tumors?
- What are the types of breast cancer? What risk factors are associated with this cancer?
- What is the basic diagnostic work-up of a breast lump and how is it treated?

BASIC SCIENCE REVIEW AND DISCUSSION

More than 1 million people are newly diagnosed with cancer every year, causing over 500,000 deaths in the year 2000. It is second only to cardiovascular disease as the leading cause of death in the United States. Yet, there are often misunderstandings about the very definitions of "tumor" and "cancer," both words eliciting strong reactions from any person. Table 6-5 is a review of tumors, the terminology used, and the histologic and behavioral aspects of tumors that define them as benign or malignant.

Benign Versus Malignant Tumors

The basic difference between these two designations is that a malignant tumor is likely to grow in a way that would eventually cause enough disruption to a person's normal physiology to cause death, whereas with a benign tumor this is unlikely to happen. These are important designations because a benign tumor is unlikely to become a malignant tumor. Benign tumors are thought to be "benign" because they behave similarly to mature, well-differentiated cells and grow in a more controlled fashion, responding to regulatory signals like "normal" cells. They grow more slowly and compress (but do not invade) adjacent tissue. They do not spread to other parts of the body and, if removed, will not recur. Malignant cells appear less differentiated, respond poorly to normal regulatory signals, invade surrounding tissue, and eventually metastasize to distant sites. Ultimately, these designations are mere predictions on the future behavior of tissue. Along with tumor markers and patients' overall clinical pictures, these histologic characteristics can provide information about patients' prognoses and help them understand what is really meant when they are told they have a tumor.

Clinical Discussion: Breast Cancer

Breast cancer is the second most common cancer and occurs in 1 of 8 American women, one third of whom succumb to the disease. Men represent less than 1% of those affected. The risk factors associated with breast cancer are those generally associated with *increased lifetime exposure to estrogen:*

1. **Increasing age:** majority of women are older than 50 years
2. **Geographic/racial influence:** common in white women, rare in Asian women
3. **History of breast cancer** in the contralateral breast or **endometrial cancer**
4. **Radiation exposure** and other mutagenic exposures
5. **Prolonged reproductive life:** early menarche and late menopause
6. **Nulliparity** or **late parity,** with first child at older than 30 years
7. **Obesity** from increased estrogen synthesis in fat deposits, lower progesterone levels, greater number of anovulatory cycles
8. **Exogenous estrogen:** hormone replacement therapy (but not oral contraceptives)
9. **Family history of breast cancer** in mother, sister, daughter, especially if bilateral or before menopause
10. **Genetic predisposition:** germ line mutations in *BRCA-1, BRCA-2,* p53, *ATM* (ataxia-telangiectasia mutation), which are tumor suppressor and DNA repair genes

A woman may present with a palpable breast mass, nipple secretion, inflammatory skin lesions, or an abnormal mammogram result during screening. A single, *nontender,* firm mass that is poorly circumscribed and fixed to the skin or chest wall is concerning for malignancy. Overall, 90% of women who present with a breast lump do not have cancer. But, ultimately, *all such women must be evaluated to rule out the possibility of cancer.* This evaluation includes a thorough history and physical, mammogram, breast ultrasound, and biopsy, either fine- or large-needle aspiration or open excisional biopsy with subsequent histologic and cytologic exam (Table 6-6).

Staging and Histologic Subtypes of Breast Cancer

Breast cancer, like many cancers, is staged according to a **TNM (tumor, node, metastasis) classification system.** Roughly speaking, T0, N0, and M0 mean no tumor, nodal involvement, or metastasis. This is carcinoma in situ, histologically malignant tissue that has not yet infiltrated the basement membrane. Tumor number increases with the tumor size. Node number also increases with progressive lymph node involvement. M1 denotes the presence of distant metastasis. Different combinations of the T, N, and M classification system categorize a woman's breast cancer into a **stage,** which is useful for prognostication and deciding definitive therapy. Higher stages of disease yield poorer prognosis. **Tumor grade** is determined by microscopic evaluation

TABLE 6-5 The Nomenclature of Tumors

Terminology	Definition
Neoplasm	"New growth:" abnormal tissue that undergoes uncontrolled or excessive growth
Tumor	"Swelling:" includes the *parenchyma,* consisting of neoplastic cells, plus *supportive stroma,* including connective tissue and blood vessels
Nonneoplastic tumors	
Hamartoma	Tumor consisting of hyperplasia of normal differentiated cells located at its normal site
Hyperplasia	Tissue growth from cellular proliferation resulting in an *increased number* of cells
Hypertrophy	Tissue growth resulting from *increased size* of each cell (e.g., muscle growth)
Metaplasia	The replacement of one type of fully differentiated cell by another type of fully differentiated cell (e.g., squamous metaplasia of Barrett esophagus in chronic GERD)
Benign tumors (-omas)	
Adenoma	Benign epithelial neoplasm that forms glandular patterns
Papilloma	Benign epithelial neoplasms forming finger-like or warty projections
Cystadenoma	Benign epithelial neoplasms forming large cystic masses
Malignant tumors/cancer	
Anaplasia	Very poorly differentiated cancers
Sarcomas	Malignant tumors arising from mesenchymal tissue (e.g., leiomyosarcoma)
Carcinoma	Malignant neoplasm of epithelial cell origin (any of three germ layers)
Adenocarcinoma	Carcinoma appearing in glandular growth pattern
Squamous cell carcinoma	Carcinoma with recognizable squamous cells
Teratoma	Mixed tumor consisting of tissue from two or three germ layers
Melanoma	Misnomer, malignant neoplasm of melanocytes

GERD, gastroesophageal reflux disease

TABLE 6-6 General Clinical Characteristic of Benign and Malignant Breast Lumps

	Benign Breast Lump	Malignant Breast Lump
History	<50 years old, premenopausal, painful, especially during premenstrual period, fluctuating size	Older (>50 years old), white, family history of breast/ovarian cancer
Physical exam	Breast mass *Fibroadenoma:* small, round, well-defined, mobile, rubbery, *tender* mass *Phyllodes tumor:* large fibroadenoma *Fibrocystic disease:* multiple or bilateral tender masses Nipple discharge Bilateral discharge *Hyperprolactinemia:* milky discharge *Oral contraceptives:* clear serous, milky *Mastitis:* purulent discharge	Breast mass Single, nontender, firm mass, poorly circumscribed, fixed to skin or chest wall Nipple discharge Green or bloody discharge Appearance Breast enlargement or asymmetry Nipple or skin retractions Axillary lymphadenopathy Peau d'orange (edematous erythematous skin)

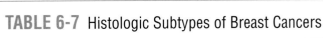

TABLE 6-7 Histologic Subtypes of Breast Cancers

Breast Cancer Type	Percentage	Characteristics
Invasive carcinoma (70–85%)		
Ductal carcinoma	—	Carcinoma arising from the intermediate ducts Increased dense, fibrous tissue stroma → hard consistency
No special type	80%	Infiltrative attachment to surrounding structures with fixation causing skin dimpling and nipple retraction
Medullary	2%	Associated with *BRCA-1* gene, better prognosis that NST cancer
Colloid	2%	Common in older women; slow-growing, well-differentiated, diploid tumor expressing hormone receptors → good prognosis
Tubular	6%	Younger women (late 40s); detected as spiculated (irregular) mass on mammography, often multifocal or bilateral; well-differentiated diploid tumors, expressing hormone receptors → good prognosis
Papillary	1%	Papillary architecture, similar to NST but better prognosis
Lobular carcinoma	10%	Often bilateral, multifocal, diffusely invasive, more likely to metastasize to CSF, ovary, uterus, and bone marrow
Inflammatory carcinoma	< 3%	Rapidly growing, painful mass that enlarges the breast with overlying skin erythema, edema, warmth; diffusely infiltrative
In situ carcinoma (15–30%)		
DCIS	80%	Malignant cells that do not infiltrate the basement membrane nor metastasize; often detected as mammographic calcifications
Paget disease	1%	Form of DCIS that extends to nipple ducts, skin, and areola, causing a fissured, ulcerated, and oozing nipple lesion
Lobular carcinoma in situ	20%	Proliferation of terminal ducts (acini), often bilateral

NST, no special type; *DCIS*, ductal carcinoma in situ

of the biopsy's histologic subtype and degree of differentiation. The presence of normal cell markers like estrogen and progesterone receptors suggest more differentiated cells and better prognosis as well as eligibility for adjuvant therapy with tamoxifen. **Aneuploidy** (abnormal number of chromosomes), changed expression of oncogenes and tumor-suppressor genes (e.g., Her2/neu, p53), and evidence of accelerated proliferation and angiogenesis are poor prognostic markers (Table 6-7).

CASE CONCLUSION

Subsequent breast ultrasound reveals a 2-cm solid mass in the upper outer quadrant of the left breast. The mammogram shows a spiculated density with clusters of microcalcifications at this same location. The breast lump is biopsied by fine-needle aspiration, which reveals no pathology. The patient undergoes open excisional biopsy of the tumor and sentinel node. Histologic exam reveals ductal carcinoma no special type (NST) with no evidence of lymph node involvement. DC is diagnosed with stage I disease and undergoes breast-conserving therapy. Five years later, she is healthy with no evidence of disease recurrence.

THUMBNAIL: Breast Cancer

Epidemiology	• >50-year-old women; white women > Asian women with breast lump
History of present illness	• Breast lump painful or painless? • Lump size fluctuating with cycle? • Nipple discharge? Color? • Skin changes? Dimpling?
Past medical history	• Prior breast cancer or other disease • Age of menarche and menopause • Use of exogenous estrogens
Family history	• Breast or ovarian cancer in mother, sister, or daughter • Known *BRCA-1, BRCA-2,* or other breast cancer genes
Physical exam **(also self-breast exam)**	• Appearance: breast dimples, asymmetry, skin changes • Palpate supraclavicular and axillary nodes • Palpate each breast superficial to deep; attempt to express discharge
Diagnostic imaging	• Mammogram: calcifications, densities • Breast ultrasound to differentiate between solid and cystic masses
Diagnostic procedures	• Fine needle/core needle biopsy • Open/excisional biopsy • Axillary dissection • Sentinel node biopsy
Treatment	• Lumpectomy + axillary dissection or sentinel node biopsy + radiation • Rare modified radical mastectomy for more extensive disease • Hormonal therapy (tamoxifen) for estrogen receptor-positive tumor • Chemotherapy

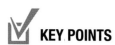

KEY POINTS

■ A malignant tumor is likely to grow in a way that would eventually cause enough disruption to a person's normal physiology to cause death, whereas a benign tumor is unlikely to behave in such a way

■ Benign tumors are better differentiated and behave like normal cells, while malignant tumors are less differentiated and do not respond well to normal regulatory signals

■ Every woman should receive a regular clinical breast exam and be taught to do monthly self-breast exams. All women with a breast lump must be evaluated to rule out the possibility of cancer.

QUESTIONS

1. A 23-year-old woman goes to her physician to ask about a tender lump in her left breast. She has no family history of cancer and is taking low-dose oral contraceptives. On exam, she has a 2-cm, rubbery, round, mobile mass. An ultrasound is performed showing a solid mass. Core needle biopsy produces a sample with benign-looking morphology. What characteristic is seen on the sample?

   A. High nucleus to cytoplasm ratio
   B. High fraction of cells with mitotic spindles
   C. Loss of glandular structure
   D. Cellular hyperplasia with glandular architecture
   E. Anaplastic cells

2. A 50-year-old woman presents with an abnormal mammogram reading showing clustered microcalcifications. She also notes recent spontaneous bloody discharge from her nipples. Her exam reveals no palpable breast, axillary, or supraclavicular masses. What is NOT a part of the appropriate diagnostic work-up for this patient?

   A. Excisional biopsy
   B. Fine-needle aspiration
   C. Sentinel node biopsy
   D. Cytology of expressed discharge
   E. Breast ultrasound

CASE 6-5   Tumor Pathogenesis

HPI: LS is a 78-year-old African American man who, during his annual checkup, is found to have a **palpable prostatic nodule** during a digital rectal exam. In addition, he noted some **tenderness on his spine.** He also noted some difficulty walking. He denied problems with urination, incontinence, numbness, weakness, or ataxia.

PE: The patient is afebrile with normal vital signs. His exam is significant for a 2-cm right-sided **prostatic nodule, spinal tenderness** at the L3 vertebra, and **mild inguinal lymphadenopathy.** He has a 4/5 left knee extensor **weakness,** and **numbness** on his left knee and inner thigh.

Labs: The patient has a markedly **elevated serum prostate serum antigen (PSA)** of 150. **Transrectal ultrasound (TRUS)** reveals a 3-cm **nodule** on the right **posterior region of the prostate** with extension into the prostatic capsule. Abdominal CT gave evidence of **lymph node involvement,** and pelvic lymphadenectomy was subsequently performed confirming malignant extension to these lymph nodes. In addition, **radionuclide bone scanning** revealed some radiopacity around the L3 vertebra. Subsequent **spinal MRI** showed impingement of the left L3 root as it exits the L3–L4 foramen.

THOUGHT QUESTIONS

- How are tumors characterized histologically?
- What is the natural history of a tumor?
- How are tumors graded and staged?
- What is prostate cancer? What are its clinical manifestations?
- How is prostate cancer screened, diagnosed, and treated?

BASIC SCIENCE REVIEW AND DISCUSSION

Now that we have reviewed the behavioral differences between benign and malignant tumors (Case 6-4), *how does one determine when a tumor is cancer?* In large part, the histologic characteristics of a tumor biopsy are used to diagnose malignancy. The characteristics that suggest **anaplasia** (or poor differentiation) are included in Table 6-8.

A neoplastic tumor begins with a single transformed cell presenting at any stage of differentiation and behavior. This cell grows to form a distinguishable mass usually confined by some anatomic capsule or basement membrane. Locally confined tumors are said to be in situ, which makes complete removal of all neoplastic tissue possible. However, if this membrane is breached, a neoplasm is said to have locally invaded adjacent tissue, which can be followed by metastasis via lymphatic or hematogenous spread.

Rate of tumor growth or **doubling time** depends on the fraction of cells in the replicative pool (**growth fraction**) and how much the rate of cell proliferation exceeds that of cell loss. The doubling time roughly correlates to the rate of clinical progression. Tumors with high growth fractions produce rapid clinical progression, if left untreated. But because such tumors have so many rapidly proliferating cells, chemotherapy quickly reduces or eliminates such tumors. On the other hand, tumors with smaller growth fractions and prolonged doubling times, while having a more indolent clinical course, are more resistant to chemotherapy.

As the tumor grows beyond 1 to 2 mm in diameter, the tumor requires neovascularization to supply the tissue with adequate oxygen and nutrients. Tumors cells stimulate **angiogenesis** by secreting angiogenic growth factors like **vascular endothelial growth factor (VEGF)** and **basic fibroblast growth factor (bFGF)**. Newly formed endothelial cells reciprocally promote tumor growth by secreting **insulin-like growth factors,** platelet-derived growth factor (PDGF), granulocyte-monocyte colony-stimulating factor (GM-CSF), and IL-1. **Neovascularization** supports not only tumor growth but also eventual metastasis.

Over time, a tumor may become more aggressive as a result of the dynamic evolution of the tumor cell population. Subpopulations may arise that divide more rapidly, are less responsive to hormonal therapy or chemotherapy, or are more prone to local invasion and metastasis. The underlying mechanisms of such shifts in behavior are thought to arise from genetic instability due to, for example, the loss of p53, which has a central role in DNA repair. If p53 is lost, the rate of spontaneous genetic mutation accelerates. With rapid negative selection of nonadvantageous genotypes, a robust, rapidly proliferating subpopulation is bound to arise.

Eventually, a tumor cell gives rise to a subpopulation that has attained the ability to metastasize. These cells adhere to and invade the basement membrane that contained the primary tumor and attach to and degrade the local extracellular matrix (ECM). The cells pass through the ECM and **intravasate** into the local vasculature. Within the circulation, it may elicit immune attack and platelet aggregation, which causes the formation of a tumor cell embolus. This embolus can adhere to endothelium at a distant site, **extravasate,** and deposit itself within that tissue. Table 6-9 lists the routes through which metastasis occurs.

Eventually, such "selfish" growth and dissemination interferes with the normal function of cells around it. Thus, it is not the mere presence of neoplastic tissue that constitutes illness. It is the dysregulation of normal physiology by the proliferation of a neoplasm that ultimately produces the disease of cancer.

Clinical Discussion: Prostate Cancer

Prostate cancer is the most common form of cancer among men, with more than 300,000 new cases per year, resulting in 41,000 deaths. Risk factors include advanced age, increased fat consumption, and family history (a few susceptibility genes have been identified). Androgen levels are suspected to contribute, as evidenced by the tumor's response to antiandrogen therapy.

Most cancers arise in the posterior gland. The cancer grows until it abuts the glandular capsule. It first invades this capsule, and then infiltrates locally to the seminal vesicles and the bladder. After this, it spreads through lymphatic vessels to the deep pelvic

TABLE 6-8 Characteristics of Anaplasia

Cellular Abnormalities	Architectural Abnormalities
Hyperchromatic DNA	Disorganized growth
↑ Nuclear-to-cytoplasmic ratio	Poor adherence to normal tissue architecture
High mitotic rate; bizarre mitotic figures	Scant vascular stroma with necrotic areas
Giant cells: large with hyperchromatic nucleus	

nodes. Finally, it spreads hematogenously to the vertebral column and visceral organs.

Most men present asymptomatically during routine screening, with a focal prostatic nodule found by **digital rectal exam (DRE)** or an **elevated PSA.** Relatively localized disease is unlikely to cause urinary symptoms, as prostate cancer is more likely to arise in the periphery within the subcapsular region away from the urethra. As the tumor grows, a patient may develop urinary problems. Back pain is an ominous sign, suggesting vertebral metastasis, and is virtually diagnostic of late-stage cancer with a very poor prognosis.

Diagnosis

1. **DRE**
2. **Serum PSA** greater than 4 ng/mL (although the specificity is poor for prostate cancer); PSA may also be elevated in benign prostatic hypertrophy (BPH) or prostatitis; adjusted for age and prostate size
3. **TRUS** for assessment of local spread
4. **Transperineal or transrectal biopsy** for histologic diagnosis of prostate cancer
5. **Radionuclide bone scan** for patients with symptoms suggestive of bony metastasis
6. **Fine-needle aspiration (FNA) of pelvic lymph nodes** for those patients with lymphadenopathy

Pathology and Staging

For prostate cancer, the **Gleason system** is used to grade tumors on a five-point scale, based on glandular pattern and degree of differentiation, scored as 1 for well-differentiated tumors and 5 for the least differentiated. There are two grades assigned, with a combined score range of 2 to 10. Staging from A to D depends on the tumor size, focal or diffuse growth, glandular capsule invasion, and metastatic spread.

Grossly, prostate cancer appears gritty and firm, classically in the posterior location in the subcapsular region. Microscopically, a well-differentiated cancer appears glandular and crowded with "back-to-back" glands lined by a single layer of cuboidal cells. This tissue architecture deteriorates to a diffuse pattern with higher-grade lesions.

Treatment

For early-stage prostate cancer, **transurethral radical prostatectomy (TURP)** and postoperative radiotherapy are performed. For those with advanced and metastatic cancer, **antiandrogen therapy** with such drugs as **finasteride** (an androgen receptor antagonist), **goserelin** (a gonadotropin-releasing hormone [GnRH] inhibitor), or **orchiectomy** (removal of testosterone-secreting testicular glands) suppresses tumor growth. However, such therapy does not induce remission, and testosterone-insensitive clones eventually arise. Such patients have a very poor prognosis.

TABLE 6-9 Methods of Metastatic Spread

Route of Spread	Metastatic Destination	Example
Direct extension	Peritoneal cavity, pleural cavity	Ovarian cancer → intraperitoneal spread
Lymphatic spread	Draining lymph nodes	Breast cancer to axillary lymph nodes
Hematogenous Spread		
Venous drainage		
Portal vein	Liver	Colon cancer metastasis to the liver
Inferior vena cava	Lungs	Renal cancer metastasis to the lungs
Paravertebral plexus	Brain or spinal column	Prostate cancer metastasis to spine or CNS
Arterial circulation[a]	Brain (depends on 1° tumor site)	Lung cancer spread via pulmonary vein → LV → aorta → internal carotid → CNS

[a]Metastasis through arterial drainage is less common, as the thick walls of arteries are more difficult to penetrate.
CNS, central nervous system; LV, left ventricle

CASE CONCLUSION

Transrectal biopsy revealed a tumor with Gleason scores of 5 and 5. With such an advanced stage cancer, LS was not considered a candidate for surgical resection. Instead, he was treated with a combination of finasteride and goserelin. He also received IV dexamethasone and a 10-day course of radiation therapy to reduce the size of the spinal tumor with the hope of decreasing the spinal root compression. He is currently stable, receiving palliative therapy for end-stage prostate cancer.

THUMBNAIL: Prostate Cancer

Identification	• >50-year-old men	• African American > Caucasian >> Asian
History of present illness	• Asymptomatic • Dysuria • Frequency	• Hematuria • Difficulty starting/stopping stream • Bone or back pain
Family history	• First-degree relatives	• Early-age onset of prostate cancer
Physical exam	• DRE • Glandular asymmetry • Palpable focal nodules	• Pelvic lymphadenopathy • Vertebral tenderness • Other bony tenderness
Diagnostic labs	• PSA > 4 age-, prostate-size adjusted	• Low free (unbound) PSA ratio
Diagnostic imaging	• TRUS	• Radionuclide bone scan
Diagnostic procedures	• Transrectal/transurethral biopsy	• FNA of lymph nodes
Grading	• Gleason system: two points 1 to 5 (from most to least differentiated)	
Staging	• Stage A to D: tumor size, capsular invasion, nodal involvement, metastasis	
Treatment	• TURP	• Hormonal therapy—finasteride • Orchiectomy

✓ KEY POINTS

■ Malignancy is diagnosed histologically by the presence of cellular and tissue abnormalities, including hyperchromatic DNA, high nuclear-to-cytoplasmic ratio, high mitotic rate, atypical or bizarre mitotic figures, and disorganized growth

■ Prostate cancer is the most common cancer among men, affecting older as well as African-American men

■ Early prostate cancer is usually asymptomatic and is picked up by DRE; late-stage prostate cancer may present with signs of local invasion and metastasis, such as dysuria and bone pain

QUESTIONS

1. Of the following, which histologic characteristics would NOT be expected in LS's Gleason 5 and 5 tumor?

   A. Hyperplastic glands of cuboidal cells arranged back to back
   B. Frequent bizarre mitotic spindles
   C. High nucleus-to-cytoplasm ratio
   D. Hyperchromatic nucleus
   E. Areas of central necrosis

2. One year after starting finasteride, LS returned, complaining of increased dysuria and urinary hesitancy. DRE revealed a larger prostatic mass than was felt several months before. His PSA was elevated several-fold higher than his previous level. What step in the pathogenesis of this new event is NOT likely to have occurred?

   A. Tumor growth was suppressed via androgen receptor antagonism by finasteride, as the relatively well-differentiated tumor cells require androgen stimulation for growth.
   B. Genetic instability led to the loss of p53 function and normal DNA repair capacity, causing acceleration in the rate of genetic mutation.
   C. A subpopulation of androgen-independent tumor cells arose against the selective pressure of finasteride therapy.
   D. A new primary prostatic tumor arose due to the selective pressure of finasteride.
   E. A subpopulation of highly proliferative tumor cells arose from spontaneous mutation, yielding a high growth fraction and accelerated tumor growth.

CASE 6-6 Molecular Oncology

HPI: MV is an 8-year-old girl who is brought in by her father after a month of markedly increasing "clumsiness." In the last month, he had noticed her frequently bumping into furniture and walls, although she denies blurry vision. She never had such symptoms before, and has no significant past medical history or any family history of any eye diseases.

PE: The patient is comfortable-appearing with normal vital signs. Her exam is significant for an **absent red reflex in the right eye,** normal visual acuity in the left eye, but **20/400 vision in the right eye.** She has a visual field consistent with **left monocular vision.** Her funduscopic exam revealed normal structures in the left eye and none in her right eye. She had no sensory or motor deficits, normal reflexes, negative Romberg sign, but a slightly ataxic gait.

THOUGHT QUESTIONS

- What are proto-oncogenes, tumor suppressor genes, apoptosis-regulating genes, and DNA repair genes, and how do these genes contribute to the development of malignancy?
- What is retinoblastoma and what are the underlying steps in its pathogenesis?

BASIC SCIENCE REVIEW AND DISCUSSION

Now that we have established the point that cancer arises from genetic mutations that promote unregulated cellular proliferation, we turn to the specific molecular events that mediate carcinogenesis. These molecular mechanisms fall under two main categories: (*a*) those that *promote growth,* and (*b*) those that *promote genetic mutation.* These two fundamental characteristics are mutually enhancing; that is, growth promotes mutation as mutation promotes growth. Under the categories of growth promotion, there are three contributing classes of genes: (*a*) **proto-oncogenes;** (*b*) **tumor suppressor genes;** and (*c*) **apoptosis-regulating genes.** In the latter category, defective **DNA repair genes,** which normally act to maintain genomic integrity, increase the chance of developing a mutation in a growth-promoting gene and thus cause tumor growth indirectly. The following is a review of these main molecular mediators of neoplasia.

Proto-Oncogenes

Proto-oncogenes can be viewed as the "green light" signal for the cell to undergo cell cycling. In a normal cell, the signal to divide is transiently released, and only after several molecular events occur. Such signals are normally tightly controlled by an elaborate system of growth-promoting and growth-inhibiting signals. But when a mutation compromises the regulation of a proto-oncogene, it can promote the uncontrolled growth of a cell (Table 6-10). The involved molecular mediators include (*a*) growth factors; (*b*) growth factor receptors; (*c*) signal transducers; (*d*) nuclear transcription proteins; and (*e*) cell cycle-regulating factors.

Growth factors are secreted proteins that bind a cell receptor and signal it to grow. Overexpression of growth factors due to a genetic mutation can promote cellular hyperplasia. **Growth factor receptors** receive the signal for growth and transmit that information to the intracellular compartment. Mutations in this class of proto-oncogenes can cause such a receptor to be *constitutively active* (i.e., it is always "on"), signaling a cell to undergo cell cycling, even in the absence of the growth factor. Alternatively, abnormal overexpression of the receptor on the cell surface may

make a cell highly sensitive to even small amounts of growth factor and can also accelerate growth.

Signal-transducing proteins include any of the proteins within the cytoplasm that transmit the external signal for growth to the nucleus. Mutations in the **ras protein,** a tyrosine kinase involved in growth signaling, is one of the most common abnormalities found in tumors. It is activated by growth factor receptors and ultimately promotes transcription and translation of *myc,* a cell cycle regulator. There are many promoters, activators, and inactivators of the ras protein, and mutations that cause dysfunction of any of these regulators can cause constitutively active *ras* and thus uninhibited cell cycling. This is present in neurofibromatosis-1, wherein a defect in the *neurofibrin-1* gene prevents proper inhibition of the *ras* gene product. **Nuclear transcription proteins** are proteins that respond to the cytoplasmic growth-promoting signals and participate in intranuclear DNA binding that either up-regulate or down-regulate expression of specific genes. Important examples of such proto-oncogenes are *myc, max,* and *mad,* which interact to either promote or inhibit cellular replication. If *max* dimerizes with *myc,* proliferation and survival is promoted. If *max* dimerizes with *mad* (forming *mad-max*), cell growth is inhibited. Dysregulation of c-*myc* expression is present in Burkitt lymphoma, breast, colon, and lung cancers.

Cell cycle-regulating proteins, or cyclins and cyclin-dependent kinases (CDKs), direct the orderly progression of the cell cycle during mitosis. CDK inhibitors inhibit cell cycle progression. Overexpression of CDKs and hypofunctioning or insufficient expression of CDK inhibitors similarly promote tumor growth.

Tumor Suppressor Genes

Tumor suppressor genes act as the "brakes" of cellular proliferation in that they inhibit the signals that promote cell cycling. The **Rb gene** is the prototypic tumor suppressor gene found in patients with retinoblastoma. **pRb** (or the *Rb* gene product) binds a transcriptional activator, the E2F protein, and keeps it from binding DNA and promoting cell cycling. Normally, pRb is present throughout a cell's nonreplicating life. But as soon as a growth factor signals a cell to grow, pRB is inactivated by cyclin or CDK, thereby releasing E2F. This allows the cell to undergo cell division. Many things can interfere with pRb's ability to inhibit E2F. For instance, HPV produces a protein that binds pRb. This can result in the development of HPV-induced **cervical cancer.**

The other important tumor suppressor gene is **p53,** also known as the "guardian of the genome" in that it acts through several mechanisms to protect the cell from genetic damage. p53

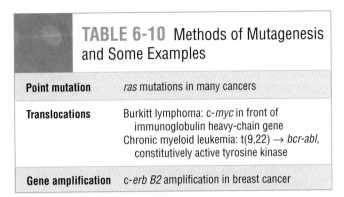

TABLE 6-10 Methods of Mutagenesis and Some Examples

Point mutation	*ras* mutations in many cancers
Translocations	Burkitt lymphoma: c-*myc* in front of immunoglobulin heavy-chain gene Chronic myeloid leukemia: t(9,22) → *bcr-abl*, constitutively active tyrosine kinase
Gene amplification	c-*erb B2* amplification in breast cancer

senses DNA damage, promotes DNA repair, delays cell cycle progression (and thereby allows time for such repair), and induces apoptosis if the DNA is inadequately repaired. It repairs damage from UV light, irradiation, and other mutagenic substances. Loss of such important functions predisposes a cell to progressive accumulation of genetic mutations that may cause it to resist death or proliferate unregulated. p53 is the most common mutation in human tumors and is present in over 50% of such cases.

Apoptosis-Regulating Genes

There are two classic regulators of programmed cell death, or **apoptosis.** *Bcl-2* inhibits apoptosis, while *bax* promotes it. Overexpression of *bcl-2* is implicated in the development of B-cell lymphoma.

DNA Repair Genes

Genetic mutations that cause defective DNA repair inherently predispose a cell to accumulating more cancer-promoting mutations. This mechanism of carcinogenesis is unique in that it does not directly promote tumor growth or survival but instead provides the condition within which a cell has an increased likelihood of acquiring a mutation in the genes that do so. This is present in **xeroderma pigmentosum,** wherein a congenital defect in DNA repair increases the risk of developing cancer due to DNA damage induced by UV light.

Two-Hit Hypothesis and Retinoblastoma

Retinoblastoma is a rare tumor of the eye, presenting in children from birth to 15 years of age. Among patients with retinoblastoma it was noted that those with the familial form of retinoblastoma were heterozygotes for a mutant *Rb* gene, despite the fact that the disease is inherited in an autosomal dominant fashion. From this, the **"two-hit" hypothesis of carcinogenesis** arose, wherein it is thought that the loss of the two copies of a tumor suppressor gene is required for malignant transformation. In those with familial retinoblastoma, a nonfunctioning *Rb* gene is inherited from a parent and is present in all somatic cells. Among those cells, particularly in the eye, one cell may acquire a genetic mutation that renders the remaining normal *Rb* gene nonfunctional. Only when this happens will one develop a retinoblastoma. Otherwise, in sporadic cases of retinoblastoma, the loss of two copies of the *Rb* gene occurs through two separate chance mutations, thus making it less likely an occurrence. This is an important concept and has been applied to many different tumors since it was first proposed for retinoblastoma.

CASE CONCLUSION

An MRI of the head is performed, which reveals a tumor localized within the right orbit with no apparent extraorbital extension. MV is diagnosed with retinoblastoma and subsequently undergoes radiation therapy. She is currently stable 2 months after therapy.

THUMBNAIL: Genes and Proteins of Carcinogenesis

Gene or Protein Type	Subtype	Examples
Proto-oncogenes	Growth factors	Fibroblast growth factor (FGF), bFGF, epidermal-derived growth factor (EDGF), transforming growth factor-α (TGF-α)
	Growth factor receptors	EDGF receptor
	Signal-transducing proteins	*ras, abl*
	Nuclear transcription factor	*myc*
	Cyclin and CDK	Cyclin D, CDK4
Tumor suppressor genes	—	p53, pRb
Apoptosis-regulating genes	Antiapoptotic	bcl-2
	Proapoptotic	bax
DNA repair genes	—	p53

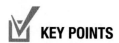

KEY POINTS

- Carcinogenesis is mediated by mutations in growth-regulating and DNA-repairing genes
- Proto-oncogenes turn into oncogenes, which promote unregulated proliferation of cells
- Tumor suppressor genes inhibit factors that promote cell proliferation
- Overexpression of antiapoptotic genes promotes cell survival and prevents the death of cells, even those normally destined for programmed cell death
- DNA repair gene defects indirectly promote carcinogenesis by increasing the likelihood of developing mutations in the above-mentioned genes

- In the "two-hit" hypothesis, homozygote loss of tumor suppressor gene function, like the *Rb* gene in retinoblastoma, is required for malignant transformation
  - Therefore, those with familial retinoblastoma inherit one defective *Rb* gene in all somatic cells, constituting the "first hit"
  - A chance acquisition of a genetic mutation causing functional loss of the other *Rb* gene in just one of those cells constitutes the "second hit"

QUESTIONS

1. AG, a 32-year-old woman with known family history of hereditary nonpolyposis colon cancer (HNPCC) syndrome, is returning for her annual screening colonoscopy. One of the biopsy samples reveals changes concerning for malignancy. HNPCC results from defects in genes involved in DNA mismatch repair (i.e., repair of mismatched base pairs during replication, e.g., C pairing to A). What step in the pathogenesis of this carcinoma is NOT likely to have occurred?

   A. AG inherited one defective DNA mismatch repair gene.
   B. One cell among all AG's colonic epithelial cells acquired a mutation that made the other copy of the repair gene nonfunctional.
   C. A chance error during replication led to a faulty pairing (e.g., G to T), which remained unrepaired.
   D. The defect in DNA mismatch repair transformed this cell into a malignant cell capable of unregulated proliferation.
   E. Accumulation of errors led to the dysfunction of several gene products involved in growth and cell cycle regulation.

2. Burkitt lymphoma is a B-cell lymphoma that results from the t(14;18)(q32;q21) translocation (32nd section of the long arm or "q" on chromosome 14 translocated upon q21 on chromosome 18). This translocation juxtaposes the site where immunoglobulin heavy-chain genes are found next to the *bcl-2* locus (on 18q21). What step in the pathogenesis of this cancer is NOT likely to occur?

   A. Chronic infection promotes B-cell differentiation into antibody-secreting plasma cells.
   B. A plasma cell with the t(14;18) translocation is stimulated to transcribe the immunoglobulin heavy-chain locus in the attempt to produce antibodies.
   C. *Bcl-2* is instead transcribed and translated to high levels of bcl-2 protein in the cytoplasm.
   D. The overabundance of *bcl-2* gene product promotes uncontrolled cellular proliferation of that transformed cell.
   E. The *bcl-2* gene product in excess forms *bcl-2* homodimers (bound pairs of bcl-2), producing an antiapoptotic signal that promotes cell survival.

CASE 6-7 Osteosarcoma

HPI: JL is a 16-year-old boy who hurt his leg snowboarding 7 months ago. Since then, he has tried splinting, rest, elevation, and ice to alleviate the pain. It has waxed and waned but has recently gotten worse. It responds partially to ibuprofen and acetaminophen. He now complains of an enlarging, firm, tender mass above the knee.

PMH: No significant illnesses. **Past surgical history (PSHx):** none. **Family history (FamHx):** Both parents alive with no significant medical illness.

Meds: Ibuprofen, acetaminophen.

PE: T 36.9°C; HR 64 beats/min; RR 14 breaths/min; BP 114/63 mm Hg.

General: Alert, oriented teenager in no distress. **Growth:** Ht 70th percentile, Wt 60th percentile. **Neck:** Supple, no masses. **Chest:** Clear to auscultation with normal respiratory effort. **GU:** Tanner IV male, descended testes. **Extremities:** The right distal femur has a tender, palpable mass about 10 cm in diameter. All extremities are warm and well perfused.

Neuro: Normal for age. **Lymph:** No enlarged lymph nodes.

An x-ray shows a lytic lesion with pronounced periosteal elevation.

THOUGHT QUESTIONS

- What are the most common malignancies of bone?
- What imaging studies are needed?
- What additional studies are required for staging a malignant bone tumor?
- What are genetic features of bone tumors?
- What is the treatment and outcome?

BASIC SCIENCE REVIEW AND DISCUSSION

Metastatic bone disease and **multiple myeloma** are far more common than primary bone tumors. Bone sarcomas are extremely rare tumors that represent only 0.2% of new malignancies. The most frequent malignant tumors of bone are osteosarcoma, chondrosarcoma, and Ewing sarcoma. The most frequent benign tumors are osteochondroma and giant cell tumor, which may be aggressive or transform into malignant tumors in certain familial syndromes.

Osteosarcoma

Osteosarcoma accounts for over 20% of primary bone malignancies. It is common in adolescence and early adulthood, occurring almost exclusively during the pubertal growth spurt. It frequently arises in the diaphyses and metaphyses of long bones, particularly of the distal femur or proximal tibia (around the knee). Genetic factors implicated in the development of osteosarcoma include the loss of the tumor suppressor genes p53 and Rb. Incidence is increased in **Li-Fraumeni syndrome** and in congenital retinoblastoma. Radiation is a major risk factor for osteosarcoma, especially in genetically susceptible individuals. Under light microscopy, osteosarcoma consists of large, primitive cells producing disorganized osteoid. On x-ray imaging, the typical appearance is called the **"sunburst effect"** or **Codman triangle,** which is created as the expanding tumor lifts the periosteum. Osteosarcoma metastasizes primarily to the lungs, via venous drainage. Therefore, lung imaging with x-ray and CT is critical for staging. Treatment is with intensive chemotherapy and surgery. Active agents are methotrexate, doxorubicin hydrochloride (Adriamycin), cisplatin, and, recently, ifosfamide. Osteosarcoma is resistant to radiation therapy.

Ewing Sarcoma

Ewing sarcoma is the second most common primary malignant bone tumor of childhood. It can present as early as age 3 years. Like osteosarcoma, Ewing can present in the long bones around the knee, but it can also be found in the pelvic bones, scapulae, and ribs. Ewing sarcoma is characterized by a t(11;22) translocation that creates a fusion gene EWS-FLI1. This creates a chimeric transcription factor that leads to malignant transformation. Histologically, Ewing sarcoma is composed of monotonous small round blue cells with little stroma. Similar to osteosarcoma, metastasis to the lungs is common.

Definitive resection with wide margins is essential to cure either of these tumors. Resection occurs after a period of induction chemotherapy to decrease the soft tissue component of the tumor. This commonly results in limb amputation; endoprostheses are in development. Radiation therapy may be used in place of surgery for Ewing sarcoma. Prognosis depends on tumor stage. Overall, localized disease has a long-term survival rate of about 70%, but metastatic tumors result in a survival rate of only about 15%. Other risk factors for relapse include poor histologic response to chemotherapy and large primary tumors.

CASE CONCLUSION

JL undergoes MRI of the leg, chest x-ray, and chest CT. These studies show four metastatic nodules in the chest. Bone biopsy reveals large malignant cells with immature osteoid, showing osteosarcoma. Immunohistochemistry for Her-2/neu is positive. No bone marrow biopsy is indicated. JL is treated with high-dose methotrexate, cisplatin, Adriamycin, and ifosfamide. The primary lesion is resected with an above-the-knee amputation after 12 weeks of chemotherapy. The surgical specimen shows tumor necrosis of only 75%, indicating a poor response. Chemotherapy lasts 9 months, after which JL has no measurable disease and good function. However, he is likely to relapse within 5 years and at that point will be a candidate for experimental therapy using anti-Her-2/neu therapeutics.

THUMBNAIL: Select Bone Tumors

Type	Location	Peak Incidence	Description
Benign osteochondroma	Metaphyses: lower femur/upper tibia	Men <25 years; most common benign bone tumor	Bony growth with cartilage cap projecting from bone surface; malignant transformation in *multiple familial osteochondromatosis*
Giant cell tumor	Epiphyses of long bones: lower femur, upper tibia	Women age 20–40 years	Multinucleated giant cells; "soap bubble" appearance on x-ray; aggressive regrowth
Malignant metastases	Variable	Variable; most common with kidney, thyroid, testes, lung, prostate, and breast primaries	Breast/prostate most common; breast: lytic and blastic; prostate: blastic; lung: lytic
Multiple myeloma	Skull, axial skeleton	Older adults	Punched-out lytic lesions associated with hypercalcemia
Osteosarcoma	Metaphyses: lower femur/upper tibia	Boys age 10–20 years; most common primary malignant bone tumor; risk factors: Paget disease, radiation, familial retinoblastoma	Bone-producing tumor; Codman triangle on x-ray; ↑↑ alkaline phosphatase; early metastases to lung, liver, brain
Chondrosarcoma	Pelvis, spine, scapula, ribs, proximal humerus	Men age 30–60 years; ↑ in *multiple familial osteochondromatosis*	Cartilaginous tumor
Ewing sarcoma	Long bones, pelvis, scapula, ribs	Boys <15 years	Small cell tumor; 11;22 chromosomal translocation

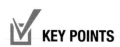

KEY POINTS

■ Metastatic bone tumors and multiple myeloma are far more common than primary bone tumors

■ Osteosarcoma is the most common primary malignant bone tumor and it affects primarily children and adolescents; it is more common in boys

■ Ewing sarcoma is the second most common primary malignant bone tumor in children

QUESTIONS

1. An otherwise healthy 9-year-old boy has a mass growing below his knee. At surgery, the mass is removed and sent to the pathology department. Sheets of hyperchromatic cells with small round blue nuclei are seen under the microscope. Cytogenic analysis reveals a t(11;22) translocation. What is the most likely diagnosis?

   A. Osteosarcoma
   B. Multiple myeloma
   C. Giant cell tumor
   D. Metastatic disease
   E. Ewing sarcoma

2. Which bone tumor(s) frequently metastasize(s) to the lungs?

   A. Osteosarcoma
   B. Ewing sarcoma
   C. Giant cell tumor
   D. A and B
   E. B and C

CASE 6-8 Acute Leukemia

HPI: PS, a 5-year-old boy, presents with 1 week of **low-grade fever,** sore throat, and persistent chest pain. The pain is localized to the sternum and is refractory to ibuprofen. His parents noted that he has not been as active during play, **bruised easily,** and had **frequent nosebleeds** in the past several months. They also noted constipation, with increased crying and distress associated with bowel movements in the past 2 days.

PMH: Monthly episodes of upper respiratory infections, including two hospitalizations for pneumonia in the past year.

PE: T 38.0°C; HR 105 beats/min; BP 100/63 mm Hg; RR 28 breaths/min; SaO_2 97%.

The patient is thin and pale. He has **multiple petechiae** in his oral mucosa with **pharyngeal erythema** and purulent exudate. **Sternal rub elicits tenderness.** The lungs are clear. Cardiac auscultation is normal. He has a **tender hepatosplenomegaly.** His extremities are cool with multiple **ecchymoses** on all extremities. Rectal exam reveals a small, tender perirectal mass compatible with an **abscess.** He is neurologically intact with no abnormalities on fundal exam.

Labs: WBC 2200/µL, Hgb 6.5 g/dL, **Hct 20%, Plt 75,000/µL,** MCV 90 fL. The differential blood count shows 15% neutrophils, **74% lymphocytes,** 2% bands, 6% monocytes, and **3% blasts.** Na 139, **K 3.5,** Cl 100, HCO_3 23, BUN 21, Cr 0.8. Throat cultures grow *Pseudomonas* sp. Given the **pancytopenia with predominance of lymphocytes,** a bone marrow aspirate and biopsy are performed showing **95% cellularity (normal 20–80%) with 75% blasts.**

THOUGHT QUESTIONS

- What is the normal differentiation of hematopoietic cells?
- What is the genetic basis of acute leukemia? What is the etiology?
- What are the clinical manifestations of acute leukemia? What is in the differential diagnosis?

BASIC SCIENCE REVIEW AND DISCUSSION

All blood cells arise from a common pluripotent stem cell via hematopoietic differentiation. The first step in hematopoiesis is the differentiation into lymphoid and myeloid stem cells. These stem cells give rise to their respective blasts cells, the precursors to the final mature cells. Mature cells from the myeloid lineage include monocytes/macrophages, erythrocytes, megakaryocytes/platelets, neutrophils, eosinophils, and basophils. Mature lymphoid cells include T lymphocytes, B lymphocytes (which further differentiate into plasma cells), and, possibly, natural killer cells (Fig. 6-3). As maturation progresses during normal hematopoiesis, there is the potential for a single cell to transform and divide unregulated by normal growth signals. In acute leukemia, malignant transformation of an immature "blast" cell with concurrent arrest of its maturation results in the rapid clonal proliferation of acute leukemia. In contrast, in chronic leukemia, the proliferating leukemic cells undergo full maturation, even though malignant transformation occurs at an earlier stage than it does in acute leukemia. The behavior of these more mature cells leads to a more indolent clinical course than that of acute leukemia. There are some conditions that predispose one to developing acute leukemia, including Down syndrome, familial syndromes (e.g., Fanconi anemia, ataxia telangiectasia), and previous exposures (e.g., cancer chemotherapy, radiation, benzene); however, most leukemias arise de novo.

Leukemia results from abberant genetic rearrangements such as translocations, additions, or deletions at the chromosomal or genetic level in hematopoietic cells. Classically, leukemia is a consequence of a nonrandom, balanced chromosomal translocation that can result in the formation of a fusion gene, or **chimeric gene,** that causes, through varying mechanisms, the inappropriate expression of specific oncogenes. This can lead to the disruption of normal cell cycle regulation and thus lead to uncontrolled clonal proliferation. The ultimate phenotype of the leukemia is dependent on the specific genetic aberration and the subsequent behavior of the proliferating cells.

Acute lymphoblastic leukemia comprises 80% of acute leukemias of childhood. Acute myelogenous leukemia (AML) occurs mostly in adults, with a median age of onset of 50 years and increasing with advanced age. Pathophysiologically, leukemic proliferation in the bone marrow leads to crowding out of normal hematopoietic cells, leading to bone marrow failure. Thus, the clinical manifestations of acute leukemia are associated with the resulting **pancytopenia** (neutropenia, anemia, and thrombocytopenia), **leukocytosis,** bone marrow expansion, as well as the infiltration of leukemic cells into the bloodstream, major organs, and other tissues (Table 6-11).

The essential diagnostic feature of acute leukemia is a **hypercellular bone marrow with greater than 30% replacement by blast cells.** Other prominent features include **pancytopenia** and **blasts** in the peripheral blood smear. Tests can also screen for evidence of soft tissue and bony infiltration as well other causes of pancytopenia or leukocytosis, such as parvovirus B19 or infectious mononucleosis from EBV, respectively. AML is categorized by morphology and histochemistry from M0 to M7, roughly correlated to the least differentiated to the most differentiated leukemia. Acute lymphocytic leukemia (ALL) is categorized by morphology into L1 (small uniform blasts of typical childhood ALL), L2 (larger, more variable-size cells), and L3 (uniform cells with basophilic or vacuolated cytoplasm). ALL is further subdivided into B-cell and T-cell lineage by the immunohistologic identification of surface antigens, as listed below. Cytogenetics provides significant prognostic information, as well (Box 6-1).

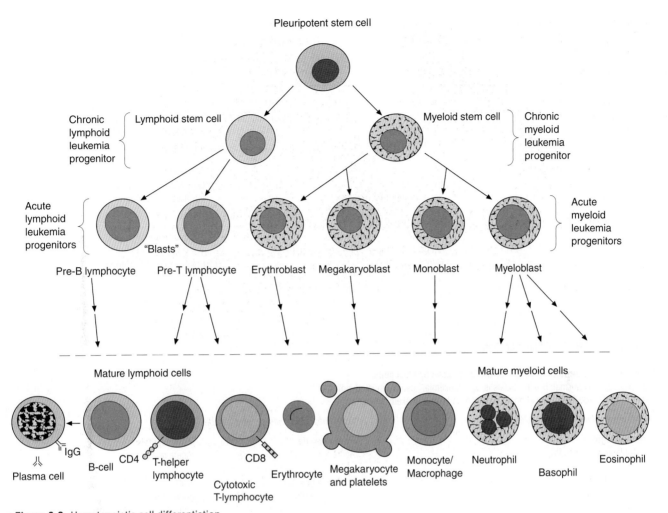

• **Figure 6-3.** Hematopoietic cell differentiation.

TABLE 6-11 Presentation of Acute Leukemias

Pathophysiology	Symptoms	Signs/Laboratory Abnormalities
Neutropenia	Frequent infection, chronic fever Anorexia Sweats Sore throat/oral sores Rectal pain	Fever, tachycardia Weight loss/thin habitus Diaphoresis Pharyngitis/dental abscess/stomatitis Rectal abscess
Anemia	Fatigue Dyspnea on exertion	Pallor Tachycardia, tachypnea, hypoxemia
Thrombocytopenia	Excess bleeding Easy bruising Epistaxis Menorrhagia	Ecchymoses/petechiae Retinal flame hemorrhages Signs of chronic bleeding from hypocoagulability
Leukostasis	Visual changes Headache/altered mental status	Leukocytosis with blasts >100,000/μL Hypoxemia
Bone marrow expansion	Bone pain	Local tenderness

(Continued)

TABLE 6-11 Presentation of Acute Leukemias *(Continued)*

Pathophysiology	Symptoms	Signs/Laboratory Abnormalities
Major organ infiltration, especially with monocytic leukemias	Early satiety Headache Vision changes Altered mental status	Tender hepatosplenomegaly Cranial nerve abnormalities Papilledema/white retinal exudate Spinal tenderness/leg weakness
Other soft tissue infiltration	Skin nodules Poor dentition Neck or inguinal masses	"Leukemia cutis" Gingival hypertrophy Lymphadenopathy
High cellular proliferation/death	Muscle weakness, constipation Gouty arthritis—joint pain Vitamin K deficiency → coagulopathy Symptoms of DIC	Hypokalemia Hyperuricemia ↑ PT, normal PTT Low or falling fibrinogen

DIC, disseminated intravascular coagulopathy; *PT,* prothrombin time; *PTT,* partial thromboplastin time

---

BOX 6-1 Diagnosis of Acute Leukemia

Definition: **30% or more of bone marrow is replaced by blast cells**
(<5% blasts is normal; 5–29% blasts is "pre-leukemia," usually myelodysplasia)
Pearl: WBC >60,000/μL is almost always some form of leukemia

Diagnostic Marker	AML	ALL	Differential diagnosis of abnormal blood count	
Morphologic			***Pancytopenia***	***Leukocytosis***
Cytoplasmic Auer rods	+	−	Acute leukemia	Acute leukemia
Histochemical			Chronic leukemia	Chronic leukemia
Myeloperoxidase	+	−	EBV, HIV, CMV, parvovirus B19	Acute infection
Nonspecific esterase	+	−	Chronic infection in marrow	Infectious mononucleosis
Immunologic			Megaloblastic anemia	Corticosteroids
TdT	−	+	Aplastic anemia	Lithium carbonate intake
			Bone marrow replacement	
ALL subtype	Surface antigens		Myelodysplasia	
Early B cell	CD10, CD19			
T cell	CD2, CD5, CD7			

CASE CONCLUSION

PS was admitted, and further cytology was performed on the bone marrow biopsy. It was determined that the child had a hyperdiploid ALL. Induction chemotherapy was initiated over 7 days. He was supported with antibiotics and red blood cell and platelet transfusions. GM-CSF was started at the 4th week, and complete remission was achieved with a neutrophil count of 2000/μL, platelets 150,000/μL, and less than 5% bone marrow blasts. Several rounds of consolidation chemotherapy followed. At the age of 30, the patient is doing well, with no evidence of leukemia.

THUMBNAIL: Acute Leukemias

Pathophysiology	Genetic translocation, addition, deletion, or inversion → aberrant expression of oncogene → cell cycle dysregulation → lymphoid or myeloid blast cell proliferation
Epidemiology	ALL: peak ages 3–7 years, 80% of childhood acute leukemias AML: more common in adults, age 15–40 years, 20% of childhood leukemias

(Continued)

THUMBNAIL: Acute Leukemias *(Continued)*

Symptoms	Short course of illness, fever, malaise, anorexia, weight loss, excessive bleeding, paleness, bone pain, sore throat, oral lesions, perirectal pain, neurologic deficits
Past medical history	Family history of AML (Fanconi, Bloom), Down syndrome Prior cancer (exposure to alkylating agents, radiation, topoisomerase II inhibitors) Occupational exposures (radiation, benzene, petroleum, smoking, paint, pesticides)
Physical findings	Fever, tachycardia, ecchymosis, papilledema, retinal hemorrhage/infiltrate, gingival hyperplasia, dental abscess, lymphadenopathy, sternal rub tenderness, hepatosplenomegaly, back tenderness, skin infiltration, neurologic deficits
Laboratory findings	**Pancytopenia** (neutropenia, anemia, thrombocytopenia) or **leukocytosis** (esp. WBC >60,000/μL), peripheral blast cells and abnormal PMNs/platelets; hypokalemia, hyperuricemia, ↑ PT, normal PTT, ↓ fibrinogen
Diagnosis	Bone marrow aspiration/biopsy: hypercellular bone marrow (normal 20–80%) **>30% blasts** (normal <5%) Differentiate between AML (Auer rods, myeloperoxidase [MPO], nonspecific esterase [NSE]) vs. ALL (terminal deoxynucleotidyl transferase [TdT]); further subtype leukemia according to morphology, surface antigen profile, and cytogenetics
Differential diagnosis	Acute or chronic leukemia, aplastic anemia, myelodysplasia, viral infection, megaloblastic anemia, mononucleosis, drug reaction, stress, infection, malignancy
Prognosis	*Favorable:* Younger Hyperdiploidy Favorable cytogenetics Moderate leukocytosis De novo leukemia <4 wks to complete remission	*Unfavorable:* Older Complex cytogenetics Unfavorable cytogenetics, e.g., t(9,22) Severe leukocytosis Secondary leukemia >4 wks to complete remission

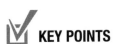

KEY POINTS

- Acute leukemia occurs from a malignant transformation and proliferation of a single leukocyte, giving rise to a monoclonal population of either myeloid or lymphoid cells

- Malignant transformation in acute leukemia occurs at the "blast" stage, with arrest in cell maturation, while in chronic leukemia it occurs at an earlier stage, with no arrest in cell maturation, thus giving rise to a pleomorphic population of "mature" leukemic cells

- The majority of the clinical manifestations arise from the pancytopenia and leukocytosis caused by the crowding out of normal bone marrow cells by proliferating leukemic cells

- Diagnosis aims to identify the leukemia by morphology and histologic and cytogenetic markers, which direct treatment and provide information on prognosis

QUESTIONS

1. A 7-year-old girl presents with a clinical picture suggestive of acute leukemia and a bone marrow biopsy performed showing greater than 30% blasts. Cytologic testing reveals Pre–B-cell ALL with L1 morphology. What diagnostic finding would not correlate with this diagnosis?

   A. TdT+ cells
   B. Small uniform blast cells
   C. CD7+ cells
   D. CD10+ cells
   E. CD22+ cells

2. A 53-year-old woman with a history of gouty arthritis presents with malaise, and bone and joint pain in the left femur

and knee. She is slightly febrile and is found to have a WBC count of 45,000/μL. What are the possible etiologies of her symptoms?

   A. Hyperuricemia from high cell turnover in acute leukemia, causing gouty arthritis
   B. Leukemic cell proliferation with bone marrow expansion
   C. Recent ingestion of contaminated meat, causing gastroenteritis
   D. Osteomyelitis from immunocompromise induced by steroid therapy
   E. All of the above

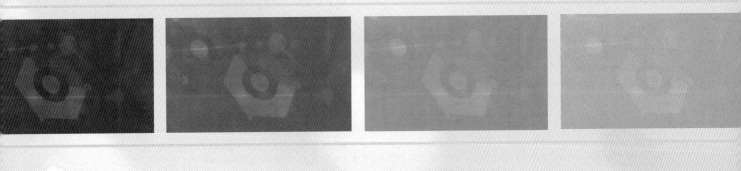

PART VII
Endocrinology

HPI: PY is a 19-year-old white man who presents to the ED with complaints of abdominal pain, nausea, and vomiting for 3 days. The patient states that he had a mild fever with chills for 1 day last week, but attributed his symptoms to "the flu." He has also noted increased thirst and urination for the past month. Patient denies diarrhea, constipation, dysuria, hematuria, headache, or flank pain, and he has not vomited any blood. He has complained of blurry vision recently, but has otherwise been free of known medical problems and is not on any medications. Systems review is significant for a 15-pound weight loss over the past 2 months and generalized fatigue for the same period.

PE: On physical exam, PY is a drowsy, thin man with an unusual fruity odor to his breath. He appears to be dehydrated, with poor skin turgor and dry mucous membranes in his mouth. The patient breathes both rapidly and heavily. He is tachycardic with normal heart sounds. He also exhibits mild epigastric tenderness, but no masses and normal bowel sounds.

Labs: Urinalysis reveals 4+ glucose and large ketones. Other significant labs include a serum glucose level of 645 mg/dL, positive ketones in serum, altered serum electrolytes, and an elevated BUN/creatinine level. Arterial blood gas (ABG) reveals an elevated anion gap metabolic acidosis, with pH 7.05, Pco_2 15 mm Hg, Po_2 = 106 mm Hg, and HCO_3^- 6 mEq/L.

THOUGHT QUESTIONS

- This is an acute presentation of what chronic disease process?
- How do insulin and glucagon function to regulate glucose metabolism?
- What is the pathogenesis behind this condition?

BASIC SCIENCE REVIEW AND DISCUSSION

PY presents to the emergency room in acute **diabetic ketoacidosis** (DKA). DKA is a metabolic complication of type 1 diabetes mellitus (DM), characterized by hyperglycemia, excess serum ketones, and metabolic acidosis. Although DKA can evolve rapidly, it is actually an acute manifestation of the chronic disease process of **type 1 diabetes.** Patients with type 1 diabetes often have a sudden onset of symptoms, commonly preceded by a viral-like syndrome. These symptoms can include polyuria, polydipsia, and polyphagia, as well as weight loss and blurry vision. In this instance, although PY attributed his condition to "the flu," laboratory studies and diagnostic signs help confirm that there is a serious underlying condition at hand.

Type 1 diabetes accounts for about 10% of all cases of diabetes. It is common in children, young adults, and people of European (especially Scandinavian) descent. The primary defect behind type 1 diabetes is a complete lack of endogenous insulin. Most commonly, this lack of insulin is caused by *autoantibodies directed against pancreatic beta-cell antigens.* These autoantibodies start a destructive cascade within the pancreatic islet (Fig. 7-1). It has been hypothesized that a precipitating event, such as a viral illness, can initiate this cascade within genetically susceptible persons. Although insulin secretion is only impaired at first, continued destruction and loss of **beta cells** eventually eliminates insulin secretion completely. This process can take years to complete, and patients can remain asymptomatic until late in the disease process. After loss of about 70% of their beta cells, however, patients become symptomatic and may develop DKA rapidly. They are *dependent on*

exogenous insulin secretion for day-to-day survival. Rarely, type 1 diabetes can occur in patients with severe insulin deficiency and no evidence of autoimmunity.

Glucose is the primary fuel source for all cells of the body. Plasma glucose levels are normally regulated by the balance of insulin and glucagon. Insulin is an anabolic hormone produced by the beta cells of the pancreas. The precursor molecule of insulin consists of a C-peptide, an A chain, and a B chain, connected by two disulfide bonds. The C-peptide portion must be cleaved off the proinsulin molecule before it becomes activated as insulin. Once activated, it promotes the burning of carbohydrate, the storage of fat, and a reduction in circulating levels of glucose, amino acids, and fatty acids.

Insulin and Glucagon

The primary stimuli for insulin secretion is an *increase in circulating glucose and amino acids.* Insulin lowers blood glucose by promoting glucose uptake and utilization by tissues that express GLUT-4 glucose transporters, namely skeletal muscle, cardiac muscle, and adipose tissue. In contrast, brain, liver, and RBCs take up glucose independent of insulin. Insulin also *suppresses hepatic glucose production* (glycogenolysis and gluconeogenesis) and *inhibits glucagon release* by the beta cells of the pancreas. **Glucagon** is a catabolic hormone that opposes the action of insulin on liver and fat, and acts to raise blood glucose. It does this by promoting the release of fatty acids from adipose tissue and promoting glycogenolysis and glucose release from the liver. A fall in plasma glucose is the main stimulus for the release of glucagon. Together, the actions of insulin and glucagon work to maintain normal glucose homeostasis. When there is an absolute or relative lack of insulin, however, DM can occur and manifests as the signs and symptoms of hyperglycemia.

Diabetic Ketoacidosis

DKA is an acutely dangerous complication of type 1 diabetes that results in a rapid spiraling sequence of events that can lead to coma and death. The diagnostic features of DKA are **hyperglycemia,**

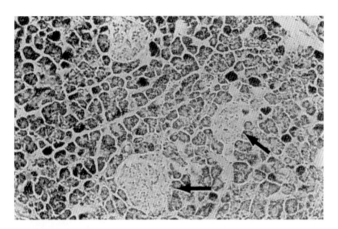

• **Figure 7-1.** The endocrine functions of the pancreas arise from the islets of Langerhans. These islets contain numerous cell types, including beta cells which secrete insulin, alpha cells which synthesize glucagon, and delta cells which produce somatostatin. The beta cells comprise about 75% of the cells in the islet and are the cells that are affected in type 1 diabetes mellitus. (Image courtesy of Joel Schechter, PhD, Keck School of Medicine at the University of Southern California.)

CASE CONCLUSION

Taking note of PY's rapidly deteriorating state, physicians in the ED immediately begin rehydrating PY with IV fluids and administer insulin therapy. As hydration is corrected and ketone overproduction is shut off by insulin, PY's anion gap slowly begins to normalize. He remains in the ED until stabilized and is transferred to the diabetes unit for further monitoring.

excess ketones (acetoacetate and β-hydroxybutyrate) in serum, and **high anion gap metabolic acidosis.** Other associated features include dehydration, electrolyte abnormalities, and severe metabolic "stress" such as infection, MI, or trauma. Because type 1 diabetics have an absolute lack of insulin, they are unable to use glucose as a source of energy. Paradoxically, this reduced glucose utilization by muscle and fat stimulates increased glucose production by the liver. Stress hormones such as epinephrine further stimulate glucose production and limit utilization, contributing to the hyperglycemia. As an alternate fuel source, increased free fatty acids are released for conversion into ketones for energy. The buildup of excess ketones in the blood results in an increased anion gap metabolic acidosis. Acidemia stimulates increased ventilation as a compensatory mechanism and thus lowers the PCO_2 of blood. Glucose excretion into the urine results in the loss of water from the body and creates an extremely dehydrated state. Correction of the hyperglycemia requires both hydration and insulin to reverse ketone production and ketoacidosis.

THUMBNAIL: Type 1 Diabetes Mellitus

Primary defect	Absolute insulin deficiency
Pathogenesis	Autoimmune attack against pancreatic beta cells
Frequency	~10% of diabetes cases
Age of onset	Usually prior to age 20
Clinical onset	Acute symptoms
HLA association	DR3/DR4
Identical twin concordance	20–30%
Islet antibodies	>90%
Islet histology	Beta cell destruction
Insulin resistance	No
Blood insulin/C-peptide levels	Low or absent
High-risk groups	European, especially Scandinavian
Primary treatment options	Exogenous insulin therapy

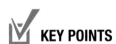 KEY POINTS

■ Autoimmune etiology: antibodies are directed against pancreatic beta cells

■ Eventually results in absolute insulin deficiency

■ **Insulin is required for treatment;** insulin secretagogues that stimulate insulin secretion (glyburide, glipizide, tolbutamide) become ineffective when all the beta cells are destroyed

■ Young age of onset, usually no family history of diabetes

QUESTIONS

1. DKA is associated with several metabolic abnormalities. These abnormalities include dehydration, hyperglycemia, and an accelerated state of lipolysis and ketone production. These metabolic imbalances are reflected in irregular laboratory values, including an altered anion gap. Using the laboratory values Na^+ 140 mEq/L, K^+ 4.0 mEq/L, Cl^- 103 mEq/L, and HCO_3^- 6 mEq/L, PY's calculated anion gap is:

   A. 12 mmol/L
   B. 20 mmol/L
   C. 31 mmol/L
   D. 35 mmol/L
   E. 44 mmol/L

2. A 26-year-old bulimic woman is found weak and lethargic in her apartment by a neighbor. Mucous membranes are dry and she is minimally responsive. The neighbor dials 911 and the woman is rushed to the nearest hospital where laboratory tests reveal blood glucose levels of 800, serum pH 7.1, Pco_2 18 mmHq, Po_2 98 mmHq, and HCO_3^- 10 meq/L. The patient is rapidly rehydrated with IV fluids and given an injection of exogenous insulin. When using exogenous insulin therapy, serum C-peptide levels are:

   A. Increased
   B. Decreased
   C. Normal
   D. Indicative of long-term glycemic control
   E. Necessary for acute therapeutic monitoring

CASE 7-2 | Diabetes Type 2

HPI: CJ is a 63-year-old African American woman who presents to her primary care physician complaining of nocturia twice nightly for the past 6 months. She states that she was reluctant to go to the doctor because she didn't think there was anything wrong, but the nocturia was beginning to interfere with her sleep. CJ states that she has felt otherwise well, but admits to being "thirsty all the time." Upon further questioning, the patient revealed that while pregnant with her daughter many years ago, she vaguely remembered her doctor mentioning that her blood sugar was "a little high." She received no medications at that time and recalls that the problem resolved shortly after delivering the baby. The patient is a pleasant and cooperative, mildly obese female. She admits to putting on "a few pounds" over the past 5 years, especially after the death of her husband. She says that the two of them used to take walks in the park together on a regular basis, but now she has no one to walk with. Patient denies any headache, visual loss, or numbness/tingling in her extremities.

PE: On physical exam, CJ appears to have scattered dot/blot hemorrhages and hard exudates in the periphery of her left eye; macula are intact bilaterally. She also exhibits reduced sensation to touch and vibration in both feet and ankles. The remainder of the exam is normal.

Labs: Blood tests reveal plasma glucose levels to be elevated at 232 mg/dL. Both BUN and creatinine are also slightly increased above normal. Urinalysis shows 3+ glucose and 2+ protein in her urine.

Upon receiving these results, the physician asks CJ to return the next morning for a fasting glucose level. Fasting results are also elevated at 170 mg/dL. The physician diagnoses CJ with type 2 DM and asks her to make an appointment to discuss her diagnosis and treatment options.

THOUGHT QUESTIONS

- What is the primary defect behind type 2 DM?
- What risk factors does CJ have for developing diabetes?
- What are the complications of this disease process?

BASIC SCIENCE REVIEW AND DISCUSSION

CJ has been diagnosed with type 2 DM. Although the symptoms of **polyuria, polydipsia,** and **hyperglycemia** are common to both type 1 and type 2 diabetes, the gradual onset, increased age of the patient, and obese body habitus suggest that type 2 DM is more likely. Type 2 DM results from a decreased sensitivity to insulin, resulting in a "relative" insulin deficiency. Although patients can produce insulin in their pancreas, they can't make enough to compensate for their increased needs. This insulin resistance is in part genetic; **central obesity, high carbohydrate diet,** and **reduced physical activity** are the most common environmental contributing factors. The condition is also most common in people of Latino, African, Native American, and Asian origin. Women with a history of gestational diabetes are at increased risk for getting type 2 DM later in life.

Pathophysiology

Physiologically, the primary defect in type 2 DM is peripheral **insulin resistance.** This resistance disturbs the delicate balance between the glucose-regulating actions of insulin and glucagon. Namely, insulin is deficient and glucagon is excessive. This imbalance results in **impaired glucose uptake and utilization by cells** (particularly skeletal muscle and fat cells), **increased protein catabolism,** and **increased lipolysis.** These changes are evident in patients as hyperglycemia and glucosuria, nitrogen loss in urine from protein breakdown, and ketonemia/ketonuria from increased fat metabolism. As the body senses decreased glucose uptake, it stimulates the pancreatic beta cells to compensate and make more insulin. However, the beta cells eventually become overworked and fail to maintain blood glucose at normal levels. Hepatic glucose overproduction occurs secondary to the perceived lack of glucose availability, further contributing to the hyperglycemia.

Acute Complications

Because type 2 diabetics make some insulin, they can suppress lipolysis and do not develop the acute, life-threatening complication of DKA seen in type 1 diabetics. Instead, type 2 patients are susceptible to a **nonketotic hyperosmolar state** that can occur with infection or other metabolic stress. Although there is no ketoacidosis, these states are characterized by **hyperglycemia, dehydration,** and **altered mental status.** With blood glucose values of greater than 600 to 800 mg/dL, a hyperosmolar coma may ensue. Electrolyte abnormalities are also common. Treatment is slow fluid rehydration to correct the hyperosmolar state.

Chronic Complications

Chronic complications of diabetes include **nephropathy, retinopathy,** and **neuropathy.** In addition, **atherosclerosis** is often present prior to the onset of symptomatic hyperglycemia, and its course is hastened and aggravated by DM. Complications are not usually present at the onset of diabetes, but develop after years of hyperglycemia. Abnormal microvascular hemodynamics and glycosylation of proteins are possible mechanisms contributing to the atherosclerosis, retinopathy, and nephropathy. In addition, individuals differ in their susceptibility to the effects of diabetes on their renal, retinal, and neural tissues.

CJ already shows signs of chronic hyperglycemia, as she has evidence of background retinopathy in her left eye (dot/blot hemorrhages from microvascular changes), although the initial changes have not yet impinged on her vision (macula are intact). Also, she may have some early symmetric polyneuropathy, as shown by the bilateral loss of touch and vibration sensation in her feet and ankles. Cells that are freely permeable to glucose, such as

169

peripheral nerves, experience a large influx of glucose during periods of hyperglycemia. This excess glucose is converted to sorbitol within the cells. Diabetic neuropathy may be caused by **sorbitol accumulation** and **myoinositol depletion** within peripheral nerves, resulting in decreased Na^+-K^+ ATPase activity and impaired nerve conduction. CJ's renal function has also been affected, as shown by the elevated BUN and creatinine. Low GFR, proteinuria, and HTN may be indicative of impending renal failure. Obesity is a risk factor for the development of type 2 DM, but it is not a result of long-term DM. More than 80% of all patients with type 2 DM are obese, because obesity is associated with resistance to the glucose-lowering effects of insulin. Weight loss often lowers elevated blood glucose in patients with type 2 DM.

Clinical Management

Because of the acute and particularly the chronic complications of type 2 DM, it is imperative that patients be followed closely and their disease carefully managed. Aggressive management can involve patients checking their blood glucose values four times per day, although this can decrease once a stable management regimen is achieved. A hemoglobin A_{1c} (**HbA$_{1c}$**), or **glycosylated hemoglobin,** can be sent to assess the average glucose values over the past 3 months, since the average lifespan of a red blood cell is 120 days. In patients who achieve tight control of their sugar levels, keeping HbA$_{1c}$ below 7%, it has been shown that they are less likely to suffer the chronic microvascular complications of diabetes.

Diet and exercise are mainstays of treatment, and patients who are actually able to maintain a low-carbohydrate diet and lose weight have been known to decrease or discontinue medications. Oral medications are commonly used, including the **sulfonylureas** (e.g., glyburide, glipizide), **biguanides** (metformin), **thiazolidinediones** (rosiglitazone, pioglitazone), and **meglitinides** (repaglinide). The most common of these medications, the sulfonylureas, act to increase insulin release from the beta cell of the pancreas. Another common medication, metformin, a biguanide, acts to decrease postprandial glucose levels, although the exact mechanism is unclear. Because these two medications operate in different ways, they can be used together to keep patients from requiring insulin. In patients who fail oral agents, insulin therapy is used. It can be used similarly to that in type 1 patients, although the risk of hypoglycemia is lower.

CASE CONCLUSION

CJ returns to her physician and is encouraged to find a new walking partner, as well as maintain a low-fat, low simple sugar, and high-fiber diet. She is also started on a regimen of glyburide to help stimulate insulin secretion by the pancreas and increase tissue sensitivity to insulin. This approach brings her glucose levels back to normal and gives CJ a chance to get more rest.

THUMBNAIL: Type 1 vs. Type 2 Diabetes Mellitus

	Type 1 Diabetes	Type 2 Diabetes
Primary defect	Absolute insulin deficiency	Peripheral insulin resistance
Pathogenesis	Autoimmune attack against pancreatic beta cells	Genetic/environmental influences
Frequency	~10% of diabetes cases	~90% of cases
Age of onset	Usually prior to age 20	>40 years old
Clinical onset	Acute symptoms	Gradual symptoms
Human lymphocytic antigen (HLA) association	DR3/DR4	None
Identical twin concordance	20–30%	60–90%
Islet antibodies	>90%	Rare
Islet histology	Beta cell destruction	Beta cells present/reduced
Insulin resistance	No	Yes
Blood insulin/C-peptide levels	Low or absent	Low for insulin resistance
High-risk groups	European, especially Scandinavian	Native American, Asian, African American, Hispanic
Primary treatment options	Exogenous insulin therapy	Weight loss, diet/exercise, insulin sensitizers/secretion enhancers, with or without exogenous insulin

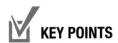

KEY POINTS

- Type 2 DM results from a combination of **insulin resistance** and a **pancreatic beta cell defect,** leading to abnormal glucose homeostasis

- Common signs and symptoms include polyuria, polyphagia, increased thirst, weight loss, sexual dysfunction, and poor wound healing

- Complications include accelerated atherosclerosis, diabetic nephropathy, diabetic retinopathy, and peripheral neuropathy

QUESTIONS

1. A 72-year-old man with a long history of type 2 diabetes treated with insulin visits his family physician for a routine checkup. He states that he administers his insulin just as the doctor ordered, but continues to present with random blood sugar levels well above 200 mg/dL. The doctor suspects the patient has not been using his insulin appropriately for some time now. What is the best way to measure long-term diabetic control of blood glucose?

   A. Glucose tolerance test
   B. Fasting serum glucose
   C. HbA$_{1c}$
   D. Urinalysis
   E. CBC

2. A 42-year-old woman is diagnosed with type 2 diabetes after two pregnancies complicated by gestational diabetes. She has never been on medications for diabetes before. Which of the following is not a first-line treatment option for type 2 DM?

   A. Metformin
   B. Insulin

   C. Glyburide
   D. Acarbose
   E. Pioglitazone

3. A 38-year-old Latina woman with borderline high glucose levels is referred to the diabetes clinic by her gynecologist. She is currently not on any diabetes medications. She is moderately overweight, eats mostly fast food, does not exercise, and smokes half a pack of cigarettes daily. The physician suggests a diabetes educational class to help her learn more about her condition and how she can take better care of herself. Her risk factors for developing overt type 2 diabetes do not include:

   A. Obesity
   B. Ethnicity
   C. Poor diet
   D. Smoking
   E. Lack of exercise

HPI: LG is a 35-year-old white woman who presents with a history of anxiety, nervousness, and difficulty sleeping for the past 3 months. She complains of feeling hot and sweaty, even in air-conditioned rooms, and has noticed her heart beating irregularly at times during the day. LG had attributed her anxiety and symptoms to increasing stress at work, but became concerned after friends and family kept commenting on her recent weight loss. She failed to notice it at first, but after stepping on the scale at the gym, LG realized she had lost some 20 lbs over the past 3 months—despite having a voracious appetite. She also complains of having puffy eyes, but thinks it is mostly due to lack of sleep. She would like a prescription for something to help calm her anxiety so she can get some rest and finally get rid of the "bags under her eyes." LG's family history is significant for her mother having a history of thyroid disease.

PE: Thin, mildly tachypneic female in no acute distress. Skin appears warm and moist. **HEENT:** Prominent eyes with lid lag, stare, and infrequent blinking. Moderate degree of periorbital edema. Patient has difficulty looking up and out but no limitation of downward gaze. **Neck:** Thyroid gland appears diffusely and symmetrically enlarged, soft, and nontender. **Cardiac:** Precordium and carotid pulses hyperdynamic to palpation. No murmurs detected. **Extremities:** Nontender, erythematous nodule on anterior aspect of left lower extremity. Brisk deep tendon reflexes.

THOUGHT QUESTIONS

- What is the likely cause of LG's symptoms and what clues lead you to this conclusion?
- What diagnostic tests would you order to confirm her diagnosis? What would these tests show?
- What is the pathophysiology of this condition?

BASIC SCIENCE REVIEW AND DISCUSSION

LG appears to have many of the classic signs and symptoms of hyperthyroidism. These include heat intolerance, weight loss, tachycardia, arrhythmias, chest pain, palpitations, anxiety, sweating, diarrhea, hyperreflexia, fine hair, and sleep disturbances. Hyperthyroidism can have multiple causes, but the most likely cause in this case is Graves disease. The combination of ophthalmopathy (proptosis, extraocular muscle swelling), pretibial myxedema, and diffuse goiter all point to the clinical diagnosis of Graves disease as the cause of LG's hyperthyroidism.

Graves Disease

Graves' disease is an **autoimmune hyperthyroidism** caused by **antibodies to the thyroid-stimulating hormone (TSH) receptor** in the thyroid gland. It has a female predilection of 5:1 and occurs in about 0.5% of the adult population. Autoantibodies (also known as thyroid-stimulating immunoglobulin) bind to and stimulate the TSH receptor, producing glandular growth and excess secretion of thyroid hormone (preferential triiodothyronine [T_3] secretion). On physical exam, the glandular growth is present as a diffuse goiter and the preferential secretion of the **active form of thyroid hormone (T_3)** produces moderate to severe thyrotoxicosis. In addition, **infiltrative ophthalmopathy** is present in about 5% of patients with Graves disease. Although LG attributes her puffy eyes to lack of sleep, the swelling and "bags under her eyes" are actually due to antibodies directed against her extraocular eye muscles. These antibodies cause a local immune response and result in inflammation of the muscles and deposition of glycosaminoglycans by orbital fibroblasts. Patients may complain of pain or double vision with

reading, burning or tearing of the eyes, and may lose the ability to look up and out. Another rare complication of Graves disease is **pretibial myxedema,** which occurs in about 1% of all cases. The nontender erythematous nodule on the anterior aspect of LG's left leg is an example of pretibial myxedema, which is caused by mucopolysaccharide infiltrate in the skin of the pretibial area.

Laboratory studies can confirm the clinical diagnosis of Graves disease. Important thyroid function tests include TSH, free thyroxine (T_4), T_3, and antithyroid peroxidase (anti-TPO) antibodies (also known as antimicrosomal antibodies). TSH from the pituitary is the best thyroid function test, as it will reveal abnormalities well before T_3 or T_4. In Graves disease, TSH levels will be markedly suppressed, while T_4 and T_3 values will be markedly elevated ($T_3/T_4 > 20:1$). Anti-TPO antibody will be positive and serves as a marker for autoimmune thyroid disease. In addition, because the gland is actively taking up iodine for thyroid hormone synthesis, administration of radioactive iodine (RAI) will show elevated and diffuse uptake, indicating a general increase in thyroid gland activity.

CASE CONTINUED

LG is diagnosed with Graves disease and treated successfully with RAI. She remains euthyroid and symptom free for the next 5 years, but slowly starts to notice increasing fatigue, muscle cramps, and weight gain. She returns to her primary care physician, hoping he may be able to help her once again.

THOUGHT QUESTIONS

- What is the most likely cause of LG's symptoms now? What are the associated symptoms of this condition?
- What would LG's lab results show?

BASIC SCIENCE REVIEW AND DISCUSSION

RAI is the most commonly prescribed treatment for Graves disease. Iodine-131 (^{131}I) is selectively absorbed by thyroid tissue, where it destroys some or all of the hyperfunctioning thyroid follicles by emitting beta particles. Unfortunately, 50 to 90% of patients with Graves disease treated this way eventually become hypothyroid. This is the most likely cause of LG's current symptoms. Other signs and symptoms associated with hypothyroidism include cold intolerance, reduced heart rate, hypoactivity, decreased appetite, decreased reflexes, constipation, cool/dry skin, myxedema (facial/periorbital), and coarse, brittle hair. Hypothyroidism can also be caused by a variety of conditions, the most common of which are RAI therapy for hyperthyroidism and Hashimoto thyroiditis. **Hashimoto thyroiditis** is a

cell-mediated autoimmune destruction of the thyroid gland. It occurs in 1 to 2% of the population, with a female predilection of 5:1. The condition begins in adolescence but is usually not evident until after 50 years of age. The result is an atrophic, fibrotic thyroid gland in a patient with the signs and symptoms of hypothyroidism. Laboratory studies for hypothyroidism will reveal an increased TSH and low T_3, free T_4 levels. Since Hashimoto thyroiditis is an autoimmune condition, anti-TPO antibody levels will be positive. All permanent forms of hypothyroidism are treated with lifelong thyroid hormone replacement.

CASE CONCLUSION

LG was started on levothyroxine 100 µg/day for treatment of her subsequent hypothyroidism. TSH levels were monitored periodically to ensure an euthyroid state.

THUMBNAIL: Hyperthyroidism vs. Hypothyroidism

	Hypothyroid	*Hyperthyroid*
Etiology	Hashimoto thyroiditis	Graves disease
	RAI therapy	Toxic multinodular goiter
	Idiopathic or atrophic thyroiditis	Iodide-induced thyrotoxicosis
	Pituitary or hypothalamic disease	Autonomous hyperfunctioning nodule
	Thyroid aplasia	Subacute thyroiditis
	Inborn defects in hormone synthesis or action	Postpartum thyroiditis
		Factitious thyrotoxicosis
Symptoms	Decreased metabolic rate	Increased metabolic rate
	Cold intolerance	Heat intolerance
	Decreased heart rate	Palpitations, irregular heart rate
	Weight gain	Weight loss
	Fatigue, lethargy	Hyperactivity
	Myxedema	Pretibial myxedema (Graves)
	Cool, dry skin	Warm, moist skin
	Coarse, brittle hair	Fine hair
	Constipation	Diarrhea
	Hyporeflexia	Hyperreflexia
Labs	Primary Hypothyroid	
	↓ total T_4	↑ TSH
	↓ free T_4	↓ TSH
	↓ T_3 uptake	↑ total T_4
	Secondary Hypothyroid	↑ free T_4
	↓ or normal TSH	↑ T_3 uptake
	↓ total T_4	
	↓ free T_4	
	↓ T_3 uptake	

☑ KEY POINTS

- The etiology of hyperthyroidism is usually autoimmune, caused by antibodies to the TSH receptor
- Signs and symptoms include increased metabolism, heat intolerance, weight loss, arrhythmias, and diarrhea
- TSH measurement is the best thyroid function test; TSH levels are markedly decreased in hyperthyroid states
- Treatment: RAI ablation of the overactive thyroid gland

QUESTIONS

1. A 33-year-old woman presents with signs and symptoms of hyperthyroidism. She complains of anxiety, tremor, nervousness, weight loss, and inability to sleep at night. Laboratory evaluation confirms hyperthyroidism with a free T_4 of 25 mg/dL and undetectable levels of TSH. Which of the following is not an appropriate option for treatment of her hyperthyroidism?

   A. Propylthiouracil
   B. RAI
   C. Levothyroxine (Synthroid)
   D. Propranolol
   E. Surgery

2. A 22-year-old woman presents to her obstetrician/gynecologist for follow-up 8 weeks after the delivery of her baby. There were no complications during her pregnancy or during delivery. On this visit, her thyroid gland is diffusely, but minimally, enlarged and nontender to palpation. The doctor decides to obtain a thyroid function panel to aid her diagnostic evaluation. In this thyroid function panel, the most sensitive indicator of thyroid function is:

   A. T_3 uptake
   B. Free T_4
   C. Total T_4
   D. T_3:T_4 ratio
   E. TSH

Cushing Disease

HPI: LS is a 31-year-old Filipino-American woman who initially presented to her gynecologist because of irregular and prolonged menses and inability to become pregnant after discontinuing birth control pills. Over the past year she has noticed increasing acne on her face and prominence of facial hair. LS complains that she can barely recognize herself in the mirror anymore—not only has her face been getting rounder, but she appears to be putting on weight in peculiar places like the back of her neck and around her abdomen. She denies any history of increased bruising or poor wound healing, but does notice that her skin appears darker and she has prominent stretch marks around her ever-enlarging abdomen.

PE: The patient is mildly hypertensive, with BP 140/90 mm Hg. Physical exam reveals an anxious but cooperative female with a full, rounded face. She has acne and excess hair over the neck. There is also excess fat over the dorsal cervical and supraclavicular areas. Skin around the waistline is significant for multiple purple striae. Musculoskeletal exam reveals slight muscle weakness.

Labs: Laboratory results demonstrate an elevated fasting glucose level, elevated 24-hour urinary free cortisol, and a slightly elevated ACTH level.

THOUGHT QUESTIONS

- Where is cortisol produced? What regulates its secretion?
- What are the clinical manifestations of excess cortisol production?
- What is the difference between Cushing disease and Cushing syndrome?
- Why do patients with Cushing disease/syndrome often have concurrent DM?

BASIC SCIENCE REVIEW AND DISCUSSION

The adrenal glands, located bilaterally above the kidneys in the retroperitoneal space, serve to produce glucocorticoids, mineralocorticoids, and androgens from the adrenal cortex. In addition, catecholamines are secreted from the medulla. The adrenal cortex itself is one of the most productive endocrine glands, responsible for much of the body's hormone production. This hormone production is regulated primarily by input from both the hypothalamus, in the form of corticotropin-releasing hormone (CRH) and the anterior pituitary, in the form of **ACTH.** CRH from the hypothalamus regulates ACTH release in response to decreased serum cortisol levels. In turn, cortisol inhibits both CRH and ACTH secretion. This negative feedback loop regulates daily glucocorticoid homeostasis. Glucocorticoid secretion normally oscillates with a 24-hour periodicity. This pattern of secretion is due to the fact that CRH and ACTH are secreted in a diurnal pattern with secretory bursts that are highest in the early morning hours. Therefore, cortisol levels are usually highest in the morning and lowest at night.

Adrenal Anatomy

The adrenal cortex is divided into three functional and histologically distinct regions (Fig. 7-2). These three regions are the (*a*) **zona glomerulosa,** the outermost layer; (*b*) **zona fasciculata,** the middle layer; and (*c*) **zona reticularis,** the inner layer. The zona glomerulosa produces aldosterone and is not dependent on the pituitary or the hypothalamus for its stimulus to secrete. Instead, aldosterone production is regulated by the renin-angiotensin system. In contrast, both the zona fasciculata and the zona reticularis are dependent on signals from the pituitary and hypothalamus. The zona fasciculata synthesizes mostly glucocorticoids (cortisol), while the zona reticularis produces mostly androgens (dehydroepiandrosterone [DHEA] and androstenedione).

Glucocorticoids

Glucocorticoids are important for the physiologic response to stress. They initiate a variety of biologic processes that relate to stress, including stimulation of gluconeogenesis, antiinflammatory reactions, and suppression of the immune response. In addition, glucocorticoids function to maintain the vascular responsiveness to catecholamines; this action is especially critical during the sympathetic "fight-or-flight" response. Cortisol increases gluconeogenesis by a number of mechanisms. There is an increase in protein breakdown and a decrease in protein synthesis; this provides more amino acids to the liver for gluconeogenesis. In addition, there is a decrease in glucose utilization and insulin sensitivity, primarily in adipose tissue. Furthermore, an increase in lipolysis provides additional glycerol to the liver for gluconeogenesis. The antiinflammatory actions of cortisol result from its inhibitory effects on prostaglandin formation. Suppression of the immune response occurs through the inhibition of IL-2 production and reduction of T lymphocytes critical for the cell-mediated immune response.

Cushing Disease

This patient's most likely diagnosis is Cushing disease. Cushing disease is an excess of adrenocortical hormones due to a **pituitary corticotroph adenoma** producing large amounts of ACTH. The disease is named after Harvey Cushing, the neurosurgeon who delineated its features in 1932. Because ACTH stimulates both the zona fasciculata and the zona reticularis, the symptoms seen in Cushing disease are due to **overproduction of both cortisol and androgens.** Clinically, patients with glucocorticoid excess present with a typical "cushingoid" appearance. There is a redistribution of adipose tissue to specific areas of the body, namely the face, abdomen, posterior neck, and supraclavicular areas. Patients are usually described as centrally obese with "moon facies" and a "buffalo hump." These patients also exhibit muscle wasting and weakness due to the increased protein catabolism. Associated DM is often present because the increase in gluconeogenesis and insulin resistance raises serum glucose levels. The excess cortisol also induces atrophic skin

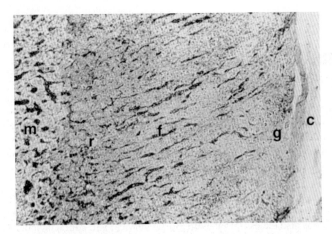

• **Figure 7-2.** H&E stain of the adrenal gland, showing the adrenal cortex, medulla, and vasculature. From left to right: the adrenal medulla (*m*), zona reticularis (*r*), zona fasciculate (*f*), zona glomerulosa (*g*), and adrenal capsule (*c*). The adrenal medulla is responsible for synthesis of the catecholamines norepinephrine and epinephrine. (Image courtesy of Joel Schecter, PhD, Keck School of Medicine at the University of Southern California.)

of glucocorticoid hormones to treat another disorder, it is best to gradually taper the dosage to the lowest dose adequate for control of that disorder. Surgical resection is the mainstay of treatment for pituitary adenomas; the procedure is called a transsphenoidal adenomectomy. If surgery is not possible in such patients, pituitary irradiation is an effective alternative. Adrenal tumors and ectopic ACTH-secreting tumors can be treated with surgery, radiotherapy, or chemotherapy. Medications such as ketoconazole, which inhibits steroid synthesis, can also be used in the treatment of Cushing.

CASE CONCLUSION

The endocrinologist orders an MRI of the head, which is read as "enlarged pituitary fossa with irregular pituitary mass." LS is immediately scheduled for surgical excision of the mass. Pathology report confirms the presence of a pituitary corticotroph adenoma.

changes such as thinning; this thinning is evident as prominent purple striae in affected areas. A history of poor wound healing and easy bruising would be consistent with the immunosuppressive effects of glucocorticoids. The increase in circulating androgens is manifested as hirsutism, acne, and virilization with menstrual irregularities. Because anterior pituitary corticotrophs are also responsible for the synthesis of **melanocyte-stimulating hormone (MSH),** many patients with Cushing disease also complain of skin darkening. This increased pigmentation is due to an increase in MSH production from the adenoma. It is particularly prominent in areas of friction (e.g., under the bra straps). Because glucocorticoids also have weak mineralocorticoid activity, excess cortisol can cause mild sodium retention and contribute to elevated blood pressures.

Cushing Syndrome

In contrast to Cushing disease, which is glucocorticoid excess specifically due to a pituitary adenoma secreting ACTH, Cushing syndrome refers to any condition in which there is an excess of glucocorticoids. This excess may be ACTH dependent or ACTH independent. ACTH-dependent glucocorticoid excess occurs with a pituitary adenoma or with paraneoplastic syndromes, in which a neoplasm (most commonly small cell lung carcinoma) produces ectopic ACTH that stimulates the adrenals. Ectopic ACTH syndrome affects men three times more frequently than women. Laboratory evaluation of ACTH-dependent conditions will demonstrate an increase in both ACTH and 24-hour urinary free cortisol. Ectopic ACTH conditions tend to have very high ACTH levels. Glucocorticoid excess due to ACTH-independent conditions results from primary adrenal neoplasms or exogenous glucocorticoid administration. In these instances, urine cortisol will be increased despite low or undetectable levels of ACTH.

Treatment for glucocorticoid excess depends on the etiology of the condition. Possibilities include surgery, radiation, chemotherapy, or the use of cortisol-inhibiting drugs. If the cause is long-term use

THUMBNAIL: Adrenal Gland

CRH (hypothalamus)

↓

ACTH (pituitary) → Androgens (zona reticularis)

↓

Cortisol (zona fasciculata)

Causes of glucocorticoid excess

ACTH dependent
Cushing disease (pituitary ACTH adenoma)
Ectopic ACTH production (paraneoplastic)

ACTH independent
Exogenous glucocorticoid administration
Adrenal neoplasm (benign or malignant)

Symptoms and signs of glucocorticoid excess

Catabolic effects on skin and muscle (striae, skin atrophy)
Classic facies and body habitus
Increased brown fat
Poor wound healing
HTN (50%)
Hypokalemia (20%)
Amenorrhea or decreased libido
Psychological disturbances
Osteoporosis
Impaired glucose tolerance
Increased pigmentation

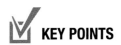

KEY POINTS

- Cushing disease = pituitary adenoma producing excess ACTH
- Cushing syndrome = nonpituitary source of excess cortisol
- Symptoms and signs include body fat redistribution (moon facies, buffalo hump), skin atrophy, poor wound healing, glucose intolerance
- Initial screen for suspected glucocorticoid excess is 24-hour urinary free cortisol measurement
- Cushing disease is treated with pituitary surgery or radiation

QUESTIONS

1. A 26-year-old man presents to his primary care physician complaining of multiple episodes of easy bruising after playing basketball. He recently started playing ball again after he noticed that he was growing a "beer belly" even though he hardly drank any alcohol. He also complains of little to no libido. Among other findings, the physician notes a plethoric, round face and skin atrophy, particularly over the pretibial areas. The most useful screening test for Cushing in this case is:

   A. Measure plasma cortisol
   B. Measure 24-hour urinary cortisol production
   C. Perform a low- and high-dose dexamethasone suppression test
   D. Perform a pituitary MRI
   E. Perform an abdominal computed axial tomography scan

2. An 11-year-old girl is prescribed oral prednisone to help control her severe, persistent asthma. Which of the following actions of cortisol is most beneficial in helping her achieve long-term control of her asthma?

   A. Increased glucose formation and release
   B. Sodium retention
   C. Increases "stress response"
   D. Inhibits T-lymphocyte proliferation
   E. Inhibits prostaglandin formation

HPI: JV is a 44-year-old Scandinavian man who presents to his family doctor with a 1-year history of fatigue, weakness, and weight loss. He states that he doesn't eat very much now, and when he does, it is usually accompanied by nausea and vomiting. His two school-aged children have been complaining that "daddy doesn't play with us much anymore." JV's response is that he simply doesn't have the energy he did in the past. Even standing up from a reclining position makes him feel dizzy and faint.

PE: On physical exam, JV is tachycardic, with blood pressures of 110/64 mm Hg supine and 92/50 mm Hg while standing. He is a thin man who appears older than his stated age. His skin exhibits peculiar areas of hyperpigmentation, most notably around his palmar creases and buccal mucosa. His eyes appear sunken, and mucous membranes are pale and dry. His verbal responses and mentation appear delayed, but the rest of his physical exam is within normal limits.

Labs: Subsequent laboratory tests are significant for hyponatremia, hyperkalemia, lymphocytosis, and marked eosinophilia.

THOUGHT QUESTIONS

- What endocrine disorder could be responsible for JV's relatively nonspecific signs and symptoms? What physical sign is most specific for this diagnosis?
- What laboratory tests would confirm your hypothesis? What would these labs show?
- What is the difference between primary and secondary adrenal insufficiency?
- How should this patient be treated for his condition?

BASIC SCIENCE REVIEW AND DISCUSSION

JV presents with many nonspecific signs and symptoms. These include a chronic history of fatigue, weakness, weight loss, anorexia, nausea, and vomiting. When taken into consideration with his significant dehydration, hypotension, and hyperpigmentation, however, one must consider the diagnosis of Addison disease. Addison disease is also known as primary adrenal insufficiency. **Primary adrenal insufficiency** is distinguished from **secondary adrenal insufficiency** in that the defect in primary disease is end organ failure of the adrenal gland itself, while secondary disease is caused by defects in the hypothalamus or pituitary resulting in decreased production of CRH or **ACTH.** The signs and symptoms of both conditions are caused by the loss of mineralocorticoid and glucocorticoid production.

Adrenal Gland

The adrenal gland is made up of two anatomically distinct regions: the outer cortex and the inner medulla. The cortex is further divided into three different hormone-synthesizing areas: the **zona glomerulosa, zona fasciculata,** and **zona reticularis.** These zones are responsible for the synthesis of mineralocorticoids (primarily aldosterone), glucocorticoids (primarily cortisol), and androgens, respectively. The fasciculata and reticularis zones of the adrenal gland are under regulatory control of the hypothalamic-pituitary axis. The hypothalamus secretes CRH, which acts on the anterior pituitary gland to produce ACTH. The action of ACTH on the adrenal gland is to stimulate the production of cortisol from the zona fasciculata. In addition, ACTH stimulates the zona reticularis to produce androgens. The zona glomerulosa is unique in that its producing

capacity is regulated by the **renin-angiotensin system (RAS).** A decrease in blood pressure sensed by decreased sodium or chloride transport to the macula densa in the kidney stimulates the juxtaglomerular cells to secrete renin. Renin catalyzes the conversion of angiotensinogen to angiotensin I, which is subsequently converted to angiotensin II in the lungs. Angiotensin II then stimulates the zona glomerulosa to secrete aldosterone. Aldosterone causes an increase in BP through sodium (and water) retention.

Primary Adrenal Insufficiency

The etiologic defect in Addison disease occurs in the adrenal gland. There are numerous causes, but an autoimmune-mediated destruction of the adrenal gland is the most common cause in the United States. Other causes include TB and other granulomatous diseases, AIDS, sarcoidosis, bacterial infections, adrenal hemorrhage, and coagulation disorders. The disease process is characterized by **atrophy of all three cortical divisions,** resulting in the complete absence of hormone production.

Secondary Adrenal Insufficiency

In contrast, secondary adrenal insufficiency occurs as a result of decreased production of CRH from the hypothalamus or ACTH from the pituitary. Atrophy of the adrenal cortex occurs as a result of **insufficient stimulation from higher regulatory centers.** The most common cause of isolated secondary insufficiency is long-term exogenous glucocorticoid therapy. Administration of exogenous cortisol decreases production of both CRH and ACTH through negative feedback regulation. Less common causes of secondary insufficiency include craniopharyngioma, empty sella syndrome, sarcoidosis, histiocytosis X, hypothalamic tumors, head trauma, and Sheehan syndrome.

Primary versus Secondary Adrenal Insufficiency

Many of the signs and symptoms of primary adrenal insufficiency are the same as those of secondary insufficiency. These common findings are caused by a lack of both aldosterone and cortisol activity. The symptoms are generally nonspecific and include tiredness, weakness, confusion, weight loss, nausea, vomiting, and, occasionally, hypoglycemia. Hyponatremia and hyperkalemia are

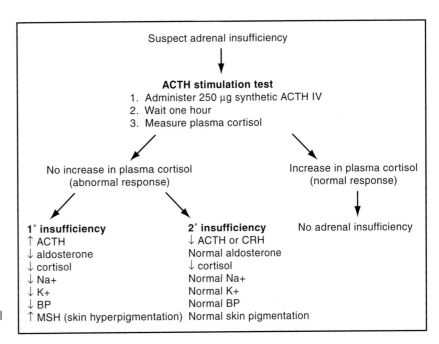

Suspect adrenal insufficiency

ACTH stimulation test
1. Administer 250 µg synthetic ACTH IV
2. Wait one hour
3. Measure plasma cortisol

No increase in plasma cortisol
(abnormal response)

Increase in plasma cortisol
(normal response)

No adrenal insufficiency

1° insufficiency
↑ ACTH
↓ aldosterone
↓ cortisol
↓ Na+
↓ K+
↓ BP
↑ MSH (skin hyperpigmentation)

2° insufficiency
↓ ACTH or CRH
Normal aldosterone
↓ cortisol
Normal Na+
Normal K+
Normal BP
Normal skin pigmentation

● **Figure 7-3.** Algorithm for diagnosis of adrenal insufficiency.

characteristic of primary disease because the absence of aldosterone causes sodium to be lost in the urine and potassium to be retained in the body. Hypotension and volume depletion are due to the inability to retain sodium, and thus water, since water follows sodium. Because the zona glomerulosa is not dependent on ACTH for stimulation, aldosterone levels are normal in secondary failure and hypotension is not a primary feature of the disease. In addition, skin pigmentation is only seen in primary adrenal failure. The hyperpigmentation (bronze skin) occurs all over the skin, but characteristically in the palmar creases and buccal mucosa. Because ACTH and MSH are formed by the same precursor, the hyperpigmentation is caused by an increase in MSH secondary to the increase in ACTH seen in primary failure. If the cause of primary failure is due to an autoimmune mechanism, patients may also present with other autoimmune conditions, such as thyroid disorders or vitiligo. Secondary failure is usually associated with the loss of gonadotropins, TSH, and/or growth hormone (GH). These deficiencies manifest as scanty secondary sex characteristics (axillary hair, pubic hair), amenorrhea in women, decreased libido/potency, delayed puberty, or hypothyroidism. Pituitary tumors may also present with headache or visual changes, while hypothalamus defects can also present with DI.

Diagnosis

Diagnosis of adrenal insufficiency is made based on the constellation of clinical signs and symptoms in combination with laboratory evaluation (Fig. 7-3). Laboratory work-up for a patient with suspected adrenal insufficiency should include a measurement of morning cortisol level and plasma ACTH. Primary adrenal insufficiency will reveal low morning plasma cortisol levels. Cortisol levels are usually highest around 8 to 9 a.m. because CRH and ACTH are secreted in a diurnal pattern with secretory bursts that are highest in the early morning hours. ACTH from the pituitary will be increased in primary insufficiency secondary to the low circulating cortisol. On the other hand, both ACTH and cortisol levels will be decreased in secondary adrenal insufficiency because the defect occurs in the pituitary or hypothalamus. An ACTH stimulation test with 250 µg of synthetic ACTH can also be used to confirm adrenal insufficiency. Administration of ACTH should increase plasma cortisol to a level >17 µg/mL within 1 hour of IV dose. Inadequate response indicates adrenal insufficiency but does not distinguish primary from secondary failure. Head CT or MRI scan may be necessary if a secondary cause of adrenal insufficiency is suspected.

CASE CONCLUSION

JV's family physician refers him to an endocrinologist, who diagnoses Addison disease based on physical evidence of hyperpigmentation, low morning plasma cortisol, and elevated ACTH. He is started on glucocorticoid and mineralocorticoid replacement therapy with rapid improvement of symptoms. JV's children are much happier now that their daddy is back to his usual playful and energetic self again.

THUMBNAIL: Adrenal Insufficiency

Primary (Addison disease)
End organ failure
Most common cause is autoimmune adrenalitis
Low plasma cortisol, low aldosterone, high ACTH
Presents with hyponatremia, hyperkalemia, hypotension, and hyperpigmentation
Hyperpigmentation is most specific sign of primary disease

Secondary
Decreased production of CRH or ACTH
Most common cause is exogenous glucocorticoid administration
Low plasma cortisol
Normal aldosterone
Normal BP, sodium, and potassium
No hyperpigmentation, but may have signs and symptoms related to loss of gonadotropins, TSH, or GH

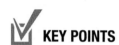

KEY POINTS

- Can be primary (adrenal gland failure) or secondary (pituitary or hypothalamic defect)
- Nonspecific symptoms and signs of fatigue, weakness, weight loss, confusion, nausea, and vomiting from lack of cortisol
- Skin pigmentation, hypotension, and hyperkalemia only present in primary disease
- Initial screen for suspected adrenal insufficiency is measurement of morning cortisol level and plasma ACTH
- Treatment with exogenous glucocorticoid and mineralocorticoid replacement

QUESTIONS

1. A 16-year-old girl is brought to see her pediatrician because her mother is concerned that she has not started her monthly periods. On physical exam, the girl is mildly obese, of short stature, and without secondary sex characteristics. Further work-up includes serum hormone levels and a CT scan of the head, which reveals a craniopharyngioma. Adrenocortical function in this patient is most likely:

   A. Absent
   B. Decreased
   C. Normal
   D. Increased
   E. Unassessable

2. A 36-year-old woman with a history of Graves disease complains of lethargy, weight loss, and feeling faint often. Her Graves disease was treated successfully with total thyroidectomy secondary to inadequate response to antithyroid medications and radioactive iodine. Physical exam reveals multiple patches of skin depigmentation and orthostatic hypotension. The physician suspects adrenal insufficiency and confirms her diagnosis with a morning cortisol level and plasma ACTH. What is the most likely cause of her adrenal insufficiency?

   A. Autoimmune adrenalitis
   B. Long-term exogenous levothyroxine therapy
   C. Undiagnosed coagulation disorder
   D. Long-term exogenous glucocorticoid therapy
   E. TB reactivation

Conn Syndrome

HPI: LW is a 47-year-old Asian American woman who presents to her primary care doctor for follow-up of her HTN. She has a 2-year history of HTN, treated unsuccessfully with multiple trials of medications. On this visit, LW's BP is elevated at 180/120 mm Hg, despite combined treatment with a beta-blocker and a diuretic. LW also complains of persistent mild frontal headaches, nocturia, and generalized weakness of her extremities.

PE: Physical exam is significant for elevated systolic and diastolic BPs, without evidence of retinopathy or abdominal bruits. LW also demonstrates normal tone, but 3/5 muscle strength in her upper and lower extremities. At this time, serum electrolyte evaluation reveals a K^+ of 2.5 mEq/L and a mild metabolic alkalosis with HCO_3^- of 32 mmol/L. LW's physician suggests that she discontinue her current medications and return in 3 weeks for further evaluation of her BP and electrolytes. On stopping her medications for 3 weeks, serum K^+ remained low at 3.0 mEq/L. Plasma renin was decreased at 0.1 ng/mL/h (normal 1–3 ng/mL/h), but plasma aldosterone was elevated at 22 ng/mL (normal 3–9 ng/mL).

THOUGHT QUESTIONS

- What are the components of the RAS?
- How does this system regulate BP?
- What are the features of primary hyperaldosteronism?
- What is the difference between primary and secondary hyperaldosteronism?

BASIC SCIENCE REVIEW AND DISCUSSION

Aldosterone is a mineralocorticoid hormone secreted by the zona glomerulosa cells of the adrenal cortex. Aldosterone acts on the distal tubule of the kidney to increase reabsorption of salt and facilitate excretion of potassium. Unlike the zona fasciculata and the zona reticularis, the zona glomerulosa is minimally regulated by ACTH from the hypothalamus. Instead, aldosterone secretion is primarily regulated via the RAS.

The Renin-Angiotensin System

The **RAS** is responsible for long-term BP regulation in the body (Fig. 7-4). The system is stimulated by a decrease in renal perfusion pressure to the kidney as sensed by the **juxtaglomerular apparatus (JGA).** The JGA consists of juxtaglomerular (JG) cells, specialized myoepithelial cells within the afferent arteriole that secrete renin, and the macula densa, cells in the distal convoluted tubule that can assess the amount of sodium that is delivered to the distal tubules per unit time. The JG cells respond to changes in stretch induced by changes in renal BP. When JG cells are stretched with increased renal BP, they respond by decreasing renin release. Conversely, a decrease in renal BP increases renal renin release.

Renin is a proteolytic enzyme that cleaves angiotensinogen to angiotensin I, an inactive intermediate in the plasma. Angiotensin I circulates to the lungs and other tissues, where it is converted to angiotensin II by ACE synthesized by pulmonary endothelial cells. Angiotensin II is the biologically active hormone that actually functions to increase BP. It does this via two primary mechanisms: (*a*) angiotensin II causes vasoconstriction of arterioles; this vasoconstriction causes increased peripheral resistance and thus leads to an increased diastolic BP; (*b*) angiotensin II also acts on the zona glomerulosa cells of the adrenal gland to release aldosterone; aldosterone then acts on the distal tubules of the kidney to increase sodium and water retention and promote potassium excretion.

Increased salt and water reabsorption increases total blood volume and mean arterial pressure.

Primary Hyperaldosteronism

This patient presents with the typical signs and symptoms of **primary hyperaldosteronism,** otherwise known as **Conn syndrome.** Jerome Conn first described primary hyperaldosteronism in 1955. Primary hyperaldosteronism occurs in 1% of all people diagnosed with HTN, with the highest incidence between ages 30 and 50 years and affecting men twice as often as women. The syndrome results from an abnormally large amount of aldosterone produced by the adrenal cortex. Most often, the excess aldosterone is due to an aldosterone-secreting adrenal adenoma in one of the adrenal glands. Less commonly, the excess can be due to idiopathic bilateral hyperplasia of the zona glomerulosa or to adrenocortical carcinomas. The syndrome is characterized by HTN, hypokalemia, metabolic alkalosis, and low plasma renin levels. Plasma renin is low because the retained sodium feeds back to the JGA and decreases renal renin release. Low renin levels are key to distinguishing primary from secondary sources of hyperaldosteronism.

Secondary Hyperaldosteronism

In contrast to primary hyperaldosteronism, which is due to an abnormality in the adrenal gland itself, **secondary hyperaldosteronism** occurs as a result of a peripheral abnormality that causes the kidney to misperceive a fall in BP. These peripheral abnormalities can include renal artery stenosis, CRF, cirrhosis, or nephrotic syndrome. In these instances, the kidney's BP regulation system is fooled into thinking that the BP is abnormally low. In response, the RAS is inappropriately activated and excess aldosterone is produced. Patients with secondary hyperaldosteronism can present in an identical manner as patients with Conn syndrome. However, patients with secondary forms of hyperaldosteronism will have **high plasma renin** in addition to high aldosterone levels (Table 7-1).

Clinical Presentation

Clinically, patients with Conn syndrome most commonly present with a history of HTN, often not responsive to medications. The excess aldosterone stimulates sodium and water retention, as well as potassium wasting. Low potassium levels are responsible for the associated symptoms of muscle weakness, neurologic changes,

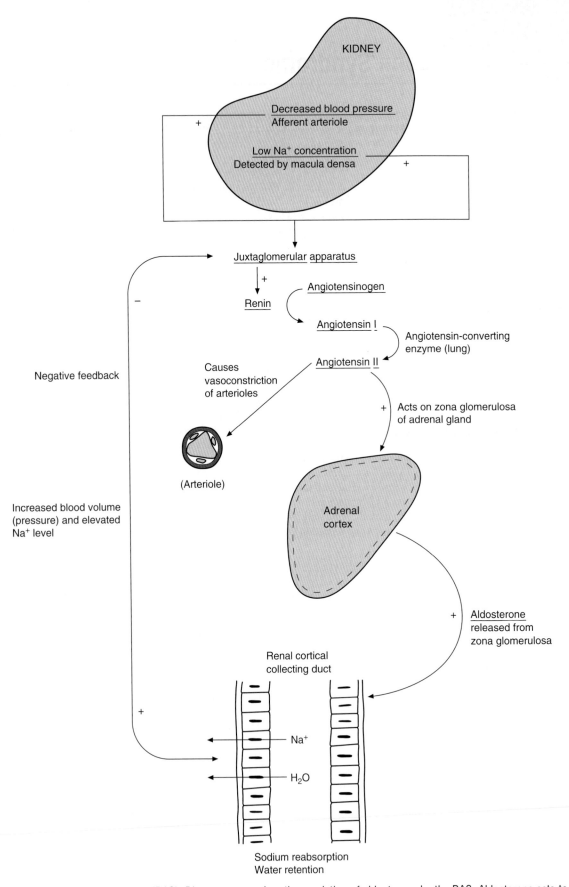

● **Figure 7-4.** Renin-angiotensin system (RAS). Diagram summarizes the regulation of aldosterone by the RAS. Aldosterone acts to increase sodium and water uptake from the renal collecting tubes.

TABLE 7-1 Primary versus Secondary Hyperaldosteronism

	Plasma Aldosterone	Plasma Renin	Plasma Na$^+$	Plasma K$^+$
Primary hyperaldosteronism	↑	↓	↑	↓
Secondary hyperaldosteronism	↑	↑	↑	↓

thirst, polydipsia, polyuria, and/or nocturia. Tachycardia can also occur without the patient feeling palpitations. Patients will have metabolic alkalosis with increased serum HCO_3^- because aldosterone also stimulates the loss of hydrogen ions from the distal tubule through the Na^+-H^+ pump. Although sodium and water retention are key features of primary hyperaldosteronism, patients remain euvolemic due to the renal escape phenomenon.

Diagnosis

Diagnosis of primary hyperaldosteronism must be made with the patient not taking any usual antihypertensive medications, which can invalidate the results. Important laboratory findings include decreased plasma renin, increased plasma aldosterone, low serum potassium, and high 24-hour urine potassium. Additional confirmatory indicators are a mild metabolic alkalosis (HCO_3^- >30 mmol/L) and a mildly elevated serum glucose level due to the hypokalemia interfering with insulin secretion and glucose regulation. CT or MRI scan of the adrenal glands can then be used to demonstrate presence of adrenal tumors or hyperplasia.

Treatment

Treatment of primary hyperaldosteronism due to an adrenal adenoma consists of removal of the affected gland (adrenalectomy). When possible, selective excision of the adenoma is attempted to preserve any functioning adrenal tissue. Medical therapy can be used as an adjunct to surgery to control BP and replenish potassium stores prior to surgery. Possible medications include spironolactone, an aldosterone antagonist, and amiloride, a potassium-sparing diuretic. These medications are also used when the source of the aldosterone excess is due to idiopathic bilateral zona glomerular hyperplasia or if the tumor is inoperable.

CASE CONCLUSION

The clinical findings of uncontrolled HTN, hypokalemia, elevated plasma aldosterone, and decreased plasma renin levels leads LW's physician to suspect primary hyperaldosteronism. The doctor orders an abdominal CT, which confirms the presence of a 6-cm round mass in the outer cortex of her left adrenal gland. LW is started on spironolactone therapy for 4 weeks before surgical excision of her tumor.

THUMBNAIL: Conn Syndrome

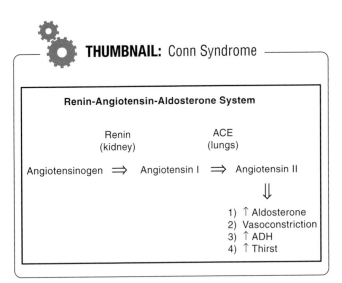

Renin-Angiotensin-Aldosterone System

Renin (kidney)   ACE (lungs)

Angiotensinogen ⟹ Angiotensin I ⟹ Angiotensin II
⟱
1) ↑ Aldosterone
2) Vasoconstriction
3) ↑ ADH
4) ↑ Thirst

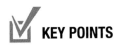 **KEY POINTS**

Functions of Aldosterone

■ ↑ renal Na^+ reabsorption
■ ↑ renal K^+ secretion
■ ↑ renal H^+ secretion

Primary Hyperaldosteronism

Due to adrenal adenoma, hyperplasia, or carcinoma producing excess aldosterone

■ ↑ plasma aldosterone
■ ↓ plasma renin
■ ↑ plasma Na^+, ↓ plasma K^+

Secondary Hyperaldosteronism

Due to renal artery stenosis, cirrhosis, nephrotic syndrome, or CHF causing overactivity of the RAS

■ ↑ plasma aldosterone
■ ↑ plasma renin
■ ↑ plasma Na^+, ↓ plasma K^+

QUESTIONS

1. A 33-year-old man complains of increased thirst, fatigue, and occasional heart palpitations unrelated to activity for the past 2 months. In the past, he has been healthy and has had no known medical conditions. BP on this visit is elevated at 158/96 mm Hg. Initial ECG evaluation is within normal limits. Key features in the diagnosis of primary hyperaldosteronism do not include:

A. Metabolic acidosis
B. Unprovoked hypokalemia
C. Low plasma renin activity
D. High aldosterone
E. HTN

2. A 50-year-old woman with a history of HTN is incidentally found to have bilateral adrenocortical hyperplasia on abdominal CT work-up for kidney stones. She is currently taking atenolol for treatment of her HTN. Appropriate treatment choices for a patient with bilateral adrenocortical hyperplasia causing primary hyperaldosteronism include:

A. Bilateral adrenalectomy
B. Loop diuretics
C. Spironolactone
D. ACE inhibitors
E. C and D

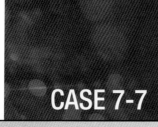

CASE 7-7 Congenital Adrenal Hyperplasia

HPI: KP is a 25-year-old white woman who has just delivered a full-term infant via normal spontaneous vaginal delivery. Immediately after delivery, the obstetrician notices ambiguous genitalia on the baby and consults the pediatricians for an evaluation.

PE: On physical exam, the infant appears to be female; however, there is moderate clitoromegaly and fusion of the labioscrotal folds. The baby is further evaluated for possible congenital adrenal hyperplasia.

THOUGHT QUESTIONS

- What is congenital adrenal hyperplasia (CAH)?
- What mechanisms regulate cortisol and aldosterone production?
- What is the common precursor to all steroid hormones? Which enzymes are important in the steroidogenic pathway?

BASIC SCIENCE REVIEW AND DISCUSSION

CAH refers to a group of autosomal recessive disorders caused by deficiencies in the adrenal enzymes that are required for cortisol or aldosterone synthesis. As a result, precursors proximal to the enzyme block accumulate and are shunted toward the formation of adrenal androgens. Affected individuals can present with a wide spectrum of clinical disease phenotypes resulting from the androgen excess. Mild enzyme deficits may be clinically unapparent, whereas complete enzyme absence can result in severe adrenal insufficiency with virilism and salt-wasting in infancy. Since the affected enzyme can be totally or partially impaired, the degree of enzyme deficiency determines the severity of the condition.

Adrenal Cortex Review

The adrenal cortex is divided into three functionally distinct areas for hormone synthesis. The zona glomerulosa, fasciculata, and reticularis are each responsible for the production of specific endocrine products. These are mineralocorticoids (aldosterone), glucocorticoids (cortisol), and androgens, respectively. Hormone synthesis in the zona fasciculata and zona reticularis is regulated by the hypothalamic-pituitary axis. More specifically, the hypothalamus secretes CRH, which subsequently stimulates the production of ACTH from the anterior pituitary. ACTH then acts on the adrenal cortex to promote synthesis of cortisol and androgens. In contrast, synthesis in the zona glomerulosa is primarily regulated via the renin-angiotensin-aldosterone (RAA) system. ACTH and CRH have minimal regulatory effects on the zona glomerulosa.

Steroid Hormone Synthesis

Cortisol and aldosterone are steroid hormones synthesized from a common precursor molecule, cholesterol. The steroid hormone synthesis pathway is depicted in Figure 7-6. Many of the enzymes involved in cortisol and aldosterone synthesis are cytochrome P450 enzymes. CAH is most commonly due to **21-hydroxylase deficiency,** accounting for more than 90% of cases of adrenal hyperplasia. Less commonly involved enzymes are **11β-hydroxylase** and **3β-hydroxysteroid dehydrogenase** (Table 7-2).

Clinical Presentation

The hallmark of CAH is **inadequate production of glucocorticoids.** The "classical" form of CAH occurs when cortisol synthesis is extremely low or absent, with the deficiency manifesting as ambiguous genitalia at birth. In affected female infants, exam of the external genitalia will reveal a phallus-like structure (smaller than a penis, but larger than a clitoris), a single opening at the base corresponding to the urogenital sinus, and varying degrees of incomplete fusion of the labioscrotal folds. Males with 21-hydroxylase deficiency are generally not diagnosed immediately after birth because their genitalia will appear normal. Rather, these male infants will present at 1 to 4 weeks of age with symptoms resulting from severe salt wasting and deficient cortisol. These may include failure to thrive, recurrent vomiting, dehydration, and shock.

Milder, "nonclassical" forms of the condition (late-onset 21- or 11β-hydroxylase deficiency) may not present until childhood or adolescence. In these instances, children will have precocious puberty in association with the laboratory abnormalities of hyponatremia and hyperkalemia. Premature closure of the epiphyseal growth plates results in short stature, even though these children grow at an accelerated rate when young. Often these children lack sufficient amounts of cortisol to mount an adequate stress response and are thus prone to frequent illnesses. Adult women with CAH may have associated signs and symptoms of androgen excess, such as hirsutism, amenorrhea, acne, and infertility.

Genetics

The defects causing CAH are autosomal recessive disorders caused by abnormalities of the gene that codes for the enzyme involved. These abnormalities include insertions, deletions, missense/nonsense codons, and point mutations. Some of these defects result in severe dysfunction of the enzyme, while others result in only partial impairment. Because the condition is inherited in a recessive fashion, both genes must carry the same mutation or deletion in order for the condition to be expressed. Carriers or heterozygotes that carry only one abnormal gene are asymptomatic.

Diagnosis

The diagnosis of CAH is suggested by clinical presentation and confirmed with laboratory evaluation to identify the deficient enzyme. For example, because 21-hydroxylase functions in both glucocorticoid and mineralocorticoid synthesis, patients may show signs of virilization and salt wasting, such as hyponatremia, hypovolemia, hyperkalemia, and hypotension. Without 21-hydroxylase, there is increased production of progesterone, 17-OH progesterone (17-OHP), and DHEA. Serum cortisol and aldosterone will be

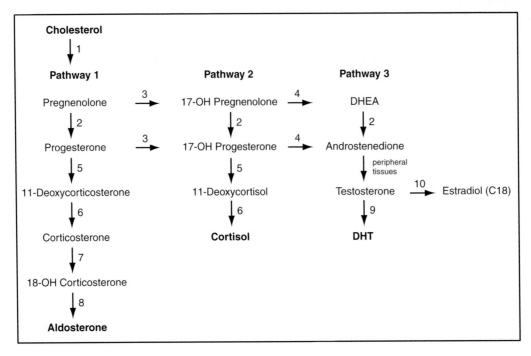

Key enzymes
1 = Desmolase
2 = 3β-hydroxysteroid dehydrogenase (3βHSD)
3 = 17α-hydroxylase
4 = C-17 Lyase
5 = 21β-hydroxylase
6 = 11β-hydroxylase
7 = 18-hydroxylase
8 = 18-oxidase
9 = 5α-reductase
10 = Aromatase

Pathway 1 = Aldosterone synthesis (C21 Mineralocorticoids)
Pathway 2 = Cortisol synthesis (C21 Glucocorticoids)
Pathway 3 = Testosterone synthesis (C19 Androgens)

• **Figure 7-6.** Pathways of steroid hormone production in the adrenal gland.

TABLE 7-2 Congenital Adrenal Hyperplasia Syndromes

Enzyme Deficiency	Accumulated Precursors	Missing Hormones
21-hydroxylase	Progesterone, 17-OHP	Cortisol, aldosterone
11β-hydroxylase	11-deoxycortisol, 11-deoxycortisosterone	Cortisol, aldosterone
3β-HSD	DHEA	Cortisol
Desmolase	Cholesterol	Cortisol, aldosterone, testosterone
17α-hydroxylase	Pregnenolone, progesterone	Cortisol, testosterone

17-OHP, 17-OH progesterone; *3β-HSD*, 3beta-hydroxysteroid dehydrogenase

TABLE 7-3 Steroid Treatment: Balance of Risks and Benefits for Treatment of CAH

Insufficient Cortisol	Excess Cortisol
Hairiness	Increased appetite
Acne	Weight gain
Greasy skin	Muscle weakness
Irregular periods	Thin skin, easy bruising
Reduced fertility	High blood pressure
Tiredness	Osteoporosis
Fatigue	Diabetes

CASE CONCLUSION

A karyotype analysis identifies the infant as a 46,XX female. Laboratory studies confirm the diagnosis of CAH and are significant for elevated serum 17-OHP and DHEA, with excess urinary pregnanetriol excretion. Metabolic abnormalities include hyponatremia and hyperkalemia, with undetectable levels of plasma cortisol and aldosterone. The family is counseled regarding treatment options and surgical correction for their daughter's ambiguous genitalia.

THUMBNAIL: Congenital Adrenal Hyperplasia

21-Hydroxylase Deficiency
Accounts for 90% of cases of CAH
Accumulation of progesterone and 17-OHP

11β-Hydroxylase Deficiency
Accounts for fewer than 10% of cases of CAH
Accumulation of 11-deoxycorticosterone and 11-deoxycortisol

Signs and Symptoms of CAH
Decreased or absent plasma cortisol and aldosterone
Androgen excess can result in virilism, hirsutism, and salt wasting

low or absent, while urinary metabolites of cortisol and aldosterone precursors (17-ketosteroids and pregnanetriol) will be increased. In addition, both plasma ACTH and renin levels will be increased due to the loss of negative feedback by cortisol and aldosterone. If the cause of CAH is 11β-hydrogenase deficiency, deoxycortisol accumulates. Deoxycortisol and its metabolites have mineralocorticoid properties and may cause pronounced HTN. An ACTH stimulation test can help identify the defective enzyme. Levels of adrenal hormone precursors are measured before and 30 minutes after 250 µg of synthetic ACTH is injected intravenously. The rise and ratio of the various precursors in response to ACTH aids in the identification of the defective enzyme.

Treatment

Treatment of CAH involves glucocorticoid replacement and possibly mineralocorticoid replacement to restore associated electrolyte abnormalities. Early recognition and treatment of CAH is important for severe enzyme deficiencies to prevent metabolic complications and irreversible growth patterns. In milder cases with few or no symptoms, the risks and benefits of long-term glucocorticoid therapy (i.e., iatrogenic Cushing syndrome) should be balanced (Table 7-3). Affected female infants may require surgical reconstruction to reverse the effects of virilization.

KEY POINTS

- Autosomal recessive disorders resulting from the absence of enzymes necessary for cortisol and/or aldosterone synthesis
- Symptoms and signs of androgen excess result from accumulation of testosterone precursors
- Treatment includes glucocorticoid and/or mineralocorticoid replacement to correct electrolyte abnormalities

QUESTIONS

1. A 14-year-old girl is brought in to see her pediatrician because her parents are concerned that her growth is stunted. Her parents state that she grew quite rapidly as a child but has remained at the same height of 4 feet 8 inches for the past 3 years. Her mother and father are 5 feet 9 inches and 6 feet 4 inches, respectively. In addition, the girl has not reached menarche yet. On physical exam, the girl is mildly obese with a husky voice and some evidence of increased facial hair. Which of the following is mostly likely to be elevated in this patient?

A. 21-hydroxylase
B. 11β-hydroxylase
C. DHEA
D. Cortisol
E. Aldosterone

2. A 1-month-old baby boy is brought in to see his pediatrician for his regularly scheduled well child checkup. Despite an uncomplicated delivery and uneventful first 2 weeks at home, his mother states that the child has become increasingly fussy and is not feeding well. He often immediately vomits up most of what he has just taken in. On physical exam, the child appears dehydrated with poor skin turgor and muscle tone. The pediatrician admits the child to the hospital on the basis of dehydration and failure to thrive. Deficiencies in which of the following could account for this child's symptoms?

A. Testosterone
B. Aldosterone
C. GH
D. Epinephrine
E. DHEA

HPI: DK is a 33-year-old white man who presents for the first time with a long history of "heartburn" not relieved by OTC medications. DK states that the heartburn occurs intermittently, is not related to meals, and is often associated with abdominal pain and diarrhea. He is concerned that he might be developing an ulcer because "ulcers tend to run in his family."

PE: On physical exam, DK is an anxious-appearing man who appears older than his stated age. His facial features appear unusually coarse, including a prominent brow and jawbone. Physical exam is significant for a palpable liver edge, 4 cm below the costal margin. DK denies smoking or excessive alcohol use.

Labs: Serum laboratory evaluation reveals elevated serum Ca^{2+} levels, but DK denies any history of kidney stones or bone pain. Other routine labs are noncontributory, and the remainder of the physical exam is within normal limits.

THOUGHT QUESTIONS

- What endocrine abnormalities could account for DK's signs and symptoms? What is his most likely diagnosis?
- How are the multiple endocrine neoplasia (MEN) syndromes inherited? What organs are affected in each syndrome?
- What are the common clinical manifestations of a patient with MEN I? MEN IIa? MEN IIb?

BASIC SCIENCE REVIEW AND DISCUSSION

The **multiple endocrine neoplasias** are inherited autosomal dominant cancer syndromes. They are categorized into MEN I and MEN II. MEN II is further subdivided into MEN IIa and MEN IIb. (Note: Some texts refer to MEN I, IIa, and IIb as MEN I, II, and III, respectively.)

MEN I involves neoplasia of the **p**arathyroid glands, **p**ancreatic islets, and **p**ituitary gland. A good mnemonic is the "**3 P's.**" MEN II syndromes consist of both medullary thyroid cancer and pheochromocytoma. Subtypes IIa and IIb differ in that IIa also has parathyroid involvement while IIb is associated with mucosal neuromas.

Genetics

The MEN syndromes arise from germline mutations in either tumor suppressor genes or oncogenes. Recently it was discovered that the mutation for MEN I occurs in a gene on chromosome 11 that codes for the protein menin. This gene is ubiquitously expressed in all cells and functions as a tumor suppressor. As a result, mutations within this gene cause loss of tumor suppressor function and uncontrolled cell cycle regulation. The gene responsible for MEN II syndromes is a proto-oncogene called *RET* on chromosome 10. In contrast to the *menin* gene of MEN I, *RET* is specifically expressed in cells derived from the neural crest. These include the C cells in the thyroid gland and the chromaffin cells of the adrenal medulla. As an oncogene, activation of *RET* leads to increased cell division and subsequent tumor formation.

MEN I

The patient described in this case presents with multiple endocrine-related findings, including a history of PUD, asymptomatic hypercalcemia, and evidence of GH excess (coarse facial features, enlarged liver). In a young patient with multiple endocrine abnormalities, the diagnosis of a MEN syndrome should be considered. In this case, MEN I is most likely because of the associated pituitary symptoms, parathyroid-related hypercalcemia, and excessive acid secretion from a pancreatic islet gastrinoma. The history is also suggestive because the patient mentions a positive family history of chronic ulcer disease.

Primary hyperparathyroidism is present in up to 90% of patients with MEN I. In contrast to the single adenomas found in idiopathic primary hyperparathyroidism, the genetic condition usually involves diffuse hyperplasia or multiple adenomas in all four parathyroid glands. Asymptomatic hypercalcemia, as in this patient, is the most common manifestation; about 25% of patients have evidence of kidney stones. Pancreatic islet cell tumors occur in about 30 to 75% of affected patients. Islet cell tumors can arise from a variety of cell types within the islet; these tumors may secret insulin, gastrin, somatostatin, ACTH, vasoactive intestinal polypeptide (VIP), serotonin, or prostaglandin. Also known as **Zollinger-Ellison syndrome,** gastrinomas are the most common islet tumor and are associated with intractable and complicated peptic ulceration. Over half of all MEN I patients have PUD, and the ulcers are often multiple and atypical in location. Although Zollinger-Ellison syndrome can also occur sporadically, some 20 to 60% of patients who first present with this condition will prove to have MEN I.

Pituitary tumors associated with MEN I arise from a variety of cells within the anterior pituitary. Pituitary adenomas are found in 50 to 65% of MEN I cases. The most common form is a hypersecreting prolactinoma, but other common products include GH that results in the signs and symptoms of acromegaly noted in DK. These include coarsening of facial features, deepening of the voice, and enlargement of internal organs (heart, spleen, liver, etc.). Like sporadic pituitary tumors, these neoplasms can cause visual disturbance, headache, and hypopituitarism if the surrounding normal tissue becomes compressed and is rendered nonfunctional.

MEN IIa

MEN IIa consists of medullary cancer of the thyroid, pheochromocytoma, and parathyroid hyperplasia. Medullary cancer of the thyroid is the most consistent and most life-threatening feature of the syndrome, followed by pheochromocytoma. In contrast to sporadic cases of pheochromocytoma, the inherited form associated with the MEN syndromes is usually bilateral and presents with paroxysmal rather than sustained HTN.

MEN IIb

Like MEN IIa, MEN IIb includes medullary cancer of the thyroid and pheochromocytoma. However, MEN IIb patients are distinguished by the presence of mucosal neuromas, which give these patients a characteristic appearance. All MEN IIb patients exhibit a marfanoid phenotype (slender body, long and thin extremities, abnormally lax ligaments), thick eyelids, and diffusely hypertrophied lips. The neuromas appear as small, shiny bumps on the lips, tongue, and buccal mucosa.

Diagnosis

Diagnosis of the MEN syndromes depends on the presentation of symptoms and the organs involved. Almost any combination of tumors and symptom complexes described is possible, and involvement of all three conditions associated with each syndrome is not necessarily required for diagnosis. For example, only 40% of patients diagnosed with MEN I actually have the complete combination of parathyroid hyperplasia, pituitary adenoma, and a pancreatic islet tumor. Diagnosis can be confirmed with genetic screening consisting of restriction fragment length polymorphism DNA analysis. Tests for the diagnosis of specific endocrine abnormalities include a 24-hour urine collection for catecholamines identifying pheochromocytoma, serum calcium and PTH levels to detect hypercalcemia, and measurement of IGF-1 to confirm acromegaly. Zollinger-Ellison syndrome is the major cause of morbidity and mortality in MEN I, while mortality in MEN II is due to the aggressive nature of medullary thyroid carcinoma. Relatives of MEN patients should be screened annually with an accurate medical history and physical exam with pertinent laboratory tests to detect early manifestations of the condition.

Treatment

Treatment of parathyroid and pituitary lesions is primarily surgical. Pancreatic islet cell tumor excision is more complex because the tumors are often small and multiple. While attempts to localize and remove the specific tumor should be made in all patients, symptomatic treatment for gastrinomas can be achieved with proton pump inhibitors and histamine-2 (H2) blockers. Prophylactic thyroidectomy should be considered in identified gene carriers of MEN II to avoid morbidity and mortality. MEN II patients undergoing surgery for medullary thyroid cancer or hyperparathyroidism should have any associated pheochromocytoma removed first because of the risk of a hypertensive crisis during surgical resection. Prognosis for patients with MEN syndromes is good if the tumors are identified and removed early in the course of the disease process.

QUESTIONS

1. A 23-year-old African American woman is advised to undergo genetic screening because her mother was recently diagnosed with a MEN syndrome. Her mother's medical history includes chronic headaches, DM, asthma, multiple kidney stones, and HTN. Screening tests to identify her mother's specific type of MEN syndrome should include:

   A. *RET* germline mutation evaluation
   B. *Menin* germline mutation evaluation
   C. Serum Ca and intact PTH measurement
   D. 24-hour urinary free catecholamines
   E. Basal and stimulated plasma calcitonin

2. An 18-year-old male college student complains of numerous episodes of headache, sweating, palpitations, and tachycardia

CASE CONCLUSION

DK is diagnosed with MEN I after further investigation confirms elevated serum IGF-1 and basal gastrin levels in association with his asymptomatic hypercalcemia. Head CT scan is significant for an enlarged sella turcica, indicative of a pituitary neoplasm. He is started on a trial of omeprazole for relief of his PUD symptoms while awaiting surgical excision of his pituitary and parathyroid neoplasms.

THUMBNAIL: MEN Syndromes

MEN I—"the 3 P's
Parathyroid hyperplasia
Pituitary adenoma
Pancreatic islet cell tumors

MEN IIa
Medullary thyroid carcinoma
Pheochromocytoma
Parathyroid hyperplasia

MEN IIb
Medullary thyroid carcinoma
Pheochromocytoma
Mucosal neuromas
Marfanoid phenotype

KEY POINTS

- All syndromes are autosomal dominant
- MEN I is characterized by a germline mutation in the *menin* gene and a tumor suppressor gene on chromosome 11. *Menin* is normally expressed in all cells. Mutations in tumor suppressor genes cause cancer through loss of function and cell cycle regulation.
- MEN II is characterized by a germline mutation in the *RET* proto-oncogene, which is expressed in neural crest-derived cells. Mutations in oncogenes cause cancer through activation of the oncogene, stimulating uncontrolled cell division.

lasting about 60 minutes each while in class. A visit to the student health center during one of these episodes reveals a BP of 200/120 mm Hg; 24-hour urinary catecholamine secretion is greater than 200 μg. The patient is tall and slender with exceptionally long fingers and toes. For which of the following conditions does this patient have the highest risk?

A. PUD
B. Hyperthyroidism
C. Osteoporosis
D. Galactorrhea
E. Thyroid carcinoma

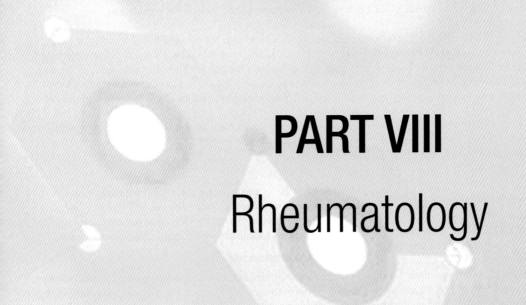

PART VIII

Rheumatology

Systemic Lupus Erythematosus

HPI: BH, a 30-year-old African American woman, presents to her primary care physician complaining of joint pain in her fingers for the past 2 months. The patient also reports associated fatigue, loss of appetite, and weight loss. Initially, BH felt it could be related to increased stress from her job at an Internet start-up company. However, her symptoms have persisted despite a recent 2-week vacation in Hawaii. She states that she felt even worse after her lazy days at the beach. Activities such as body surfing and snorkeling were less enjoyable because she found herself sensitive to the bright sunshine. Moreover, BH complains of an unusual "sunburn" that has continued to bother her since her return. The patient is concerned and feels that now she has turned 30 everything in her body is going awry. "My hair seems to be falling out and even brushing my teeth seems to give me trouble as my gums are always seeming to bleed!" she exclaims. She recalls her mother having arthritis and always being sickly and fears that soon she will be the same way. The patient denies any past medical history. She has no drug allergies, and is currently taking birth control pills and multivitamins. Both of her parents have hypertension and, in addition to arthritis, BH's mother is currently receiving dialysis for renal failure.

PE: The patient is noted to have a low-grade fever of 38.1°C. Her vital signs are otherwise within normal limits. She is noted to be a thin, athletically built woman who is anxious but in no acute distress. A butterfly rash with scaling is noted on her face, and discrete macular lesions are observed on her arms and legs. Ocular exam reveals acute sensitivity to having a light shined into her eyes. Oral ulcers are seen on the hard palate. The patient has no lymphadenopathy and her thyroid is noted to be normal. Cardiac, pulmonary, and abdominal exams are unremarkable. Extremity exam reveals swelling and tenderness of her distal interphalangeal (DIP) joints in both hands.

Labs: WBC 5.0; RBC 38.0; Plt 75,000; Cr 0.9; ESR, 120; rheumatoid factor positive; antinuclear antibody (ANA) positive; urinalysis 1.012, negative protein, negative ketones, no WBC, no RBC

THOUGHT QUESTIONS

- What is the *most likely* diagnosis for this patient?
- What is *immunologic tolerance* and how is it achieved?
- How would you describe the proposed mechanisms for autoimmunity?
- If BH's mother's renal failure was caused by systemic lupus erythematosus (SLE), what would you expect to see on a biopsy of her kidney and how would you follow her disease?
- What is the mechanism underlying this patient's thrombocytopenia?

BASIC SCIENCE REVIEW AND DISCUSSION

Clinical Features and Epidemiology

This young woman most likely has **SLE,** an autoimmune disorder. This disease is seen predominantly in women with a 9:1 female-to-male ratio. There is also a higher prevalence in black women, 1:250 versus 1:1000 for Caucasian women. The onset is typically between age 16 and 55 years. SLE can affect nearly every organ system in the body and is therefore a disease with varying presentations. BH has a typical presentation with vague constitutional symptoms of fatigue, anorexia, weight loss, and fever in conjunction with arthritis (seen in 95%) and abnormalities of the skin, hair, and mucous membranes (seen in 85%).

The **arthritis** associated with this disorder is usually symmetric and involves the small joints of the hands and feet. The two most common skin manifestations of SLE are (*a*) a classic malar butterfly rash that is an erythematous, confluent macular rash with fine scaling covering both cheeks and the bridge of the nose and frequently sensitive to sunlight; and (*b*) discrete discoid erythematous plaques on the face, scalp, forearms, fingers and toes. Diffuse alopecia and painless mucosal ulcers are also commonly seen. Other organs that can be affected include the kidneys, lung pleura, pericardium, cardiac valves, and CNS. These patients are

also noted to have hematologic disorders, including hemolytic anemia, thrombocytopenia, lymphopenia, and leukocytopenia.

Because this disease can vary widely in its presentation, criteria for diagnosis were established in 1982 and are outlined in Box 8-1.

Tolerance and Autoimmunity

Immunologic tolerance is unresponsiveness of a functioning immune system to certain antigens. It prevents the immune system from attacking self tissues and what allows a fetus to develop in the womb without being rejected by the maternal immune system. Immunosuppressive drugs given following organ transplantation enhance tolerance, preventing rejection of the foreign organs. **Clonal deletion** is the main process by which self-reactive **T cells** are eliminated. During fetal development, T lymphocytes are exposed to self antigens, primarily self major histocompatability complex (MHC) proteins. Those **T lymphocytes** that react with self antigens are "negatively selected" and die via programmed cell death. In the thymus, tolerance acquired in this way is termed **central tolerance.** The exact molecular mechanisms of this process are not as yet known or documented. **Clonal anergy** is tolerance that is acquired outside of the thymus. This process involves functional inactivation of T cells. Tolerance acquired in this fashion may be transient and change over time. Like clonal deletion, the exact mechanism of clonal anergy is unknown. It is, however, suspected to be related to suppressor cells or inappropriate presentation of antigen and thus a failure of co-stimulatory signals. **B-cell** tolerance likely develops in a similar fashion with clonal deletion occurring in the bone marrow and clonal anergy in the periphery. However, B-cell tolerance is less complete and shorter lasting than that in T cells as evidenced by the fact that most autoimmune diseases are mediated by antibodies.

Autoimmune disorders such as SLE occur when tolerance is lost. These diseases can involve humoral or cell-mediated reactions. However, most are **antibody mediated.** Three general mechanisms of autoimmunity have been suggested. The first involves release of sequestered antigens. According to this theory, the body

BOX 8-1 Criteria for the Classification of SLE*

1. Malar rash

2. Discoid rash

3. Photosensitivity

4. Oral ulcers

5. Arthritis

6. Serositis

7. Renal disease
   a. >0.5 gm/day proteinuria or
   b. =3+ proteinuria on dipstick or
   c. cellular casts

8. Neurologic disease
   a. seizures or
   b. psychosis (without other cause)

9. Hematologic disorders
   a. hemolytic anemia or
   b. leukopenia (<4000/μL) or
   c. lymphopenia (<1500/μL)
   d. thrombocytopenia (<100,000/μL)

10. Immunologic abnormalities
    a. positive LE cell preparation or
    b. antibody to native DNA or
    c. antibody to Sm or
    d. false-positive serologic test for syphilis

11. Positive ANA

*To meet the diagnosis, a patient needs to have any four of the 11 criteria listed.

possesses immunologically privileged sites that contain tissues that are not exposed to the immune system. When these antigens are accidentally released into the circulation, an immune response is triggered. A second possible mechanism underlying autoimmunity involves T-cell loss of tolerance. T-cell tolerance is maintained by continued presence of self antigen as well as the presence of suppressor T cells that provide important co-stimulatory signals. Exposure to foreign antigens that are similar to self antigens may terminate tolerance and lead to an autoimmune response. Also, decreased suppressor T-cell function may lead to loss of T-cell tolerance. A third general mechanism of autoimmunity involves a loss of B-cell tolerance. This type of tolerance is far more readily lost than that of T cells. Activated T cells can produce interleukins and co-stimulatory proteins like CD28, which in turn stimulate anergic B cells to produce antibodies against self antigens.

Pathophysiology of Systemic Lupus Erythematosus

SLE is a multisystem autoimmune disease that varies widely in presentation. Almost every organ in the body can be affected. The disease itself is characterized by the production of autoantibodies. Autoantibodies directed at components of the cell nucleus, known as ANAs, are most commonly seen. However, at this time the exact pathophysiology of all the various manifestations is not clearly understood. Exam of affected tissues at autopsy reveals minimal pathologic changes, including nonspecific inflammation, vessel abnormalities, or no changes at all. The best characterized pathology is that observed in the kidney, because biopsies of this organ are often performed in the course of the disease.

The renal damage caused by SLE is mediated by **immune complexes.** Autoantibodies, primarily ANAs and anti–double-stranded DNA (dsDNA) antibodies react with antigens in the circulation and are deposited in the glomerulus. These complexes subsequently set off the complement cascade, leading to the release of inflammatory mediators from circulating leukocytes. The resulting inflammation causes damage to the glomerular structure and glomerulonephritis results. Lupus patients with renal disease therefore have proteinuria, casts, and WBCs in their urine. On renal biopsy, five histologic patterns have been described (Table 8-1).

TABLE 8-1 Renal Disease in SLE

Class	Pathologic Diagnosis	Prevalence	Distinguishing Features
Class 1	Normal	Rare	No abnormalities
Class 2	Mesangial lupus glomerulonephritis	25%	Mildest Slight to moderate increase in the intercapillary mesangial matrix Granular mesangial deposits of immunoglobulin and complement are present
Class 3	Focal proliferative glomerulonephritis	20%	Focal lesion affects <50% of glomeruli Swelling and proliferation of endothelial and mesangial cells Infiltration with neutrophils ± fibrinoid deposits and intracapillary thrombi
Class 4	Diffuse proliferative glomerulonephritis	35%–40%	Most serious Most or all glomeruli involved Proliferation of endothelial, mesangial, and sometimes epithelial cells; crescents filling Bowman space + Fibrinoid necrosis and hyaline thrombi
Class 5	Membranous glomerulonephritis	15%	Widespread thickening of capillary walls

Given that BH's mother has renal failure, the most likely lesion found on this patient's renal biopsy would be class 4. Patients with this lesion on biopsy are usually symptomatic with microscopic or gross hematuria, proteinuria severe enough to cause nephritic syndrome, HTN, and mild to severe renal insufficiency. Once a biopsy is performed and the baseline level of disease is determined, serum complement and anti-DNA antibodies are followed serially. Decreasing complement and/or increasing anti-DNA antibodies can thus be used as early indicators of disease exacerbation or progression. Treatment consists of corticosteroids or immunosuppressive agents, such as cyclophosphamide,

depending on the severity of the lesions and progression. Such therapy can be effective. However, it is important to realize that opportunistic infections as well as lupus nephritis are the leading causes of death in SLE patients.

In addition to forming ANAs, patients with lupus form autoantibodies against red cells, white cells, and platelets. Cell destruction is the result of type II hypersensitivity in which autoantibodies bind antigens on the blood cell or platelet and the cell is either lysed through activation of the complement cascade and membrane attack complex or more commonly becomes susceptible to phagocytosis via fixation of the antibody or C3b to the cell surface.

CASE CONCLUSION

The differential diagnosis is SLE, rheumatoid arthritis, and discoid lupus. One month after diagnosing this patient with SLE and starting her on NSAIDs to relieve her joint pain and having her avoid sun exposure, BH returns for follow-up. She reports that her skin rash is much improved and that she has less joint pain.

THUMBNAIL: Autoantibodies and Associations with Connective Tissue Diseases

Autoantibody	Main Disease Association	Other Disease Associations	Comments
ANA	SLE	Rheumatoid arthritis Scleroderma Sjögren syndrome Discoid and drug-induced lupus	Screening test for SLE, high sensitivity (95%), low specificity, titers do not correlate with disease severity
Anti-dsDNA antibody	SLE	Rheumatoid arthritis Connective tissue disease (low titers)	Good confirmatory test for SLE, high positive predictive value if high titers
Anti-Smith antibody (anti-Sm)	SLE	None	Low sensitivity, high specificity
Rheumatoid factor	Rheumatoid arthritis	SLE, chronic infections, elderly patients, some healthy patients	Low sensitivity, titers do not correlate with disease severity
Anti-ribonucleoprotein (RNP) antibody	Scleroderma, mixed connective tissue disease (MCTD)	SLE, Sjögren syndrome, rheumatoid arthritis, discoid lupus	High sensitivity for MCTD (>95%)
SSA/Anti-Ro Antibody SSB/Anti-La Antibody	Sjögren's syndrome	SLE, rheumatoid arthritis, vasculitis	Positive test associated with neonatal SLE and congenital heart block
Anticentromere antibody	CREST syndrome	Scleroderma, Raynaud disease	High positive predictive value for scleroderma
ANCA	Wegner granulomatosis	Polyarteritis nodosa	Titers do not correlate with disease activity

KEY POINTS

- Immunologic tolerance occurs when the immune system fails to mount an immune response to a specific antigen. Loss of this immunologic tolerance can result in autoimmune disease.

- The two primary mechanisms of self-tolerance are **clonal deletion** and **clonal anergy. Clonal deletion** is the loss of self-reactive T and B lymphocytes that occurs in the process of maturation. **Clonal anergy** is

functional inactivation of lymphocytes that occurs in the periphery after encountering specific antigens.

- SLE is a multisystem autoimmune disease with multiple clinical presentations. The primary affect of this disease is a failure to process regulating self-tolerance, which results in the production of numerous autoantibodies.

QUESTIONS

1. BH's younger sister now presents 3 weeks postpartum with fevers, arthritis, and fatigue. She denies any health problems except for some elevated blood pressures noted at the time of delivery that have been treated with hydralazine. What is the *most likely* diagnosis?

   A. Postpartum arthritis
   B. Rheumatoid arthritis
   C. Lupus
   D. Discoid lupus
   E. Drug-induced lupus-like syndrome

2. You suspect that one of your patients has SLE. Which of the following is the *most specific* laboratory test that will help confirm your diagnosis?

   A. ESR
   B. Rheumatoid factor
   C. ANA
   D. Anti-dsDNA antibody
   E. Lupus anticoagulant

3. A patient presents with a malar rash, oral ulcers, pleuritis and psychosis. ANA titers are notably elevated. Which of the following *best* describes the mechanism underlying her disease?

   A. Clonal deletion of self-reactive T cells
   B. Release of a sequestered antigen
   C. Primary enzyme deficiency
   D. Failed clonal anergy
   E. Molecular mimicry

4. A patient with severe long-standing SLE dies of renal failure. On autopsy, which of the following is *unlikely* to be observed?

   A. Erosive changes in joints
   B. Pleural effusion
   C. Verrucous lesions on the mitral valve
   D. "Onion skin lesions" in the central arteries of the spleen
   E. Fibrinoid necrosis and hyaline thrombi affecting more than 50% of glomeruli

HPI: RS, a 38-year-old man, presents with a chief complaint of pain and stiffness of his hands, wrists, and knees that is most pronounced in the morning. He reports he hasn't really felt right for the past year following his divorce. Initially, he thought the fatigue, malaise, anorexia, and weight loss were all related to the lifestyle adjustments he had to make. However, now that his life is in order and he is enjoying himself more he continues to be bothered by his symptoms. Moreover, the problem with his hands and knees is starting to impair his ability to work as a plumber.

RH states that he has been healthy without any history of prior medical problems. He has never been hospitalized, has no drug allergies, and is currently taking no medications. RH is active and enjoys the outdoors. However, he admits that it has been increasingly difficult to hike and fish due to the pain in his joints. He denies tobacco use but does report consuming one or two beers after work and on the weekends.

PE: T 37.0°C; BP 132/78 mm Hg; HR 88 beats/min; RR 18 breaths/min; SaO_2 99%; **Gen:** Thin. NAD **CVR:** RRR, chest CTA bilaterally. **Abdomen (Abd):** Soft, nontender + BS (bowel sounds); **Extremities (Ext.):** + swelling, tenderness, and warmth over proximal interphalangeal (PIP) joints of both hands and knees.

Labs: WBC 7.5; Hct 42; Plt 360; ESR 98; ANA 1:250; rheumatoid factor 1:400.

THOUGHT QUESTIONS

- Who is most likely to get rheumatoid arthritis (RA)? What are the most common clinical manifestations?
- How would you describe the changes that occur in the joints with RA? Which characteristic joint deformities develop after progressive joint destruction?
- How would you describe the autoimmune reaction that occurs in the joints in RA? What are the key mediators of joint damage?
- What is rheumatoid factor? What is the general structure of immunoglobulins? What are the different classes of immunoglobulins and what roles do they play in the immune response?

BASIC SCIENCE REVIEW AND DISCUSSION

Clinical Features

RA is a chronic, inflammatory disease that can affect multiple organ systems, including skin, blood vessels, heart, lungs, and muscles. The most common manifestation is destruction of articular cartilage. RA's global prevalence is approximately 1 to 2% in the general population. This disease is more common in women, with a 3:1 female to male predominance. The typical age of onset is the 20s and 30s. Initial symptoms are usually insidious with vague prodromal symptoms of malaise, weight loss, and joint stiffness. The stiffness is most pronounced in the morning and after periods of inactivity. Symmetric joint swelling, warmth, tenderness, and pain are noted. The most commonly affected joints include the PIP and metacarpophalangeal (MCP) joints as well as the wrists, knees, ankles, and toes. Subcutaneous "rheumatoid" nodules located over bony prominences are seen in approximately 20% of patients with RA. Other less common extra-articular manifestations include pericarditis, pleural disease, and vasculitis.

Histopathology of the Joint in Rheumatoid Arthritis

In RA the joint undergoes characteristic changes as the disease progresses. Initially, the synovium becomes edematous, thickened, and hyperplastic. An inflammatory infiltrate made up of CD4 cells, plasma cells, and macrophages fills the synovial stroma, and increased vascularity is noted. This inflamed synovium assumes a polypoid form producing a pannus that then erodes into the underlying articular cartilage. Inflammatory cells release mediators that increase osteoclastic activity, thereby allowing the synovium to further erode into the subchondral bone. The result is juxta-articular erosions and subchondral cysts. Over time, the articular cartilage is totally destroyed and the pannus expands, bridging the distance between the opposing bones of the joint, and forms a fibrous ankylosis that eventually ossifies. This process correlates with the clinical joint symptoms. Initially, joints are inflamed and painful. With time, the inflammation resolves as the normal anatomy of the joint is completely destroyed. This progressive joint destruction leads to characteristic deformities, including radial deviation of the wrist, ulnar deviation of the fingers, **boutonniere** deformity of the fingers (hyperextension of the DIP joint with flexion of the PIP joint), and **swan neck** deformity of the fingers (flexion of the DIP joint with extension of the PIP joint).

Pathophysiology

The exact initiating event for the synovitis characteristic of RA is currently unknown. However, it is postulated that this disease is triggered by an exposure of an immunogenetically susceptible host to an arthritogenic microbial antigen. A majority of patients with this disease have class II MHC molecules alleles HLA-DR4 and/or HLA-DR1 and thus have a shared binding site that predisposes them to development of synovial inflammation. Initiation of this inflammation is thought to occur with exposure to a microbial agent that has not yet been identified. This exposure triggers an autoimmune reaction within the synovial membranes. It is the inflammatory mediators of this reaction that ultimately cause joint destruction.

T cells play the primary role in the immune reaction in RA, in particular, CD4 memory T cells. Shortly after the onset of joint symptoms, large numbers of these cells are seen in the synovial fluid of the affected joints. The endothelial cells of the synovial vessels are subsequently activated and there is an increase in the expression of intracellular adhesion molecules-1 (ICAM-1). As a result, other inflammatory cells such as neutrophils, plasma cells, and macrophages are recruited to the joint. Activated T cells, B cells, and macrophages then release numerous cytokines, including **TNF-a** and **interleukin-1** (IL-1), which stimulate the release of **collagenases** from synovial cells and inhibit synthesis of proteoglycans in cartilage, thus leading to destruction of cartilage. Neutrophils release **proteases** and **elastases** that further contribute to the alteration of the normal structure of the joint.

Rheumatoid factor is an IgM autoantibody that reacts with the Fc portion of autologous IgG molecules. It is found in about 3% of healthy persons and its incidence increases with age. More than 75% of persons with RA will have this autoantibody present in their serum. High levels of the antibody are commonly associated with severe disease. However, this autoantibody is not unique to RA; it is also observed in other conditions, including sarcoiditis, TB, leprosy, parasitic infections, sarcoidosis, and other autoimmune diseases, such as SLE. In RA, these autoantibodies form immune complexes with autologous IgG molecules. These immune complexes are found in the serum, synovial fluid, and synovial membranes. Those found in the serum are believed to be responsible for the extra-articular manifestations of RA.

Antibodies Antibodies are proteins that react with specific antigens and thus play an important role in humoral immunity. They make up 20% of serum proteins and are produced by plasma cells. Structurally, these globular proteins are composed of four polypeptide chains, two identical heavy chains and two identical light chains that form a "Y" shape. The variable regions of the light and heavy chains are located at the tips of the Y and are where antigen binding occurs. In contrast, the constant regions of these chains are responsible for complement activation and binding to cells' surface receptors. If treated with proteolytic enzymes, antibodies are broken into three pieces: two identical **Fab fragments** containing the antigen-binding sites and one Fc fragment that is made up of the constant regions of the heavy chains. It is this **Fc fragment** that rheumatoid factor binds to.

There are five classes of antibodies: IgG, IgM, IgA, IgE, and IgD. **IgG** is the predominant class and is made up of immunoglobulin monomers (two heavy chains/two light chains). This antibody class plays an important role in the secondary host defense response against bacteria and viruses through opsonization and complement fixation. It is the only antibody that can cross the placenta. **IgM** is the antibody produced in a primary immune response. It is a pentamer made up of five immunoglobulin monomers connected by a J (joining) chain. This class of antibody has a total of 10 antigen-binding sites and is the most efficient immunoglobulin in agglutination and complement fixation and therefore plays a key role in host defenses against bacterial and viral infections. **IgA** is the primary antibody found in secretions, including saliva, tears, intestinal/GI/genital secretions, and colostrum. IgA molecules are made up of two immunoglobulin monomers connected by one J chain. This class of antibodies prevents attachment of microorganisms to mucous membranes. **IgE** antibodies are found in only trace amounts in the serum. These are made up of immunoglobulin monomers. Their primary roles are (*a*) in the host defenses against parasitic infections and (*b*) in mediating type I (anaphylactic) hypersensitivity reactions. **IgD** is an antibody found bound to the surface of B cells as well as in serum. It exists as an immunoglobulin monomer. The function of this class of antibodies is not presently well understood.

CASE CONCLUSION

Differential diagnosis: RA, ankylosing spondylitis, Reiter syndrome, SLE, osteoarthritis, gout, chronic lyme disease, polymyalgia rheumatica. The patient is diagnosed with RA and counseled extensively on the chronic nature and likely course of the disease. A program of physical and occupational therapy combined with stretching, exercise, and rest is initiated. NSAIDs are prescribed for symptomatic relief. Despite this treatment regimen, RH's symptoms continue to worsen and, after 7 months, he is started on gold salts.

THUMBNAIL: Immunoglobulin Classes

	Percent of Ig in Serum	Structure	Crosses Placenta	Main Functions
IgG	75%	Monomer	Yes	Main antibody in secondary response against bacteria and bacterial toxins Opsonizes bacteria Fixes complement Crosses the placenta
IgA	15%	Monomer or dimer	No	Found in secretions Prevents attachment of microorganisms to mucous membranes
IgM	9%	Monomer or pentamer	No	Main antibody in primary response to antigen Fixes complement Antigen receptor on surface of B cells

(Continued)

THUMBNAIL: Immunoglobulin Classes *(Continued)*

	Percent of Ig in Serum	Structure	Crosses Placenta	Main Functions
IgD	0.2%	Monomer	??	Unknown function Found on surface of B cells as well as in serum
IgE	0.004%	Monomer	No	Mediates immediate hypersensitivity reactions by causing degranulation of mast cells and basophils Important in host defenses against helminthic infection through triggering the release of enzymes from eosinophils

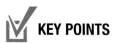

KEY POINTS

■ RA is a chronic, inflammatory disease that primarily affects the PIP and MCP joints bilaterally

■ Inflammation in the joint is characterized by a synovitis that is progressive and eventually leads to joint destruction and deformities

■ RA is more common in women (3:1 female-to-male ratio); age of onset is the 20s and 30s

■ Patients with RA often have HLA-DR4 and/or HLA-DR1 alleles and have rheumatoid factor in their serum

■ Rheumatoid factor is an IgM autoantibody to the Fc portion of autologous antibodies

QUESTIONS

1. Analysis of fluid removed from one of this patient's affected joints would reveal:

   A. Fragments of *Chlamydia trachomatis*
   B. Turbid fluid with high levels of WBCs
   C. Birefringent crystals seen with polarized light microscopy
   D. Bloody fluid
   E. High levels of rheumatoid factor

2. After failing treatment with NSAIDs and gold salts the patient is started on a new medication. Three weeks later he notes oral ulcers and nausea. He is seen again in your office and you send him to the lab to have blood tests drawn. Which of the following abnormalities is *most likely* to be found?

   A. Decreased levels of rheumatoid factor
   B. Decreased RBCs
   C. Decreased WBCs
   D. Increased RBCs
   E. Increased RBCs
   F. Elevated creatinine
   G. Elevated AST

3. Despite treatment this patient's disease progresses. He develops joint deformities and has increasing difficulties at work secondary to limited range of motion and pain. X-rays are done and reveal:

   A. Global demineralization of the ulnar and radius
   B. Increased bony cortex, with increased bone density
   C. Joint space narrowing, osteophytes, and dense subchondral bone
   D. Calcification of the anterior and lateral spinal ligaments with squaring and demineralization of the vertebral bodies
   E. Multiple lytic lesions
   F. Joint space narrowing and erosions

4. A 30-year-old woman presents to the office complaining of facial swelling and urticaria that developed after eating barbecued shrimp for the first time. This reaction is *most likely* caused by which of the following?

   A. IgG-mediated immune complexes deposited in the skin
   B. IgG-mediated complement lysis
   C. IgE-induced mast cell degranulation
   D. IgA-mediated histamine release
   E. IgD-mediated histamine release

CASE 8-3   Reiter and Sjögren Syndromes

HPI: FR, a 31-year-old Caucasian male, presents to the acute care clinic complaining of urinary frequency and burning. He states that he hasn't felt right since returning from a vacation in Thailand a couple of weeks ago. Initially, FR thought he was merely experiencing some jet lag with fatigue and general malaise. However, over the past 2 weeks he has developed pain in his right heel and knee as well as in his back. Overnight he noted the onset of urinary symptoms. The patient denies any prior medical problems. However, he does describe having a week of bloody diarrhea while in Thailand.

PE: The patient is afebrile. He is mildly ill appearing, with red, itchy eyes. Painless oral ulcers are noted on his buccal mucosa and palate. Extremity exam reveals sausage-shaped toes, tenderness of the heels and low back, and swelling of the right knee. The remainder of the exam is unremarkable.

Labs: First void urine is positive for WBCs; however, it is negative for both gonorrhea and chlamydia.

THOUGHT QUESTIONS

- What is the most likely diagnosis? Who is at most risk for this disease?
- Which infectious agents are associated with this disorder?
- Describe the concept of molecular mimicry and how it could explain the mechanism of Reiter syndrome.
- Which gene is associated with this form of arthritis? What are the two classes of HLA or MHC molecules and what role do they play in the immune system?
- Which other spondyloarthropathies are associated with HLA-B27 and how do they compare to Reiter syndrome?

BASIC SCIENCE REVIEW AND DISCUSSION

Clinical Features of Reiter Syndrome

The combination of arthritis, conjunctivitis, urethritis, and mucocutaneous lesions is classic for Reiter syndrome, which most commonly affects young men in their 20s and 30s. The arthritis is characteristically polyarticular and asymmetric. The most common joints affected are the knees, ankles, feet, wrists, and spine. Inflammation of the tendinous insertions on the bone is unique to Reiter syndrome and the associated spondylopathies. In the fingers and toes this inflammation leads to a "sausage digit" appearance, whereas in the ankles it is seen as heel pain.

The onset of Reiter syndrome typically follows a genitourinary tract infection with *Chlamydia trachomatis* or a GI infection with *Salmonella, Shigella, Yersinia,* or *Campylobacter.* Synovial fluid cultures are negative for these organisms. However, fragments of these bacteria have been identified in synovial tissues.

Pathophysiology of Reiter Syndrome

The exact pathophysiology of this disease is not clearly understood at this time. However, the association of Reiter syndrome with specific infections suggests that **molecular mimicry** may be a mechanism underlying this autoimmune disorder. Normally, the immune system exhibits tolerance toward self tissues. When this tolerance is lost, the immune system mounts an attack against native tissues, resulting in autoimmune disease. Molecular mimicry is one proposed mechanism used to explain how tolerance is lost. According to this theory, an environmental trigger—in this case *Chlamydia, Salmonella, Shigella, Yersinia* or *Campylobacter*—resembles or "mimics" self antigens. These self antigens are therefore viewed as "foreign" and are subject to immune attack. The result is inflammation of tissues in the joints, urethra, and mucous membranes.

Genetics of Reiter Syndrome

There is a genetic predisposition to Reiter syndrome. Most affected individuals carry the gene for **HLA-B27.** HLA molecules were initially identified as antigens that triggered rejection of transplanted organs and so were named **MHC** molecules. There is tremendous within-species variations in these proteins; therefore, these molecules play an important role in the recognition of self and non-self. The genes coding for these proteins are found on chromosome 6 and 15. Three of these genes—HLA-A, HLA-B, and HLA-C—code for class I MHC proteins, whereas the HLA-D genes code for class II MHC proteins. These genes contain hypervariable regions that lead to a high degree of polymorphism in the proteins that are produced, thereby accounting for the vast differences between individuals within the same species.

Sjögren Syndrome

Sjögren syndrome is also an **autoimmune disorder,** and is characterized by chronic inflammation of the exocrine glands. It may be primary and seen in the absence of other diseases, or may be secondary and associated with RA, SLE, systemic sclerosis, myositis, biliary cirrhosis, chronic hepatitis, cryoglobulinemia, vasculitis, or thyroiditis. The disease progresses slowly and can be limited to lacrimal and salivary glands or may involve multiple organs, including the lungs, kidneys, blood vessels, and muscles. Signs and symptoms may include dry eyes, xerostomia, dental caries secondary to decreased saliva with its antibacterial properties, epistaxis, dry throat with hoarseness, dysphagia, bronchitis, pneumonia, reduced gastric acid output, constipation, pancreatic insufficiency, and vaginal dryness.

Autoantibodies are common in Sjögren syndrome, the most specific being those directed against RNA, **anti-SS-A (Ro),** and **anti-SS-B (La).** However, elevated levels of ANAs as well as rheumatoid factor can also be seen. Additionally, autoantibodies directed against specific tissues, such as gastric parenchyma, thyroid, smooth muscle, and salivary duct, can be found. The presence and levels of these autoantibodies have not been found to correlate with disease severity or activity. However, the presence of anti-SS-A (Ro) antibodies has been associated with the development of neonatal SLE and congenital heart block or arrhythmias in babies of mothers who have these antibodies.

Lymphocytes and the Immune System The body's ability to mount a specific immune response is due primarily to the functions of **lymphocytes.** There are two main types of lymphocytes: B and T lymphocytes. These two types differ in their immune function, where they mature, how they interact with antigen, and their specific surface markers. Although both types have their origin in the bone marrow, **B cells** develop and become immunocompetent in the bone marrow, whereas **T cells** develop and become immunocompetent in the thymus. In the absence of antigen, a population of lymphocytes forms with a unique antigen receptor that is capable of responding to a wide variety of antigens. Self-reactive lymphocytes are eliminated through clonal deletion during this process of development. The next stage of development occurs in peripheral lymphoid regions, lymph nodes, the spleen, and lymphoid aggregates such as Peyer patches and tonsils. Immunocompetent lymphocytes are exposed to foreign antigens that trigger division and differentiation. Division results in the formation of a clone of lymphocytes with the same antigen specificity. Differentiation leads to the development of effector cells that perform the actual immune function and memory cells that circulate for years and maintain the ability to respond rapidly to re-exposure to a specific antigen.

T lymphocytes play a primary role in **cell-mediated immunity.** There are two main populations of T cells: **helper T cells,** which are distinguished by the cell surface marker **CD4;** and **cytotoxic T cells,** which are distinguished by the cell surface marker **CD8.** Both types have CD3 and T-cell receptors as characteristic cell surface molecules. CD4 helper T cells (*a*) assist in

B-cell development and differentiation into antibody-producing plasma cells; (*b*) help CD8 T cells become activated cytotoxic T cells; and (*c*) enhance macrophage action in delayed hypersensitivity reactions. This type of T cell can be further subdivided into T_h1 cells and T_h2 cells. T_h1 cells produce IL-2 and γ-interferon, both of which enhance the delayed hypersensitivity response. T_h2 cells produce IL-4 and IL-5, both of which assist in B-cell activation. CD8 cytotoxic T cells kill virus-infected cells, tumor cells, and allograft cells via the release of perforins that damage cell membranes or via induction of programmed cell death. T cells are activated by recognition of polypeptide antigens associated with major histocompatability molecules on APCs. CD4 T cells interact with MHC class II-associated antigen, and CD8 T cells interact with MHC class I-associated antigen. Both cell types interact with MHC molecules through T-cell receptor molecules. T lymphocytes are subsequently activated by signals transmitted by CD3.

B lymphocytes play a key role in **humoral immunity.** These cells are distinguished by the cell surface markers CD19, CD20, and surface IgM and/or IgD. The two primary functions of these cells is antibody production and antigen presentation. Once exposed to antigen, these cells differentiate into plasma and memory cells. Plasma cells secrete antibodies specific to the antigen responsible for its activation. B-cell activation is enhanced by helper T-cell interaction with antigen presented by activated B cells on MHC class II molecules. This interaction leads to the production of stimulating cytokines IL-2, IL-4, and IL-5 by these helper T cells.

THUMBNAIL: B and T Lymphocytes

	T Cells	B Cells
Primary immune function	Cell-mediated immunity Host defense against fungal, viral, and TB infections Regulate the immune response (CD4 cells) Kill virus-infected cells, tumor cells, and allografts (CD8 cells)	Humoral immunity Host defense against bacterial, viral, and parasitic infections Production of antibodies APCs
Site of maturation	Thymus	Bone marrow
Cell surface markers	CD4, CD8, CD3, TCR (T-cell receptor)	CD19, CD20, IgM
Antigen recognition	T-cell receptor + CD3 recognize antigen bound to MHC molecules on APCs CD4 cells—class II MHC CD8 cells—class I MHC	Surface IgM binds free-floating antigen
Response to antigen activation	CD4 cells: T_h1—production of γ-interferon and IL-2 T_h2—production of IL-4 and IL-5 CD8 cells kill infected/abnormal cells	Production of antibodies Antibody presentation

Major Histocompatibility Molecules

In addition to their role in recognition between self and non-self, HLA molecules play an important role in shaping the body's immune response. The primary function of these molecules is to bind peptide fragments of foreign proteins and present them to the appropriate T cells, leading to a T-cell mediated immune response. **Class I MHC** molecules are found on all cells and are

composed of a long α-chain and a short β-chain. These MHC molecules present peptides from proteins synthesized within the cell and are therefore important in immune surveillance and destruction of virus-infected or otherwise altered body cells, such as tumor cells. The antigen/MHC complexes of these abnormal cells are recognized and killed by CD8 T cells. **Class II MHC** molecules, on the other hand, are only found on specific cells of the immune

TABLE 8-2 Spondylopathies Associated with HLA-B27

	Reiter Syndrome	Ankylosing Spondylitis	Psoriatic Arthritis	Enteropathic Arthritis
Age at onset	Young to middle-aged adult	Young adult <age 40	Young to middle-aged adult	Young to middle-aged adult
Sex ratio	Male:female 3:1	Male:female 10–15:1	Male:female 1:1	Male:female 1:1
Arthritis	Peripheral arthritis > sacroiliitis/spondylitis	Sacroiliitis > spondylitis >> peripheral arthritis	Peripheral arthritis >> sacroiliitis/spondylitis	Peripheral arthritis > spondylitis > sacroiliitis
Disease associations	Chlamydia infection, dysentery (*Shigella/Salmonella*)	None	Psoriasis	Crohn disease, ulcerative colitis
Extra-articular manifestations	GU, oral/GI, eye	Eye, heart	Skin, eye	GI, eye
Clinical course	Acute > chronic	Chronic	Chronic	Acute or chronic
Triggered by infection	Yes	No	No	No

system, such as B cells, macrophages, Langerhans cells, and dendritic cells. These molecules are made up of two intrinsic membrane proteins that are approximately equal in length. Exogenous foreign peptides that are phagocytosed by cells expressing these molecules are digested and then presented by class II MHC molecules. These complexes are, in turn, recognized by CD4 T cells, leading to either a type II delayed hypersensitivity reaction or production of antibodies through a T cell-dependent humoral response.

It has recently been learned that certain HLA types are associated with specific diseases. Even though the exact pathophysiology underlying these disorders has not yet been elucidated, the HLA associations have led to speculation on possible disease mechanisms. Diseases related to class I MHC include ankylosing spondylitis and Reiter syndrome; those diseases related to class II MHC include RA, Graves disease, and SLE (Table 8-2).

CASE CONCLUSION

Differential diagnosis: Reiter syndrome, enteropathic arthritis, ankylosing spondylitis, RA. FR is diagnosed with Reiter syndrome and is treated with NSAIDs. Over the following few weeks his symptoms gradually resolve.

THUMBNAIL: Differences Between Class I and II MHC

	Class I MHC	*Class II MHC*
Genes	HLA-A, HLA-B, HLA-C	HLA-D
Type of cells on which they are located	All nucleated cells	Macrophages B cells Dendritic cells of the spleen Langerhans cells of the skin
Structure	α-chain, which is an intrinsic membrane protein, and a short β-chain	α- and β-chains are intrinsic membrane proteins of approximately the same length
Site of the genes	α-chromosome 6 β-chromosome 15	α-chromosome 6 β-chromosome 6

(Continued)

THUMBNAIL: Differences Between Class I and II MHC *(Continued)*

	Class I MHC	Class II MHC
Antigen-binding domain	Composed of the α1 and α2 domains of the α-chain	Composed of the α1 domain of the α-chain and the β domain of the β-chain
Antigens presented	Peptides from proteins synthesized within the cell	Exogenous proteins that are ingested and degraded in lysosomes
Type of T cell involved in recognition of antigens presented	CD8	CD4
Consequences of T-cell recognition	Cytotoxic T-cell killing of APC	Induction of helper T cells and antibody production or delayed hypersensitivity reactions
Disease associations	HLA-B27; ankylosing spondylitis and Reiter syndrome	HLA-DR4; RA, insulin-dependent diabetes HLA-DR3; Sjögren syndrome

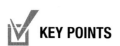

KEY POINTS

- Reiter syndrome is a reactive arthritis that is seen following urethritis or dysentery. Symptoms include arthritis, urethritis, conjunctivitis, and mucocutaneous lesions.

- Reiter syndrome is just one of a group of interrelated disorders including ankylosing spondylitis, psoriatic arthritis, and enteropathic arthritis. These disorders are characterized by (*a*) arthritis affecting the spine, sacroiliac joints, and peripheral joints; (*b*) extra-articular inflammation involving the eye, intestines, urethra, skin, or heart; (*c*) association with HLA-B27.

- Sjögren's syndrome is another autoimmune disorder, which primarily affects the exocrine glands and includes the presence of anti-ribonuclear protein anti-SS-A (Ro) and anti-SS-B (La) autoantibodies.

- Molecular mimicry is one proposed mechanism explaining autoimmune disease. According to this theory there may be homology between certain infectious agents and host proteins. Thus, infection with these microorganisms generates an immune response that cross-reacts with autologous body constituents.

- The broad diversity of antibodies found in the human repertoire is the result of the organization of the immunoglobulin genes and the mechanisms by which they are rearranged and combined into immunoglobulin molecules.

QUESTIONS

1. Which of the following is *not* typically seen in Reiter syndrome?

   A. Diarrhea
   B. Arthritis
   C. Macular papular rash with scaling
   D. Urethritis
   E. Conjunctivitis

2. Which of the following findings is associated with Reiter syndrome?

   A. HLA-DR4 positive
   B. Urethral culture positive for *Chlamydia*

   C. Urethral culture positive for gonorrhea
   D. Synovial fluid culture positive for *Chlamydia*
   E. Synovial fluid culture positive for gonorrhea

3. Class I MHC molecules:

   A. Are found only on B cells and macrophages
   B. Present antigen to CD4 cells
   C. Such as HLA-DR4 are associated with autoimmune disorders
   D. Play an important role in cytotoxic T-cell killing of abnormal host cells
   E. Trigger the complement cascade

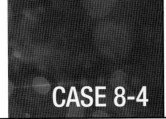

CASE 8-4 Kawasaki Disease

HPI: MA, a 3-year-old Filipino boy, presents to your office with an 8-day history of high fevers and rashes. His mother reports that at first they thought it was the flu and gave him ibuprofen and soup, but then he developed a rash on his chest and hands. Normally quite a calm boy, MA has been unusually fussy according to his grandmother. He is refusing to eat and cries, saying that his mouth hurts. MA's mother denies vomiting, headaches, vision changes, bowel, or bladder changes. He has a 5-year-old sister who has a cold. The patient has no known drug allergies. He is taking ibuprofen and traditional herbal remedies. The patient has a normal developmental history and his vaccines are up to date except for second hepatitis A vaccine.

PE: T 39.3°C; RR 32 breaths/min; HR 174 beats/min; BP 120/60 mm Hg.

Gen: Screaming loudly in his mother's arms. **HEENT:** Bilateral injected conjunctivae, erythematous oropharynx and tongue with dry, cracked lips. **Neck:** Two anterior cervical lymph nodes of 1–2 cm each on right side. **Chest:** CTA B no signs of respiratory distress. **Cor:** Hyperactive precordium, II/VI SEM at LUSM, normal S1 but extra S2 sound. **Abd:** + BS, soft, nontender, nondistended, no hepatosplenomegaly. **Ext:** Warm, well perfused. **Skin:** Fine maculapapular rash on chest, hands, and feet. **Neurologic (Neuro):** Very agitated but grossly intact.

Labs: WBC 14.8; Hgb 12.2; Plt 605; ESR 84; monospot negative, rapid strep antigen negative.

THOUGHT QUESTIONS

- What is the differential diagnosis of this child's ailment?
- What is the epidemiology of this disease?
- What tissue types seem to be specifically targeted in this disease?
- Why is early recognition so vital?
- Which other disorders are characterized by inflammation of the blood vessel? What is the typical epidemiology of these related disorders?

BASIC SCIENCE REVIEW AND DISCUSSION

Kawasaki disease (KD; also known as mucocutaneous lymph node syndrome) is an **autoimmune** vasculitis characterized by inflammation of the mucous membranes, lymph nodes, lining of the blood vessels (vascular endothelium), and heart. This acute self-limited disease is the most common cause of acquired heart disease in the pediatric population. At least 3000 cases are diagnosed annually in the United States with an incidence of 6 to 11 cases per 100,000. The disease is most prevalent in Japan, where it was first described. Most children who acquire the disease are younger than age 2 years and 80% are younger than age 5 years. It occurs somewhat more frequently in boys than in girls (ratio 1.5:1). Approximately 20% of children with KD will develop coronary artery abnormalities resulting in aneurysm, thrombosis, and MI if left untreated.

The exact etiology of KD remains unclear, but epidemiologic evidence and clinical presentation both point to an infectious cause. Although a direct infectious- or antigen-mediated response has not been clearly characterized, an exaggerated inflammatory response is mostly responsible for its pathophysiology. It is postulated that secreted cytokines somehow target vascular endothelial cells, producing cell-surface neoantigens. KD-associated vasculitis is most severe in medium-sized arteries and is pathologically indistinct from **infantile periarteritis nodosa.** Inflammatory cells of the blood vessels are initially neutrophils and later monocytes and possibly T cells. These cells produce the numerous cytokines responsible for the clinical manifestations of the illness. Of these, **IL-6** has been associated with the acute febrile illness and increased acute phase reactants. IL-2, TNF-α, IL-1a appear to be responsible for the acute cutaneous responses. The presence of **IgA**-producing cells in the vascular wall suggests an antigen-driven immune response to an etiologic agent with either a respiratory or GI port of entry.

Diagnosis and Treatment

The differential diagnosis of KD includes scarlet fever, staphylococcal toxic shock syndrome (TSS), Stevens-Johnson syndrome (erythema multiforme), leptospirosis, EBV, juvenile rheumatoid arthritis, measles, acrodynia, polyarteritis nodosa, Rocky Mountain spotted fever, drug reaction, and scalded skin syndrome. Classically, KD is diagnosed after at least 5 days of fever plus four of five of the following clinical criteria:

1. Rash primarily on the trunk (maculapapular, erythema multiforme, or scarlatiniform, but not vesicular)
2. Changes in the hands and feet (swelling and redness in the acute phase, periungual desquamation in the subacute phase)
3. Bilateral conjunctival injection
4. Changes in the oral mucosa (may be irritation or inflammation of mouth mucous membranes, lips, and throat with erythematous dry, fissured lips, erythema of the pharynx, and the so-called strawberry tongue)
5. Cervical lymphadenopathy (node diameter >1.5 cm).

Fever usually subsides within 1 to 2 weeks and subacute disease may follow with arthritis, arthralgias, and thrombocytosis. Atypical disease is more common among younger children and may only involve two or three of clinical criteria. The cardiac findings in KD include pericardial effusion, myocardial inflammation (with nonspecific ECG changes), coronary artery abnormalities, and signs of ischemia. Approximately 25% of children present with an aseptic meningitis during the acute phase of KD.

Laboratory abnormalities typically involve an elevated ESR, neutrophil count, and platelet count but are otherwise highly variable and nonspecific. Treatment for KD involves early recognition, supportive care, and initiation of aspirin and IV immunoglobulin. Clinical suspicion should be followed by rapid ascertainment via two-dimensional echocardiogram to rule out coronary aneurysms.

Other Vasculitides

There is a heterogenous group of disorders characterized by inflammation of the blood vessel wall. Vessels of any size in any location may be affected. The affected vessels determine the symptoms of each of these syndromes. There are a number of pathologic mechanisms underlying the various vasculitides. The two most common are direct injury to vessels by infectious pathogens, and physical or chemical injury or immune-mediated inflammation. Immune-mediated vascular inflammation may be caused by immune complexes or direct antibody attack. Some of the vasculitides are associated with **ANCA.** Cytoplasmic or **C-ANCA** is seen in Wegener granulomatosis and microscopic polyangiitis. Perinuclear or **P-ANCA** is seen in polyarteritis nodosa. The exact role of these antibodies in the pathogenesis of these disorders is as yet unclear. However, it is clear that the levels of the antibodies are associated with disease activity. Both C-ANCA and P-ANCA are directed against myeloperoxidase in the primary granules of neutrophils. One proposed mechanism is that these antibodies activate neutrophils, causing a respiratory burst and degranulation and release of toxic oxygen-free radicals and lytic enzymes. This results in endothelial cell damage. The etiology of some vasculitides is still undetermined (Box 8-2).

Blood Vessel Structure All blood vessels—regardless of size—share the same basic structure: They are made up into three layers. The innermost **tunica intima** is made up of the endothelium, the basal lamina, and subendothelial connective tissue. An arterial internal elastic lamina is included in this layer. The next layer is the **tunica media,** which is made up of connective tissue elements including elastic fibers, collagen fibers, and proteoglycans, as well as a varying number of smooth muscle cells layered in a circular fashion. The outer layer is the **tunica adventitia** that is made up primarily of connective tissue, which functions to stabilize the blood vessel in its surrounding connective tissue environment. In larger vessels, smooth muscle fibers and the **vasa vasorum,** or vessels of the vessel, are included in this layer. These three layers are best developed and most distinct in arteries. These are less prominent in veins and capillaries.

BOX 8-2   Vasculitides by Pathogenesis

Infectious
Bacterial (*Neisseria*)
Rickettsial (Rocky Mountain spotted fever)
Spirochetal (syphilis)
Fungal (herpes)

Direct Vascular Injury
Mechanical trauma (iatrogenic)
Radiation

Immunologic
Immune complex-mediated
Henoch-Schönlein purpura
Essential cryoglobulinemic vasculitis
Lupus vasculitis
Direct antibody attack-mediated
KD
Goodpasture syndrome

ANCA* associated
Wegener granulomatosis
Microscopic polyangiitis
Churg-Strauss syndrome
Polyarteritis nodosa

Unknown
Giant cell arteritis
Takayasu arteritis

---

*Unclear whether or not ANCA directly involved in pathogenesis

---

Classification of Vasculitides by Type of Vessel Affected Systemic vasculitis may be classified by the size of the vessels affected as well as the histologic characteristics of the lesions. There is considerable overlap among these disorders. Those affecting large vessels include giant cell (temporal) arteritis and Takayasu arteritis. Medium-sized vessels are the primary target in polyarteritis nodosa and KD. Disorders affecting the small vessels include Wegener granulomatosis, Churg-Strauss syndrome, microscopic polyangiitis, and Henoch-Schönlein purpura. Both medium and small arteries and veins are affected in thromboangiitis obliterans (Winiwarter-Buerger disease).

CASE CONCLUSION

After admitting MA and starting him on high-dose aspirin and IV immunoglobulin, an ECG reveals mild ST segment depression. An echocardiogram reveals multiple large coronary aneurysms along the LAD coronary artery, and the boy was started on antithrombotic therapy.

THUMBNAIL: The Vasculitides

Vasculitides	Vessels Involved	Pathogenesis	Histopathology of Lesions	Other Organs Affected	Incidence	Age at Onset
Giant cell (temporal) arteritis	Large and medium muscular arteries Temporal arteries	Unknown	Granulomatous arteritis or aorta and branches	Renal ischemia related to renal artery involvement, granulomatous hepatitis	15-30 per 100,000	60s
Takayasu arteritis	Large elastic and some muscular arteries, including **aorta**	Unknown, but immune complex-mediated occlusion of vessels	Granulomatous inflammation with decreased tunica media leading to dissection and aneurysms	Ocular disturbances and weakened pulses of the upper extremities secondary to fibrous changes and narrowing of the aortic arch and origin of great vessels	0.26 per 100,000	20s
Polyarteritis nodosa	Small and medium muscular arteries	Unknown, but lymphocytic infiltration of vessel	Necrotizing vasculitis, often at bifurcations, leading to aneurysms	Renal-segmental necrotizing glomerulonephritis	1.8 per 100,000	40s and 50s
KD	Medium muscular arteries but can affect all, including **coronary arteries**	Direct antibody attack on vascular endothelium	Inflammation, endothelial proliferation, and thrombosis	Mucous membranes, lymph nodes, cardiac	Rare	Children
Wegener granulomatosis	Small arteries and veins	ANCA associated with likely abnormal proteinase 3 activity	Granulomatous inflammation and necrotizing vasculitis	Upper and lower respiratory tract (lung necrosis/granulomas), renal-necrotizing glomerulonephritis	Rare	40s
Churg-Strauss syndrome	Small- and medium-sized arteries, veins	ANCA associated	Necrotizing vasculitis, eosinophil-rich, and granulomatous inflammation	Lungs, viscera, cardiac, muscle and renal-focal segmental necrotizing glomerulonephritis	Rare History (Hx) of atopy	40s and 50s
Henoch-Schönlein purpura	Small arterioles and venules as well as capillaries	Immune complex mediated	IgA immune complex deposition, fibrinoid necrosis	Purpuric skin lesions, abdominal pain, arthralgias, and renal-proliferative glomerulonephritis	14 per 100,000 Hx of atopy and recent upper respiratory infection (URI)	Children and teenagers
Thromboangiitis obliterans	Medium- and small-sized arteries and veins	Unknown	Acute or chronic inflammation with segmental thrombosis	Extremities	Primarily in heavy smokers	20s to 30s

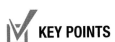

KEY POINTS

- KD is a rare vasculitis that primarily affects children; key features of the disease include inflammation of medium-sized vessels, including coronary arteries associated with inflammation of the mucous membranes and lymph nodes

- ANCA target myeloperoxidase located in the primary granules of neutrophils; **P-ANCA** is associated with polyarteritis nodosa and primary glomerular disease; **C-ANCA** is associated with Wegener granulomatosis and microscopic polyangiitis

- Blood vessels are composed of three layers: the innermost **tunica intima,** composed of endothelium, basal lamina, and connective tissue; the **tunica media,** composed of elastic fibers and smooth muscle; and the **tunica adventitia,** composed of connective tissue and, in large vessels, smooth muscle and the **vasa vasorum**

QUESTIONS

1. Which part of the patient's blood vessels are *most likely* the primary target of the inflammation?

   A. Endothelium
   B. Intima
   C. Elastic fibers
   D. Tight junctions
   E. Epithelium

2. In a patient with KD, the elevated ESR is best explained by the:

   A. Increased weight of individual erythrocytes
   B. Decreased impedance by fewer leukocytes
   C. Increased platelet aggregation
   D. Increased acute-phase proteins
   E. Decreased rouleaux formation

3. A 28-year-old Japanese woman presents to her doctor complaining of malaise, arthralgias, and double vision. She has no past medical history and is not taking any medications at this time. The patient smokes a pack of cigarettes a day. On physical exam the patient is noted to have mildly elevated BP and her pulses are noted to be asymmetrically decreased. Which of the following is the best test to confirm her diagnosis?

   A. ESR
   B. P-ANCA
   C. EKG
   D. Arteriography
   E. Renal biopsy

4. A 45-year-old man with asthma presents to the ER for an acute asthma exacerbation. He has a long history of asthma that, until recently, has been relatively well controlled. On further questioning the patient reveals that he has also experienced fever, malaise, and weight loss over the past year. CBC shows slightly increased WBCs with increased numbers of eosinophils. A chest x-ray is obtained and reveals patchy, nodular infiltrates. What of the following is the *most likely* diagnosis?

   A. Pneumonia
   B. Churg-Strauss syndrome
   C. Goodpasture disease
   D. Polyarteritis nodosa
   E. Winiwarter-Buerger disease

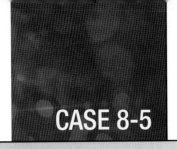

CASE 8-5 Osteoarthritis

HPI: TD, a 66-year-old woman, presents to your office complaining of right knee and hip pain. The patient states that the pain started shortly after she began a daily weight-loss exercise program 3 months ago. Initially, the pain was intermittent, occurring once or twice a week. Since then the pain has become increasingly frequent. It worsens with activity and improves with rest. Ibuprofen has provided some relief but causes stomach discomfort. TD is quite distressed and states, "It's hopeless. After years of trying to work up the motivation to improve my health through exercise, I get started on a program and am now forced to quit because of this pain." The patient denies any recent trauma. She has no other symptoms. Her past medical history is significant for asthma, GERD, elevated cholesterol, and obesity. She has no drug allergies. Her current medications include albuterol, omeprazole, and simvastatin. Family history is significant for mother and grandmother with "rheumatism."

PE: TD is an obese woman weighing 230 pounds. She is in no acute distress. Lungs are clear to auscultation bilaterally. Extremity exam reveals a normal-appearing right knee without swelling, erythema, tenderness, or warmth. There is slight limitation in the range of motion and crepitus on palpation. Other joints are unremarkable.

THOUGHT QUESTIONS

- What are the characteristic features of osteoarthritis? Which joints are most commonly affected? What are the risk factors for the development of this kind of arthritis?
- How would you describe the structure and primary functions of cartilage?
- What is the pathophysiology of osteoarthritis?
- What changes are noted in the bones of joints affected by osteoarthritis?
- How would you describe the process of bone remodeling that underlies these changes?

BASIC SCIENCE REVIEW AND DISCUSSION

Clinical Features

Osteoarthritis, a degenerative joint disease, is the most common form of arthritis. It is characterized by the slow progressive loss of articular cartilage, the formation of new bone at the appositional surfaces of the joint, as well as the formation of osteophytes at the joint margins. There are no systemic manifestations of this type of arthritis. Disease is often asymmetric and localized to just a few joints. The most commonly affected joints are weight-bearing joints, such as the hips, knees, and spine. However, small joints of the hands (first carpometacarpals, proximal and distal interphalangeals) and feet (metatarsophalangeals) can also be affected. Joint pain in osteoarthritis typically worsens with activity and is relieved by rest. Stiffness is most pronounced after periods of immobility. The pain may initially be intermittent and mild but worsens as the disease progresses. With severe disease there is decreased range of motion in the affected joints as well as nocturnal pain.

Etiology

Osteoarthritis is seen most commonly in older people (>50–60 years) with more than 60% of the population having some degree of cartilage abnormality in their joints. Heredity and mechanical factors play a role in pathogenesis. There are two types of osteoarthritis. The most common is primary, in which the joint degeneration occurs insidiously without any obvious initiating cause. Secondary osteoarthritis is less common and can be seen in younger individuals (<40–50 years). It is usually associated with joint injury such as a fracture; chronic overuse of a joint due to sports or occupational activity; metabolic disease such as hyperparathyroidism, hemochromatosis, and ochronosis; or increased mechanical stress on joints caused by obesity. Regardless of the initiating cause of the degenerative joint disease, the disease process is the same: progressive loss of cartilage and bony remodeling in the joint.

Molecular Pathogenesis

Articular cartilage is connective tissue that serves two primary purposes: (*a*) as a shock absorber and (*b*) as a wear-resistant smooth surface for joint movement. This type of cartilage lacks blood supply, innervation, or lymph drainage. Articular cartilage is made up of hyaline cartilage that is composed of cells (chondrocytes) and extracellular matrix (fibers and ground substance). Type II collagen fibers form the skeleton of hyaline cartilage. These fibers are arranged in arches, providing resistance to tensile stresses and allowing for transmission of vertical loads. The ground substance of articular cartilage is made up of proteoglycan aggregates. **Proteoglycans** are molecules composed of numerous hydrophilic polysaccharide chains (chondroitin sulfate and keratan sulfate) that are covalently linked to a protein backbone. In hyaline cartilage, proteoglycans form aggregates with hyaluronic acid. The hydrophilic portions of the proteoglycans attract water, giving this type of cartilage its elasticity and turgor. Chondrocytes are responsible for the maintenance of the extracellular matrix.

Chondrocytes play a key role in the cartilage destruction found in osteoarthritis. Early in the disease, they are noted to be actively dividing and producing increased quantities of collagen, proteoglycans, and hyaluronic acid. However, these new products do not aggregate well and are not adequately stabilized in the extracellular matrix. Next, proteolytic and collagenolytic enzymes are released from chondrocytes and the extracellular matrix is degraded. IL-1 is believed to be the mediator initiating this process. TNF-α, TGF-β, and prostaglandins are thought to perpetuate this process through induction of the release of lytic enzymes from chondrocytes and inhibition of matrix synthesis.

Over time, remodeling and hypertrophy of the bone occur, leading to appositional bone growth and sclerosis. At the margins of the joints there is further growth of bone and cartilage, resulting in osteophytes or bone spurs. X-rays reveal narrowed joint spaces with sharp articular margins, osteophytes, and thickened, dense subchondral bone at the articular surfaces.

This remodeling and hypertrophy of the bone that occurs at affected joints is a direct result of osteoclast and osteoblast activity. **Osteoclasts** are multinucleated cells that contain lysosomal enzymes and acid phosphatase. Their primary role is bone resorption. This function is controlled by local **cytokines,** such as IL-1, TNF-α, and IL-6, as well as systemic hormones, such as parathyroid hormone and 1,25-dihydroxyvitamin D. **Osteoblasts** originate from stromal cells and are responsible for the production of bone matrix proteins including type I collagen, as well as proteins and particles that lead to bone mineralization. Formation of new bone is regulated by systemic hormones such as 1,25-dihydroxyvitamin D, as well as growth factors including TGF-β, IGF I and II, and PDGF, which are stored in bone and likely released during the process of osteoclastic resorption. The signal responsible for initiating this process is unknown; however, it is clear that increased stress on the bone is one trigger. Therefore, in osteoarthritis, increased repetitive stress on the articular surfaces of the bones of affected joints leads to the start of this remodeling process. The final result is thicker, denser bone that can better withstand the increased forces that occur once the cartilage has been lost.

CASE CONCLUSION

Differential diagnosis: rheumatoid arthritis, SLE, seronegative spondylopathies (ankylosing spondylitis, Reiter syndrome, psoriatic arthritis), gout, pseudogout, and septic arthritis.

Labs are done and TD is found to have a normal WBC count and ESR. She is rheumatoid factor negative and ANA negative. The patient is then referred to a physical therapist who designs a low-impact exercise and stretching program that focuses on strengthening muscles surrounding the affected joints and increasing flexibility and range of motion. TD is instructed to discontinue the ibuprofen and take acetaminophen and celecoxib as needed for pain.

THUMBNAIL: Comparison of Different Types of Arthritides

Type of Arthritis	Epidemiology	Pathophysiology	Joints Affected; Extra-articular Manifestations	Symptoms	Physical Findings	Signs
Osteoarthritis	Increase with age, in those with obesity, repetitive joint injury/stress	Degenerative Abnormal stresses on normal cartilage or normal stresses on abnormal cartilage	**Asymmetric** Hips, knees, spine, DIP, PIP; none	Joint pain worse after activity, better with rest	Crepitus, joint enlargement, osteophytes, Bouchard and Heberden nodes	Synovial fluid: clear, minimal WBCs, glucose normal, Gram stain and culture negative
Septic arthritis	**Non-gonococcal (GC):** prior trauma, IV drug users **GC:** young women	Infectious (*Staphylococcus. aureus*, *streptococcus*, GC)	**Monoarticular** Non-GC: none **GC:** skin rash	**Non-GC:** sudden-onset joint pain, fever, chills **GC:** prodromal migratory polyarthralgias, joint pain	Joint inflammation **GC:** skin rash; necrotic pustules palms and soles	+ blood cultures in 40-50% Synovial fluid: turbid, markedly elevated WBCs, mostly PMNs, decreased glucose, + Gram stain and culture
Rheumatoid arthritis	Women > men Age 30s–40s	Autoimmune Progressive synovitis leading to pannus formation and eventual erosion of articular cartilage, bone, and tendon	**Symmetric** Wrists, MCP, PIP, ankles, knees, shoulders, hips, elbows, spine Subcutaneous nodules, vasculitis, eye, pleuritis, pericarditis	Joint pain and swelling worse after rest/ inactivity, better with activity Fatigue, malaise, anorexia, weight loss	Early swelling, warmth, erythema, pain Late deformities: hammer toe, swan neck, boutonniere	Elevated rheumatoid factor, Elevated ESR Synovial fluid: cloudy, elevated WBCs with a slight increase in percentage of PMNs, decreased glucose, negative Gram stain and culture

(Continued)

THUMBNAIL: Comparison of Different Types of Arthritides *(Continued)*

Type of Arthritis	Epidemiology	Pathophysiology	Joints Affected; Extra-articular Manifestations	Symptoms	Physical Findings	Signs
SLE	Women >> men African American ages 15–40 yrs	Autoimmune	**Symmetric** Small joints of hands, wrists, and knees Skin rashes, oral ulcers, pleuritis, pericarditis, seizure, psychosis, anemia, leukopenia, lymphopenia, thrombocytopenia	Joint pain, anorexia, fever, weight loss, photosensitivity Oral ulcers	Malar rash, joint tenderness, and inflammation Deformities rare	+ ANA + dsDNA Cloudy, elevated WBCs with a slight increase in percentage of PMNs, decreased glucose, negative Gram stain and culture
Seronegative spondylopathies	Men > women Age 20s–30s	Noninfectious, inflammatory	**Asymmetric Monoarticular** Sacroiliac, spine, shoulders, hips, and knees Urethritis, conjunctivitis, psoriasis, IBD	Mid and low back stiffness, pain, enthesopathy	Spondylitis, sacroiliitis, enthesopathy, conjunctivitis, uveitis, psoriatic rash	Elevated ESR, HLA-B27 Synovial fluid: cloudy, elevated WBCs with a slight increase in percentage of PMNs, decreased glucose, negative Gram stain and culture
Gout/ pseudogout	Men >> women Pacific Islanders Age 40–50 yrs	Noninfectious, inflammatory	**Asymmetric Monoarticular** First metatarsophalangeal, midfoot, knees, ankles, wrist Tophi with chronic disease	Acute onset of severe pain, typically nocturnal ± fever	Early swollen, tender, red joints Late deformities due to tophaceous invasion of joints	Elevated uric acid level, increased ESR Synovial fluid: cloudy, elevated WBCs with a slight increase in percentage of PMNs, decreased glucose, negative Gram stain and culture **Urate or calcium oxalate crystals**

 KEY POINTS

■ Articular cartilage is made up of chondrocytes, type II collagen, and proteoglycans; chondrocytes maintain the cartilage by producing the extracellular matrix as well as enzymes that digest it

■ The cytokines that stimulate chondrocyte dysfunction and increased breakdown of cartilage in osteoarthritis are IL-2, TNF-α, and TGF-β

■ Bone remodeling is a direct result of osteoblast and osteoclast activity; **osteoclasts** are responsible for bone resorption, whereas **osteoblasts** produce proteins that lead to bone formation

QUESTIONS

1. TD returns to your office 7 years later complaining of increasing difficulty using her hands, which has forced her to give up knitting. Exam of her hands reveals:

   A. Swelling, erythema, warmth, and tenderness over the distal metatarsophalangeal joints
   B. Swelling, erythema, warmth, and tenderness over the DIP joints
   C. Bony enlargement of the PIP joints
   D. Rheumatoid nodules over the DIP joints
   E. Hyperextension deformity of the PIP joints

2. TD's 45-year-old daughter, LM, has accompanied her on this visit. LM has no joint symptoms at this time but is concerned about developing osteoarthritis. Which of the following contributes the most to the elastic nature of LM's healthy articular cartilage?

   A. Osteoclasts
   B. Type II collagen
   C. Chondrocytes
   D. Proteoglycans
   E. Synovial fluid

3. In a patient with advanced osteoarthritis of the hip who is about to undergo hip replacement, which of the following cells is most active in the affected joint?

   A. Chondrocytes
   B. Neutrophils
   C. CD8 T cells
   D. Osteophytes
   E. Osteoblasts

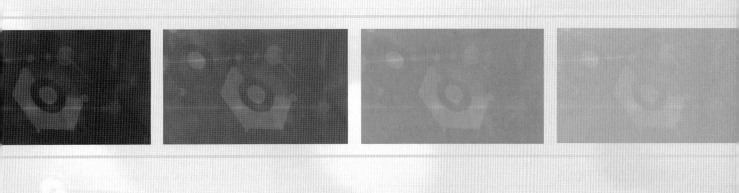

PART IX

Reproduction

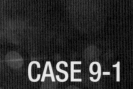

Male and Female Development:
CASE 9-1 Internal and External Genitalia

HPI: HS is a newborn boy who was born at 39-2/7 weeks' gestational age. On routine newborn exam, he is found to have a small defect on the ventral surface of the distal penis. His prenatal and labor histories are both unremarkable. The patient's parents are quite disturbed by the penile defect and are concerned about his ability to have sex and conceive when he grows up.

PE: On physical exam, he is a 3725-g male infant. On inspection of his genitalia there is a small opening on the ventral surface of the penile shaft in the midline from which urine is expelled. He has a normal scrotum and both testes are descended and appear normal on palpation.

THOUGHT QUESTIONS

- What are the steps of genital duct differentiation in males and females?
- What are the steps of external genitalia development in males and females?
- Discuss hypospadias.
- What abnormalities of genital duct differentiation can affect females?

BASIC SCIENCE REVIEW AND DISCUSSION

Parallel to gonadal development, the male and female internal genitalia develop from separate duct systems in the fourth embryonic week. Initially, both **wolffian (mesonephric) ducts** and **müllerian (paramesonephric) ducts** are present in the embryo (see Thumbnail below). The wolffian duct is originally part of the **primordial kidney (mesonephros)** and grows toward the urogenital sinus to eventually contact the primitive sex cords. Meanwhile, the müllerian duct develops laterally to the wolffian duct from an invagination of the coelomic epithelium of the urogenital ridge. Further differentiation of the duct systems is dependent on the presence of testicular secretory products. Therefore, a female phenotype will develop in the absence of these secretory products. Depending on the genetic sex of the fetus, the other duct system disappears by the third fetal month.

In genetic males, the sex-determining region of the Y chromosome (SRY) induces the production of **müllerian-inhibiting substance (MIS)** from Sertoli cells. As its name suggests, MIS causes the müllerian ducts to regress. The Leydig cells secrete testosterone, which then induces development of the wolffian ducts to form the **epididymis, vas deferens,** and **seminal vesicles.** Under the influence of **dihydrotestosterone (DHT)** formed locally from the **5-α-reductase**–mediated conversion of testosterone, the tissue at the base of the regressing müllerian tubercle develops into the **prostate gland.**

In contrast to male embryos, the müllerian duct system persists in female embryos due to the absence of MIS and eventually gives rise to the **fallopian tubes, uterus,** and **upper one third of the vagina.** The cranial portion of the müllerian duct remains patent to the coelomic cavity and becomes the fimbria portion of the fallopian tube. The caudal portion of the müllerian duct crosses the wolffian duct ventrally and contacts the müllerian duct from the opposite side. These eventually fuse to form

the uterine canal. Uterine and cervical anomalies can occur when these ducts do not develop or fuse properly. When the combined müllerian ducts reach the posterior wall of the urogenital sinus, the formation of a **paramesonephric or müllerian tubercle** is induced. The upper one third of the vagina develops from the uterine canal and the lower portion develops from the urogenital sinus. Finally, the wolffian duct system regresses in the absence of testosterone.

Development of male or female external genitalia is dependent on the presence or absence of testicular testosterone, which is locally converted to DHT by the enzyme 5-α-reductase. While the differentiation of external genitalia due to hormone exposure begins in the fifth embryonic week, it is not until the eighth embryonic week that the structures of the indifferent external genitalia become apparent. These structures include the **genital tubercle, urogenital slit, lateral genital folds,** and **labioscrotal swellings.** Under the influence of DHT, the penis develops when the genital folds fuse around the urethra and the genital tubercle develops into the glans penis. As the labioscrotal swellings enlarge, they fuse to form the **scrotum.** The **prostate gland** and **bulbourethral glands** arise from the urogenital sinus. Testicular descent into the scrotum is mediated by fetal gonadotropins and the **gubernaculum,** a fibrous cord that connects each testis to the developing scrotum. As the embryo grows, the testes are gradually pulled down toward the scrotum. Final descent of the testes through the bilateral inguinal rings occurs in the last 3 months of pregnancy. Failure of the inguinal canals to narrow after testicular descent can lead to the eventual descent of abdominal contents into the scrotum, resulting in inguinal hernias.

In the absence of testosterone and irrespective of the presence or absence of ovaries, the folds of the urogenital slit do not fuse in the female embryo. The anterior portion of the urogenital sinus becomes the urethra, above which the genital tubercle develops into the **clitoris.** Meanwhile, the posterior portion develops into the lower two thirds of the vagina. The **labia minora** and **labia majora** develop from the lateral genital folds and the labioscrotal swellings, respectively. In females, the gubernaculum attaches to the ovary and cornua of the uterus, ultimately forming the **ovarian and round ligaments.** Prior to the end of pregnancy, connective tissue obliterates the gubernacular attachments to the labioscrotal swellings.

Hypospadias results when the distal urethra does not develop appropriately and the urethral meatus is found anywhere along the ventral surface in the midline of the penile shaft,

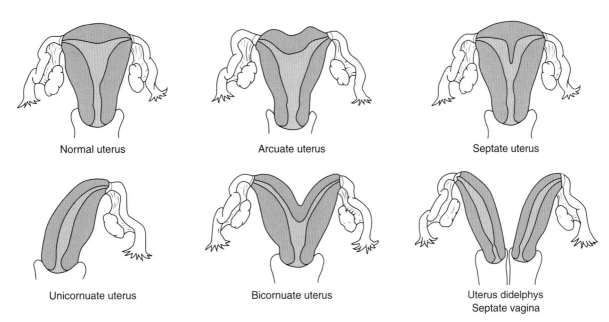

Normal uterus   Arcuate uterus   Septate uterus

Unicornuate uterus   Bicornuate uterus   Uterus didelphys / Septate vagina

• **Figure 9-1.** Anatomic anomalies of the uterus. (Reprinted from Blueprints Obstetrics and Gynecology. 4th Ed. Philadelphia: Lippincott Williams & Wilkins, 2007.)

scrotum, or perineum. It is the most common congenital anomaly of the penis. Because it is associated with hernias and undescended testes, detailed exam of the genitals is important when hypospadias is identified. When hypospadias occurs proximally, curving of the penis known as **chordee** can result. Surgical repair to extend the urethral meatus to the tip of the glans penis involves usage of preputial tissue, making circumcision contraindicated in cases of hypospadias. Distal lesions have an excellent prognosis, whereas proximal lesions may require multiple revisions to create a normal-appearing penis.

As previously mentioned, vaginal, cervical, and uterine abnormalities can occur when the two müllerian ducts do not fuse properly (Fig. 9-1). This can result in a range of abnormalities, including **uterus arcuatus,** in which the uterus is only slightly indented in the middle, and **uterus didelphys,** in which the uterus, cervix, and sometimes vagina are duplicated entirely.

CASE CONCLUSION

A pediatric urologist is consulted and examines HS and meets with his parents. He reassures them that the surgical repair should be relatively straightforward, and that HS will most likely have a normally functioning penis. The patient is discharged home on day of life 2 with his mother and given follow-up appointments for the surgical repair.

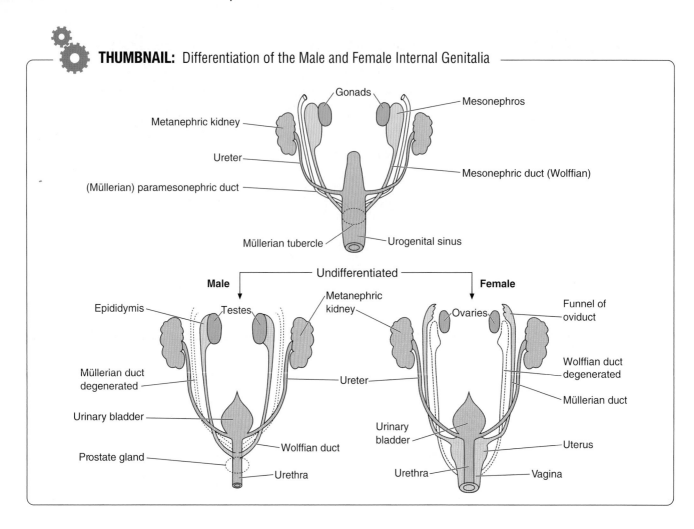

THUMBNAIL: Differentiation of the Male and Female Internal Genitalia

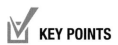 **KEY POINTS**

■ Various gene products influenced by SRY mediate wolffian duct differentiation in genetic males; absence of these gene products leads to the development of female internal genitalia from the müllerian duct system

■ DHT mediates the development of male external genitalia; in its absence, female external genitalia develop

■ Abnormalities in fusion of the urethral folds can lead to varying degrees of hypospadias

■ Uterine, cervical, and vaginal anomalies can arise from absent or improper fusion of the müllerian duct system

QUESTIONS

1. A 16-year-old girl comes to your clinic because she is concerned that she has not begun to menstruate yet. Her prenatal, birth, and childhood histories are all benign. Physical exam is significant for normal breast development, average height, a short vagina, and absence of the uterus and cervix on bimanual exam. Which of the following conditions does this patient most likely have?

   A. Hermaphroditism
   B. Turner syndrome
   D. Klinefelter syndrome
   C. Female pseudohermaphroditism
   E. Testicular feminization syndrome

2. Which structures arise from the wolffian duct system?

   A. Fallopian tubes, uterus, vagina
   B. Epididymis, seminal vesicle, vas deferens
   C. Fallopian tubes, uterus, vagina, clitoris
   D. Epididymis, seminal vesicle, vas deferens, gubernaculum
   E. Fallopian tubes, uterus, vagina, clitoris, Bartholin glands

HPI: PP is a 5-year-old girl who is brought to your office by her mother who is concerned that her daughter has begun developing breasts and pubic hair. Her prenatal and birth histories were significant only for neonatal jaundice, and to date she has been healthy.

PE: On physical exam, you confirm that the child has indeed undergone thelarche (onset of breast development) and pubarche (onset of pubic hair growth) and also note multiple brown skin patches on the child's buttocks, back, and extremities, which her mother states have been there since birth.

Labs: Concerned for McCune-Albright syndrome, you order plain x-rays of the femur and pelvis as well as check estrogen, follicle-stimulating hormone (FSH), and luteinizing hormone (LH) levels.

THOUGHT QUESTIONS

- What are the key changes observed in female puberty?
- What are the key changes observed in male puberty?
- Discuss precocious puberty.

BASIC SCIENCE REVIEW AND DISCUSSION

Puberty is the series of events leading to sexual maturity. This process includes the development of behavioral and physical characteristics that ultimately lead to adult reproductive function. While there is some variance in mean age of each stage of puberty, age 5 is certainly far outside the norm of age ranges of puberty.

Puberty In Girls

In girls, the stages of puberty include adrenarche, gonadarche, thelarche, pubarche, and menarche. **Adrenarche,** which is the increase in adrenal hormone synthesis as a result of regeneration of the zona reticularis, occurs between the ages of 6 and 8 years, before any visible signs of puberty are evident. DHEA, dehydroepiandrosterone sulfate (DHEAS), and androstenedione are the adrenal androgens responsible for initial development of pubic and axillary hair.

Pulsatile secretion of GnRH from the hypothalamus around the age of 8 years marks the beginning of **gonadarche.** The gonadotrophs in the anterior pituitary are stimulated to secrete LH and FSH, which eventually lead to stimulation of the ovary and estrogen secretion.

The first visible sign of puberty occurs with **thelarche,** the development of breasts. This typically occurs around age 11 years in response to rising estrogen levels and continues throughout adolescence, as described by Tanner (Fig. 9-3). The vaginal mucosa, uterus, and labia minora and majora also grow in response to estrogen.

Pubarche is the growth of pubic hair in response to circulating androgens and usually occurs in conjunction with axillary hair growth around age 12 years. The onset of menstruation, **menarche,** typically occurs 1 to 3 years after thelarche, around age 12 to 13 years. Menstrual cycles are irregular and anovulatory for the first 6 months to 2 years, and can take up to 5 years to develop regular, ovulatory cycles.

Somatic growth is most noticeable during the growth spurt, which is an acceleration in growth rate around age 9 or 10 years in response to GH and IGF-1. Excess levels of estrogen, as seen in precocious puberty, can lead to short stature via decreased secretion of GH and insulin-like growth factor 1 (IGF-1), as well as premature fusion of the epiphyseal plate in long bones.

Despite the orderly fashion described above, it is not unusual for some girls to experience a different order of the presenting signs and symptoms of puberty. The ages at which (some) girls go through the different stages can vary (quite a lot) as well.

Puberty In Boys

The stages of puberty in boys include adrenarche, pubarche, testicular maturation, and further development of secondary sexual characteristics. Adrenarche occurs similarly to girls except that the adrenal steroids DHEA, DHEAS, and androstenedione are converted peripherally to the more potent androgens, testosterone, and DHT. These, in turn, promote pubic and axillary hair development. Along with enlargement of the testes, these are the first visible signs of puberty and usually begin between ages 9 and 14 years.

Testicular maturation is mediated by the pulsatile release of GnRH, which stimulates the diurnal secretion of FSH and LH approximately 1 year prior to testicular enlargement. These gonadotropins initiate androgen production by Leydig cells, growth of the seminiferous tubules, and spermatogenesis.

Although the growth spurt typically occurs 2 years after that in girls, the mechanism of somatic growth and eventual epiphyseal plate closure is similar. Other somatic changes that occur during puberty include deepening of the voice, increase in bone and muscle mass, increase in laryngeal size, and development of facial and trunk hair.

Precocious Puberty

True precocious puberty involves the premature maturation of the hypothalamic-pituitary-gonadal axis and is considered when puberty occurs before age 8 years. Precocity is five times more frequent in girls than in boys, with over 70% of cases being idiopathic. In addition to nonorganic causes of precocity such as drug ingestion, neoplastic etiologies such as intracranial, gonadal, and adrenal tumors should be ruled out. Finally, hypothyroidism can rarely cause precocious puberty possibly via stimulation of the FSH receptor by elevated levels of TSH.

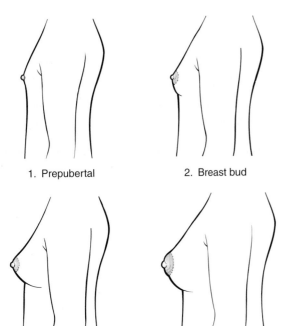

1. Prepubertal   2. Breast bud

3. Breast elevation   4. Areolar mound

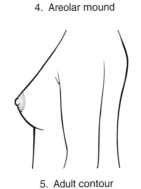

5. Adult contour

• **Figure 9-3.** Tanner stages of thelarche. (Reprinted from Blueprints Obstetrics and Gynecology. 4th Ed. Philadelphia: Lippincott Williams & Wilkins, 2007.)

McCune-Albright syndrome, also known as polyostotic fibrous dysplasia, is considered precocious pseudopuberty since sexual maturation occurs via early production of estrogen by the ovaries rather than from maturation of the hypothalamic-pituitary-gonadal axis. It accounts for 5% of female precocity and manifests as multiple cystic bone lesions prone to fracture, café au lait skin spots, and sexual precocity. It is caused by a mutation during embryogenesis and is not hereditary. While there is no cure for McCune-Albright syndrome, management of endocrine and metabolic abnormalities can result in achievement of normal stature, fertility, and lifespan.

CASE CONCLUSION

The labs reveal an elevated estrogen level and decreased levels of gonadotropins. The x-rays reveal multiple lytic lesions with scalloped borders in the cortex and ground-glass pattern centrally. You diagnose PP with McCune-Albright syndrome and send her for immediate endocrinology consultation.

KEY POINTS

- Puberty is initiated by pulsatile GnRH released from the hypothalamus in both sexes
- The effects of GnRH are mediated by FSH and LH and their actions on the gonads
- The range in timing of the stages of puberty is more varied in males than in females
- McCune-Albright syndrome is considered precocious pseudopuberty because rather than early maturation of the hypothalamic-pituitary-gonadal axis, it involves early estrogen secretion from the ovaries, leading to acceleration of many of the phenotypic changes of puberty

THUMBNAIL: Puberty

Stage	Age of Onset (yrs)	Description
Girls		
Adrenarche	6–8	Adrenal gland secretion of adrenal androgens
Gonadarche	8	Gonadotropin stimulation of ovarian hormone secretion
Thelarche	11	Breast development
Pubarche	12	Pubic hair development
Menarche	12–13	Onset of menses
Somatic growth	9–10	Growth spurt
Boys		
Adrenarche	8	Adrenal gland secretion of adrenal androgens
Pubarche	9–14	Pubic hair development
Gonadarche	9–14	Gonadotropin stimulation of testicular maturation, testosterone secretion, spermatogenesis
Somatic growth	11–16	Growth spurt, deepening of voice, facial/trunk hair, increased bone and muscle mass

QUESTIONS

1. It is still unclear exactly what occurs on the molecular level to initiate puberty. However, we do know how a variety of the changes are mediated. Which of the following hormones is correctly paired with its role in puberty?

   A. Increased estrogen—increased hepatic enzyme activity
   B. DHEAS—primarily responsible for pubic and axillary hair in males and females
   C. LH—stimulation and maturation of breast tissue
   D. FSH—maturation of secondary sexual characteristics
   E. GnRH—constant release of this hormone increases its effects

2. LB is a 13-year-old girl who presents to your office. She has had breast development for over 2 years, but has not begun menstruating and is quite concerned. You discuss that the typical order of the stages of puberty in a female are:

   A. Gonadarche, adrenarche, pubarche, thelarche, menarche
   B. Adrenarche, gonadarche, thelarche, pubarche, menarche
   C. Gonadarche, adrenarche, menarche, thelarche, pubarche
   D. Adrenarche, gonadarche, menarche, thelarche, pubarche
   E. Pubarche, adrenarche, gonadarche, thelarche, menarche

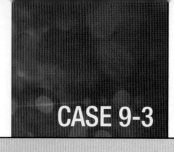

CASE 9-3 Menstrual Cycle

HPI: NM is a 17-year-old gravida 0 competitive gymnast who comes to your office because she has not had her period for approximately 2 years. She began menstruating at age 13 but never had regular periods. She has always been thin and physically active but increased her level of activity at age 14 when she left school to train as a professional gymnast. Approximately 6 months later, her periods stopped entirely. She denies current sexual activity or galactorrhea and does not take any medications.

PE: On physical exam, she is slim but muscular. Her exam is entirely within normal limits, and there are no signs of pregnancy.

THOUGHT QUESTIONS

- What are the steps of the menstrual cycle?
- What are the causes of amenorrhea?
- How is amenorrhea evaluated?

BASIC SCIENCE REVIEW AND DISCUSSION

Most women of child-bearing age experience ovulatory menstrual cycles every 24 to 35 days (average 28 days). The menstrual cycle involves the hypothalamus, pituitary, ovaries, and endometrium all working in concert to coordinate ovulation and prepare the endometrium for implantation should fertilization occur. It is divided into four phases: menstrual, follicular, ovulatory, and luteal (Fig. 9-4).

Menstrual Phase

The first day of menstruation is considered day 1 of the menstrual cycle. The endometrium that was built up from the previous cycle is shed in response to the loss of progesterone support from the corpus luteum. While bleeding typically lasts 3 to 7 days, the start of the follicular phase begins prior to the cessation of menses.

Follicular/Proliferative Phase

The **follicular phase** starts around day 4 of the cycle and lasts until ovulation occurs approximately at mid-cycle (day 14 of an average 28-day cycle). Differences in cycle length can generally be attributed to variations in this phase of the menstrual cycle. Levels of **FSH** from the anterior pituitary begin to rise in response to hypothalamic **GnRH,** which is stimulated by the decrease in estrogen and progesterone during the luteal phase of the prior cycle. FSH stimulates the growth of 5 to 15 primordial follicles that continue to develop until one becomes a dominant follicle that will be ovulated. The dominant follicle produces estrogens that enhance its own maturation as well as increase the production of FSH and **LH** receptors. In response to the rising estrogen levels, the endometrium begins to proliferate and thicken. LH begins to rise late in the follicular phase, stimulating the synthesis of androgens that are converted to estrogen.

Ovulation

When the dominant follicle secretes a sustained critical level of estrogen, this positively feeds back to the anterior pituitary, which responds by secreting a surge of LH, causing the dominant follicle to rupture and release the mature **ovum** approximately 24 to 36 hours later. The ovum is then swept into the fallopian tube and makes its way toward the uterus.

Luteal/Secretory Phase

The **luteal phase** begins after ovulation. Under stimulation by LH, the **corpus luteum** forms from the granulosa and theca interna cells lining the wall of the empty follicle. The corpus luteum then synthesizes progesterone to both stabilize the endometrium and make it more glandular and secretory to prepare it for possible implantation. If implantation does not occur, the corpus luteum degenerates, leading to a rapid decline in progesterone and onset of menses (as described above). The decreasing levels of estrogen and progesterone release the negative feedback mechanism, and the pituitary begins to secrete FSH again to start a new cycle.

If fertilization does occur, the trophoblast produces **human chorionic gonadotropin** (hCG), which is very similar to LH, to maintain the corpus luteum. Endometrial support via progesterone production shifts from the corpus luteum to the placenta by 7 to 9 weeks' gestational age.

Evaluation of Amenorrhea

Amenorrhea is the absence or cessation of menses. It is generally categorized as either primary or secondary amenorrhea to guide the evaluation process. **Primary amenorrhea** is the absence of **menarche** (onset of menses) by age 16 and can be caused by anatomic abnormalities resulting in outflow tract obstruction, hypothalamic dysfunction, gonadal failure, chromosomal abnormalities, enzyme or hormonal deficiencies, and other rare causes. **Secondary amenorrhea** is the absence of menses for 6 months or three menstrual cycles in a previously menstruating woman and can be caused by hypothalamic dysfunction, polycystic ovarian syndrome (PCOS), pituitary or thyroid disease, abnormal prolactin secretion, premature ovarian failure, or anatomic abnormalities.

The evaluation of primary amenorrhea is guided by the absence or presence of the uterus and breasts (see Thumbnail below). If both uterus and breasts are absent, the karyotype is usually 46,XY. When the uterus is present but the breasts are absent, **hypergonadotropic hypogonadism** (e.g., gonadal dysgenesis) must be differentiated from **hypogonadotropic hypogonadism** (e.g., hypothalamic dysfunction) by checking serum FSH levels, which will be low in the latter situation. Additionally, a karyotype may be necessary to rule out gonadal agenesis in a 46,XY individual. If breasts are present but the uterus is absent, a karyotype is necessary to differentiate between testicular feminization and müllerian agenesis. Finally, patients with both uterus and breasts should be evaluated as patients with secondary amenorrhea.

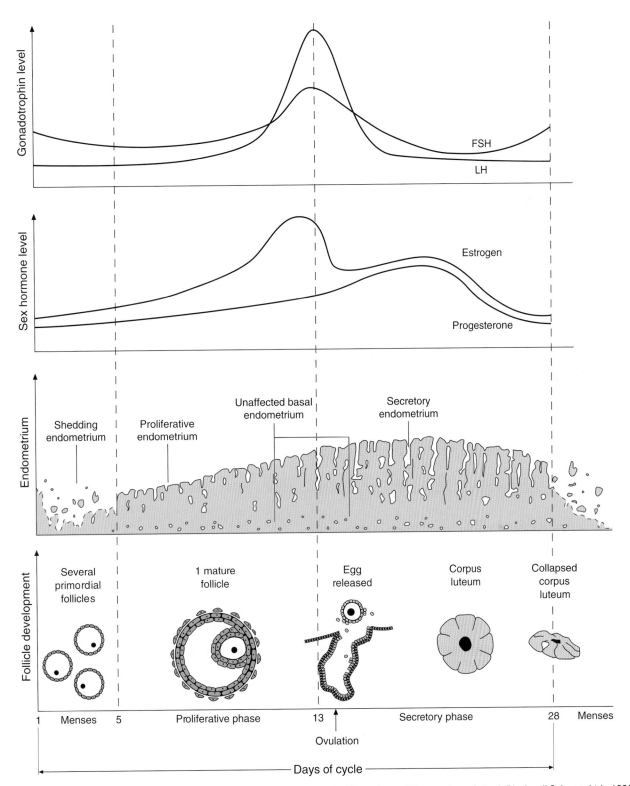

• **Figure 9-4.** Normal menstrual cycle. (Adapted with permission from Impey L. Obstetrics and Gynaecology. Oxford: Blackwell Science, Ltd., 1999.)

The most common cause of secondary amenorrhea is pregnancy. When this has been ruled out, anatomic abnormalities that can disrupt the patency of the outflow tract such as cervical stenosis and Asherman syndrome (intrauterine synechiae or adhesions) should be investigated.

Several endocrine abnormalities can lead to secondary amenorrhea, either via hypogonadotropic hypogonadism or hypergonadotropic hypogonadism. High levels of prolactin are known to cause galactorrhea and amenorrhea via interference in gonadotropin secretion, resulting in hypogonadotropic hypogonadism. Treatment of **hyperprolactinemia** ranges from medication to surgery depending on the etiology. Hypothyroidism can cause amenorrhea via elevated levels of TSH and TRH that, in turn, can cause hyperprolactinemia. Treatment of the hypothyroidism usually corrects the amenorrhea. Nonendocrine factors that lead to hypothalamic dysfunction and hypogonadotropic hypogonadism include anorexia nervosa and extreme levels of stress and exercise. Hypergonadotropic hypogonadism etiologies of secondary amenorrhea include menopause and premature ovarian failure. In these two conditions, the ovaries no longer produce estrogen and progesterone. In addition to clinical signs and symptoms consistent with menopause, diagnosis is confirmed by an abnormally elevated FSH level.

Secondary amenorrhea can be seen in patients with obesity and PCOS. In these patients, chronically elevated estrogen levels secondary to peripheral aromatization of adrenal androgens to estrogens by adipose cells leads to a disruption in the feedback loop and anovulation. Patients may have only several menses per year and can present with amenorrhea. This can be differentiated from hypogonadism by performing a **progesterone challenge.** If a withdrawal bleed occurs after administration of progesterone for 10 days, anovulation with normal gonadal estrogen production is the likely cause of amenorrhea. These patients can be placed on oral contraceptives to regulate their cycles.

CASE CONCLUSION

A pregnancy test is negative, and prolactin and TSH levels both return within normal limits. You prescribe a progesterone challenge and the patient subsequently reports a withdrawal bleed, indicating that she has an intact, estrogen-primed uterus and is likely experiencing amenorrhea as a result of hypothalamic dysfunction due to excessive exercise. You place her on oral contraceptives and schedule a follow-up appointment in several months.

THUMBNAIL: Etiology of Primary Amenorrhea

	Uterus Absent	Uterus Present
Breasts absent	Gonadal agenesis in 46,XY *Enzyme deficiencies in testosterone synthesis*	Gonadal failure/agenesis in 46,XX Disruption of hypothalamic-pituitary-gonadal axis
Breasts present	Testicular feminization	Hypothalamic, pituitary, or ovarian pathogenesis similar to that of secondary amenorrhea
	Müllerian agenesis or Mayer Rokitansky Kuster Hauser Syndrome	Congenital abnormalities of the genital tract

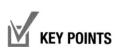

KEY POINTS

- Menstruation is the cyclical shedding of the endometrium experienced by women of reproductive age
- The menstrual cycle is driven by a feedback loop between the hypothalamus (GnRH), pituitary gland (FSH and LH), and ovaries (estrogen)
- Primary amenorrhea is the absence of menarche by age 16 or 4 years after thelarche

- Evaluation of primary amenorrhea is guided by the presence or absence of the breasts and uterus
- Secondary amenorrhea is the absence of menses for more than 6 months or the equivalent of three menstrual cycles in a previously menstruating woman

QUESTIONS

1. A 16-year-old girl presents to your office complaining of primary amenorrhea. On physical exam, she has both breasts and a uterus. A pregnancy test returns positive and explains the patient's amenorrhea. Which of the following does not lead to primary amenorrhea?

   A. Testicular feminization
   B. Imperforate hymen
   C. Transverse vaginal septum
   D. Intense physical activity since age 8
   E. Removal of left ovary secondary to torsion at age 8

2. A 24-year-old woman presents to your office with complaints of secondary amenorrhea since age 22. She had regular menses from age 13 to age 21, but only four periods during her last year of college. She reports no sexual intercourse since age 18. She gained 110 pounds during college, increasing from 140 to 250 pounds. Since age 22, she has lost 40 pounds, and is back down to 210 pounds. During this time she has increased her exercise to five times per week, 1 to 1½ hours each time. Which of the following is the most likely cause of her secondary amenorrhea?

   A. Elevated hCG leading to maintenance of her corpus luteum
   B. Elevated circulating estrogen leading to a disruption in FSH/LH production by the pituitary
   C. Sudden weight loss leading to hypogonadotropic hypogonadism

   D. Excessive exercise leading to hypogonadotropic hypogonadism
   E. Testicular feminization

3. A 34-year-old woman is undergoing evaluation for secondary amenorrhea of 8 months' duration. She also reports occasional hot flushes. She has never been pregnant before. Her physical exam is within normal limits and a pregnancy test is negative. Prolactin (PRL) and TSH values are also within normal limits. You schedule her for a progestin challenge. Which of the following results is correctly matched to a plausible etiology of her secondary amenorrhea?

   A. Withdrawal bleed seen with progestin challenge—Asherman syndrome
   B. Withdrawal bleed seen with progestin challenge—premature ovarian failure
   C. Withdrawal bleed seen only with estrogen/progestin challenge and FSH abnormally low—PCOS
   D. Withdrawal bleed seen only with estrogen/progestin challenge and FSH abnormally elevated—premature ovarian failure
   E. Withdrawal bleed seen only with estrogen/progestin challenge and FSH abnormally elevated—testicular feminization

CASE 9-4   Maternal Physiology in Pregnancy

HPI: A 22-year-old G3P0 recent immigrant from Mexico presents to the ER complaining of shortness of breath, fatigue, palpitations, and cough, especially at night, for the past 2 weeks. She denies night sweats, weight loss, or exposure to TB. She also reports that she is approximately 25 weeks pregnant and has not received any prenatal care during this pregnancy. Her past medical history is significant for recurrent strep throat infections as a child. She works as a nanny and does not smoke.

PE: On physical exam, she is tachycardic and appears to be in moderate distress. Her neck veins are distended and she has a diastolic rumble heard best in the left lateral decubitus position, an opening snap, and an S_3 gallop. Her fundal height is 26 cm, and she has 2+ bilateral lower extremity edema. CXR shows bilateral pulmonary edema.

THOUGHT QUESTIONS

- What pathophysiologic process is most consistent with this patient's symptoms?
- What are the key changes of maternal physiology in pregnancy?
- How would these changes affect cardiac valvular disease?

BASIC SCIENCE REVIEW AND DISCUSSION

The findings of distended neck veins (JVD), 2+bilateral edema, pulmonary edema, and a diastolic murmur are most consistent with CHF, particularly in the setting of mitral stenosis. There are other etiologies of CHF, and certainly an echocardiogram to determine cardiac function should be done. Although unlikely, the patient should also be evaluated for recent MI. This patient with no known prior disease may have a history of a valvular heart disease that is now exacerbated by the physiologic changes of pregnancy. Pregnancy places new demands on the mother that require physiologic adaptations in almost every organ system in order to meet these demands. These changes are reviewed by system below.

Cardiovascular

Elevated progesterone levels during pregnancy lead to smooth muscle relaxation, which results in decreased systemic vascular resistance (SVR) and BP. The decrease in BP nadirs at 24 weeks' gestation and slowly returns to prepregnancy levels by term. Any further increases in BP are abnormal and should be evaluated. Because preload increases via the increase in blood volume, cardiac output increases by 30 to 50%.

Pulmonary

Because the enlarging uterus elevates the diaphragm, the TLC is decreased by 5% during pregnancy. Nevertheless, the tidal volume increases by 30 to 40% and the RR stays the same, which leads to a 30 to 40% increase in the minute ventilation and a concomitant decrease in arterial PCO_2. However, bicarbonate decreases to maintain the pH and results in a compensated respiratory alkalosis.

Renal

The GFR increases by 50% during pregnancy, resulting in 25% decreases in both serum creatinine and BUN. The increased GFR also leads to decreased resorption of glucose, leading to glycosuria in approximately 15% of normal pregnancies. High progesterone levels lead to dilatation of the ureters and mild hydronephrosis, which can be further exacerbated by mechanical compression by the enlarging uterus. Increased sodium filtration also occurs due to the increased GFR, but plasma levels of sodium do not increase because of a concomitant increase in aldosterone to resorb this sodium.

Gastrointestinal

Progesterone relaxation of GI smooth muscle leads to delayed gastric emptying, decreased tone of the gastroesophageal sphincter, and decreased large bowel motility. These changes lead to the symptoms of increased reflux and constipation. Nausea occurs in more than 70% of pregnancies and tends to resolve by 17 weeks' gestation. While this phenomenon has been termed "morning sickness," it can occur at any time of the day.

Heme

The red cell mass also increases during pregnancy (20–30%), although proportionally less than the increase in blood volume (50%). Thus, a mild dilutional anemia results. A leukocytosis also occurs but should not affect the differential count. Approximately 10% of women experience a mild thrombocytopenia (<150,000 platelets/mL), but this is rarely of clinical significance. Increased levels of factors I (fibrinogen), VII, VIII, IX, and X, as well as increased stasis, make pregnancy a hypercoagulable state.

Endocrine

Elevated levels of estrogen in pregnancy stimulate production of thyroid-binding globulin by the liver. However, levels of free T_3, T_4, and TSH remain unchanged in pregnancy due to increased production of T_3 and T_4 via the thyroid-stimulating properties of placental hormones such as hCG. While PRL levels increase during pregnancy, they paradoxically decrease after delivery and then rise again in response to suckling.

Cardiac Valvular Disease in Pregnancy

Preexisting maternal heart disease that does not compromise function in the nonpregnant state can worsen during pregnancy as a result of its associated cardiovascular changes. Specifically, cardiac output is relatively fixed in cases of tight mitral stenosis. Elevation of preload and cardiac output in normal pregnancy can lead to ventricular failure and pulmonary HTN. Additionally, worsening LA enlargement can lead to arrhythmias and thrombus formation. As such, tachycardia and heart failure from fluid overload can be seen in mitral stenosis during pregnancy. Since 25% of women with mitral stenosis have cardiac failure for the first time in pregnancy, mitral stenosis can be confused with idiopathic peripartum cardiomyopathy.

CASE CONCLUSION

The patient has heart failure likely from undiagnosed rheumatic heart disease resulting in mitral stenosis. You admit her to the hospital for diuresis, bed rest, and start her on a low-dose beta-blocker to control her HR and prevent rate-related heart failure. Echocardiography confirms mitral stenosis. She responds well to this regimen and is eventually discharged home on a diuretic and beta-blocker with instructions to limit her activity and adhere to a low-salt diet.

THUMBNAIL: Maternal Adaptations in Pregnancy

Maternal Adaptations in Pregnancy

Organ system	Changes
Heme	Red cell mass increases 20–30% Plasma volume increases 50% Leukocytosis Thrombocytopenia (mild) Elevated factors I, VII–X
Endocrine	Estrogen increases Progesterone increases Thyroid-binding globulin increases Prolactin increases
Renal	GFR increases 50% BUN and creatinine decrease 25% Mild hydronephrosis and hydroureter
Gastrointestinal	Gastric emptying times prolonged Gastroesophageal sphincter tone decreases Large bowel motility decreases
Pulmonary	Total lung capacity decreases 5% Respiratory rate stays the same Tidal volume increases 30–40% Expiratory reserve volume decreases 20% Minute ventilation increases 30–40%
Cardiovascular	SVR and BP decrease Cardiac output increases 30–50%

KEY POINTS

- Pregnancy induces maternal physiologic adaptations in almost every organ system
- Blood volume increases by approximately 50%, leading to an increase in cardiac output of approximately 30 to 50%
- While TLC is decreased by the enlarging uterus, tidal volume and minute ventilation both increase by 30 to 40%
- GFR increases by 50%, resulting in decreased levels of both serum creatinine and BUN
- Elevated progesterone levels in pregnancy cause decreased esophageal sphincter tone, leading to increased gastroesophageal reflux

QUESTIONS

1. A 28-year-old woman presents for a routine prenatal appointment at 24 weeks' gestation. Which of the following cardiovascular and/or hematologic indices are elevated?

   A. Systemic vascular resistance
   B. Cardiac output
   C. Platelets
   D. Blood pressure
   E. Hematocrit

2. A 30-year-old woman presents for a routine prenatal appointment at 22 weeks' gestation. Which of the following pulmonary and/or renal indices are decreased?

   A. Tidal volume
   B. GFR
   C. RR
   D. BUN and serum creatinine
   E. Minute ventilation

Maternal-Fetal Circulation

HPI: HF is a 32-year-old G2P1 pregnant woman at 10-2/7 weeks' gestation who presents for her initial prenatal visit. On review of her prenatal labs, you notice that her blood type is A-negative and that her antibody screen for rhesus factor (Rh) is positive with a titer of 1:16. Her past obstetric history is significant for an uncomplicated spontaneous vaginal delivery of a term infant 2 years ago in South America. She recalls getting one dose of RhoGAM mid-pregnancy but not at delivery. The blood type of the father of the baby is A-positive and the first child's blood type is also A-positive. Her past medical history is otherwise noncontributory.

You repeat the antibody screen and confirm that the titer is correct. You advise the patient that she has been alloimmunized to fetal D antigen and that this pregnancy is at risk for hydrops fetalis if the blood type of the fetus is confirmed to be Rh-positive. You schedule her for serial antibody titers and amniocentesis to determine fetal blood type.

THOUGHT QUESTIONS

- Discuss maternal-fetal circulation and the fetal adaptations that facilitate fetal oxygenation.
- What is Rh D alloimmunization?
- What is the management of a pregnant Rh-negative woman who has been sensitized to Rh antigen?
- What is RhoGAM and how is it used?

BASIC SCIENCE REVIEW AND DISCUSSION

Fetal circulation is designed to maximize fetal oxygenation. Because the fetal lungs are functionally inactive until birth, the fetus is dependent on the placenta for oxygen and nutrition. The placenta also facilitates clearance of fetal waste. It consists of fetal villi that are bathed in maternal blood contained in the intervillous spaces and have a large surface area for exchange.

Oxygenated blood reaches the fetus from the placenta via the umbilical cord, which consists of one **umbilical vein** and two **umbilical arteries.** The umbilical vein transports maternally oxygenated blood, half of which passes through the fetal liver and the remainder of which bypasses the liver to the inferior vena cava (IVC) via the **ductus venosus.** In the vena cava, blood from the ductus venosus, hepatic veins, and lower trunk and extremities combines. This blood then travels to the RA, where the majority is shunted to the LA via the **foramen ovale,** which separates the two atria and allows oxygenated blood to bypass the pulmonary system. In fact, only one tenth of RV output goes to the lungs because of the large pulmonary resistance. The remainder of the blood bypasses the pulmonary system by traveling from the pulmonary artery through the **ductus arteriosus** to the aorta. Blood returns from the lungs to the LA and is subsequently pumped to the aorta and the rest of the body via the LV. Deoxygenated blood and fetal waste then return to the placenta via the umbilical arteries (Table 9-1).

Fetal blood is also designed to maximize fetal oxygenation. Fetal hemoglobin (**hemoglobin F**) has a higher affinity for oxygen than does adult hemoglobin (hemoglobin A). Additionally, the fetal oxyhemoglobin dissociation curve is shifted to the left to favor fetal over maternal oxygenation. Sites of fetal hematopoiesis change with gestational age (GA), starting with the yolk sac and transitioning to the fetal liver, spleen, lymph nodes, and, finally, bone marrow.

At birth, the umbilical vessels are clamped and ligated, resulting in increased total peripheral resistance and BP. Additionally, the umbilical vessels, ductus arteriosus, and ductus venosus constrict. With the infant's first breath, pulmonary vascular resistance decreases to about one tenth of its previous level. This reverses the pressure gradient between the left and right atria and causes the foramen ovale to close and eventually fuse. Additionally, the pressure in the pulmonary artery falls to about half its previous level, facilitating the reversal of flow through the ductus arteriosus, which proceeds to constrict and close over the course of 1 to 2 days.

Rh D Alloimmunization

The **D antigen,** also known as **rhesus factor,** is the most antigenic protein on the surface of erythrocytes. Rh incompatibility occurs when an Rh-negative woman (i.e., a woman who does not possess the D antigen on her erythrocytes) carries an Rh-positive fetus and is exposed to Rh-positive fetal blood during the pregnancy or labor. If the exposure is significant, she can form antibodies to D antigen and become alloimmunized. These antibodies can then cross the placenta and attack fetal erythrocytes that possess the D antigen in subsequent pregnancies, resulting in hemolysis, anemia, and possibly **hydrops fetalis.** Aside from death, fetal hydrops is the most severe sequela of Rh D alloimmunization and consists of a hyperdynamic state resulting in fetal heart failure, diffuse edema, and ascites. Alternatively, if the fetus is Rh-negative, it will not be affected by circulating anti-D antibodies. In general, the pregnancy that causes the sensitization is not affected because the initial immune response is IgM, which does not cross the placenta. It is only with subsequent pregnancies that an IgG response is triggered.

Rh D alloimmunization can be prevented in unsensitized Rh-negative women by administration of **RhoGAM,** which is anti-D immunoglobulin that destroys fetal erythrocytes before a maternal immune response can be mounted. To be effective, RhoGAM must be administered any time fetal-maternal hemorrhage is a potential, including pregnancy, miscarriage, invasive procedures (e.g., amniocentesis), delivery, and abortion. Additionally, mismatched blood transfusion can also cause alloimmunization. Prior to administration of RhoGAM to an Rh-negative woman, an antibody screen and titer, if appropriate, should be performed to confirm that she has not already been sensitized. Once this is confirmed, routine prophylaxis includes administration of RhoGAM at 28 weeks' GA and again within 72 hours of delivery if the infant's blood type is undetermined or found to be Rh-positive. A standard dose of RhoGAM is 300 µg, which should cover maternal exposure to 30 mL of fetal blood. However, if

TABLE 9-1 Fetal Circulatory Adaptations

Structure	Purpose	Adult Structure
Umbilical vein	Transport oxygenated blood to fetus	Ligamentum teres
Umbilical arteries	Return deoxygenated blood from fetus to placenta	Umbilical ligaments
Ductus venosus	Bypass oxygenated blood from liver to IVC	Ligamentum venosum
Foramen ovale	Bypass pulmonary system (RA to LA)	Closed foramen ovale
Ductus arteriosus	Bypass pulmonary system (pulmonary artery to aorta)	Ligamentum arteriosum

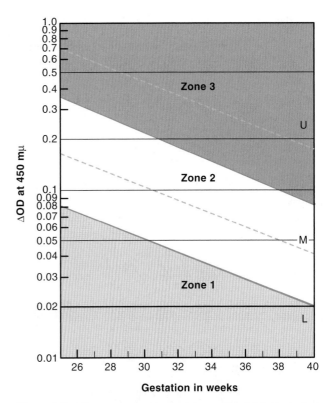

• **Figure 9-5.** Liley curve used to depict severity of fetal hemolysis with red cell isoimmunization.

maternal-fetal hemorrhage is suspected to exceed this amount, a **Kleihauer-Betke test** can be performed to quantitate the amount of fetal erythrocytes in the maternal circulation and allow for adjustment of RhoGAM dosing.

Management of the Rh D alloimmunized woman during pregnancy depends on the blood type of the fetus, which can be determined by amniocentesis. Alternatively, if paternity is certain and paternal blood type is Rh-negative, the fetus must therefore be Rh-negative as well and will not be affected. If fetal blood type is unknown or confirmed to be Rh-positive, maternal antibody titers should be followed serially. Pregnancies with titers less than 1:16 can be managed expectantly. However, because titers of 1:16 or greater have been associated with fetal hydrops, serial amniocentesis should be performed in these pregnancies starting at 16 to 20 weeks to obtain amniotic fluid samples. Fetal hemolysis releases bilirubin into the amniotic fluid, which can then be analyzed by a spectrophotometer to measure the light absorption by bilirubin (ΔOD_{450}) (Fig. 9-5). Fetuses should also undergo frequent ultrasound exams to look for signs of hydrops, such as ascites, pericardial effusion, and pleural effusion. Additional invasive therapeutic procedures can be performed if the fetus is severely affected. These procedures include intraperitoneal transfusion and **percutaneous umbilical cord sampling** (PUBS) during which time the PUBS needle can be used to transfuse the fetus if necessary. Premature delivery may be indicated in cases where the risk of remaining in utero exceeds that of prematurity. If premature delivery is likely and the fetus is beyond 24 weeks' GA, a course of antenatal corticosteroids can be administered to promote fetal lung maturity.

Of note, several other erythrocyte antigens can also cause alloimmunization. These include ABO blood type, C, E, Kell, Duffy, and Lewis. The sequelae range from immune hydrops to mild hemolysis and anemia. These antigens are managed in a similar fashion to Rh D alloimmunization with the exception of RhoGAM administration.

CASE CONCLUSION

At 16 weeks' GA, the patient undergoes amniocentesis, which unfortunately confirms a fetal blood type of A-positive. During the amniocentesis, amniotic fluid is sampled to test for ΔOD_{450}. This returns a result in zone 1 of the Liley curve. The patient subsequently undergoes serial amniocentesis every 2 weeks. At 26 weeks' GA, the ΔOD_{450} level enters zone 3 and fetal ultrasonography shows ascites. The patient is given a course of corticosteroids in anticipation of premature delivery and starts undergoing weekly PUBS transfusions. At 28 weeks' GA, fetal ultrasound indicates worsening ascites as well as the presence of a pericardial effusion. The risk of fetal harm is determined to exceed that of maintaining the pregnancy and the patient undergoes delivery via cesarean section.

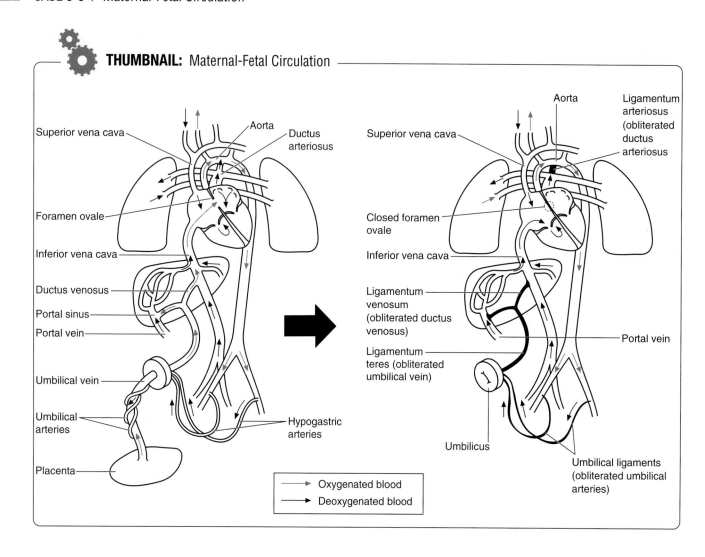

THUMBNAIL: Maternal-Fetal Circulation

KEY POINTS

■ Fetal adaptations such as the foramen ovale, ductus arteriosus, and ductus venosus allow maximal fetal oxygenation by bypassing functionally inactive structures

■ The decrease in pulmonary vascular resistance caused by lung inflation at birth reverses the pressure gradient between the atria and causes the foramen ovale to close

■ The umbilical vessels, ductus arteriosus, and ductus venosus constrict at birth

■ Fetal hemoglobin and the fetal oxyhemoglobin dissociation curve favor fetal over maternal oxygenation

■ D antigen, or Rh, is the most antigenic protein found on erythrocytes and can cause immune fetal hydrops when maternal antibodies cross the placenta and cause fetal hemolysis and anemia

QUESTIONS

1. Which of the following is not an absolute indication for RhoGAM administration in an Rh D-negative woman?

   A. An Rh D-negative woman at 28 weeks' GA
   B. An Rh D-negative woman who has just delivered at 37 weeks' GA

   C. An Rh D-negative woman who has just experienced a spontaneous abortion at 10 weeks' GA
   D. An Rh D-negative woman undergoing an amniocentesis
   E. An Rh D-negative woman with a ruptured ectopic pregnancy

2. You have been following an Rh D-negative woman with antibody titers of 1:32 at her intake obstetric visit and a prior history of a mildly affected infant requiring no interventions except performing serial amniocenteses for ΔOD_{450} values. Her prior ΔOD_{450} values have resided within Liley zone 1 but have slowly been increasing. Today at her 29-week prenatal visit, she is found to have a ΔOD_{450} value within Liley zone 3. However, ultrasonography shows no signs of fetal hydrops. What is the next step in the management of this patient?

A. Immediate delivery
B. PUBS to determine severity of fetal disease and possible IV transfusion if indicated
C. Confirm presence of fetal lung maturity and deliver as soon as it is achieved
D. Short course of antenatal corticosteroids followed by immediate delivery
E. Continued serial amniocenteses to assess ΔOD_{450} value trends and PUBS and transfusion as indicated

3. Which of the following can be an indication of severe fetal disease?

A. ΔOD_{450} value in Liley curve zone 3
B. Fetal ascites
C. Fetal pericardial effusion
D. Fetal pleural effusion
E. All of the above

4. Which of the following fetal structures is correctly matched to its purpose in fetal circulation?

A. Ductus arteriosus—bypass liver by shunting blood from umbilical vein to the IVC
B. Ductus venosus—bypass lungs by shunting blood from the pulmonary artery to the aorta
C. Foramen ovale—bypass lungs by shunting blood from the RA to the LA
D. Umbilical vein—transport deoxygenated fetal blood back to the placenta
E. None of the above

HPI: PB is a 47-year-old G5P2 woman who recently immigrated from China and presents to your office for her first pelvic exam. She reports recurrent postcoital bleeding for several months and now has irregular menses. She is sexually active with her husband only, and her gynecologic history includes two spontaneous vaginal deliveries, three therapeutic abortions, and regular menses until 5 months ago. Her past medical history is significant for hepatitis B infection and tubal ligation at age 37.

PE: On physical exam, she is found to have a large, friable lesion involving the right side of her cervix. No adnexal masses are palpated, and rectovaginal exam reveals that the mass does not involve the parametria or cul-de-sac. You suspect cervical cancer and refer the patient to gynecologic oncology for further evaluation and treatment.

THOUGHT QUESTIONS

- What is the incidence of cervical cancer, and what are the associated risk factors?
- How can we screen for cervical cancer?
- Discuss cervical dysplasia.
- How is cervical cancer staged?
- Discuss the treatment of cervical cancer.

BASIC SCIENCE REVIEW AND DISCUSSION

An estimated 15,000 women are diagnosed with cervical cancer in the United States every year. With approximately 4600 deaths per year, cervical cancer is the sixth leading cause of death from cancer in women in the United States. In undeveloped countries where screening is unavailable, cervical cancer is the leading cause of cancer deaths in women.

Infection with **human papilloma virus (HPV)** causes over 90% of cervical cancer cases, especially infections due to genotypes 16, 18, and 31. Other risk factors for cervical cancer include cigarette smoking, early onset of sexual activity, large number of sexual partners, and history of sexually transmitted diseases, especially human immunodeficiency virus (HIV).

Because the natural history of cervical cancer is typically slow and predictable, starting with dysplasia and moving to **cervical intraepithelial neoplasia (CIN)** and finally invasive disease, early detection can lead to improved outcomes. The **Papanicolaou smear,** or Pap smear, was implemented in the 1950s to screen for cervical dysplasia and cancer. It involves scraping cells from the cervix to sample the squamocolumnar junction, or transformation zone. Pap smears should be performed annually in all sexually active women and those older than age 18 years. Screening frequency can be adjusted depending on risk factors and presence of dysplasia.

Cervical cytology is evaluated using the Bethesda System, which classifies epithelial cell abnormalities in the following manner: atypical squamous cells of undetermined significance (**ASCUS**); low-grade squamous intraepithelial lesion (**LGSIL**) or **CIN I;** or high-grade squamous intraepithelial lesion (**HGSIL**), which encompasses **CIN II** and **CIN III.** ASCUS can be due to inflammation or preinvasive lesions. Determination of CIN grade is dependent on the depth of epithelial involvement. In CIN I, the lower one third of cells are abnormal, while CIN II involves the lower two thirds, and CIN III is full-thickness involvement. **Colposcopy** is the microscopic evaluation of the transformation zone to identify abnormal areas that may display acetowhite epithelium, mosaicism, punctation, or atypical vessels.

While the classic presentation of cervical cancer is postcoital bleeding, other symptoms include watery discharge, rectal or urinary tract symptoms, abnormal vaginal bleeding, and pelvic pressure or pain. Findings consistent with cervical cancer on physical exam are an exophytic, ulcerative, papillary, or necrotic lesion involving the cervix and possibly vagina, and/or palpable lesions that extend from the cervix to the vagina, adnexa, or cul-de-sac. Suspicious lesions should be examined via biopsy for histologic diagnosis.

Staging of cervical cancer is clinical rather than surgical and is determined by the degree of invasion into adjacent structures and the presence of distant metastasis. Formal staging involves exam under anesthesia, chest x-ray, cystoscopy, proctoscopy, and, occasionally, IV pyelography, barium enema, or CT scan.

Stage IA1 (microinvasive disease) can be treated with cone biopsy excision, if the patient wishes to retain fertility, or with simple hysterectomy. **Cone biopsy** excision is the removal of a wedge-shaped portion of the cervical stroma and endocervical canal. Depending on the patient's medical status and age, hysterectomy or radiation can be performed if the cancer has not spread beyond the cervix, uterus, and vagina (stage IIA or less). With more advanced disease (stage IIB to IV), the treatment is chemoradiation, which involves weekly cisplatin and external beam radiation followed by brachytherapy (local application of radiation). Chemoradiation is also used for palliative purposes.

Ovarian Cancer

Ovarian cancer is the fourth leading cause of cancer deaths in women, with approximately 15,000 deaths and 26,000 new cases diagnosed annually in the United States. The lifetime risk of developing ovarian cancer is roughly 1.5% in the general population. However, this risk is 10- to 20-fold higher in the 5 to 10% of ovarian cancers that are hereditary and due to **BRCA1** or **BRCA2** mutations. Ovarian cancer has a greater incidence in industrialized countries and in women of low parity. Age appears to be the most important risk factor, with the median age of diagnosis being 61 years. Alternatively, factors that decrease the number of lifetime ovulations, such as multiparity, breast-feeding, oral contraceptive use, and chronic anovulation, appear to be protective against ovarian cancer.

Unfortunately, early signs of ovarian cancer are rare. As such, many women are diagnosed with advanced disease by the time they present with complaints of abdominal discomfort, increasing abdominal girth, and early satiety. Evaluation of suspected ovarian cancer should include a complete history and physical exam, as well as ultrasonography to characterize any pelvic masses and confirm the presence of ascites. Masses that are larger than 8 cm, solid, multilocular, and bilateral are suspicious for malignancy. Serum **CA-125** (a tumor marker) levels may be elevated, but are usually not useful in premenopausal women because other conditions can elevate CA-125 levels (e.g., endometriosis, pancreatitis).

Ovarian cancer staging involves pelvic washings; abdominal exploration of peritoneal surfaces, liver, bowel, and lymph nodes; biopsy of the omentum; possible appendectomy; and usually total abdominal hysterectomy and bilateral salpingo-oophorectomy (TAH-BSO). Removal of all gross disease should be attempted. Chemotherapy is usually recommended for stages IC and higher, with the typical regimen being six cycles of **carboplatin** and **paclitaxel.** Frequent follow-up evaluation during the first 2 years is critical, because the majority of recurrences will appear during this time. History, physical exam, and serial serum CA-125 levels should be evaluated. The most important prognostic factor is surgical stage, but other factors include patient age, extent of residual disease after debulking surgery, and volume of ascites. The overall 5-year survival rate for ovarian cancer is 35%.

Many histologic subtypes of ovarian cancer exist (see Thumbnail below). However, the majority (85–90%) of ovarian cancers are epithelial in origin. The epithelial subtypes include **serous** (50–70%), **mucinous** (10–15%), **endometrioid, undifferentiated,** and **clear cell.** Additionally, there are tumors of low malignant potential known as **borderline ovarian tumors** that constitute 10 to 15% of epithelial ovarian cancers. **Germ cell tumors** (5–7%) are another group of ovarian cancers, and **sex cord stromal tumors** (5–7%) include **granulosa cell tumors** (70%) and **Sertoli-Leydig tumors** (rare).

Endometrial Cancer

Ninety-five percent of uterine cancers are endometrial in nature, and the remaining 5% are uterine sarcomas. **Endometrial cancer** is the most common gynecologic cancer, with 36,100 new cases diagnosed in the United States each year. Despite being the most curable of the gynecologic malignancies, it still has a mortality rate of 6500 women per year. Endometrial cancer is primarily a disease of postmenopausal women, with a median age at diagnosis of 60 years.

Risk factors for endometrial cancer tend to involve increased exposure to unopposed estrogen such as nulliparity, chronic anovulation, obesity, early menarche, late menopause, history of breast or ovarian cancer, or use of tamoxifen or exogenous estrogen. Additionally, women with hereditary nonpolyposis colorectal cancer syndrome (Lynch type II) are at increased risk for endometrial cancer. Conversely, factors that reduce exposure to estrogen or increase progesterone levels are protective, such as oral contraceptives, high parity, pregnancy, and smoking.

Fortunately, endometrial cancer tends to be diagnosed in its early stages because 90% of women will have abnormal vaginal bleeding. As a rule, vaginal bleeding of any type in a postmenopausal woman must be evaluated for malignancy. In premenopausal women, prolonged, heavy, or intermenstrual bleeding should be investigated. Evaluation of abnormal bleeding includes a thorough history and physical exam, including a pelvic exam. Additionally, a Pap smear should be done because it will be abnormal in 30 to 40% of patients with endometrial cancer.

Finally, the endometrium must be sampled by endometrial biopsy or dilatation and curettage, the former of which is a simpler procedure yielding comparable results. **Endometrial biopsy** provides a tissue diagnosis and allows grading of tumor based on the percentage of solid (non–gland-forming) growth pattern. Eighty percent of endometrial cancers are adenocarcinoma. The remaining histologic types of carcinoma include adenosquamous (7%), clear cell (6%), uterine papillary serous (5%), and secretory (2%).

Uterine sarcomas comprise 5% of uterine cancers. They include leiomyosarcomas, mixed müllerian tumors, and endometrial stromal sarcomas. In general, these tumors are aggressive, have a poor prognosis, and are treated surgically. **Leiomyosarcomas** are uterine smooth muscle tumors that must be differentiated from benign **leiomyomas,** otherwise known as fibroids, which are much more common. **Mixed müllerian tumors** (MMTs) are composed of both carcinoma and sarcoma, and the malignant components can include bone, cartilage, or skeletal muscle. **Endometrial stromal sarcomas** (ESSs) protrude into the endometrial cavity and can be low or high grade depending on the number of mitoses.

In addition to malignancy, endometrial biopsy can identify **endometrial hyperplasia,** which represents abnormal endometrial gland proliferation. Similarly to endometrial cancer, endometrial hyperplasia usually manifests as abnormal vaginal bleeding. It is usually a result of prolonged exposure to unopposed estrogen and is a premalignant lesion if atypia is present.

CASE CONCLUSION

The patient is evaluated by gynecologic oncology and determined to have stage IIA disease. She subsequently undergoes radical hysterectomy with negative surgical margins and is scheduled for frequent follow-up appointments.

THUMBNAIL: International Federation of Gynecology and Obstetrics (FIGO) Staging for Cervical Cancer

Stage	Findings
Stage 0	Carcinoma in situ, intraepithelial carcinoma
Stage I	The carcinoma is strictly confined to the cervix
Stage IA	Invasive cancer identified only microscopically and limited to a maximum depth of 5 mm and no wider than 7 mm
Stage IA1	Invasion ≤3 mm depth and no wider than 7 mm
Stage IA2	Invasion 3–5 mm depth and no wider than 7 mm
Stage IB	Clinical lesions confined to the cervix or preclinical lesions more extensive than stage IA
Stage IB1	Clinical lesions ≤4.0 cm in size
Stage IB2	Clinical lesions >4.0 cm in size
Stage II	The carcinoma extends beyond the cervix but has not extended to the pelvic wall; vaginal involvement does not reach the lower third
Stage IIA	No obvious parametrial involvement
Stage IIB	Obvious parametrial involvement
Stage III	The carcinoma has extended to the pelvic wall; no cancer-free space between tumor and pelvic wall on rectal exam; lower one third of vagina involved; hydronephrosis or nonfunctioning kidney
Stage IIIA	No extension to the pelvic wall
Stage IIIB	Extension to the pelvic wall and/or hydronephrosis or nonfunctioning kidney
Stage IV	The carcinoma has extended beyond the true pelvis or involves the mucosa of the bladder or rectum
Stage IVA	Spread to adjacent organs
Stage IVB	Spread to distant organs

THUMBNAIL: Summary—Cervical, Ovarian, and Uterine Cancers

	Risk Factors	Presentation	Staging	Main Histologic Type	Tumor Markers
Cervical cancer	HPV especially 16, 18, and 31; cigarette smoking, early onset of sexual activity, large number of sexual partners, history of sexually transmitted diseases	Postcoital bleeding, watery discharge, rectal/urinary symptoms, abnormal vaginal bleeding, pelvic pressure/pain	Clinical	Squamous cell	None
Ovarian cancer	Age, family history, especially BRCA1 and 2 carriers; protective (by reducing the number of lifetime ovulations): multiparity, OCP use, chronic anovulation	Early signs rare; advanced disease: abdominal discomfort, increasing abdominal girth, early satiety	Surgical	Epithelial (serous or mucinous)	Epithelial —CA-125, dysgerminomas —LDH, endodermal sinus —alpha-fetoprotein (AFP)
Uterine cancer	Unopposed estrogen exposure: nulliparity, chronic anovulation, early menarche, late menopause, use of tamoxifen or exogenous estrogen	Postmenopausal bleeding or prolonged, heavy, or intermenstrual premenopausal bleeding	Surgical	Adenocarcinoma	None

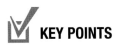

KEY POINTS

Cervical cancer

■ Risk factors for cervical cancer include HPV infection, early age of first sexual activity, large number of sexual partners, cigarette smoking, and history of sexually transmitted infections

■ Pap smears are used to screen for cervical cancer and should be performed annually in all sexually active women or women older than age 18 years

■ Without treatment, cervical dysplasia typically progresses slowly to CIN and finally to invasive cervical cancer

■ Treatment of cervical dysplasia and cancer varies depending on desired fertility and degree of invasion

Ovarian cancer

■ Protective factors for ovarian cancer include multiparity, breast-feeding, oral contraceptive use, and chronic anovulation

■ The majority (85–90%) of ovarian cancers are epithelial in origin

■ Early symptoms of cervical cancer are rare, and diagnosis of disease in advanced stages is not uncommon

■ Ovarian cancer is surgically staged and treated with surgery and platinum-based chemotherapeutic agents

Endometrial cancer

■ Endometrial cancer is the most common gynecologic malignancy and usually results from prolonged exposure to estrogen without progesterone (unopposed estrogen)

■ The median age of diagnosis is 60 years, but any patient presenting with irregular bleeding, particularly postmenopausally, should be evaluated for endometrial cancer or hyperplasia

■ Approximately 80% of endometrial cancer is adenocarcinoma

QUESTIONS

1. A 20-year-old woman presents for routine pelvic exam. She is sexually active and uses condoms occasionally. She began sexual activity at age 13 and has had seven lifetime partners. She has been treated for both chlamydia and gonorrhea over the past 3 years and experiences five to six UTIs per year. She started menstruating at age 13 and continues to have irregular menses. Which of the following is not a risk factor for cervical dysplasia or cancer?

   A. Chlamydial infection
   B. Multiple sexual partners
   C. Recurrent UTIs
   D. Cigarette smoking
   E. Early age of first sexual activity

2. In the process of performing an endometrial biopsy on a 56-year-old woman with postmenopausal bleeding, you notice an exophytic mass on the posterior portion of her cervix. A biopsy of this area shows squamous cell carcinoma. Which of the following is used to stage her disease?

   A. MRI
   B. Physical exam
   C. Margins from hysterectomy specimen
   D. Lymph node dissection
   E. All of the above

3. A 32-year-old woman is diagnosed with CIN II on Pap smear. Which of the following would not be appropriate management?

   A. Hysterectomy
   B. Cervical conization
   C. Loop electrosurgical excision procedure
   D. Cryotherapy
   E. Radiation

4. A 20-year-old virginal woman presents complaining of abdominal fullness and pain that started 2 months ago. Her menses are regular and she does not have any other medical problems. Your pelvic exam reveals a large right-sided mass that is suspicious for malignancy on ultrasonography. Which of the following tumor markers is matched to the correct neoplasm?

   A. Dysgerminomas—LDH
   B. Endodermal sinus tumor—CA-125
   C. Immature teratoma—hCG
   D. Embryonal carcinoma—LDH
   E. Choriocarcinoma—AFP

5. Rank the following types of cancer in women in the United States in order of decreasing incidence.

   A. Breast cancer, endometrial cancer, cervical cancer, lung cancer, ovarian cancer
   B. Breast cancer, lung cancer, endometrial cancer, ovarian cancer, cervical cancer
   C. Breast cancer, lung cancer, endometrial cancer, cervical cancer, ovarian cancer
   D. Lung cancer, endometrial cancer, breast cancer, cervical cancer, ovarian cancer
   E. Lung cancer, ovarian cancer, breast cancer, endometrial cancer, cervical cancer

6. Rank the following cancers in decreasing order of annual deaths in women in the United States.

   A. Breast cancer, lung cancer, ovarian cancer, endometrial cancer, cervical cancer
   B. Breast cancer, lung cancer, cervical cancer, ovarian cancer, endometrial cancer
   C. Lung cancer, breast cancer, endometrial cancer, cervical cancer, ovarian cancer
   D. Lung cancer, breast cancer, ovarian cancer, endometrial cancer, cervical cancer
   E. Lung cancer, breast cancer, cervical cancer, ovarian cancer, endometrial cancer

7. A 54-year-old G3P2 woman presents to your office complaining of vaginal bleeding for the past few months despite being menopausal for 3 years. Her medical history is significant only for HTN. On further history, the patient reveals that she stopped taking her replacement estrogen and progesterone several months ago because of concerns about heart disease. You perform an endometrial biopsy, which returns negative for cancer or hyperplasia. You reassure the patient that her bleeding is likely due to hormone withdrawal and advise her to return for repeat biopsy if the bleeding is persistent. Which of the following is a potential cause of postmenopausal bleeding?

   A. Vaginal atrophy
   B. Cervical cancer
   C. Endometrial atrophy
   D. Endometrial polyps
   E. All of the above

8. A 63 year-old G0P0 woman presents for her first pelvic exam since becoming menopausal at age 55. On reviewing her history, you discover that she has been experiencing occasional vaginal bleeding for almost a year. On physical exam, she has a slightly enlarged uterus but no adnexal masses, although exam is limited by her obesity. You perform an endometrial biopsy, which returns grade 3 adenocarcinoma. The patient undergoes TAH-BSO and surgical staging, revealing stage IIIC endometrial cancer, for which she receives postoperative radiation treatment. Which of the following is not a risk factor for endometrial cancer?

   A. Obesity
   B. Nulliparity
   C. Chronic anovulation
   D. Early age of first intercourse
   E. Late menopause

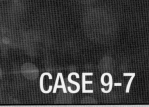

CASE 9-7 · Gestational Trophoblastic Disease

HPI: MP is a 15-year-old G1P0 girl at 9-5/7 weeks' gestation who presents to the ED complaining of severe nausea, vomiting, and inability to tolerate any oral intake for several days. She also reports that she has had vaginal spotting for the past week but was going to wait until her first prenatal appointment tomorrow to discuss it with a clinician. She denies fever, chills, pain, or loose stools.

She has no significant past medical history and is enrolled in the 10th grade at a local high school, where she is a "B" student and plays field hockey. She is sexually active with her boyfriend with occasional condom use. Although this was an unplanned pregnancy, they have decided to move into her parents' home and raise the child together.

PE: Her physical exam is significant for a moderate amount of blood in the vagina coming from the cervix. Her uterus is approximately 12 weeks' size, and she has bilateral adnexal masses that are small and minimally tender to palpation.

You check a quantitative β-hCG level and blood type and Rh. Pelvic ultrasonography reveals no identifiable fetus or cardiac motion. Instead, you see bilateral theca lutein cysts and a uterus filled with swollen chorionic villi resembling a "snow storm" pattern.

THOUGHT QUESTIONS

- What conditions are included in gestational trophoblastic disease (GTD)?
- Compare and contrast complete and partial hydatidiform moles.
- Discuss malignant GTD.
- Discuss the treatments for the various GTDs.

BASIC SCIENCE REVIEW AND DISCUSSION

Gestational trophoblastic disease is an umbrella term for a group of histologically distinct neoplastic diseases that arise from the placenta. Also referred to as gestational trophoblastic tumors (GTTs) and gestational trophoblastic neoplasia (GTN), GTD encompasses the following diseases: partial and complete hydatidiform moles, invasive moles, placental site trophoblastic tumors, and choriocarcinomas. While the latter three diseases are considered malignant GTD, the hydatidiform moles are considered benign unless they are invasive.

The incidence in the United States of the various GTDs varies, with hydatidiform moles being the most common (1:1200 pregnancies). The incidence of choriocarcinoma is approximately 1:20,000 to 40,000 pregnancies. Finally, placental site trophoblastic tumors are very rare. Approximately 80% of GTDs are hydatidiform moles. Invasive moles account for 10 to 15% of GTD, and choriocarcinoma represents 2 to 5% of GTD. Fortunately, GTD is exquisitely chemosensitive and considered to be the most curable gynecologic malignancy. In addition, β-hCG is a useful tumor marker to monitor disease in all the GTDs.

Benign Gestational Trophoblastic Disease

Hydatidiform moles, also referred to as molar pregnancies, can be either partial or complete. They vary in karyotype, clinical presentation, and pathology (Table 9-2). **Partial hydatidiform moles** usually contain 69 chromosomes from three haploid sets of chromosomes (two paternal and one maternal) and arise when a normal ovum is fertilized by two sperm at once. They also contain a nonviable fetus, a minimal amount of trophoblastic hyperplasia, and focally edematous chorionic villi. In contrast, **complete hydatidiform moles** contain 46 chromosomes that are paternally derived and arise when a single sperm fertilizes an empty ovum and then duplicates its chromosomes (90%), or when two sperm fertilize an empty ovum (10%). Complete moles do not contain

fetal tissue and have severe trophoblastic hyperplasia in addition to diffusely edematous chorionic villi that are often described as "grape-like" vesicles and appear as a "snow storm" pattern on ultrasonography (Fig. 9-7). Clinically, complete moles tend to present with abnormal vaginal bleeding (85% of patients). Additional signs and symptoms of complete mole include excessive uterine size (28%), hyperemesis gravidarum (8%), anemia (5%), and preeclampsia before 24 weeks (1%). Patients may also report or be found to have expulsion of grape-like molar clusters into the vagina, bilateral theca lutein cysts, and hyperthyroidism. Additionally, β-hCG levels will be extremely elevated (>100,000 mIU/mL) and the characteristic snow storm appearance may be evident on ultrasonography. While patients with partial moles can have similar signs and symptoms, they can also be asymptomatic and diagnosed with a missed abortion when fetal heart tones are not detectable and pathology specimen after suction curettage subsequently returns positive for molar gestation. The differential diagnosis for molar pregnancy includes multiple gestation pregnancy, erythroblastosis fetalis, fibroids, threatened abortion, ectopic pregnancy, or normal intrauterine pregnancy.

Both complete and partial moles can be 95 to 100% cured with suction evacuation and gentle curettage of the uterus. Additionally, IV oxytocin can be administered after uterine evacuation to stimulate contractions and minimize blood loss. Alternatively, if the patient has completed child-bearing, hysterectomy can also be performed. Because the risk for persistent disease is 15 to 25% with complete moles and less than 4% with partial moles, close follow-up with weekly and then monthly β-hCG levels for 1 year is essential. Reliable contraception must also be provided to the patient during this time to prevent misinterpretation of β-hCG levels. After successful treatment of molar gestation, the risk for developing GTD in subsequent pregnancies is less than 5%.

Malignant Gestational Trophoblastic Disease

There are three histologic types of malignant or persistent GTD: invasive moles, gestational choriocarcinoma, and placental site trophoblastic tumor. Prognosis is more dependent on clinical presentation than on histologic type. Evaluation of metastases should include physical exam and chest x-ray at the minimum with possible CT scan of the head, chest, and abdomen. Multiple classification systems exist for malignant GTD. The WHO's system allows the computation of a prognostic score based on the patient's age, the time interval between and type of antecedent

TABLE 9-2 Partial and Complete Hydatidiform Moles

Feature	Partial Mole	Complete Mole
Karyotype	69,XXX (20%) or 69,XXY (80%)	46,XX (90%) or 46,XY (10%)
Pathology		
Fetus	Often present	Absent
Amnion, fetal RBCs	Often present	Absent
Trophoblastic proliferation	Variable, focal, slight to moderate	Variable, slight to severe
Clinical presentation		
Diagnosis	Missed abortion Small for dates	Molar gestation
Uterine size	Rare	50% are large for dates Occur in 25–30%
Theca lutein cysts	Rare	Frequent
Medical complications	<5–10%	20%
Postmolar GTD		

pregnancy, β-hCG levels, size of tumor, sites and number of metastases, and prior chemotherapy used. The National Institutes of Health (NIH) has a system that categorizes patients based on the presence of metastases because most nonmetastatic disease can be cured using single-agent chemotherapy (usually methotrexate) and, depending on fertility preferences, can also be treated with hysterectomy. Those patients with metastatic disease are further subdivided into low risk/good prognosis and high risk/poor prognosis disease. Patients with poor prognosis disease are treated initially with multiagent chemotherapy (usually EMA/CO: etoposide, methotrexate, and dactinomycin alternating with cyclophosphamide and vincristine). Like the approach to benign GTD, follow-up should continue until serial β-hCG levels become undetectable, and concomitant reliable contraception is essential.

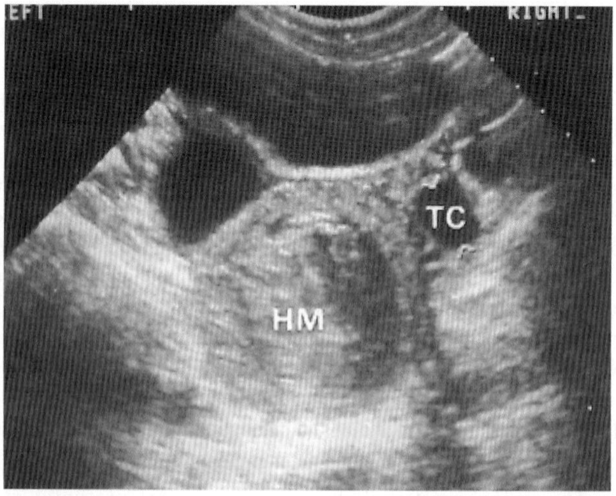

Invasive moles arise when villi and trophoblasts penetrate into the myometrium or even reach the peritoneal cavity. They result from persistent molar pregnancy (75%) or from recurrent GTD (25%) and are usually detected during the follow-up period when β-hCG levels plateau or rise after uterine evacuation. The incidence of invasive moles is approximately 1:15,000 pregnancies. Diagnosis is similar to that for molar gestation. Fortunately, invasive moles rarely metastasize and are sensitive to single-agent chemotherapy, with a cure rate of 95 to 100%.

Gestational choriocarcinoma can arise weeks to years after molar gestations (50%), normal pregnancies (25%), or other gestations such as miscarriage or ectopic pregnancy (25%). It has an incidence of 1:40,000 pregnancies in the United States and is considered a pure epithelial neoplasm, consisting of syncytiotrophoblasts and cytotrophoblasts without chorionic villi. Early hematogenous spread to the lung, vagina, pelvis, brain, and liver can occur; therefore, patients should undergo thorough metastatic evaluation. Single or multi-agent chemotherapy is utilized depending on the presence of metastases. Surgery is not generally a part of choriocarcinoma treatment.

Placental site trophoblastic tumor (PSTT) is a variant of choriocarcinoma that arises from the placental implantation site and consists of cytotrophoblasts and no chorionic villi. Patients can present weeks to years after an antecedent pregnancy with bleeding. These tumors produce chronic low levels of β-hCG and human placental lactogen. Although PSTT is resistant to chemotherapy, it rarely metastasizes beyond the uterus and can be treated with hysterectomy.

• **Figure 9-7.** Complete molar pregnancy on ultrasonography. Note the hydropic villi (seen as black lucent areas) and the general snow storm appearance. *HM,* hydatiform mole; *TC,* theca lutein cyst. (Reprinted with permission from Chamberlin G. Lecture Notes on Obstetrics. 7th ed. Oxford: Blackwell Science, 1996.)

CASE CONCLUSION

The patient's β-hCG returns 256,000 mIU/mL and her blood type is B-negative. Given this and your ultrasound findings, you confirm the diagnosis of complete hydatidiform mole and treat the patient with suction curettage of uterine contents and administer RhoGAM to prevent Rh sensitization. A chest x-ray to evaluate for metastases is normal. The patient is also given oral contraceptives for birth control and subsequently undergoes regular monitoring of β-hCG levels until they go to zero.

THUMBNAIL: FIGO Staging for Gestational Trophoblastic Disease

Stage	Findings
Stage I	Disease confined to the uterus
Stage IA	Disease confined to the uterus with no risk factors
Stage IB	Disease confined to the uterus with one risk factor
Stage IC	Disease confined to the uterus with two risk factors
Stage II	GTT extends outside of the uterus but is limited to the genital structures (e.g., adnexa, vagina, broad ligament)
Stage IIA	GTT involving genital structures with no risk factors
Stage IIB	GTT extends outside of the uterus but limited to the genital structures with one risk factor
Stage IIC	GTT extends outside of the uterus but is limited to the genital structures with two risk factors
Stage III	GTT extends to the lungs with or without known genital tract involvement
Stage IIIA	GTT extends to the lungs with or without genital tract involvement and with no risk factors
Stage IIIB	GTT extends to the lungs with or without genital tract involvement and with one risk factor
Stage IIIC	GTT extends to the lungs with or without genital tract involvement and with two risk factors
Stage IV	All other metastatic sites
Stage IVA	All other metastatic sites with no risk factors
Stage IVB	All other metastatic sites with one risk factor
Stage IVC	All other metastatic sites with two risk factors

Risk Factors:
1. β-hCG >100,000 mIU/mL
2. Duration from termination of antecedent pregnancy to diagnosis >6 months

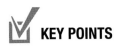

KEY POINTS

- GTD can be classified as benign (partial and complete moles) or malignant (invasive moles, choriocarcinoma, and PSTT)
- The GTDs tend to produce β-hCG, which is used to follow therapy and monitor for recurrence
- Ninety percent of molar pregnancies are complete moles, which commonly have a 46,XX karyotype and no associated fetus
- Malignant GTD is classified as nonmetastatic or metastatic; nonmetastatic GTD can often be treated with single-agent chemotherapy

to preserve fertility, while metastatic GTD can be treated with either single- or multi-agent chemotherapy depending on the presence of risk factors

- Invasive moles are diagnosed when β-hCG levels plateau or rise during the postmolar follow-up period, are generally not metastatic, and can be treated with single-agent chemotherapy, with a 95 to 100% cure rate

QUESTIONS

1. Rank the following GTDs in order of decreasing incidence.

   A. Complete mole, partial mole, invasive mole, choriocarcinoma, placental site trophoblastic tumor
   B. Complete mole, invasive mole, partial mole, placental site trophoblastic tumor, choriocarcinoma
   C. Partial mole, complete mole, choriocarcinoma, invasive mole, placental site trophoblastic tumor
   D. Invasive mole, complete mole, partial mole, choriocarcinoma, placental site trophoblastic tumor
   E. Choriocarcinoma, complete mole, partial mole, invasive mole, placental site trophoblastic tumor

2. Which of the following are potential sites of metastases for choriocarcinoma?

   A. Vagina
   B. Liver
   C. Lungs
   D. Brain
   E. All of the above

3. Which of the following correctly matches the disease with its components?

   A. Complete hydatidiform mole—69,XXY
   B. Partial hydatidiform mole—46,XY

   C. Invasive mole—chorionic villi
   D. Choriocarcinoma—cytotrophoblasts and syncytiotrophoblasts
   E. Placenta site trophoblastic tumor—cytotrophoblasts and chorionic villi

4. A 42-year-old G3P1 presents with vaginal bleeding and is concerned she may have endometrial cancer. Her past gynecologic history is significant for a vaginal delivery of an infant with a neural tube defect 13 years ago, a first trimester miscarriage 10 years ago, and a ruptured ectopic pregnancy for which she underwent surgery 4 years ago. Her β-hCG level is elevated, but you cannot visualize a fetus or a snow storm pattern on ultrasonography. The patient is diagnosed with PSTT and undergoes successful hysterectomy. Which of the following are considered risk factors for GTD?

   A. Age younger than 20 or older than 40 years
   B. Diets low in beta-carotene and folic acid
   C. History of prior molar pregnancy
   D. Women with blood type A married to men with blood type O
   E. All of the above

PART X

Neuroscience

HPI: RS is a 66-year-old right-handed smoker who had sudden onset of right-hand clumsiness 2 hours ago. He initially thought nothing of this problem, but it has progressed to the point that he can barely move his right upper extremity. He presents for further evaluation.

PE: He is awake and alert. His vital signs are stable. He is able to understand your instructions and follow commands but is frustrated by not being able to express himself adequately. He has a halting, stuttering speech pattern. He has trouble finding words. He is not able to repeat words or phrases. He cannot sustain his right arm against gravity and he has a weak grip on the right side. His strength is otherwise intact. His coordination is appropriate to his strength. Sensation and reflexes are normal.

THOUGHT QUESTIONS

- What is the structural implication of impaired speech?
- What cortical areas mediate language?
- Is this patient right-handed or left-handed?
- Where is the lesion?

BASIC SCIENCE REVIEW AND DISCUSSION

When evaluating a patient with impaired speech, one must distinguish between dysarthria and the aphasias. Dysarthria implies a slurring speech quality. It is associated with disruption of motor control to the muscles of speech. Dysarthria is an important feature of lower cranial nerve dysfunction. Upper motor neuron lesions of the corticobulbar pathways innervating the cranial nerve nuclei also can be associated with dysarthria. The aphasias, on the other hand, represent disruption of the cortical language system that can be independent of motor function.

Perisylvian Language Areas

The processing of language requires input of sensory information, processing of that information, integration of that information with previously acquired data, coordination of language output, and language expression. Disruptions of language function are called *aphasias*. The primary language areas involved in this series of functions are all located around the lateral (sylvian) sulcus, in the **dominant hemisphere**. Perisylvian aphasias are associated with disruption of these key structures and are all **characterized by an inability to repeat language.**

Wernicke Area for Receptive Language

Receptive aphasias involve Wernicke area, which is located at the border of the temporal and parietal lobes (parts of Brodmann areas 22 and 39). Patients with **Wernicke aphasia** are unable to understand or repeat language but have fluent, albeit nonsensical, speech. They may make paraphasic errors, substituting words or syllables during relatively fluent speech. **Pure word deafness** is a variant of Wernicke aphasia limited to verbal language, with intact written language. The pathways connecting the auditory cortex to Wernicke area are affected. **Alexia without agraphia** is a variant of Wernicke aphasia limited to written language, with intact spoken language.

Broca Area for Expressive Language

Expressive aphasias involve Broca area, which is located in the inferolateral frontal lobe (Brodmann areas 44 and 45). Broca area is involved in coordinating the motor programs needed to generate language. Like the current patient, patients with **Broca aphasia** have a stuttering speech pattern. They may not be able to name objects. They are unable to repeat or produce fluent language, but they have intact comprehension of language. The **arcuate fasciculus** connects Wernicke area to Broca area. Patients with lesions of the arcuate fasciculus have a **conductive aphasia;** they can understand and produce language but cannot repeat. When all of these areas are affected, patients present with **global aphasia.** Comprehension, repetition, and fluent speech all are lost.

Transcortical Language Pathways

The primary language areas must communicate with higher-order associative cortical regions for language to be integrated into complex cognitive functions. Disruption of these connections results in **transcortical aphasias.** Transcortical aphasias are all **characterized by intact repetition** because Wernicke area, the arcuate fasciculus, and Broca area are all intact. Patients with **transcortical sensory aphasias** generally have lesions in the pathways connecting Wernicke area to the higher-order associative cortex. They have poor comprehension with intact repetition and fluent speech. Patients with **transcortical motor aphasias** generally have lesions of the pathways connecting associative cortical areas to Broca area. They have intact comprehension and repetition with nonfluent speech. In **mixed transcortical aphasia,** repetition is the only language function left intact.

Nondominant Hemisphere

The comparable cortical regions in the contralateral (nondominant) hemisphere mediate prosody. **Prosody** refers to the melodic emotional content of language. Patients with lesions of Brodmann area 44 in the nondominant hemisphere have **aprosodic speech** (monotonic, unemotional). Patients with lesions of Brodmann area 22 in the nondominant hemisphere are not able to detect speech inflection. For example, they cannot detect the difference between a statement of fact and a question, if both are similarly phrased (if you hold out an apple toward them and say "Apple?" they may reply "Yes, it is."). As a general rule, one is more likely to see apraxia with nondominant hemispheric lesions and aphasia with dominant hemispheric lesions.

CASE CONCLUSION

RS was evaluated through an acute stroke protocol that included routine laboratory studies and CT imaging on an emergent basis. He was determined to be a good candidate for thrombolytic therapy, which he tolerated without incident. His symptoms fluctuated over the following days but ultimately stabilized to a moderate right upper extremity hemiparesis. His speech became more fluent, although he continued to have some difficulty with naming. MRI of the brain confirmed a small acute left frontal ischemic infarction. A definitive etiology could not be identified. He was started on an antiplatelet agent and was discharged with arrangements for outpatient therapies.

THUMBNAIL: Frontal Cortex and Language Function

Perisylvian Aphasias

Syndrome	Spontaneous Speech	Comprehension	Repetition
Broca	Nonfluent	Good	Poor
Wernicke	Fluent	Poor	Poor
Conduction	Fluent	Good	Poor
Global	Nonfluent	Poor	Poor

Transcortical Aphasias

Syndrome	Spontaneous Speech	Comprehension	Repetition
Transcortical motor	Nonfluent	Good	Good
Transcortical sensory	Fluent	Poor	Good
Mixed	Nonfluent	Poor	Good
Anomic	Fluent	Good	Good

KEY POINTS

- Broca area for expressive language is in Brodmann areas 44 and 45
- Wernicke area for receptive language is in Brodmann areas 22 and 39
- Pure word deafness is a variant of Wernicke aphasia limited to verbal language, with intact written language
- Alexia without agraphia is a variant of Wernicke aphasia limited to written language, with intact spoken language
- **Prosody** refers to the melodic, emotional content of language

QUESTIONS

1. You evaluate a right-handed patient who is brought in by his family for evaluation of confusion. He has fluent speech but often uses "made-up" words or inappropriate words. When you try to speak to him, he repeats everything you say but does not interact. Where is his lesion?

   A. Right parietal lobe
   B. Left parietal lobe
   C. Wernicke area
   D. Broca area
   E. Left arcuate fasciculus

2. The family of the patient you have just evaluated would like to know the cause of his transcortical sensory aphasia. You explain that he has had a stroke. Compromise of which of the following vascular territories would lead to his deficit?

   A. Right middle cerebral artery (MCA)
   B. Left MCA
   C. Left MCA/anterior cerebral artery (ACA) border zone
   D. Left MCA/posterior cerebral artery (PCA) border zone
   E. Left PCA

3. You evaluate a 67-year-old right-handed gentleman who has had a stroke. He reports that he is having trouble reading. He took some notes while on the telephone but cannot read them even though they appear quite legible. Which of the following regions is likely to be affected?

   A. Left occipital cortex
   B. Right occipital cortex
   C. Left frontal cortex
   D. Right frontal cortex
   E. Left supplementary motor area

4. You are asked to evaluate a patient who was admitted for a cardiovascular evaluation following an episode of chest pain.

The nurse tells you that the patient became aphasic about 20 minutes before your arrival. The patient is somewhat disoriented. He has normal speech rhythm but slurs his words as though intoxicated. He cooperates with your exam and is oriented to his name and the fact that he is in a hospital. He cannot state the year, month, or day of the week. Which of the following structures is implicated?

   A. Broca area
   B. Wernicke area
   C. Arcuate fasciculus
   D. Left parietal cortex
   E. None of the above

HPI: TR is a 65-year-old man who was in good health until approximately 9 months ago. His family reports that they did not notice any problems at the time, but in retrospect, they note that he became more withdrawn. When he does become involved, he seems confused and often interjects inappropriate comments. He also has become increasingly unsteady on his feet and has had several falls. Most recently, he has become incontinent of urine. This has prompted a referral to your office. His only remarkable medical history consists of an episode of meningitis several years ago. His family does not recall the details. Alcohol use is denied.

PE: You note that TR does appear confused at times. He knows the day but makes errors on naming the month and year. It is difficult to engage him in conversation during the exam. He has difficulty with naming, remote memory, and recall. His exam is unremarkable, except for a marked abnormality of gait. He walks with a wide base, seems very unsteady, and slides his feet across the floor as though being held down by magnets.

THOUGHT QUESTIONS

- What is the nature of this patient's confusion?
- Does he have altered perception?
- What cognitive processes are affected?
- What brain regions might be implicated in this case?
- What brain regions are involved in cognition?

BASIC SCIENCE REVIEW AND DISCUSSION

TR presented with a chronic deterioration of cognition and gait with subsequent development of incontinence. This clinical triad (wacky, wobbly, and wet) is the hallmark of **normal-pressure hydrocephalus** (NPH). **Hydrocephalus** is a relative increase in the volume of CSF resulting in dilatation of the ventricles of the brain. Two major categories of hydrocephalus are recognized, either **communicating** or **noncommunicating.** The latter is generally associated with a structural process that obstructs the normal flow of CSF. Examples include tumors in the third or fourth ventricles. In communicating hydrocephalus, the normal flow of CSF is preserved, but, most commonly, the reabsorption of CSF through the arachnoid granulations is slowed. This may be related to previous injury to the arachnoid granulations, as may be seen with meningitis or hemorrhage. Hydrocephalus can present either acutely or chronically, depending on the mechanics of flow disruption. Essentially, NPH is a chronic manifestation of communicating hydrocephalus in adults. Imaging confirms enlargement of the ventricular system out of proportion to any cerebral atrophy that may be present. Imaging is also important to exclude any other structural processes, such as previous extensive ischemia or tumor, which can present similarly. If all other reversible causes are excluded, then ventricular shunting has been reported to be helpful in some cases of NPH. This intervention can be supported by a favorable response to large-volume lumbar puncture, suggesting that some of the deficits may be reversible.

The signs and symptoms illustrated in this patient can be localized to the frontal lobes in general and to the prefrontal cortex in particular. From a clinical standpoint, it is important to note that structural frontal lesions and more generalized processes such as hydrocephalus, metabolic encephalopathy, and dementia can all present similarly. This is related to the fact that the frontal lobes mediate those higher functions that define human behavior. The ventricular system is discussed in more detail separately. Here, we focus on the prefrontal cortex and to a lesser extent on the manifestations of dementia. Note that the dementias are not localized uniquely to the prefrontal cortex. However, the prefrontal manifestations of dementing disorders are particularly striking.

Organization of the Prefrontal Cortex

From a clinical standpoint, the distinction between frontal and prefrontal lesions is somewhat blurred. The **prefrontal cortex** refers to the most anterior portion of the frontal lobe, including the frontal pole. It corresponds to Brodmann areas 9, 10, 11, and 46. The prefrontal cortex is involved in higher order cerebral functions. It facilitates complex tasks that require **integration of information over time.** It is involved in **affective behavior, judgment, creativity,** and **planning of complex movements.**

Given the diverse nature of prefrontal cortical function, it is not surprising that this region is extensively interconnected with other brain areas. The prefrontal cortex receives input from and sends output to other associative cortical areas, the limbic system, the hypothalamus, the thalamus (mainly the dorsomedial nucleus), and the basal ganglia (mainly the head of the caudate nucleus). The prefrontal cortex also receives modulatory input from aminergic brainstem and basal forebrain nuclei. These latter pathways are discussed separately.

The complex nature of prefrontal cortical function makes it difficult to categorize different functional components on an anatomic basis. Much of what is known about the function of the prefrontal cortex is derived from animal studies or anecdotal reports of prefrontal lesions. One of the best known examples is the case of **Phineas Gage,** a 19th century railroad worker. An accidental explosion sent an iron rod through his skull, destroying most of his left prefrontal cortex. He survived and lived another 13 years but had dramatic personality changes. He was noted to have become moody, impulsive, and irresponsible.

Some gross generalizations can be made about prefrontal cortex function on the basis of these kinds of observations. Two major types of syndromes can be identified, although considerable overlap can be seen in the clinical setting. **Dorsolateral prefrontal lesions** tend to be associated with **behavioral apathy.** On the other hand, **orbitofrontal lesions** tend to be associated with **impulsive behavior** and **disruption of normal mood and affect.**

Dorsolateral Prefrontal Cortex

The **dorsolateral prefrontal cortex** seems to be important **for working memory.** This is a temporary storage area for information that is only needed in the moment, like keeping track of the location of other cars while driving. This area also seems to cooperate with the medial temporal lobe in learning new facts. When this area is injured, patients are noted to have **psychomotor retardation,** difficulty with organization of complex tasks, and relative **indifference** to their environment. On exam, they may be noted to have **perseverative behavior,** difficulty generating word lists, and difficulty with repetitive or complex motor tasks. They may not be able to follow multistep commands. Performance of alternating or rhythmic tasks may be impaired. These last deficits also can be associated with extrapyramidal disorders, but remember that the prefrontal cortex is connected to the basal ganglia.

Patients whose lesions extend more medially may become **incontinent** of urine. Their **apathy** may be so profound that they are indifferent to their incontinence. The apathy associated with prefrontal lesions has been used to clinical advantage in the past. The prefrontal lobotomy was a surgical procedure that severed the connection between the prefrontal cortex and the **dorsomedial nucleus of the thalamus.** It was used to treat psychotic patients in the era before the introduction of neuroleptics. It also was used to treat patients with intractable pain. These patients did not experience less pain after the procedure, but they cared less about their pain.

Orbitofrontal Prefrontal Cortex

The **orbitofrontal cortex** is extensively interconnected with the **limbic system.** Patients with lesions in this area tend to have problems with **behavioral control.** They become disinhibited, impulsive, and distractible. They may be emotionally labile and euphoric, and they may have an inappropriate or jocular affect.

Clinical Manifestations of Prefrontal Disease

The clinical manifestations of frontal lobe disease can be quite varied. The features of orbitofrontal and dorsolateral syndromes often overlap. Other characteristic findings are difficult to localize to a specific anatomic location. Patients with prefrontal lesions may have difficulty with **abstract reasoning,** such as proverb interpretation. They may exhibit **poor judgment,** requiring close supervision. **Paratonia (gegenhalten)** may be found during the motor exam. This is a characteristic increase in tone that can seem as though the patient is intentionally resisting the examiner. Primitive reflexes, normally present only in infants, may reemerge. These **frontal release signs** include the grasp, suck, rooting, and snout reflexes. Finally, these patients often have a shuffling **magnetic gait** that can predispose to falls.

Initial screening evaluations of patients with altered mental status are performed to identify potentially reversible causes. These studies include a careful exam to look for localizing clues and neuroimaging to identify structural disturbances or hydrocephalus. Routine laboratory studies include metabolic and hematology panels, thyroid function, and vitamin B12 level, as well as studies to identify infectious or inflammatory processes either systemically or localized to the CNS. EEG is used to identify nonconvulsive seizures and to confirm generalized encephalopathy.

Dementia and Delirium

Although the aforementioned features are commonly associated with frontal lobe lesions, it is important to note the broad range of generalized disorders that can present similarly. The cognitive changes in patients like TR are often seen in the setting of dementia. When assessing such patients, confusion often arises between the diagnosis of delirium and dementia. **Delirium** is an acute state of confusion associated with altered perception. **Dementia,** on the other hand, is a term used to describe chronic deterioration of cognitive function. The two conditions are not mutually exclusive. In fact, patients with dementia often are more susceptible to acute confusional states. Both conditions are commonly encountered as the consequence of general medical problems. Infections, metabolic disturbances, deficiency states, endocrine abnormalities, and toxin exposure (including alcohol and illicit drugs) can all be associated with altered mentation. Dementia, in particular, is often associated with clinical manifestations resembling the frontal lobe syndromes described earlier in this case. This does not mean that the frontal lobe is the primary site of pathology in dementing illnesses. The dementias generally lack specific neuroanatomic localization. The key features of some of the most common forms of dementia are discussed later in this case (see Thumbnail below).

CASE CONCLUSION

TR was admitted to the hospital for evaluation of his deteriorating neurologic function. Initial screening laboratory studies were performed to exclude metabolic, endocrine, nutritional, and toxic causes for his symptoms. No evidence of systemic disease was found. An MRI of the brain did not reveal any structural causes. The ventricular system appeared to be enlarged. A large-volume lumbar puncture was performed and a normal opening pressure was documented. Several hours after the procedure, the family noted some improvement in TR's condition. His condition, however, deteriorated again over several days. Arrangements were made for ventricular shunt placement to treat his NPH.

THUMBNAIL: Prefrontal Cortex

Syndromes	Characteristics	Causes
Broad categories		
Cortical dementias	Memory problems, getting lost, aphasia, apraxia, agnosia, executive problems	Degenerative, vascular, infectious, inflammatory
Subcortical dementias	Bradyphrenia, poor attention and motivation apathy, irritability, depression	Degenerative, vascular, infectious, inflammatory, often reversible general medical conditions

(Continued)

THUMBNAIL: Prefrontal Cortex *(Continued)*

Syndromes	Characteristics	Causes
Dementia plus	Dementia with associated pyramidal, extrapyramidal, or cerebellar signs	Dementia with Lewy bodies; Huntington disease; Parkinson disease; corticobasal degeneration; Creutzfeldt-Jakob disease
Specific syndromes		
Alzheimer disease	Most common dementia; initially cortical dementia pattern with gradually broadening and worsening symptoms	Cerebral atrophy; neuronal loss; amyloid plaques; neurofibrillary tangles; both sporadic and hereditary forms are recognized
Vascular dementia	Second most common dementia; cause, stigmata of multiple infarctions such as hemiparesis, hemianesthesia, or visual field deficits may be seen	Multiple cerebral infarctions
Binswanger syndrome	A vascular dementia syndrome; subcortical dementia features, prominent frontal lobe features	Extensive subcortical white matter ischemic disease
Dementia with Lewy bodies	Intermittent psychosis, parkinsonian features, second most common primary dementia	Intraneuronal Lewy body inclusions—more extensive than Parkinson disease
Frontotemporal dementias	Prominent frontal lobe features	Anterior frontal and/or anterior temporal atrophy can be asymmetric
Pick disease	A frontotemporal dementia; prominent frontal lobe features	Neuronal loss in cortical layers 1 through 3, Pick bodies (neuronal inclusion bodies)
Creutzfeldt-Jakob disease and other spongiform encephalopathies	Rapidly progressive, aggressive dementing illnesses	Prion diseases; mostly sporadic, some hereditary Spongiform cerebral changes; may have elevated 14-3-3 protein in CSF
Pseudodementia	Variable features	Depression

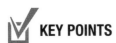

KEY POINTS

- The prefrontal cortex facilitates the integration of information over time
- The prefrontal cortex is involved in affective behavior, judgment, and creativity
- Dorsolateral prefrontal lesions are associated with behavioral apathy
- Orbitofrontal prefrontal lesions are associated with impulsive behavior and disruption of normal mood and affect
- Medial prefrontal lesions are associated with incontinence
- Paratonia (gegenhalten) is a characteristic increase in tone associated with frontal lesions
- Frontal release signs include the grasp, suck, rooting, and snout reflexes
- Delirium is an acute state of confusion associated with altered perception
- **Dementia** is a term used to describe chronic deterioration of cognitive function

QUESTIONS

1. A 50-year-old man with a known history of meningioma is being evaluated for worsening leg weakness and new-onset urinary incontinence. Where is his tumor?

   A. Over the dorsolateral prefrontal cortex, on the left
   B. Over the dorsolateral prefrontal cortex, on the right
   C. Near the orbitofrontal prefrontal cortex, in the midline
   D. Along the falx cerebri, in the midline
   E. Near the pineal gland, in the midline

2. A 36-year-old woman has suffered a rupture of an aneurysm on the anterior communicating artery. She survives and the lesion is clipped. However, she sustains injury to the prefrontal cortex and has marked personality changes. She is noted to be profoundly apathetic to her condition. The connection between her prefrontal cortex and which thalamic nucleus has been affected?

   A. Anterior nucleus of the thalamus
   B. Dorsomedial nucleus of the thalamus
   C. Ventral posterior nucleus of the thalamus
   D. Ventral lateral nucleus of the thalamus
   E. Medial geniculate nucleus (MGN) of the thalamus

3. What are the cardinal manifestations of NPH?

   A. Gait disturbance, snout reflex, and confusion
   B. Incontinence, rooting reflex, and gegenhalten
   C. Incontinence, grasp reflex, and gait disturbance
   D. Gait disturbance, incontinence, and confusion
   E. Confusion, suck reflex, and incontinence

4. You evaluate a patient with an orbitofrontal lesion. Which of the following behaviors is most likely to be seen?

   A. Difficulty organizing complex tasks
   B. Impulsivity
   C. Poor working memory
   D. Apathy
   E. Perseveration

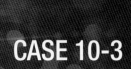

CASE 10-3 Occipital Cortex and Visual Processing

HPI: BS is a 69-year-old right-handed male who presents to the ED with acute onset of vision loss and mental status changes 2 hours ago.

PE: His vital signs are stable. He has a history of atrial fibrillation, but only takes his medications intermittently. He is somewhat somnolent, but he is able to answer orienting questions and follows commands during the exam. His cranial nerve exam reveals a left homonymous hemianopia. His cranial nerve function is otherwise spared. There are no abnormalities noted on testing of motor or sensory function. Coordination is appropriate to the remainder of his exam. He has symmetric reflexes and no long tract signs.

THOUGHT QUESTIONS

- What is the anatomic basis for visual processing?
- What structures are associated with hemianopia?
- What structures are associated with quadrantanopia?
- What other signs and symptoms might one expect in such a case?
- What clues do the acute manifestation and medical history give concerning etiology?

BASIC SCIENCE REVIEW AND DISCUSSION

The acute manifestation of neurologic deficits should always bring to mind the possibility of a vascular cause, particularly in the setting of cardiovascular disease. This patient's symptoms are localized to the occipital lobe. This area is supplied by the PCA, which branches from the posterior circulation of the CNS. Associated symptoms could include vertigo, cranial nerve deficits, motor and sensory deficits, thalamic dysfunction, and peduncular hallucinosis. The clinical manifestations of cerebral vascular disease are discussed in further detail separately. This case focuses on the functional implications of occipital lobe injury. The main function of the occipital lobe is the processing of visual information. Different regions within the occipital lobe process units of information of varying complexity.

Organization of the Occipital Lobe

The **occipital lobe** extends anteriorly from the occipital pole. The anterior boundary of the occipital lobe on the lateral surface of the brain is poorly defined. In this region, the occipital lobe merges with the parietal and temporal lobes. On the medial surface of the brain, the **parieto-occipital sulcus** defines the anterior boundary of the occipital lobe. The **calcarine sulcus** is perpendicular to the parieto-occipital sulcus and extends posteriorly to the occipital pole. These two sulci, together, look like a capital letter *T*.

Visual Cortex and Visual Processing

Remember that visual input to the cortex originates in the **lateral geniculate nucleus** of the thalamus and terminates in the fourth cortical layer of the primary visual cortex. A key point, however, is that visual information processed in one hemisphere represents input from both eyes pertaining to the contralateral visual field. Thus, a cortical lesion involving the occipital lobe on one side, as in the current case, would be expected to result in a **contralateral homonymous hemianopia.** However, there is usually a degree of **macular sparing** in these lesions. This may

be related to an abundant collateral vascular supply of the primary visual cortex and to some bilateral cortical representation of central vision.

The **primary visual cortex,** or calcarine cortex, is contained within and around the calcarine sulcus. It corresponds to **Brodmann area 17.** It is also called the **striate cortex** because it has a striped histologic appearance. This is because the fourth cortical layer in the primary visual cortex is divided by a visible line of white matter, called the **line of Gennari.**

As we have seen in other sensory systems, the organization of the visual cortex is **retinotopic.** This means that adjacent retinal areas and adjacent regions in the visual field are processed in adjacent calcarine cortical areas. The cortical areas responsible for central vision are located most posteriorly in the calcarine cortex, near the **occipital pole.** The amount of cortical area devoted to central vision is disproportionately large, reflecting the importance of the information being received from the **macula.** The remaining retinal areas are represented by cortical areas extending anteriorly from the occipital pole like a collapsed spiderweb. Throughout this cortical system, the regions of cortex responsible for processing information from the upper retina (and lower visual field) are located superior to the calcarine sulcus, in an area called the **cuneus.** The regions of cortex responsible for processing information from the lower retina (and upper visual field), on the other hand, are located inferior to the calcarine sulcus, in an area called the **lingual gyrus.**

Primary Visual Cortex

The processing of visual information has several layers of complexity. Visual processing in the primary visual cortex is concerned primarily with basic visual units that respond preferentially to specific stimuli. Electrical stimulation of the primary visual cortex results in the perception of flashes of light, rather than formed image. Neurons within the primary visual cortex have **receptive fields** that respond preferentially to specific linear visual stimuli (horizontal, vertical, etc.). Neurons that respond to a particular orientation in a particular region of the retina are grouped together within **simple units.** Within each unit, some neurons may respond preferentially to either onset or cessation of illumination. **Complex units** receive information from multiple simple units. Groups of units concerned with a particular stimulus type are called *columns.* **Ocular dominance columns** respond preferentially to input from a given eye. **Orientation columns** respond preferentially to stimuli in a particular orientation in space. Higher-order visual cortex areas are involved in further processing of these basic components of visual input.

Secondary Visual Cortex

The primary visual cortex is generally designated as V1. Subsequently higher orders of visual processing occur in cortical areas designated V2–V5. The **main secondary visual cortical regions** are V2 and V3, which respectively correspond to **Brodmann areas 18 and 19**. Like V1, V2 is organized retinotopically. Neurons in this area have more complex receptive fields. The remaining areas of visual cortex are more concerned with specific aspects of vision. V3 appears to be associated with the processing of more **complex forms.** The localization of V4 and V5 is less precise. Both areas are located in the border area between the occipital and temporal lobes. V4 appears to be associated with the processing of **color information.** V5 has been implicated in the processing of information regarding **the motion of objects in the visual field.** These cortical regions, in turn, project to higher-order associative cortical areas where visual input is integrated with information from other sensory modalities.

The disruption of cortical sensory function can manifest clinically as agnosia. **Agnosia** is a modality-specific inability to recognize sensory input, often localized near the junction of the parietal, occipital, and temporal lobes. The agnosias are summarized later in this case (see Thumbnail below). Note that the visual system plays an important role in many of these clinical manifestations. Output from the visual association cortex to **Brodmann area 7** in the posterior parietal cortex is thought to mediate the **perception of depth and movement.** Output to the associative parietal cortex in **Brodmann areas 39 and 22** is implicated in the visual **recognition of objects and symbols.** Patients with lesions in these areas may not be able to identify objects **(visual agnosia)** and may not be able to read **(alexia).** Output to **Brodmann area 37,** at the occipitotemporal border, is involved in the **recognition of faces.** The loss of this function is called **prosopagnosia.** Output to **Brodmann areas 20 and 21** in the inferior and middle temporal gyri is thought to be associated with the **analysis of form and color.** Stimulation of these areas is associated with complex visual hallucinations.

CASE CONCLUSION

BS was initially evaluated under an acute stroke pathway because of the nature and abrupt onset of his symptoms, as well as his cardiac risk factors. Stat routine laboratory studies, including a coagulation panel, were normal. A CT scan of the head revealed no evidence of hemorrhage or subacute changes. Thrombolytics were initiated and were tolerated without complications. An MRI of the brain confirmed the diagnosis of a right occipital lobe infarction in the distribution of the right PCA. The area of infarction was wedge shaped and consistent with an embolic cause. A cardiology consultation was obtained and, eventually, warfarin therapy was restarted. BS regained some vision in the left half of his visual fields, but it was incomplete. He was also troubled by visual illusions, suggesting a residual impairment of higher-order visual processing.

THUMBNAIL: Occipital Cortex and Visual Processing Agnosias

Subtypes	Manifestations	Localization
Visual		
Apperceptive agnosia	Picture, object, or color not perceived	Parieto-occipital associative cortex
Simultanagnosia	Recognize the parts but not the whole	Parieto-occipital associative cortex
Associative agnosia	Objects perceived but devoid of meaning	Parieto-occipital associative cortex
Prosopagnosia	Inability to recognize faces	Occipitotemporal border
Alexia without agraphia	Pure word blindness; hemianopia; inability to read; writing is spared	Dominant primary visual cortex and splenium of corpus callosum; part of Dejerine syndrome
Alexia with agraphia	Inability to read or write	Dominant angular gyrus
Acalculia	Inability to do math	Parieto-occipital associative cortex; part of Gerstmann syndrome
Auditory		
Verbal agnosia	Pure word deafness	Disconnection of auditory cortex from Wernicke area
Sound agnosia	Impaired recognition of nonverbal sounds	Associative auditory cortex
Sensory amusia	Inability to recognize music	Dominant temporal cortex in musicians Nondominant in nonmusicians
Tactile		
Astereognosia	Inability to recognize objects by touch	Contralateral parietal cortex
Asymbolia	Inability to associate objects to their meaning	Contralateral parietal cortex

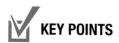

KEY POINTS

- The primary visual cortex is contained within and around the calcarine sulcus
- Unilateral occipital injuries result in contralateral homonymous hemianopia
- Neurons in the visual cortex have receptive fields that respond preferentially to specific linear visual stimuli
- Neurons that respond to a particular orientation in a particular region of the retina are grouped together within simple units

- Complex units receive information from multiple simple units
- Ocular dominance columns respond preferentially to input from a given eye
- Orientation columns respond preferentially to stimuli in a particular orientation in space
- Agnosia is a modality-specific inability to recognize sensory input

QUESTIONS

1. You evaluate a patient with a visual field deficit. You determine that she has a homonymous left superior quadrantanopia. Where is her lesion?

   A. Right occipital lobe
   B. Right parietal lobe
   C. Right temporal lobe
   D. Right optic tract
   E. Right lateral geniculate nucleus of the thalamus

2. You evaluate a patient with known epilepsy. His seizures are associated with vivid visual hallucinations, followed by secondary generalization. Which of the following is most likely to contain his seizure focus?

   A. Posterior parietal cortex
   B. Inferior temporal cortex
   C. Occipitotemporal junction
   D. Angular gyrus
   E. Calcarine cortex

3. You evaluate a woman who has lost color vision. Which region of the visual cortex is most likely to be affected?

   A. V1
   B. V2
   C. V3
   D. V4
   E. V5

4. You evaluate a man who has developed visual illusions in the wake of an ischemic stroke. He states that as he is talking with you, your head appears to be floating away from your body. Which region of the visual cortex is most likely to be affected?

   A. V1
   B. V2
   C. V3
   D. V4
   E. V5

CASE 10-4 Hypothalamus

HPI: HR is an 8-month-old male infant who is being evaluated because of altered level of consciousness and poor feeding. He has had an upper respiratory tract infection and poor oral intake for a few days. He has also had an associated decrease in urine output and has become progressively lethargic. He was noted to be microcephalic at birth but has not been evaluated further for this. He has missed developmental milestones, but his medical history and family history are otherwise unremarkable.

PE: His vital signs are stable. He is sleepy, but easy to arouse, with a good cry. He is microcephalic but has no other prominent dysmorphic features. He is less interactive than his stated baseline. His tone and reflexes are somewhat increased, but he moves all extremities well.

Labs: He has a serum sodium level of 180 mEq/L with a serum osmolality of 350 mOsm/kg.

THOUGHT QUESTIONS

- What type of brain disorders present with altered autoregulation?
- What other functions are mediated by this area?
- To what other brain regions is this area connected?
- What type of developmental problem might be implicated?

BASIC SCIENCE REVIEW AND DISCUSSION

The regulation of salt and water balance is mediated by a hormonal interaction between the hypothalamus, pituitary gland, and kidneys. This case highlights the important role of the hypothalamus in regulation of water balance. **ADH (arginine vasopressin [AVP] in humans)** is produced in the supraoptic and paraventricular nuclei of the **hypothalamus.** It is stored in the **posterior pituitary gland.** The hypothalamus is also involved in monitoring **serum osmolality.** The release of AVP from the posterior pituitary gland is normally triggered by increased serum osmolality, resulting in reabsorption of water in the distal convoluted tubule of the kidney. HR's dehydration from poor oral intake did not trigger an appropriate autoregulatory response. This failure of antidiuresis could be either central or renal. In this case, a **central DI** is suggested by the noted microcephaly and developmental delay. Central DI can be related to impaired osmoreceptor function or to impaired AVP production. However, both etiologies implicate the hypothalamus. This chapter focuses on the structure and function of the hypothalamus. The pituitary gland is discussed separately. Endocrine function and renal function are covered in other volumes in this series.

Organization of the Hypothalamus

The **lamina terminalis** defines the anterior border of the hypothalamus. Structures rostral to this border include the septal nuclei and basal forebrain. The **mammillary bodies** are the most posterior nuclei of the hypothalamus and are rostral to the midbrain. The **internal capsule** forms the lateral border of the hypothalamus. Fibers of the internal capsule come together in this area to form the **cerebral peduncles.** The hypothalamus makes up the floor of the **third ventricle.** The **tuber cinereum** is the most ventral portion of the hypothalamus. The **median eminence** is the most central part of the tuber

cinereum. The **infundibulum** (pituitary stalk) emerges from the median eminence.

Many different nuclei make up the hypothalamus. They can be broadly divided into anterior, tuberal, and posterior groups. Each group can be divided further into medial and lateral zones. The hypothalamic nuclei receive input from a wide variety of brain regions. The most important input sources include brainstem nuclei, the limbic system, intrinsic hypothalamic sensors for autoregulation, and feedback from hypothalamic target areas. Output from the hypothalamus can be divided into a neural division and an endocrine division. **Neural output** from the hypothalamus controls the function of the autonomic nervous system (ANS) and contributes to the limbic system and projects to many other brain regions. The **endocrine function** of the hypothalamus includes both the release of regulatory hormones that influence anterior pituitary gland function and the production of hormones that are transported to and released from the posterior pituitary gland. Pituitary gland function is discussed separately in Case 10-5.

Anterior Hypothalamic Nuclei The anterior hypothalamus includes the anterior hypothalamic area and the supraoptic, suprachiasmatic, and paraventricular nuclei. The anterior hypothalamus monitors serum osmolality, produces the neuropeptides oxytocin and AVP, regulates autonomic function, and helps regulate sleep and circadian rhythms. The **anterior hypothalamic area** and the adjacent **lamina terminalis** contain the receptors that monitor serum osmolality. These **osmoreceptors** regulate the release of **ADH** (i.e., AVP) and help mediate **thirst.** In the present case, HR may have had osmoreceptor dysfunction. He was not able to dilute his serum by reabsorbing water and concentrating the urine (all mediated by AVP). He also did not seem to have increased thirst despite his high serum osmolality. While the anterior hypothalamic area regulates the release of AVP, it is not produced here. AVP is produced in the **supraoptic** and **paraventricular nuclei.** These nuclei are also located in the anterior hypothalamus. They produce oxytocin and AVP. Note that the hormones produced by these anterior hypothalamic nuclei are stored in and released from the **posterior pituitary gland.**

The anterior hypothalamus has two other important functions. Some neurons in the **paraventricular nuclei** project to autonomic nuclei in the brainstem and spinal cord where they help regulate **autonomic function.** In addition, the anterior hypothalamus is involved in regulation of sleep and circadian rhythms. The **suprachiasmatic nucleus** receives input from the retina. It projects to other hypothalamic nuclei, the pineal gland, and several other areas. This system is thought to mediate **circadian rhythms.** A role for the anterior hypothalamic area in the **regulation of sleep** has also been proposed.

Tuberal Hypothalamic Nuclei The tuberal portion of the hypothalamus refers to the central portion of the hypothalamus directly superior to the tuber cinereum. This region includes the lateral, dorsomedial, ventromedial, and arcuate nuclei. The tuberal hypothalamus helps regulate feeding, emotional behavior, and endocrine function. The **lateral nuclei** are interconnected with the reticular formation and other brainstem nuclei. They have been implicated in **feeding behavior and arousal.** Lesions in the lateral hypothalamus are associated with **anorexia and weight loss.** The **dorsomedial** and **ventromedial nuclei** are closely related both anatomically and functionally. They also are involved in regulating **feeding (satiety center)** and **emotional behaviors.** Lesions in this area result in obesity and violent behavior. The ventromedial nuclei, in particular, receive considerable input from the amygdala.

The **arcuate nuclei** are located at the base of the hypothalamus, adjacent to the median eminence. The **median eminence** itself is located in the most proximal portion of the **infundibulum.** This is one of the few areas in the CNS where the **blood–brain barrier is compromised.** Humoral feedback on hypothalamic function is detected here. This is the area where all of the **releasing hormones** that act on the anterior pituitary gland are made. These endocrine interactions are covered in more detail separately. This is also an area where emotional experience can influence endocrine function.

Posterior Hypothalamic Nuclei The posterior hypothalamus can be broadly divided into the posterior nuclei and the mammillary bodies. The posterior hypothalamus is involved in temperature regulation and participates in limbic and memory functions. The **posterior nuclei** are essentially continuous with the **periaqueductal gray matter of the midbrain.** Most neurons in this area project to brainstem nuclei. This area is thought to be important in **temperature regulation.** This area mediates reactions to cold ambient temperature, such as shivering and vasoconstriction. This area may also be involved in maintaining **arousal.**

The **mammillary bodies** have been discussed within the context of the limbic system. The nuclei of the mammillary bodies are the main target of axonal fibers in the **fornix.** Remember that the fornix is made up of fibers projecting from the **subiculum** and the **CA1 region of the hippocampal formation** to the hypothalamus. The mammillary nuclei are divided into medial and lateral groups, both of which receive input from the hippocampus. The medial **mammillary nuclei** subsequently project to the **anterior nucleus of the thalamus** along the **mammillothalamic tract.** This is a component of the main limbic circuitry. The lateral mammillary nuclei project to nuclei in the midbrain and the pons. This pathway may be involved in memory and autonomic systems.

CASE CONCLUSION

The patient was admitted to the hospital for further evaluation. Supportive measures were initiated to treat the osmolality disturbance. The serum sodium level was stabilized with desmopressin (DDAVP). An MRI of the brain revealed holoprosencephaly, which is a failure of cerebral hemisphere separation. **Holoprosencephaly** is the most common developmental defect to involve the forebrain and midface, although the face may not be involved in all cases. This disorder is characterized by developmental delay, disruption of autoregulation, hydrocephalus, abnormal tone, and poor feeding. A variety of hypothalamic disturbances can be seen because the hypothalamus is a midline structure. These include dysautonomia, central DI, and other endocrine deficiencies. Nearly half of all cases have been linked to one of several genetic abnormalities. **Trisomy 13** is the most commonly encountered clinically. **Mutations of the Sonic hedgehog gene** are also an important association. Survival is correlated with cause. Few of these infants survive beyond the first year if a chromosomal abnormality is found. Survival at 1 year is as high as 50% in the absence of a documented chromosomal abnormality. HR ultimately returned to baseline and was discharged with arrangements for follow-up in the endocrinology and neurology clinics. Appropriate genetic testing was performed and counseling was provided to the family.

THUMBNAIL: Developmental Malformations of the CNS

A complete review of embryology and developmental disorders is beyond the scope of this text. However, several key elements from these disciplines should be emphasized. The manifestations of major CNS malformations can be divided on the basis of developmental stages. These categories are summarized in the following table:

Developmental Period	Likely Abnormality	Clinical Manifestations
1–4 weeks' gestation	Failure of neural tube closure	Anencephaly Encephalocele Meningomyelocele
4–8 weeks' gestation	Midline malformations of prosencephalon	Holoprosencephaly Callosal agenesis Arrhinencephaly Septo-optic dysplasia Colpocephaly
8–20 weeks' gestation	Disruption of cortical organization	Lissencephalies Heterotopias
After 20 weeks' gestation	Predominantly secondary events, ischemia, etc.	Schizencephaly

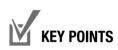

KEY POINTS

- The hypothalamus has both neural and endocrine functions
- Hypothalamic nuclei can be divided into anterior, tuberal, and posterior groups
- The anterior hypothalamus monitors serum osmolality, regulates autonomic function, and helps regulate sleep and circadian rhythms
- The anterior hypothalamus produces the neuropeptides oxytocin and vasopressin (AVP), which are stored in the posterior pituitary gland

- The tuberal hypothalamus helps regulate feeding, emotional behavior, and endocrine function
- The posterior hypothalamus is involved in temperature regulation and participates in limbic and memory functions

QUESTIONS

1. A 52-year-old woman presents with acute confusion and memory difficulties. You suspect a nutritional deficiency may be related to her condition. Which of the following anatomic findings is most likely to be seen?

   A. Hypertrophy of the pituitary gland
   B. Atrophy of the paraventricular nuclei
   C. Atrophy of the mammillary bodies
   D. Hypertrophy of the mammillary bodies
   E. Arcuate nucleus degeneration

2. You evaluate a 12-year-old boy with intractable epilepsy. His seizures are characterized by episodes of uncontrollable laughter with retained consciousness. After the spells, he reports that he does not find anything particularly funny. He is rather scared during his spells. Which of the following regions is likely to be affected?

   A. Amygdala
   B. Hypothalamus
   C. Hippocampus

   D. Parahippocampal cortex
   E. Entorhinal cortex

3. You see a patient who is suspected of having a rare lesion involving his anterior hypothalamus. Which of the following is an unlikely manifestation of his lesion?

   A. Osmotic instability
   B. Disruption of circadian rhythm
   C. Dysautonomia
   D. Poor temperature regulation
   E. Trouble sleeping

4. You see another patient who is suspected of having a rare lesion. This one involves the posterior hypothalamus. Which of the following is an unlikely manifestation of his lesion?

   A. Disruption of appetite control
   B. Impaired arousal
   C. Poor memory performance
   D. Impaired vasoconstriction
   E. Poor temperature control

HPI: A 36-year-old woman presents to your gynecology practice complaining of amenorrhea for the past 8 months. With the exception of her one normal pregnancy at age 23, she reports having normal menses from age 13 until a year ago, when her periods became irregular and then ceased altogether. She has not lost any weight in this time but notes she has been having headaches with increasing frequency. Upon questioning, she notes a recent episode of galactorrhea, although she has not been pregnant or breast-feeding for more than 10 years. A pregnancy test in your office is negative.

THOUGHT QUESTIONS

- Disease in what part of the CNS could produce this constellation of symptoms?
- What pathways does the brain use to affect endocrine function?
- What specific hormones are directly regulated by the brain, through which mechanisms?

BASIC SCIENCE REVIEW AND DISCUSSION

This patient describes symptoms of a **prolactinoma,** one type of tumor of the pituitary gland. To make this diagnosis and properly treat the tumor, one must understand the normal anatomy and function of the pituitary gland.

The pituitary gland lies at the **sella turcica,** inferior to the hypothalamus and just next to the optic chiasm. It is connected to the hypothalamus by the **pituitary stalk,** which allows for hypothalamic signals to directly regulate pituitary function. The pituitary gland has two parts: the anterior lobe (adenohypophysis) and the posterior lobe (neurohypophysis) (Fig. 10-1).

The **anterior lobe** of the pituitary is the largest portion, making about three fourths of the mass of the pituitary. It receives hypothalamic input via a portal vascular system—vessels pass from the hypothalamus directly to the anterior lobe. Embryologically, the anterior lobe arises from the Rathke pouch and is connected to the brain by these blood vessels. Hypothalamic-releasing hormones pass through the portal vessels to the anterior pituitary, where they stimulate the release of pituitary hormones. These include **GH, ACTH, MSH, TSH, FSH,** and **LH. Prolactin** is the major exception to the positive effect of hypothalamic hormones; dopamine released by the hypothalamus *inhibits* prolactin secretion from the anterior pituitary. Some of these hormones have similar structures. For example, TSH, LH, and FSH share an α subunit and are only different in their β subunit. Likewise, ACTH and MSH have similar precursors. Nonetheless, each of these hormones is made by specific cells with certain histologic characteristics. Acidophilic staining indicates somatotrophs, which make GH, or lactotrophs, which make prolactin. Basophilic staining indicates corticotrophs, which make ACTH; thyrotrophs, which make TSH; or gonadotrophs, which make FSH and LH. To further distinguish cell types, special antibody stains are used. Knowing the general staining patterns is useful in distinguishing which type of pituitary adenoma is present in a given histology sample from a pituitary biopsy (both clinically and on the USMLE).

The **posterior lobe** of the pituitary is the smaller portion, made of modified glial cells and direct axonal projections from the hypothalamus (as contrasted with the portal vascular system to the anterior pituitary). Embryologically, the posterior lobe arises from a budding of tissue from the floor of the third ventricle of the brain. Hypothalamic projections from the paraventricular nuclei to the posterior lobe release **oxytocin,** and those from the supraoptic nuclei release vasopressin (or **ADH**). Oxytocin is important in some smooth muscle contractions, particularly uterine contractions, whereas ADH acts on the collecting duct to allow the kidney to concentrate urine.

Clinical Correlates

The pituitary gland can cause disease through either hyperpituitarism or hypopituitarism. **Hyperpituitarism,** or too much hormone secretion, is usually the result of a hormone-secreting pituitary adenoma. **Prolactinomas** are the most common type of anterior pituitary adenoma, constituting 30% of these tumors. In advanced cases, pituitary adenomas can cause visual changes such as **bitemporal hemianopia.** In these instances, the enlarged pituitary compresses the optic chiasm, causing a loss of visual fields. Most typically this affects the vision in the lateral (temporal) fields of each eye. Before mass effects such as headaches or visual changes occur, pituitary adenomas will generally manifest through endocrine hyperfunction. For example, prolactin secretion is necessary in pregnancy for normal lactation. High prolactin levels also inhibit ovulation and normal menstruation. Therefore, a woman with a prolactinoma will present earliest with a loss of menses and sometimes galactorrhea caused by the end organ effects of prolactin. Likewise, adenomas that secrete TSH can present with symptoms of hyperthyroidism, those that secrete ACTH can present with cushingoid features, and so on.

Hypopituitarism can be the result of ischemia in times of blood loss, radiation, inflammation, or tumors that do not actively secrete hormones but cause destruction of normal functioning tissue. In these cases, disease generally becomes apparent through the absence of hormone activity. As such, ischemic damage to the pituitary may not be immediately apparent but may manifest through chronic amenorrhea or hypothyroidism. Likewise, damage to the posterior pituitary may become apparent as **diabetes insipidus (DI),** a problem of decreased ADH activity in the kidney. Patients with DI lose the ability to concentrate their urine; they present with symptoms of polyuria and polydipsia.

The **pituitary stalk** is a common site of injury in certain types of trauma, such as motor vehicle accidents. Shearing momentum of the brain against the skull in a jarring stop causes transection of the thin stalk, disrupting hypothalamic signaling to the pituitary. In these cases, panhypopituitarism may present acutely along with elevated prolactin levels. This is because most pituitary hormones have lost the stimulation of releasing factors from the hypothalamus, and prolactin has lost the inhibition of dopamine.

Pituitary disorders are often treated medically by supplementing hormone levels as needed. For example, glucocorticoids or

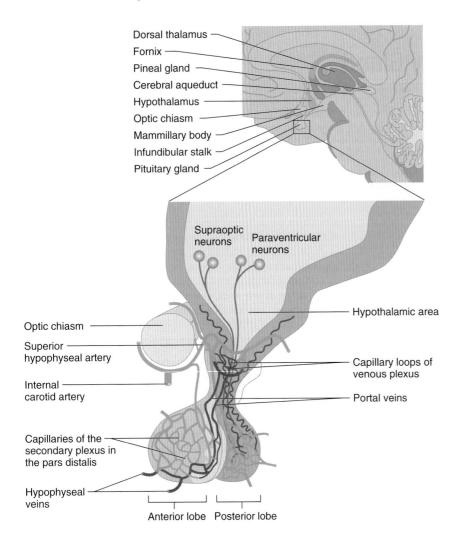

• **Figure 10-1.** Anatomy of the pituitary gland. Note the location of the pituitary in relation to the hypothalamus, mammillary bodies, and optic chiasm. The anterior lobe of the pituitary is connected to the hypothalamus via a portal system of veins. These carry hormone signals to the anterior lobe. The posterior lobe receives signals through direct axonal inputs from the hypothalamus running through the infundibular stalk.

thyroid hormone can be given to compensate for low levels of ACTH or TSH, respectively. Hyperpituitarism can be treated medically in the case of prolactinoma; bromocriptine is a dopamine agonist that can be taken to inhibit prolactin secretion.

In other cases, surgery may be required to remove the adenoma. In these cases, transsphenoidal surgery of the pituitary can remove the entire adenoma with minimal disruption of brain anatomy.

CASE CONCLUSION

Given the patient's symptoms, you refer her for blood work and a CT to determine whether there might be a common cause of her headaches, galactorrhea, and amenorrhea. Indeed, CT reveals an enlarged pituitary gland, which corresponds with her elevated blood prolactin levels. You begin treatment with oral bromocriptine, which soon provides relief from her galactorrhea, and within months, normal menses return. Her adenoma is able to be well controlled by medical therapy alone at this time, but you plan regular follow-up to ensure no new symptoms arise and the adenoma does not grow further.

THUMBNAIL: Characteristics of Pituitary Hormones

Pituitary Hormone	Released by Which Lobe?	Produced by Which Cells?	Cell Appearance	Hormone Effects
Prolactin	Anterior	Lactotrophs	Acidophilic	Lactation, inhibits menstruation
GH	Anterior	Somatotrophs	Acidophilic	Growth

(Continued)

THUMBNAIL: Characteristics of Pituitary Hormones *(Continued)*

Pituitary Hormone	Released by Which Lobe?	Produced by Which Cells?	Cell Appearance	Hormone Effects
TSH	Anterior	Thyrotrophs	Basophilic	Thyroid function
ACTH	Anterior	Corticotrophs	Basophilic	Cortisol release
FSH, LH	Anterior	Gonadotrophs	Basophilic	Ovulation, menstruation
Oxytocin	Posterior	Paraventricular hypothalamic projections	N/A	Uterine contraction
ADH	Posterior	Supraoptic hypothalamic projections	N/A	Urine concentration

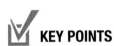

KEY POINTS

- The pituitary gland has two components: the anterior lobe and the posterior lobe
- The anterior lobe is stimulated by releasing hormones from the hypothalamus, which are delivered via the portal vascular system
- The anterior lobe releases prolactin, GH, ACTH, TSH, FSH, and LH

- All anterior lobe hormone release is stimulated by hypothalamic-releasing hormones; the only exception is prolactin, which is under inhibitory control by dopamine
- The posterior lobe has direct axonal connections from the hypothalamus
- The posterior lobe releases oxytocin and ADH

QUESTIONS

1. A patient develops significant blood loss after childbirth, causing massive ischemic damage to the anterior pituitary. This condition, known as Sheehan's syndrome, would cause which of the following sets of hormone levels?

	Cortisol	FSH	T_4	Prolactin	ADH
A.	decreased	decreased	decreased	decreased	decreased
B.	decreased	decreased	decreased	increased	normal
C.	decreased	decreased	decreased	increased	decreased
D.	decreased	decreased	decreased	decreased	normal
E.	normal	normal	normal	increased	decreased

2. A 40-year-old patient presents with a hormone-secreting pituitary adenoma. Biopsy of the tumor shows proliferation of a single type of acidophilic cells. Which of the following signs and symptoms are most likely?

   A. Hypertension, obesity, diabetes
   B. Heat intolerance, weight loss, tachycardia
   C. Inability to breast-feed, menorrhagia, headache
   D. Enlarged jaw, diabetes, increased hand size
   E. Polyuria, increased thirst, low urine-specific gravity

3. A patient comes to her primary care provider complaining of fatigue, cold intolerance, weight gain, and hair loss. Suspecting possible hypothyroidism, the provider orders blood tests to assess her thyroid function. The assay for TSH must be specific for the β subunit, because TSH shares an α subunit with which of the following other hormones?

   A. FSH, LH
   B. FSH, ACTH
   C. ACTH, MSH
   D. MSH, LH
   E. FSH, MSH

4. A patient with central DI begins therapy with a vasopressin nasal spray. This medication replaces the hormone usually secreted by which set of pituitary cells?

   A. Acidophilic cells of the anterior lobe
   B. Basophilic cells of the anterior lobe
   C. Cells of the posterior lobe receiving projections from the paraventricular hypothalamus
   D. Cells of the posterior lobe receiving projections from the supraoptic hypothalamus
   E. Cells of the posterior lobe receiving signals through the hypothalamic portal vein

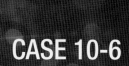

CASE 10-6 Autonomic Nervous System

HPI: TD is a 68-year-old man who has been undergoing physical therapy for left shoulder pain over the past year. He has otherwise been in relatively good health despite a significant smoking history. He is being evaluated because of his persistent shoulder problems.

PE: On meeting him, you notice that his left pupil is somewhat smaller than the right one. His left eyelid also seems somewhat drooped. An extensive exam does not reveal any other deficits. Of incidental note, TD found his exam somewhat strenuous and had broken into a sweat. You notice that he seems to be sweating more on the right side of his face than on the left.

THOUGHT QUESTIONS

- Which system regulates the identified abnormalities?
- Where in the brain does this system begin?
- What path does the system follow to its targets?
- What types of problems might be implicated?

BASIC SCIENCE REVIEW AND DISCUSSION

TD has the triad of **ptosis, miosis,** and **anhydrosis.** These are the classic features of **Horner syndrome,** which results from disruption of sympathetic innervation to the face and eye. A lesion anywhere along the course of the sympathetic nervous system from the hypothalamus down to the upper thoracic spinal cord and back up along the carotid circulation can cause this syndrome. A CNS process can be excluded by the absence of any other neurologic deficits. The involvement of the face along with the eye on the left helps localize the lesion between the extra-axial thoracic spine and the carotid artery on the left. Combined with the smoking history and shoulder pain, the most likely explanation is a **Pancoast tumor** (involving the apex of the lung) with compression of the superior cervical ganglion.

Anatomy of the Autonomic Nervous System

The ANS mediates control of **homeostasis,** influencing critical functions such as BP, HR, and temperature regulation. The motor component of this system can be distinguished from the somatic motor system in several ways. Unlike somatic motor function (striated muscles), autonomic motor function is largely involuntary (smooth muscle and cardiac muscle). Somatic motor output from the CNS is monosynaptic (lower motor neuron projecting to target). Autonomic motor output is disynaptic (preganglionic neuron to postganglionic neuron to target). In the somatic system, motor output is always excitatory, and inhibition occurs centrally via interneurons. In the ANS, output to a given target can be either excitatory or inhibitory. The ANS is separated into **sympathetic** and **parasympathetic** divisions that often exert opposing influences on a given target. The varying effects of sympathetic and parasympathetic function are summarized later in this case (see Thumbnail below).

Control of autonomic function occurs largely below the level of consciousness and is regulated by the **hypothalamus.** Changes in homeostasis are detected in the hypothalamus and appropriate responses are generated to help maintain homeostasis. Hypothalamic function is reviewed in Case 10-4. The hypothalamus influences the activity of **autonomic preganglionic neurons** (located in the brainstem or spinal cord). The axons of these neurons exit the CNS and make synaptic contact with postganglionic neurons located in **autonomic ganglia.** The location of the postganglionic neurons differs between the two divisions. Postganglionic neurons in the two divisions also use different neurotransmitters.

Sympathetic Nervous System

Sympathetic control descends from the level of the hypothalamus to preganglionic neurons in the **intermediolateral cell columns** in the **thoracolumbar spinal cord.** Preganglionic axons, which are myelinated, leave the spinal cord and enter the adjacent sympathetic chain ganglia via the **white communicating rami** (**white** because the axons within are myelinated). Once in the sympathetic chain, these axons may ascend or descend briefly before making synaptic contact with **postganglionic neurons.** The postganglionic axons exit the sympathetic chain via the **gray communicating rami** (**gray** because the axons within are unmyelinated) and join peripheral nerves to get to their targets. For example, sympathetic innervation to the head originates in the **superior cervical (stellate) ganglion,** which is at the top of the **sympathetic chain.** These sympathetic nerves travel along the **carotid arteries,** their branches, and then join branches of various cranial nerves to reach their targets.

Outflow from the sympathetic chain to target organs is divergent. This means that many different target organs will be stimulated "in sympathy" (i.e., will all be influenced at the same time) by sympathetic activity. This ability to react in concert is important for those behaviors mediated by the sympathetic system **(fight or flight).** The sympathetic system mediates rapid responses to environmental stressors. Sympathetic effects include increased cardiac output, pupillary dilation, increased energy availability, and maintenance of temperature by shivering, piloerection, and vasoconstriction. Sympathetic innervation to the adrenal medulla is unique in that it is only preganglionic.

Parasympathetic Nervous System

Parasympathetic control descends from the level of the hypothalamus to preganglionic neurons in brainstem nuclei and the sacral spinal cord. The parasympathetic system is also called the **craniosacral system,** based on the distribution of its preganglionic neurons. The preganglionic axons exit the CNS along cranial or peripheral nerves. They reach postganglionic neurons contained within peripheral parasympathetic ganglia, which are located close to the target organs. Postganglionic axons in the parasympathetic system then travel to their final target. The parasympathetic system is less divergent than the sympathetic system. The parasympathetic system is concerned with maintaining baseline conditions such as

TABLE 10-1 Major Functions Mediated by Adrenoreceptors and Muscarinic Receptors

	α_1-Receptors	α_2-Receptors	β_1-Receptors	β_2-Receptors	ACh$_{muscarinic}$
BP	Increased	—	Increased	—	Decreased
Cardiac output	—	—	Increased	—	Decreased
Heart rate	—	—	Increased	—	Decreased
Blood vessels	Vasoconstriction	—	—	Vasodilation in skeletal and cardiac muscle	—
Lungs	—	—	—	Bronchodilation	Bronchoconstriction
Pupils	Mydriasis	—	—	—	Miosis
Metabolism	—	Decreased insulin release	Increased lipid utilization	Increased glycogen utilization	Promotes glucose storage

basal HR, respirations, and metabolic activity **(rest and digest).** **Cranial nerves III, VII, IX,** and **X** all have a parasympathetic component. Cranial parasympathetic functions include pupillary constriction, lens accommodation, lacrimation, salivation, and control of cardiac function. The **sacral component** of the parasympathetic system innervates the urinary tract, bladder, distal large intestine, and reproductive organs. Autonomic functions in various organs are reviewed later in this case (see Thumbnail below).

Enteric Nervous System

Both the sympathetic and parasympathetic divisions of the ANS contribute to the innervation of the GI tract. The **enteric nervous system** is considered by many to be a third autonomic division. Sympathetic preganglionic fibers contributing to this system bypass the sympathetic chain ganglia and terminate in several **splanchnic ganglia** within the abdomen. Postganglionic sympathetic fibers from these ganglia then contribute to a meshwork of nerve fibers within the intestinal walls. The sympathetic contribution to the enteric nervous system inhibits motility and secretion.

Parasympathetic preganglionic fibers contributing to this system originate in both the cranial and the sacral portions of the parasympathetic system. They terminate in **enteric ganglia** located within the intestinal walls. The enteric ganglia, their postganglionic projections, and associated contributions from the sympathetic system make up the enteric nervous system. This system is further divided into a **submucosal (Meissner) plexus** and a **myenteric (Auerbach) plexus.** The parasympathetic contribution to the enteric nervous system promotes motility and secretion.

Autonomic Neurotransmitters

All autonomic preganglionic neurons use **acetylcholine (ACh)** as their primary neurotransmitter. A variety of **neuropeptides** can be co-secreted with ACh. The two divisions of the autonomic system differ in their postganglionic neurotransmitters.

Postganglionic parasympathetic neurons also use **ACh** as their primary neurotransmitter. Again, several neuropeptides also can be released as secondary neurotransmitters. **Postganglionic sympathetic neurons** use **norepinephrine (NE)** as

their primary neurotransmitter and use neuropeptides as secondary neurotransmitters.

ACh acts through both nicotinic and muscarinic cholinergic receptors. The binding of ACh to **nicotinic receptors** triggers a fast excitatory postsynaptic potential (EPSP). This interaction often results in an **action potential.** It should be noted that autonomic nicotinic receptors are structurally different from the receptors found at the neuromuscular junction in striated muscle. The binding of ACh to **muscarinic receptors** may trigger either slow EPSPs or **slow inhibitory postsynaptic potentials (IPSPs).** The release of **neuropeptides** also can result in slow EPSPs. In addition, the release of neuropeptides can act through second-messenger systems to modify the efficiency of the co-secreted primary neurotransmitter. **NE** acts through several **different adrenoreceptors** (α_1, α_2, β_1, and β_2). Some of the major functions mediated by the different adrenoreceptors and muscarinic cholinergic receptors are summarized in Table 10-1.

Autonomic Dysfunction

Autonomic disorders are broadly divided into primary and secondary syndromes. The etiology of **primary dysautonomia** is often unclear. Both sympathetic and parasympathetic systems are usually involved. The most commonly encountered acute primary dysautonomia is vasovagal **syncope** (fainting), which is caused by increased parasympathetically mediated bradycardia in the setting of decreased sympathetic vasoconstrictor tone. The most commonly encountered chronic primary dysautonomia is **orthostatic hypotension** (in the absence of dehydration or other neurologic disease). Multiple system atrophy (MSA) describes a combination of dysautonomia, parkinsonism, and cerebellar dysfunction. Three forms of this disorder are recognized (parkinsonian, cerebellar, and mixed). The term Shy-Drager syndrome also has been used to describe dysautonomia in combination with other neurologic deficits.

The list of conditions resulting in **secondary dysautonomia** is extensive. As seen in TD's case, a structural lesion anywhere along the course of the ANS can disrupt its function. Diseases of the brainstem and spinal cord, such as infarction (as in **Wallenberg syndrome**), demyelinating lesions, trauma, and tumors, can all be associated with dysautonomia. Many conditions can also be associated with neuropathy causing peripheral dysautonomia. The most common of these include **diabetes mellitus (DM)** and the toxic effects of drugs or **alcohol.** Disorders of neuromuscular transmission can also result in impaired autonomic function.

Synkinesis is another interesting manifestation of autonomic dysfunction in which functions not usually associated with each other become linked. This usually occurs as a result of aberrant reinnervation following injury to a nerve. For example, lacrimation may become linked to salivation **(crocodile tears)** following facial nerve injury.

CASE CONCLUSION

TD was suspected of having a Pancoast tumor. A chest x-ray film was unrevealing. A CT scan of the chest confirmed a large, left apical lung mass with extension into the adjacent soft tissues. Biopsy confirmed a non–small cell carcinoma. TD was referred for an oncology evaluation and further management of his carcinoma. Arrangements were made for presurgical irradiation and subsequent resection and chemotherapy.

THUMBNAIL: Autonomic Nervous System

	Sympathetic Effects	Parasympathetic Effects
Pupils	Mydriasis	Miosis
Ciliary muscle (lens shape)	—	Contraction (accommodation for near vision)
Lacrimation	—	Promotes tearing
Salivation	Thick secretions	Thin secretions
Cardiac output	Increased	Decreased
Blood vessels	Vasoconstriction and vasodilation	—
Lungs	Bronchodilation	Bronchoconstriction; increased secretions
GI tract	Decreased motility; decreased secretions	Increased motility; increased secretions
Urinary bladder	Relaxes detrusor (promotes retention)	Contracts detrusor (promotes excretion)
Sphincter muscles (bowel and urinary)	Contracts sphincters	Relaxes sphincters
Adrenal medulla	"Preganglionic" cholinergic fibers trigger epinephrine release	—
Sweat glands	"Preganglionic" cholinergic stimulation	—
Reproduction	Ejaculation; uterine relaxation	Erection
Metabolism	Promotes energy use	Promotes energy storage

KEY POINTS

- Horner syndrome is characterized by sympathetic dysfunction, resulting in ptosis, miosis, and anhydrosis
- Preganglionic sympathetic neurons are located in the intermediolateral cell columns of the thoracolumbar spinal cord
- Sympathetic output is divergent, allowing target organs to react simultaneously to environmental stressors
- The parasympathetic system is also called the **craniosacral system,** based on the distribution of its preganglionic neurons
- The parasympathetic system is concerned with maintaining basal conditions

- The most common acute primary dysautonomia is vasovagal syncope
- The most common chronic primary dysautonomia is orthostatic hypotension
- Neuropathy, as seen in DM, can be associated with peripheral dysautonomia
- In synkinesis, functions not usually associated with each other become linked as a result of aberrant regeneration following nerve injury

QUESTIONS

1. A 52-year-old woman presents with a left internal carotid artery dissection and associated right-sided hemiparesis. Which of the following might be an associated finding?

   A. Mydriasis on the left
   B. Mydriasis on the right
   C. Increased sweating on the left side of the face
   D. Miosis on the right
   E. Miosis on the left

2. A 63-year-old man has been diagnosed with a right-sided posterior communicating artery aneurysm. Which of the following might be an associated finding?

   A. Mydriasis on the left
   B. Mydriasis on the right
   C. Increased sweating on the left side of the face
   D. Miosis on the right
   E. Miosis on the left

3. You evaluate a newborn for excessive vomiting. He was born 48 hours ago and still has not passed any meconium. His abdomen is distended. You are able to appreciate colonic peristalsis and note a palpable fecal mass. You are able to determine that several family members have had similar problems. What neurons are affected?

   A. Preganglionic sympathetic neurons
   B. Postganglionic parasympathetic neurons
   C. Preganglionic parasympathetic neurons
   D. Postganglionic sympathetic neurons
   E. Neurons in the splanchnic ganglia

4. You evaluate a 34-year-old man who is recovering from a spinal cord injury sustained in a motorcycle accident. He confides in you that he has not been able to achieve an erection since his accident. Which of the following neurons is most likely to have been affected?

   A. Preganglionic sympathetic neurons
   B. Neurons in the splanchnic ganglia
   C. Cranial preganglionic parasympathetic neurons
   D. Postganglionic sympathetic neurons
   E. Sacral preganglionic parasympathetic neurons

HPI: A 25-year-old man is brought to the hospital after being shot in the back. He is conscious and shouts that he is unable to walk and cannot feel his left leg. He is taken to the neurosurgical suite where the bullet and bone fragments are removed. You are able to examine him after he has been stabilized and the anesthesia has worn off. He is now able to tell you that he still cannot feel his left leg and cannot move it, but he does note that his left toes feel cold.

PE: T 100.4°F; HR 105 beats/min; BP 155/85 mm Hg; RR 14 breaths/min; SaO$_2$ 94% on room air

Previous medical history (PmHx): The patient had an appendectomy 14 years ago. **Medication (Rx):** He did not take any medications before this incident.

Sensation to pressure and light touch is absent on the left side up to and including the T10 dermatome. Surprisingly, sensation to temperature and pain is absent on the *right side* up to the T10 dermatome. He cannot feel pain or temperature bilaterally in the T10 dermatome itself. Strength is absent in the left leg and hip muscles, but upper extremity strength is intact bilaterally. He has a clean and dry dressing over the surgical site in the lower thoracic region of the back.

THOUGHT QUESTIONS

- How can this constellation of symptoms be explained?
- Where is the likely lesion?
- What is the prognosis?

BASIC SCIENCE REVIEW AND DISCUSSION

The Somatosensory System: From Nerve Endings to the Cortex

Nerve Endings, Types of Sensation Somatic sensation, using the skin, muscles, and joints as sensory organs, begins at the level of the receptor, usually located within or just deep to the dermis. The viscera also have receptors, which are not discussed here. Each different receptor type allows for a slightly different type of sensation. A few major types are highlighted here, although there are many other types of receptors.

- *Pacinian corpuscles:* the largest receptors, "onion skin" structure, detect deep pressure
- *Muscle spindle and Golgi tendon organ:* provide proprioceptive information by recognizing stretch on muscles and tendons, respectively
- *Nociceptors:* simple free nerve endings that detect pain
- *Meissner corpuscles:* smaller receptors that detect light touch

Peripheral Sensory Nerves Once an action potential has been generated with the appropriate stimulus at a nerve ending, it is transduced to the spinal cord via the afferent peripheral nerves, which come in various nerve fibers. Pain fibers are either **unmyelinated** or **thin myelinated** fibers. On the other hand, fine touch may be transmitted via thick myelinated fibers.

Spinal Cord Tracts Afferent input from the somatosensory system arrives at the spinal cord via the **dorsal nerve root** (Fig. 10-2). Action potentials transverse the **dorsal root ganglion** along this pathway, as peripheral sensory nerves are **pseudounipolar** neurons (there is no synapse at the ganglion, merely the transition from dendrite to axons). The dorsal root transmits action potentials to the **dorsal horn** of the spinal cord.

There are three major somatic sensory systems, each of which is discussed separately. The **dorsal columns system** governs sensation of fine touch, conscious proprioception, and vibratory sense. The **spinothalamic system** governs sensation of pain and temperature, as well as crude touch. The **spinocerebellar system** governs sensation of unconscious proprioception.

Dorsal Columns System Afferent fibers from the periphery arrive via the dorsal nerve root and synapse onto cell bodies located in the dorsal columns of the spinal cord (hence the name). Axons from the sacral and lumbar nerve roots run directly into and up (without synapsing) the **medial** dorsal column of the spinal cord, more specifically named the **fasciculus gracilis.** Thoracic and cervical dorsal root axons run up the other (more lateral) dorsal column, the **fasciculus cuneatus.** These fascicular axons synapse on the **nucleus gracilis and nucleus cuneatus,** respectively, in the ipsilateral medulla. Second-order neurons located in these nuclei collectively project fibers that cross the midline to form the **medial lemniscus,** which projects onto the **ventral posterolateral nucleus of the thalamus.** Finally, third-order neurons located in the thalamus project to the **postcentral gyrus** of the cortex, where all sensation is brought to consciousness.

Spinothalamic System The spinothalamic system crosses at the level of the dorsal root, unlike the dorsal column system. Multiple modulatory factors are in place throughout the spinothalamic system, which explains why the same stimulus may be mild or excruciating, depending on the context.

The initial stimulus must excite a receptor in the periphery, be it for temperature, crude touch, or free nerve endings (nociceptors) for pain. Free nerve endings are stimulated by the local release of bradykinins, prostaglandins, histamine, and particularly **substance P** (a polypeptide that is one of the major neurotransmitters and stimulants in the pain pathway) secondary to inflammation or tissue damage.

The afferent impulse arrives via the dorsal nerve root. These axons first run up or down several spinal levels in **Lissauer tract** of the dorsal horn before synapsing in the **substantia gelatinosa** (also of the dorsal horn). Second-order neurons then cross the midline in the **ventral commissure** to form the **medial** (crude touch) and **lateral** (pain, temperature) **spinothalamic tracts,** which run superiorly to synapse (again) in the ventral posterolateral nucleus

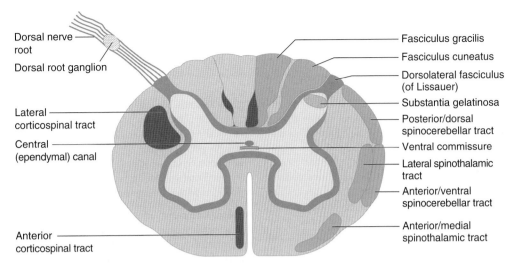

Dorsal nerve root

Dorsal root ganglion

Lateral corticospinal tract

Central (ependymal) canal

Anterior corticospinal tract

Fasciculus gracilis

Fasciculus cuneatus

Dorsolateral fasciculus (of Lissauer)

Substantia gelatinosa

Posterior/dorsal spinocerebellar tract

Ventral commissure

Lateral spinothalamic tract

Anterior/ventral spinocerebellar tract

Anterior/medial spinothalamic tract

• **Figure 10-2.** Spinal cord in cross-section.

of the thalamus. The spinothalamic tracts run contralateral to the afferent nerve ending due to decussation at the ventral commissure, unlike the dorsal columns system. Third-order neurons again project to the postcentral gyrus of the cortex, bringing pain, temperature, and crude touch to consciousness.

Spinocerebellar Tract The spinocerebellar tracts, dorsal and ventral, receive unconscious proprioceptive input via the dorsal horn and transmit it to the ipsilateral anterior lobe of the cerebellum. The **dorsal** tract remains ipsilateral and travels via the inferior cerebellar peduncle, whereas the **ventral** tract crosses the midline at the level of the dorsal root and crosses back again in the pons to arrive at the anterior lobe of the cerebellum via the superior cerebellar peduncle. This system allows the cerebellum to modulate balance and fine motor activity by recognizing limb placement. Because these tracts do not run to the cerebral cortex, they are not brought to consciousness.

Modulation of Pain Sensation and the Gate Control Theory

As experience tells us, a stimulus that may seem painful while lying in bed at night may not even be recognized when sufficiently distracted. The perception of pain at the level of the postcentral gyrus may be modified at almost every step in the sensory system, including the receptor, the sensory nerve, and, in particular, within the spinal cord and brain. Medications and the environment play a role in affecting pain perception, as described later in this case.

Peripheral nociceptors, which are stimulated by the release of prostaglandins and substance P, may be relieved by **NSAIDs,** which decrease local prostaglandin production. **Capsaicin** (the active ingredient in hot pepper spray) may deplete stores of substance P to deaden the sensation of pain. **Peripheral nerves,** which rely on sodium channels to propagate action potentials, may be deadened by using sodium channel blockers such as **lidocaine.**

The **spinal cord** modifies pain input at the level of the dorsal horn in the **substantia gelatinosa.** Second-order spinothalamic neurons are excited by input from nociceptive peripheral nerves. At the same time, they are inhibited by input from certain nonnociceptive peripheral nerves (specifically thick myelinated fibers). This inhibition explains why rubbing or massaging a tender area may decrease the sensation of pain via the competitive interaction of pain fibers versus dorsal column fibers. Finally, feedback

interneurons from the brain also project onto the substantia gelatinosa to modify neuronal activity in accordance with emotional state, anxiety, and so on. This complex "gating" function of the substantia gelatinosa is referred to as the **gate control theory.**

The **brain** also has numerous sites that modify the perception of pain, including the periaqueductal gray matter, the thalamus, and the reticular formation and limbic system. Opioid receptors in these locations, stimulated by endogenous opiates (called **endorphins** or **enkephalins**) as well as prescribed **opiates** (such as morphine or methadone), act to decrease the sensation of pain.

Pathologic States of the Somatosensory System

The list of diseases that affect the sensory system is far too long to go over in detail. A few important conditions that are specific or particularly significant to the sensory system are described in the following sections.

Brown-Séquard's Syndrome Brown-Séquard's syndrome refers to the constellation of symptoms seen with hemisection of the spinal cord: **ipsilateral paresis, ipsilateral dorsal column** sensory loss, and **contralateral spinothalamic** sensory loss. Patients will present with loss of fine touch ipsilateral to the lesion but will lose sensation to pain and temperature contralateral to the lesion. They may lose pain and temperature bilaterally at the site of the lesion because entering pain fibers may be obliterated within the dorsal root. The most common causes of Brown-Séquard's syndrome are trauma and compression secondary to tumor. As with all spinal cord lesions, recovery is usually minimal, unless decompression is an option.

Tabes Dorsalis Tabes dorsalis ("dorsal softening") refers to the syndrome seen in neurosyphilis of sensory loss due to selective destruction of the dorsal roots and dorsal columns of the spinal cord. The spirochete *Treponema pallidum* disproportionately involves the dorsal columns system, which results in **sensory ataxia** (a "staggering gait" may be seen), loss of proprioception (positive Romberg sign), and potential loss of reflexes. Dysesthesias may also present, often described as "lightning pains." The autonomic fibers may also be involved and may cause urinary incontinence, impotence, and constipation. Penicillin will cure the infection, but the symptoms may persist because of permanent spinal cord damage.

Subacute Combined Systems Degeneration Subacute combined systems degeneration refers to the subacute involvement of multiple neurologic systems seen in **vitamin B12** (cobalamine) **deficiency.** Vitamin B12 is a cofactor used by methyltransferases, which in turn play a role in fatty acid metabolism and myelin synthesis. Vitamin B12 deficiency leads to inadequate myelin production and the accumulation of abnormal fatty acids, causing demyelination and axonal degeneration in the peripheral nerves, dorsal columns, and spinocerebellar and corticospinal tracts. This initially presents **with distal paresthesias,** followed by distal numbness, then a **sensory ataxia** with gait difficulty, and finally **distal weakness** as the corticospinal tracts become involved. As is the case with most peripheral neuropathies, long nerves are most susceptible, resulting in hand and foot involvement initially in a "glove and stocking" distribution. Vitamin B12 repletion is curative if started within a few months of symptom onset, but otherwise, some of the CNS effects may be permanent.

Syringomyelia The spontaneous formation of a "syrinx" (tube) within the spinal cord white matter (an enlargement of the central canal) is known as **syringomyelia.** The cause is not entirely clear; patients with anatomic abnormalities such as the **Arnold-Chiari malformation** (elongated brainstem with downward displacement of the cerebellar tonsils into the foramen magnum) are at greater risk. A syrinx is most often found in the **low cervical cord.** Central cord fibers are initially affected, with the decussating spinothalamic fibers in the ventral commissure being most vulnerable, initially causing **pain** and discomfort in the **hands/upper extremities** bilaterally. This may progress to a **"cape-like" distribution** of insensitivity to pain and temperature of the upper extremities and

torso (the legs are not involved because their spinothalamic fibers are crossed in the lumbosacral cord, well inferior to the syrinx). Treatment usually involves medical pain management, with severe cases leading to surgical drainage of the syrinx, which has limited benefit in arresting syrinx progression.

Multiple Sclerosis Multiple sclerosis (MS) is a disease of unclear origin, which causes spotty demyelination in apparently random areas of the CNS white matter, both brain and spinal cord. It may result in **patchy** areas of **anesthesia/dysesthesia,** as well as **weakness.** Symptoms usually flare at varying intervals, although they predictably flare in warmer weather. Medical treatment is employed with varying success.

Peripheral Neuropathy Various diseases cause peripheral neuropathies. As a general rule, nerve fibers are more susceptible to any ischemic, inflammatory, or demyelinating process in proportion to their length. Sensory fibers are generally smaller and more susceptible than motor fibers. Peripheral neuropathies thus selectively involve the hands and feet and progress proximally as the disease progresses in what is often referred to as a **glove-and-stocking distribution. Diabetes** causes an ischemic neuropathy that usually presents with **distal sensory loss.** Vitamin **B deficiency** (in addition to vitamin **B12 deficiency**) and **folic acid deficiency** cause a demyelinating neuropathy with similar symptoms. **Alcohol abuse** (possibly secondary to nutritional deficiencies) and lead poisoning may cause sensory loss. **HIV** neuropathy may cause bilateral foot pain on the soles of the feet. Finally, familial peripheral neuropathies have also been reported.

CASE CONCLUSION

An operative report from this patient's surgery indicates that the bullet transected the left half of the spinal cord before lodging in the T10 vertebral body. Destruction of the left half of the spinal cord at the level of the T10 spinal nerves was essentially complete, but the right side was relatively unaffected. The functional consequence is hemisection of the spinal cord on the left side, resulting in **Brown-Séquard syndrome.** Regrettably, the prognosis for spinal cord lesions is poor, and it is anticipated that he will not regain motor function of the left lower extremity, which will require him to use a wheelchair.

THUMBNAIL: Sensory Systems and Pathologic States

Anatomic Location	Disease	Function or Symptoms
Dorsal columns		Fine touch, vibration, proprioception
	Tabes dorsalis	Sensory ataxia, staggering gait
	Subacute combined systems degeneration	Distal paresthesias/sensory loss, distal numbness, distal weakness
Spinothalamic		Contralateral pain/temperature/crude touch
	Syringomyelia	"Cape-like" loss of pain sensation in arms/torso
Spinocerebellar		Unconscious proprioception
Peripheral nerves		Peripheral sensation or motor function
	Peripheral neuropathy	Distal glove-and-stocking loss of fine touch, may progress to involve proximal areas or pain sensation
Other		
	Brown-Séquard syndrome (cord hemisection)	Ipsilateral plegia and loss of fine touch with contralateral pain and temperature loss
	MS	Patchy areas of weakness and sensory loss

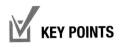

KEY POINTS

■ The somatosensory system is divided into three major systems based on spinal cord tracts: the dorsal columns (fine touch and proprioception), spinothalamic (crude touch, pain, and temperature), and spinocerebellar (unconscious proprioception)

■ Sensation of pain is affected by various factors, including medications and neuronal feedback, as shown in the gate control theory; substance P is the major transmitter of pain

■ A number of diseases affect sensation by interfering with nerves and sensory tracts, including trauma (Brown-Séquard syndrome), neurosyphilis, alcohol abuse, nutritional deficiencies (particularly vitamin B12, folic acid), MS, and syringomyelia

QUESTIONS

1. A patient has a spinal cord tumor that has affected the dorsal horn only on the right side at the C7 level. Which of the following symptoms should be seen on exam?
   A. Right-sided pain and temperature loss of the right C7 dermatome only
   B. Right-sided fine touch/vibratory loss of the right C7 dermatome only
   C. Right-sided fine touch/vibratory loss, left-sided pain/temperature loss of the C7 dermatome
   D. Right-sided fine touch/vibratory loss, right-sided pain/temperature loss of the C7 dermatome
   E. Left-sided pain/temperature loss of the C7 dermatome only

2. A 45-year-old male is brought to the hospital for difficulty walking and appearing confused. He does not have any significant medical history. He has diminished sensation to light touch bilaterally involving the upper and lower extremities and looks at his feet while walking. Proprioception is markedly diminished, with a positive Romberg sign. Reflexes are almost completely absent, including no pupillary reflex to light. What is the most likely diagnosis?
   A. Peripheral neuropathy
   B. Syringomyelia
   C. Neurosyphilis
   D. Subacute combined systems degeneration
   E. Brown-Séquard syndrome

3. A 32-year-old woman develops diffuse burning pain in her right arm that is now beginning to affect the left arm as well. On exam, sensation to pinprick and pain is markedly diminished across her upper torso and arms but is intact beneath the shoulder blades and around the neck. She is otherwise intact. What might an MRI of the brain and spinal cord be expected to show?
   A. Bilateral foraminal stenosis of the cervical spine
   B. Downward displacement of the cerebellar tonsils into the foramen magnum and central syrinx in the low cervical/upper thoracic cord
   C. Diffuse patchy demyelination bilaterally throughout brain white matter
   D. Normal
   E. Low cervical disc herniation with cord compression

4. A homeless patient visits the clinic for the first time for a routine physical. He does not have any complaints and is not aware of previous medical history. On exam, you note numerous cuts on his feet and markedly reduced sensation to pain and light touch up to the ankles and wrists bilaterally. The scent of alcohol is noticeable on his breath. His neurologic exam is otherwise intact. What is the most likely diagnosis?
   A. Peripheral neuropathy
   B. Subacute combined systems degeneration
   C. Syringomyelia
   D. Tabes dorsalis
   E. Multiple sclerosis

HPI: RK is a 33-year-old woman who has been in good health until 5 days ago when she developed tingling in her feet. A sensation of numbness then gradually ascended up her legs. She has also noted worsening back pain. There is no history of trauma. She did not seek medical attention initially but has now developed bilateral leg weakness. She reports that the weakness came on gradually and was subtle yesterday. This morning she awoke to find she could not stand or even get out of bed. She has been unable to urinate. She denies any other medical problems. She had the flu a few weeks earlier. She has never had anything like this before.

PE: Her vitals signs are all within normal parameters. Her neurologic exam reveals marked paraparesis. Reflexes are somewhat brisk in the lower extremities only. Toes are up-going bilaterally. She appears to have a T8 sensory level to all modalities. She is neurologically intact above the T8 level and her general exam is unremarkable.

THOUGHT QUESTIONS

- Does this patient have a peripheral or a central lesion?
- What structure(s) is(are) affected?
- What pathways are affected?
- What is the significance of the brisk reflexes?

BASIC SCIENCE REVIEW AND DISCUSSION

If this patient had presented earlier in the course of her syndrome, consideration might have been given to the possibility of a peripheral process. At this point, however, her syndrome represents central dysfunction. **Upper motor neuron (UMN) signs** including **brisk reflexes** and **extensor plantar (Babinski)** responses accompany her leg weakness. She also has a **sensory level,** which helps to localize her lesion to the midthoracic spinal cord. This is further supported by her inability to void, evidence of **autonomic dysfunction.**

This **acute myelopathy** most likely represents an inflammatory, infectious, or parainfectious process (given her recent viral syndrome). Spinal cord ischemia, spinal vascular malformations, and spinal tumors would be important differential considerations. However, vascular processes manifest more acutely with maximum deficits reached within the first few hours. Tumors, on the other hand, tend to present more insidiously. Trauma is an important consideration but is excluded by history.

This chapter focuses on the **motor pathways.** Sensory systems, the ANS, spinal anatomy, and spinal nerves are all discussed separately. Other structures are also critically involved in motor function. The basal ganglia and cerebellum are also integral to normal motor function. Lesions in these areas result in various movement disorders. These regions are also discussed further in other chapters.

Motor System Organization

The execution of movement begins in the **frontal cortex. Premotor** and **supplementary motor** areas contribute to the preparation of movement. The **primary motor cortex (Brodmann area 4)** initiates movement. Cortical output is carried by the axons of pyramidal neurons in cortical layer V, which make up the pyramidal tract. The **pyramidal tract** is a more generic term that reflects all of the **corticofugal pathways.** The **corticospinal tract** is the main motor output pathway and is part of the pyramidal tract. However, the majority of pyramidal axons actually end at targets within the brainstem. These latter pathways include the **corticopontocerebellar pathway** and several **corticobulbar pathways.** Each of these systems is also part of the pyramidal tract. The motor cortex of each hemisphere controls movement of the contralateral side of the body via the corticospinal system. To reach contralateral targets, these fibers cross the midline at the **pyramidal decussation** in the caudal medulla.

Corticospinal Tract

The main motor output pathway is a two-neuron system, consisting of an **UMN** and a **lower motor neuron (LMN).** The large **pyramidal neurons** of **cortical layer V** in the **primary motor cortex** are the UMNs of this system. The **corticospinal tract** primarily contains the axons of these pyramidal neurons. However, this pathway also contains some axons originating in premotor, supplementary motor, and primary sensory cortical areas. Together, these fibers make up the **corona radiata** of the subcortical white matter. This name reflects the cone-shaped appearance of these fibers as they funnel together to pass between the **deep gray nuclei** and through the **diencephalon.** Of course, the corona radiata also contains ascending sensory fibers. Within the corona radiata, fibers mediating motor function of the face, arm, and leg are relatively separated from each other. Thus, focal lesions in this area are not likely to cause complete hemiparesis of the face, arm, and leg. However, as these fibers pass between the basal ganglia and the thalamus, they become more densely packed within the **internal capsule.** Lesions of the internal capsule (such as from **lenticulostriate** ischemia) are more likely to manifest as hemiparesis involving the face, arm, and leg contralateral to the lesion.

The corticospinal tract remains tightly packed together as it passes though the **cerebral peduncles** of the **midbrain.** As these fibers reach the **pons,** they become more dispersed, passing between clusters of **pontine nuclei.** Fibers making up the **corticopontocerebellar pathway** end here while the corticospinal fibers continue caudally. The corticospinal tracts are visible on the ventral surface of the **medulla,** where they are called the **pyramids.** The **pyramidal decussation** is also visible in the caudal medulla. This is where the majority of corticospinal fibers cross the midline.

Throughout the brainstem, **corticobulbar fibers** that innervate various **cranial nerve nuclei** also branch of from the pyramidal tract and terminate at their corresponding brainstem levels. Most of the corticospinal fibers (about 80%) cross the midline at the pyramidal decussation and descend through the spinal cord as the **lateral corticospinal tract** within the contralateral **lateral**

funiculus of the spinal cord. The remaining fibers descend ipsilaterally through the **ventromedial corticospinal** tract in the **anterior funiculus** of the spinal cord. Most of these fibers ultimately cross the midline when they reach their terminal spinal cord level. A very small percentage of these fibers terminate on ipsilateral targets. Lesions of UMNs can occur anywhere from the cortical surface to the spinal cord. They usually manifest as weakness at first. UMN lesions are subsequently characterized by **pathologic reflexes** (such as **Babinski sign**), **hyperreflexia, clonus,** and ultimately by **spasticity** and **increased tone.**

Alpha Motor Neurons

The primary targets of the descending UMN fibers include both **LMNs (alpha motor neurons)** and **interneurons** located in the **ventral horns** of the spinal cord. The **somatotopic organization** found at higher levels is maintained within the spinal cord. LMNs innervating axial and proximal muscles are located more medially in the spinal cord gray matter. LMNs innervating distal muscles, on the other hand, are located more laterally with the spinal cord gray matter of the ventral horns. Alpha motor neurons that innervate muscles in the **upper extremities** are clustered together at several cervical spinal levels where the spinal cord becomes enlarged. This is called the **cervical enlargement.** Alpha motor neurons that innervate muscles in the **lower extremities** are similarly arranged in the **lumbosacral enlargement.** Axons of the alpha motor neurons exit the spinal cord through the ventral roots to join peripheral nerves. Most muscles are innervated by neurons from multiple spinal levels. However, some muscles receive their innervation predominantly from one prominent spinal level. Weakness in these muscles can aid in the localization of lesions. These muscles are summarized later in this case (see Thumbnail below).

Spinal nerve anatomy is discussed further in Case 10-9. Gamma motor neurons are similar to alpha motor neurons but innervate muscle spindles, which are involved in mediating spinal reflexes. Spinal reflex mechanisms are discussed within the context of sensory systems. **LMN lesions**, such as peripheral nerve compressions and radiculopathies, manifest as **weakness** with **diminished reflexes. Muscle wasting** and **fasciculations** ultimately develop.

Corticopontocerebellar and Corticobulbar Tracts

Many of the axons contained within the pyramidal tract terminate on brainstem targets. The most prominent example of this is the **corticopontocerebellar tract.** The axons in this tract outnumber the axons in the corticospinal tract by nearly 20:1. They terminate on **pontine neurons** in the **pontine nuclei.** Axons from the pontine neurons cross the midline to enter the **contralateral middle cerebellar peduncle.** These pontocerebellar fibers are a major source of **mossy fibers** to the cerebellum.

Remember that the function of the cranial nerve nuclei in motor and sensory systems of the head is analogous to that of the spinal cord for the rest of the body. Similarly, the function of the **corticobulbar tract** is analogous to that of the **corticospinal tract.** Although some corticobulbar fibers project directly onto their associated **brainstem LMN,** most influence their targets via **reticular interneurons.** One important difference between the corticobulbar system and the corticospinal system is that many of the cranial nerve nuclei receive **bilateral cortical input** via corticobulbar fibers. However, these two systems essentially mediate the same motor functions albeit for different muscle groups.

Bulbospinal Tracts

Some brainstem nuclear groups act as regions of intermediate processing for the motor system or provide feedback information to the motor system through various modalities. These brainstem regions give rise to several **bulbospinal pathways** that influence the interaction between UMNs and LMNs. Four major tracts are reviewed. The locations of the major motor pathways within the spinal cord are summarized in Figure 10-3.

Rubrospinal Tract The **red nucleus** is a venue for integration of information coming from the **cerebral cortex** and information coming from the **cerebellum.** Lesions in this area result in **tremor.** Two major red nucleus output pathways are recognized. The first pathway projects to the **inferior olivary nucleus** on the same side. This is the major pathway in humans. It provides feedback to the **contralateral cerebellum.** The second is the **rubrospinal tract.** The rubrospinal tract is, in essence, an indirect corticospinal pathway. Axons of neurons in the red nucleus

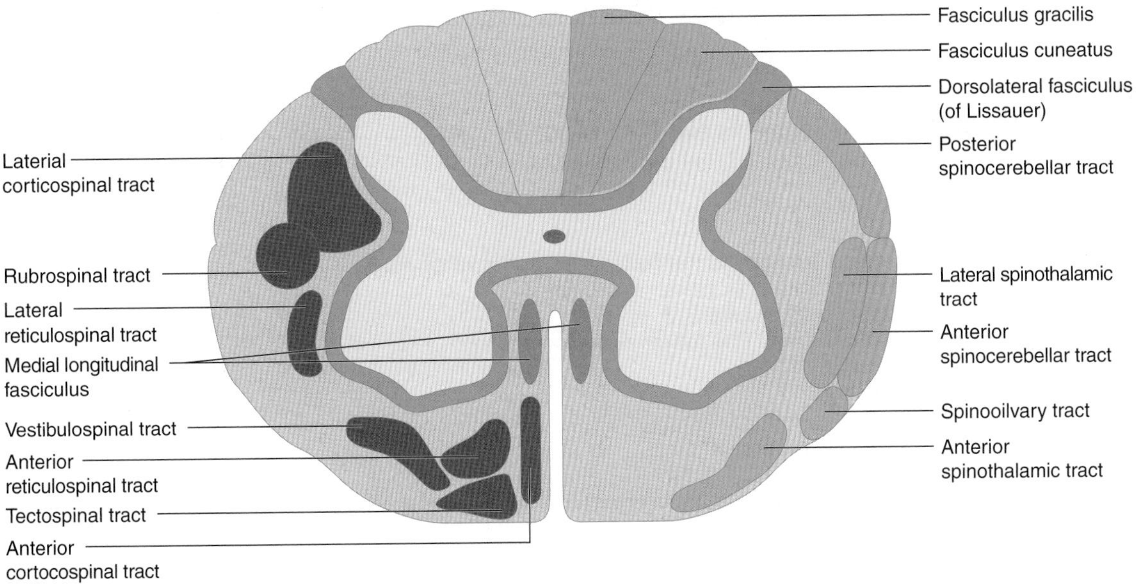
Fasciculus gracilis
Fasciculus cuneatus
Dorsolateral fasciculus (of Lissauer)
Posterior spinocerebellar tract
Laterial corticospinal tract
Rubrospinal tract
Lateral reticulospinal tract
Medial longitudinal fasciculus
Vestibulospinal tract
Anterior reticulospinal tract
Tectospinal tract
Anterior cortocospinal tract
Lateral spinothalamic tract
Anterior spinocerebellar tract
Spinooilvary tract
Anterior spinothalamic tract

• **Figure 10-3.** Principal fiber tracts of the spinal cord.

cross the midline in the **ventral tegmentum,** course through the central tegmental tract, then through the lateral funiculus of the spinal cord to their target level.

Tectospinal Tract The **tectospinal tract** originates in the **superior colliculi.** These fibers cross the midline within the midbrain and descend medially through the brainstem to the spinal cord. In the medulla, it joins with the **medial longitudinal fasciculus.** The function of this system in humans is not clear. However, given the visual function of the superior colliculi and the vestibular function of the medial longitudinal fasciculus, this system may be involved in orienting movements of the head and body to visual cues.

Reticulospinal Tract The **reticular formation** makes up a central core through much of the brainstem. It contains many different nuclear groups. Many of these nuclei use monoamine neurotransmitters. These systems are discussed further in subsequent chapters. As a general rule, the **rostral reticular formation** is concerned with **consciousness and vigilance.** More **caudal reticular formation** regions are involved in regulating **cardiovascular and respiratory tract mechanisms.** Several **pontine and medullary reticular nuclei** project to the spinal cord and **influence motor function** (voluntary and reflexive movements, muscle tone).

Vestibulospinal Tract The **vestibular system** detects motion in several planes. This information is conveyed to brainstem vestibular nuclei by the **vestibulocochlear nerve** (CN VIII). The vestibular nuclei (superior, lateral, medial, and inferior) are interconnected with medial cerebellar structures, the oculomotor nuclei, and the cervical spinal cord. The **lateral and medial vestibular nuclei** give rise to descending fibers that project to

the spinal cord as the **vestibulospinal tract.** This complex system helps coordinate eye, head, and neck movements.

Clinical Correlation

Acute transverse myelitis (ATM) is focal inflammation of the spinal cord. The inflammation is evident on MRI studies and in the spinal fluid. Prompt diagnosis is very important. The first goal of therapy is to minimize further injury. **IV steroids** are the standard of care. Plasma exchange, IV immunoglobulin (IVIG), and immunosuppressive agents also have been used. Primary ATM is the result of an autoimmune process. Secondary ATM can be seen in the setting of acute infection, during the postinfectious period, and after immunizations. **Molecular mimicry,** a similarity between an extrinsic antigen and a self-antigen, may be involved in these cases. ATM can also be encountered within the context of the connective tissue diseases.

ATM affects people of all ages but is most often seen in the second and fourth decades. Its clinical manifestation is characterized by sensory, motor, and autonomic symptoms. The sensory symptoms are usually associated with a distinct spinal sensory level. As a general rule, about one third of patients will recover with little or no residual deficit. One third will be left with more moderate disability. One third will be left with severe disability.

ATM can represent the first clinical manifestation of what will ultimately become **multiple sclerosis** (MS). Patients who have white matter lesions on their MRI scan of the brain at the time of their ATM are much more likely to develop MS than those who have normal brain MRI studies. Of course, a history of demyelinating disease in another CNS region supports the diagnosis of MS.

CASE CONCLUSION

RK was admitted to the hospital. An MRI of the thoracic spinal cord confirmed a focal inflammatory lesion involving the T7 and T8 spinal levels. MRI scans of the brain, cervical spine, and lumbosacral spine did not reveal any other areas of abnormality. A lumbar puncture revealed mild inflammatory changes with no evidence of infection. The patient received a 5-day course of high-dose IV steroids followed by an oral tapering dose. She was ultimately transferred to the rehabilitation service where she gradually regained most of her function. In follow-up at 1 year, she was self-ambulatory with only mild residual weakness.

THUMBNAIL: Spinal Segments and Their Major Muscles

Roots	Muscles
C3, C4	Levator scapulae
C5 > C6	Deltoid, supraspinatus, infraspinatus, rhomboids, biceps, brachioradialis, supinator
C6 + C7	Flexor carpi radialis, pronator teres, extensor carpi radialis
Mostly C7	Triceps, extensor digitorum, anconeus
Mostly C8	Extensor indicis proprius, most other forearm extensors and flexors
C8 + T1	Intrinsic hand muscles
L2 + L3	Iliopsoas, rectus femoris
L3	Adductor longus
L3 + L4	Gracilis, vastus medialis and lateralis
L4 + L5	Tibialis anterior
Mostly L5	Extensor hallucis longus, extensor digitorum longus and brevis, peroneus longus and brevis, posterior tibial, flexor digitorum longus, medial hamstrings, gluteus medius
Mostly S1	Abductor hallucis, abductor digiti quinti, soleus, gastrocnemius, lateral hamstrings, gluteus maximus
S2, S3	Sphincter ani

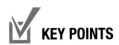
KEY POINTS

- Many of the axons contained within the pyramidal tract terminate on brainstem targets

- The corticospinal tract is the main motor output pathway and part of the pyramidal system

- Corticospinal fibers cross the midline at the pyramidal decussation in the caudal medulla

- Approximately 80% of corticospinal fibers cross the midline at the pyramidal decussation and descend as the lateral corticospinal tract

- The remaining fibers descend ipsilaterally through the ventromedial corticospinal tract

- UMN lesions are characterized by pathologic reflexes (such as Babinski sign), hyperreflexia, clonus, and spasticity

- LMN lesions manifest as weakness with diminished reflexes and eventual muscle wasting and fasciculations

QUESTIONS

1. You evaluate a patient whose right arm is markedly weak. Reflexes in the arm are diminished. However, you note that reflexes are rather brisk in the right leg and the patient has an up-going toe on the right. Reflexes are normal on the left. What structure is involved?

   A. Peripheral nerves
   B. Ventral roots
   C. Spinal cord
   D. Brainstem
   E. Alpha motor neurons

2. You evaluate a 63-year-old patient who has developed progressive muscle weakness and wasting over several months. Muscle fasciculations are diffusely evident on exam. Reflexes are rather brisk. Which structure is most likely affected?

   A. Peripheral nerves
   B. Ventral roots
   C. Muscles
   D. Neuromuscular junction
   E. Alpha motor neurons

3. You evaluate a 38-year-old acutely myelopathic female. She has previously been treated for optic neuritis. Which of the following tissues is most likely affected in her spinal cord?

   A. White matter only
   B. Gray matter only
   C. Both gray and white matter
   D. Small caliber vasculature
   E. All of the above

4. You evaluate a patient who has a spinal cord injury and note very brisk reflexes in the lower extremities. Which of the following is responsible?

   A. Increased sensory input to alpha motor neurons
   B. Increased corticospinal axon function
   C. Decreased alpha motor neuron function
   D. Decreased corticospinal axon function
   E. Increased alpha motor neuron function

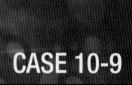
Spinal Nerves and Nerves of the Upper Extremity

HPI: An elderly female 78-year-old friend of the family is brought to your attention for recurrent arm and neck pain. She recalls no trauma or inciting event, but for the past 6 months she has noted a recurrent sharp pain originating in the back of her neck, which shoots down her right arm to her thumb. This is often brought about when she coughs or turns her head and is minimized when she lies down. She has a history of HTN and has had bilateral hip replacements. She takes Tylenol and occasional Motrin for joint pains and hydrochlorothiazide for high BP.

PE: T 36.7°C; HR 72 beats/min; BP 135/85 mm Hg

On neurologic exam, she has diminished sensation to pinprick on her right lateral arm and forearm, as well as the thumb. Right biceps strength and reflex is diminished, though still present. She has some neck pain on palpation throughout. On turning her head, the shooting pain from her neck to her right arm is reproduced.

Labs: WBC 7; Hct 35; Na 136; K 3.6

THOUGHT QUESTIONS

- What nervous structure is the likely source of the problem?
- What adjacent anatomic structures are contributing?
- What about this patient has likely placed her at risk?

BASIC SCIENCE REVIEW AND DISCUSSION

The spinal cord gives off a tetrad of nerve roots (left and right, ventral and dorsal) at each spinal level. The motor nerve root (ventral) and sensory nerve root (dorsal) come together to form a unified **spinal nerve.** The spinal nerves are grouped into basic categories by the vertebrae they accompany, namely cervical, thoracic, lumbar, and sacral. Each spinal nerve is named for the vertebrae that it runs adjacent to (C5, T1, etc.). Cervical spinal nerves are named for the vertebrae that they run superior to (i.e., C5 nerve root runs just superior to the C5 vertebral body), whereas all other nerve roots are named for the vertebrae they run inferior to (the T6 nerve root runs inferior to the T6 vertebral body, in the T6–T7 intervertebral space).

As the nerve roots emerge from the spinal cord, the dorsal and ventral roots coalesce and the single nerve runs laterally toward the "neural foramina," the intervertebral openings through which the spinal nerve passes out of the bony spine. It is in the foramina, surrounded by bone (namely, the bony pedicle of the vertebra), that the nerve root is most vulnerable to compression. Once outside of the foramina, spinal nerves either intertwine to form the cervical, brachial, and lumbosacral plexuses or run solitary as the intercostal nerves.

Compression of these nerve roots or spinal nerves is referred to as a **radiculopathy** (*radiculo-* refers to a root).

Cervical Spinal Nerves

The cervical spinal nerves are of particular note for a variety of reasons. For one, because there are in fact eight cervical nerves and seven cervical vertebrae, the C8 nerve root deserves special mention as running in the C7–T1 intervertebral space. They are of particular importance because they innervate the upper extremities. The brachial plexus (Fig. 10-4) is comprised of branches from the C5–T1 roots and gives rise to the five major nerves of the upper extremity, whose function may be summarized into broad categories (with some minor exceptions). Each of these nerves run different anatomic courses, generally running close to the muscles and cutaneous regions that they innervate. Injuries involving the ulnar and median nerves are most common because they have the longest courses and have anatomically vulnerable spots.

The **axillary** nerve supplies the deltoid and teres minor muscles and provides sensation of the shoulder. It runs adjacent to the shoulder (glenohumeral) joint en route to the deltoid muscle. It is thus sometimes injured with **shoulder dislocation.**

The **radial** nerve supplies motor function to the extensor (dorsal) compartments of the arm and forearm, as well as sensation of the dorsal hand. It runs around the humerus (in the **radial** or **spiral groove**) as it innervates the triceps, then forms the posterior interosseous nerve of the forearm. It is the most likely nerve to be injured by **humerus fracture.** Injury to the radial nerve results in unopposed wrist flexion, sometimes described as the characteristic **waiter's tip.**

The **musculocutaneous** nerve supplies motor function to the flexor (ventral) compartment of the arm, as well as sensation of the ventral arm and part of the ventral forearm. This nerve runs anteromedially to the humerus and is sometimes injured by a **humerus fracture.**

The **ulnar** nerve supplies motor function to the bulk of the intrinsic hand muscles (except the thumb), as well as sensation of the ulnar aspect of the hand (fifth and medial fourth digits). It runs posterior to the humerus prior to passing through the **ulnar canal** of the medial epicondyle (here the nerve is colloquially called the *funny bone*), then runs in the anterior compartment of the forearm to the hand. It is thus injured by **elbow dislocation,** or **entrapment** in the ulnar canal. This results in an **ulnar neuropathy,** which results in denervation of the hand musculature, particularly the muscles of the fourth and fifth digits, resulting in **hypothenar atrophy** and the characteristic **ulnar claw.** The ulnar claw is caused by denervation of the lumbricals of the fourth and fifth digits, preventing extension of the phalanges against the preserved flexor tension of the flexor digitorum (median nerve).

The **median** nerve supplies motor function to the flexor (ventral) compartment of the forearm and the thumb, as well as sensation of the ventral (or palmar) hand. This nerve runs in

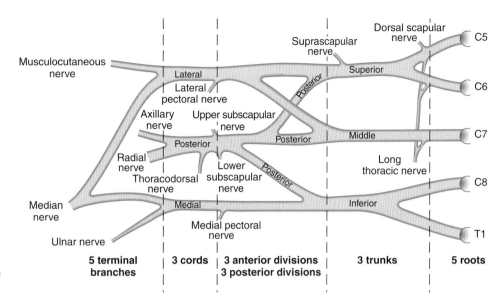

- **Figure 10-4.** Brachial plexus. (Note: Smaller nerve branches have been omitted for simplicity.)

the anterior compartment of the arm en route to forming the **anterior interosseous nerve** of the forearm, where it innervates the majority of the muscles in the anterior forearm compartment. It sends its most distal branch through the flexor compartment of the wrist, the **carpal tunnel.** The carpal tunnel is the narrow channel defined by the carpal bones and the ventral fibrous band known as the **flexor retinaculum,** or **transverse carpal ligament.** It contains the flexor tendons of the hand and the median nerve, with little room to spare. As a result, the majority of median neuropathies occur by compression in this tunnel causing **carpal tunnel syndrome.**

Carpal Tunnel Syndrome Carpal tunnel syndrome results from median nerve dysfunction secondary to mechanical compression or enlargement of structures in the carpal tunnel. Only the fibers in the median nerve present in the carpal tunnel will be affected; all branches that diverged from the median nerve proximally are spared. **Tinel sign** elicits wrist pain by striking the midline anterior wrist with a reflex hammer on the irritated median nerve. **Phalen maneuver** also elicits wrist pain by holding the wrist in 90-degree palmar flexion for 60 seconds.

By the time the median nerve reaches the carpal tunnel, it has already innervated the anterior forearm and given off the **recurrent median nerve,** which passes outside of the carpal tunnel to provide thumb sensation. Thus, only sensation of the palmar second, third, and lateral fourth digits are affected by carpal tunnel syndrome. The motor innervation of the thumb (opponens pollicis, abductor pollicis brevis, and flexor pollicis brevis) may also be affected. These muscles begin to atrophy from the relative denervation, and **thenar atrophy** develops.

Carpal tunnel syndrome is most often found in women and is often associated with **repetitive motions** that involve pressure on the ventral surface of the wrist, such as **typing.** Various medical conditions also may contribute by causing swelling of the nerve, connective tissue, or tendons within the carpal tunnel. Hypothyroidism is a relatively common and correctable ailment that is often associated with carpal tunnel syndrome (presumably through water retention).

Cervical Radiculopathy Because the cervical vertebrae are relatively small with relatively small neural foramina to match, the stage is set for nerve root compression (radiculopathy). As the spinal nerves run toward neural foramina, they run tangentially and adjacent to the intervertebral discs. Lateral protrusion or **herniation** of the discs will, in turn, compress the nerve root against the bony pedicle, resulting in radiculopathy. It is worth noting that posterior herniation of the disc (the notorious "slipped disc") will potentially compress the cord itself, resulting in spinal cord compression, or **myelopathy.**

Radiculopathy may also be caused by alterations in the bony architecture of the neural foramen, as is seen with degenerative joint disease—that is, osteoarthritis. In this case, hypertrophy and/or degeneration of the bony facet joints will contort the foramina. This is referred to as **foraminal encroachment,** and it causes the majority of cervical radiculopathy. In rarer cases, a mass, fracture, localized infection, or other process may also compress a spinal nerve root.

Foraminal encroachment occurs most often in the joints that receive the most wear and tear, namely the C4–C7 vertebral joints (they have greater rotational and flexional mobility). As a result, C5, C6, and C7 cervical radiculopathies are the most common.

Cervical radiculopathy is often manifested by particular symptoms, namely a sharp, shooting pain running from the neck along the dermatomal distribution of the affected nerve root, which is usually along the arm. Paresthesias and numbness also often occur. Weakness and loss of reflexes may occur in muscle groups that are innervated by the affected nerve root. Movements that promote further impingement or movement of the nerve in the restrictive foramen tend to make this worse: coughing, straining, and turning the head. Conversely, lying down with the neck in a neutral position often affords relief. Management is usually conservative, involving relative immobilization of the neck and decreased use of the involved extremity, which is generally effective.

Lumbar Radiculopathy The lumbar region deserves special mention because it is a region of particular strain, as it supports the weight of the spinal column and is thus most prone to disc herniation. Disc herniation, or **lumbar disc prolapse,** usually occurs laterally and thus leads to radiculopathy (posterior herniation, on the other hand, poses a risk for cord compression or cauda equina compression). Lumbar radiculopathy is symptomatically similar to cervical radiculopathy. It often presents with sharp pain radiating down the leg, paresthesias, numbness, and potential weakness and loss of reflexes in the segmental distribution pertaining to the affected nerve root. The L4, L5, and S1 nerve roots are most often affected.

CASE CONCLUSION

On account of thumb paresthesias, biceps weakness, and reduced biceps reflex, this patient's C6 radiculopathy became apparent. She was started on conservative management with a soft neck collar to minimize turning of her head for 3 days, which reduces her symptoms. NSAIDs such as ibuprofen may also be used for pain. She is able to use her arm with only occasional twinges thereafter. Should her symptoms recur and cervical immobilization or traction prove ineffective, she may become a candidate for **foraminectomy,** or surgical enlargement of the offending neural foramen.

THUMBNAIL: Selected Spinal Nerves: Key Functions and Resulting Deficits

Note: It is important to recognize that the functions stated in the following table are by no means all inclusive. They merely reflect key functions to aid memorization; more specific details have been omitted.

Nerve	Function	Presentation with Injury
C5	Biceps strength and reflex; sensation lateral arm	Biceps weakness; paresthesias/pain lateral arm; pain referred to scapula
C6	Biceps strength and reflex; sensation lateral forearm, thumb	Biceps weakness; paresthesias/pain in forearm/thumb
C7	Triceps strength and reflex; sensation second, third digits (lateral fingers)	Triceps weakness; paresthesias/pain to lateral fingers
L4	Quadriceps strength and reflex; gluteal strength; sensation kneecap, medial calf	Quads weakness, decreased knee jerk; pain/paresthesias kneecap, medial calf
L5	Extensor hallucis longus (EHL)/foot dorsiflexor strength; gluteal and hamstring strength; sensation lateral calf, dorsal foot	EHL, foot dorsiflexor weakness; moderate gluteal/hamstring weakness; pain/paresthesias lateral calf, dorsal foot
S1	Gastrocnemius strength, ankle jerk; gluteal and hamstring strength; sensation lateral foot and sole	Gastrocnemius weakness, reduced ankle jerk; moderate gluteal/hamstring weakness; pain/paresthesias
Axillary nerve	Shoulder sensation and innervation	Deltoid weakness, shoulder anesthesia
Radial nerve	Extension and posterior sensation of upper extremity	**Waiter's tip,** loss of triceps reflex, posterior anesthesia
Musculocutaneous nerve	Flexion of arm, anterior arm sensation	Biceps weakness, loss of biceps reflex
Ulnar nerve	Innervation of hand, sensation of ulnar hand	Ulnar claw
Median nerve	Flexion of wrist and fingers, thumb innervation, sensation of palm	Thenar wasting, palmar anesthesia (**carpal tunnel syndrome**)
Cervical nerve root	Myotomal innervation, dermatomal sensation	Weakness of one nerve root (which usually affects multiple nerves), dermatomal anesthesia, may lose reflexes
Myelopathy	Unilateral/bilateral strength and sensation at and below compression; autonomic functions (bowel/bladder)	Weakness or paralysis at or below lesion; pain/paresthesia/anesthesia; bowel/bladder incontinence
Spinal cord injury	Motor function and sensation at and below level of injury	Hyperreflexia, clonus, possible loss of bowel/bladder function, may lose strength/sensation at and below level of lesion

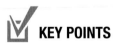

KEY POINTS

■ The spinal nerve roots emerge from the spinal cord in segmental tetrads, with the dorsal and ventral roots coalescing to form pairs of spinal nerves (left and right)

■ The five major nerves of the upper extremity are the axillary, radial, musculocutaneous, ulnar, and median nerves; each nerve's function may be generalized into sensation and motor function of a part of the upper extremity

■ The more common injury syndromes include ulnar neuropathy (usually due to entrapment at the ulnar canal) and carpal tunnel syndrome

■ Spinal nerves and nerve roots are vulnerable to compression, resulting in partial or complete dysfunction; the dysfunction is specific to the myotome (motor function) and dermatome (sensation) of the affected nerve or nerve root

■ Compression usually occurs as a result of bony deformation of the spine and neural foramina but may also result from disc prolapse and/or herniation; other processes are also possible

■ Treatment usually involves rest and immobilization, although surgical decompression may be warranted in severe cases

QUESTIONS

1. On a radiology rotation, you are given a cervical spine x-ray film of a 35-year-old man. You can detect only mild congenital narrowing of the cervical spinal canal. The only clinical information available is that the patient has been experiencing neck pain worsened by movement, radiating along the left arm to "some of his fingers." Triceps reflex is reduced on the left. What is the most likely diagnosis?

   A. Radial nerve injury
   B. C7 radiculopathy
   C. Musculocutaneous nerve injury
   D. C6 radiculopathy
   E. Cervical cord compression

2. On examining an older male patient, you discover complete anesthesia on the sole of the left foot. The patient tells you that this has been the case since sustaining a grenade blast in Vietnam, with shrapnel hitting his back in multiple locations. He has healed since surgical removal of the shrapnel and is not bothered by this lack of sensation. What might explain this finding?

   A. Sciatic nerve injury
   B. Left dorsal L4 nerve root transection
   C. Left ventral S1 nerve root transection
   D. Left dorsal L5 nerve root transection
   E. Left dorsal S1 nerve root transection

3. Routine exam of a 69-year-old man demonstrates relative weakness of the left EHL muscle (big toe extension is weakened). Ankle jerk and plantar flexion are intact. He appears to have decreased sensation on the dorsum of the left foot and mentions a history of low back pain with occasional "shooting pain" down the side of the left leg. What is the most likely diagnosis?

   A. Left L4 radiculopathy
   B. Left L5 radiculopathy
   C. Left S1 radiculopathy
   D. Left S2 radiculopathy
   E. Lumbar myelopathy

4. After an automobile accident, a 35-year-old man is placed on a backboard and transported to the hospital. Although he remains conscious, you note that sensation to pinprick is reduced but present bilaterally over the kneecaps and below. As the ambulance goes over bumps, you note that he transiently loses continence of stool. What is the best explanation?

   A. Bilateral L4 radiculopathy secondary to acute nerve root compression
   B. Bilateral L4 spinal nerve transection
   C. High cervical cord transection
   D. Diffuse lumbar radiculopathies bilaterally secondary to lumbar vertebral fractures
   E. Lumbar cord compression causing myelopathy

5. A 55-year-old man is found to have new difficulty moving his left arm hours after a car accident in which both the left humerus is fractured in the diaphysis (midshaft) and the left elbow is dislocated. On exam, he has inability to extend the wrist or fingers, anesthesia in the posterior forearm and dorsal hand, and wasting of the thenar eminence, all on the left. His fourth and fifth fingers are flexed more so than the others. He tells you that he has had tingling in his left fingers before. What is the most likely constellation of injury?

   A. Acute radial nerve injury, acute median nerve injury (carpal tunnel syndrome)
   B. Acute ulnar nerve injury
   C. Acute radial and ulnar nerve injury, chronic median nerve injury (carpal tunnel syndrome)
   D. Acute median nerve injury, chronic ulnar and radial nerve injury
   E. Acute axillary and ulnar nerve injury

6. You are asked to see a 72-year-old woman with several weeks of spontaneous neck pain and pain in the area of the right scapula. She has no history of trauma or arm/shoulder injury. She describes occasional numbness running down her right arm anterolaterally, which stops proximal to the wrist. On exam, you appreciate slight biceps weakness and deltoid weakness on the right. X-ray film of the right shoulder and humerus shows no evidence of fracture or bony deformity other than degenerative changes in the cervical spine. What is the most likely diagnosis?

   A. Median nerve injury
   B. C5 radiculopathy
   C. Axillary nerve injury
   D. Musculocutaneous nerve injury
   E. Upper brachial plexus injury

Nerves of the Lower Extremity

HPI: A 55-year-old male runner is seen at the doctor's office for worsening right leg pain brought on with running. He describes the pain as "shooting" down the back of his leg, running sometimes all the way down to his toes and the bottom of his foot. There is no history of trauma. He noted small fleeting episodes of this pain while running over the past couple of weeks, which have gradually worsened. He currently is not experiencing the pain, although it does intermittently occur when he walks as well. Previous medical history is unremarkable.

PE: T 37.1°C; HR 52 beats/min; BP 130/75 mm Hg

He appears to have full strength of the hamstring muscles. He does have minimally decreased sensation on the lateral aspect of the right leg. When the right leg is passively raised to an angle of 30 degrees while he is lying on the table (straight leg raise test), he re-experiences the shooting pain.

THOUGHT QUESTIONS

- Which nerve is most likely to be affected?
- What about the history and physical is suggestive that this nerve is involved?
- What anatomic structures are most likely to cause the problem?
- What is the prognosis?

BASIC SCIENCE REVIEW AND DISCUSSION

Much as was the case in the upper extremity, the nerves of the lower extremity are derived from a plexus of spinal nerves. The **lumbosacral plexus** is composed of spinal nerve segments L2–S3 and is discussed in greater detail in its own section. It gives rise to the three major peripheral nerves of the lower extremity: the femoral nerve, the obturator nerve, and the sciatic nerve, which are discussed in this case. The sciatic nerve, by far the largest of the three, divides into the tibial and common peroneal nerves.

The Femoral Nerve

Function The femoral nerve is an upper lumbosacral plexus nerve, generated by the L2–L4 nerve roots. It runs along the iliopsoas muscle, exits the pelvis via the **femoral canal** (with the femoral artery and femoral vein) and then runs along the femur as it innervates the **quadriceps muscles.** The quadriceps muscles include the four major muscles of the anterior thigh: the vastus medialis, vastus intermedius, vastus lateralis, and the rectus femoris. The quadriceps extends the knee. The femoral nerve also flexes the hip via the sartorius and iliopsoas muscles. It provides sensation for the anterior thigh, proximal medial thigh, and medial leg (via the **saphenous nerve,** a pure sensory branch).

Dysfunction The femoral nerve is most often affected by changes in the iliopsoas, pelvis, or femur, such as an iliopsoas abscess or hematoma, hip dislocation or surgery, or femoral fractures. This often presents with quadriceps weakness and possibly atrophy, as well as weakness of thigh flexion. Sensation of the anteromedial thigh and medial leg may be affected. The knee jerk or **patellar reflex** will be lost in the presence of significant quadriceps weakness.

The Obturator Nerve

Function The obturator nerve is also an upper lumbosacral plexus nerve originating from the L2–L4 nerve roots. It runs through the **obturator canal** or **obturator foramen** of the pelvis and along the medial thigh to innervate the major **adductor muscles,** namely the adductor magnus, adductor longus, and gracilis muscles. It also serves to externally rotate the thigh via the obturator externus muscle (and the superior gemellus muscle). It determines sensation of the distal medial thigh (the proximal inner thigh being innervated by the femoral nerve).

Dysfunction The obturator nerve is most vulnerable to compression against the bony pelvis within the obturator foramen, which occurs most commonly in women during labor. It may also be affected by pelvic fractures and many of the same factors that can damage the femoral nerve. Obturator nerve palsy predictably results in adductor weakness and weakness of external rotation of the thigh. Patients may note an inability to cross the affected leg onto the other and/or anesthesia of the distal inner thigh. The **adductor reflex** (jerk of adductor muscles when their tendons are struck proximal to the medial epicondyle of the femur) may be lost.

The Sciatic Nerve

Function The sciatic nerve is the largest and the most significant nerve of the lower extremity. It is involved in the most common neuropathies of the lower limb: foot drop and sciatica. It is derived from the lower lumbosacral plexus, L4–S3, and emerges from the posterior pelvis via the greater sciatic foramen. It is joined in this foramen by the posterior femoral cutaneous nerve, a pure sensory branch of the sciatic nerve, which serves the buttocks and posterior thigh. As the sciatic nerve runs within the pelvis, it abuts the **ischial tuberosity,** which may compress the nerve and result in **sciatica.** The sciatic nerve then runs down the posterior compartment of the thigh and innervates the **hamstring muscles,** which include the semimembranosus, semitendinosus, biceps femoris, and adductor magnus (also innervated in part by the obturator nerve). The hamstring muscles extend the hip joint and flex the knee joint. Within the popliteal fossa, the sciatic nerve divides into two major branches: the tibial nerve and common peroneal nerve.

Dysfunction: Sciatica and Other Causes The sciatic nerve is most vulnerable to compression at the sciatic notch of the pelvis, immediately adjacent to the ischial tuberosity. Its close proximity to the ischium may result in friction and irritation with repetitive hip joint flexion/extension, which may be seen in athletes (especially runners) but may present in any patient spontaneously.

This irritation of the sciatic nerve is known as **sciatica.** It usually presents with "shooting pain" along the posterior leg as far as the sole and even the plantar toes, following the cutaneous innervation of the sciatic nerve. Weakness resulting from sciatica is uncommon. It is usually treated by conservative management, including rest and anti-inflammatory medications.

Localized trauma in the area of the ischium may also result in sciatic nerve damage. For this reason, it is essential to administer IM gluteal injections in the upper outer quadrant of the gluteal muscles. Injections placed in the medial inferior gluteal quadrant place the sciatic nerve at risk and have been known to produce permanent sciatic nerve injury.

However, it is worth noting that L5 or S1 radiculopathy (often from a herniated disc) may also present with pain similar to that seen in sciatica. It may be very difficult to clinically distinguish L5 or S1 radiculopathy from sciatic nerve entrapment. Radiculopathy, however, is more likely to result in demonstrable weakness. Both radiculopathy and sciatica may produce a **positive straight leg raise test,** which is pain in the sciatic nerve distribution when passively raising the patient's leg into the air. This maneuver places tension on the affected nerve roots and sciatic nerve, exacerbating the pain.

The Tibial Nerve

Function The tibial nerve is served by all of the nerve roots within the sciatic nerve, L2–S3. The tibial nerve (also referred to as the **posterior tibial nerve**) runs posterior to the tibia as it innervates the plantar flexor muscles of the leg. It then runs posterior and inferior to the medial malleolus, splitting into the **medial and lateral plantar nerves** on the sole of the foot. It provides for **plantar flexion** via the muscles of the posterior leg (gastrocnemius, soleus, plantaris, and tibialis posterior muscles) and toe flexion (flexor digitorum longus and flexor hallucis longus). The medial and lateral plantar nerves innervate the intrinsic foot muscles.

Sensation of the sole of the foot is also provided by the medial plantar nerve (medial sole) and lateral plantar nerve (lateral sole of the foot). The tibial nerve otherwise has no cutaneous sensation.

Dysfunction The tibial nerve is most vulnerable to popliteal fossa trauma and tibial fractures, resulting in an inability to plantar flex and intrinsic foot muscle weakness. Sensation on the sole of the foot may be lost. The ankle jerk (reflexive plantar flexion upon jerking the Achilles tendon) may be diminished or absent. **Tarsal tunnel syndrome** refers to entrapment of the tibial nerve against the medial malleolus of the tibia. It is compressed as it runs in the tarsal tunnel deep to the flexor retinaculum of the ankle, very much analogous to carpal tunnel syndrome of the median nerve. Tarsal tunnel syndrome results in a burning sensation of the sole of the foot and may also cause weakness of the intrinsic foot muscles. Surgery may be required to relieve the nerve compression.

The Common Peroneal Nerve

Function The common peroneal nerve is the other major branch of the sciatic nerve, diverging laterally from the tibial nerve to run over the head of the fibula. This overlap allows for a common nerve compression palsy to arise in various circumstances, namely **peroneal nerve palsy or foot drop.** The peroneal nerve remains in the lateral compartment of the leg where it innervates the peroneal muscles, which control eversion, as well as the tibialis anterior, the major muscle involved in **dorsiflexion of the foot.**

Sensation of the anterolateral leg and foot is likewise controlled by the common peroneal nerve.

Dysfunction **Foot drop** is the common name given to peroneal nerve palsy, as the inability to dorsiflex makes the foot "drop" or hang limp with each step, which makes the patient likely to trip. Patients with a foot drop develop a circumducting gait to avoid tripping on the dragging foot. It may be caused by trauma to the fibular head or compression injury from lying on one side (during anesthesia or during critical illness). It may also arise spontaneously with predisposing factors such as poor nutrition, alcohol abuse, rapid weight loss, and so on. Patients usually recover some function over a period of weeks, although complete palsies are at greatest risk for permanent foot drop. There is no treatment. Patients may wear a boot or brace that holds the foot perpendicular to the ankle to minimize dragging while walking.

CASE CONCLUSION

The runner is advised that he has likely developed a case of sciatica. He admits that he had increased his mileage last week, which may have precipitated the episode. He is advised to abstain from running for several days and then gently resume as his symptoms permit. After taking a week off, he notes improvement in his symptoms. He is counseled that the sciatica may recur and that he should decrease his running if the symptoms recur or worsen.

THUMBNAIL: Nerves of the Lower Extremity

Peripheral Nerve	Motor Function	Sensation	Dysfunction Syndromes
Obturator nerve	Thigh adduction	Distal inner thigh	Inability to cross legs
Femoral nerve	Quadriceps	Anteromedial thigh; medial leg	Inability to extend knee
Sciatic nerve	Hamstrings, all leg muscles	Posterior thigh and lateral leg, foot	Sciatica
Common peroneal nerve	Dorsiflexion, eversion of foot	Lateral leg	Foot drop (peroneal nerve palsy)
Tibial nerve	Plantar flexion, intrinsic foot muscles	Posterior leg, sole	Tarsal tunnel syndrome

☑ KEY POINTS

■ The lower extremity is innervated by three major peripheral nerves: the obturator, the femoral, and the sciatic nerve; the sciatic nerve divides into the tibial and common peroneal nerves

■ The most common neuropathies of the lower extremity include foot drop, sciatica, and tarsal tunnel syndrome; these may present spontaneously and usually are managed conservatively

■ Sciatica is difficult to differentiate from L5 or S1 radiculopathy, although cases with significant weakness are usually due to neuropathy

QUESTIONS

1. After what appears to be an uneventful spontaneous vaginal delivery with epidural anesthesia of a healthy female infant, a previously healthy 35-year-old woman is surprised to discover that she has difficulty crossing her right leg onto her left, and she cannot dorsiflex her right foot. Her epidural anesthesia has by now worn off. What nerve(s) is(are) most likely to be involved?

   A. Right sciatica
   B. Right femoral nerve injury
   C. Right common peroneal nerve injury
   D. Right sciatica and femoral nerve injury
   E. Right obturator and common peroneal nerve injury

2. A 70-year-old male patient presents with pain running along the back of his left lower extremity to the ankle. The left ankle jerk is diminished. Straight leg raise reproduces the pain on the left leg. He has weakness of plantar flexion. He notes that the pain started after lifting heavy boxes around the house. What is the most likely cause?

   A. Left sciatica
   B. Left S1 radiculopathy
   C. Left common peroneal nerve palsy
   D. Left tarsal tunnel syndrome
   E. Left femoral nerve palsy

3. After being struck on the head of the right fibula by a riot policeman's club, a now sober demonstrator discovers that he cannot run because his right foot is dragging. He is able to limp away and eventually pursue medical attention, where no fracture is seen on x-ray film. Over the next few hours, he regains the ability to walk normally. What is the most likely explanation?

   A. Transient tarsal tunnel syndrome due to tibial nerve injury
   B. Acute sciatica secondary to trauma
   C. Hairline fibular head fracture not seen on x-ray film
   D. Femoral nerve palsy secondary to trauma
   E. Common peroneal nerve palsy secondary to trauma

4. A 46-year-old woman on anticoagulation develops spontaneous abdominal pain. Abdominal CT scan shows a large retroperitoneal hematoma adjacent to the left iliopsoas muscle. She begins to complain of left thigh numbness. On exam, she has new profound weakness of the hip flexors and quadriceps muscles on the left. What has most likely happened?

   A. Left femoral nerve compression secondary to hematoma
   B. Left sciatic nerve compression secondary to hematoma
   C. Left obturator nerve compression secondary to hematoma
   D. Left L2 radiculopathy secondary to hematoma
   E. Left S2 radiculopathy secondary to hematoma

HPI: AF, a 23-year-old right-handed woman, presents to the ED with sudden onset of vision disturbance. She reports that the previous day, she noticed some pain in the right eye, especially when looking around. This morning she awoke and realized she was unable to see on the right. She has never experienced anything like this before. She is otherwise in good health, does not take any daily medications, and reports no significant illnesses in first-degree relatives.

PE: Her examination is remarkable for complete vision loss in her right eye with an absent pupillary response. She is noted to have a Marcus Gunn pupil on the right. She denies eye pain at this time. Her extraocular movements are full. Her visual field is intact in the left eye. CNs, fundi, power, sensation, coordination, and reflexes are otherwise intact.

THOUGHT QUESTIONS

- How is what we see represented in the brain?
- Where is this patient's lesion?
- What other structures could be involved?
- What is the most likely diagnosis?
- What is the most potentially dangerous diagnosis?

BASIC SCIENCE REVIEW AND DISCUSSION

Acute **optic neuritis** can occur in isolation or can be a harbinger of future demyelinating disease. It is the most likely diagnosis in light of the examination and available data. Patients commonly present with monocular vision loss sometimes preceded by pain with movement of the eye. An afferent pupillary defect **(Marcus Gunn pupil)** can be found in the affected eye. The light input cannot be transmitted across the lesion, so the pupil of the affected eye does not constrict in response to light. However, it does constrict when light is presented to the intact eye because pupillary constriction is consensual (via bilateral third CN innervation). When the examiner swings a flashlight back and forth between the eyes, the pupil of the affected eye appears to dilate "paradoxically" in response to light. This is not active dilation but passive relaxation because the light is moving away from the intact eye.

Visual Fields

The "visual field" is an image of everything the patient sees with the eyes at rest in the central position and is the sum of the visual fields of both eyes. Each eye has its own visual field and the two fields are mostly overlapped (spatial separation of the eyes and obstruction by the nose are the reasons for this incomplete overlap). Each visual field is projected onto its corresponding **retina** by light passing through the **cornea** and **lens.** In this process, the image is reversed and turned upside down. It is important to remember that the upper right portion of a visual field projects (upside down and backward) to the lower left portion of the corresponding retina. So, an object in the upper right quadrant of the "visual field" is "seen" by the lower left quadrant of each retina (the medial or nasal portion of the right retina and the lateral or temporal portion of the left retina). This relationship is maintained throughout the retina and the optic nerve.

Innervation of the Eye

The control of extraocular movement is mediated by CNs III, IV, and VI. The **superior oblique muscle** is innervated by the fourth or **trochlear nerve** (SO4).

The cell bodies of the neurons whose axons make up CN IV are located in the trochlear nucleus. The nerve passes through the cavernous sinus and enters the orbit through the superior orbital fissure. It is responsible for intorsion ("top" of iris rotates toward the nose) and helps direct downward gaze when the eye is adducted. Patients with fourth nerve palsies have vertical diplopia.

The **lateral rectus muscle** is innervated by the sixth or **abducens nerve** (LR6). The cell bodies of the neurons whose axons make up CN VI are located in the abducens nucleus. The sixth nerve courses through the cavernous sinus and enters the orbit through the superior orbital fissure. Its only target is the ipsilateral lateral rectus muscle, which is responsible for directing lateral gaze.

The third or **oculomotor nerve** innervates all of the other extraocular muscles, including the levator palpebrae muscle, and also provides parasympathetic innervation to the eye. The cell bodies of the axons that make up the third nerve are in a cluster of nuclei located near the midline in the **midbrain tegmentum.** The third nerve passes between the **superior cerebellar and posterior cerebral arteries** adjacent to the **posterior communicating artery,** then through the cavernous sinus, and enters the orbit through the superior orbital fissure. **Infarction of the third nerve** classically presents as a **painful pupil-sparing third nerve palsy,** but **third nerve palsy** from compression by a **posterior communicating artery aneurysm** or **uncal herniation** does not spare pupillary function (extrinsic compression of the third nerve affects the most superficial parasympathetic fibers first and causes the pupil to dilate).

The eye receives **parasympathetic** autonomic innervation from the **Edinger-Westphal nucleus.** Preganglionic parasympathetic axons originating in the Edinger-Westphal nucleus travel along the **surface of CN III** and terminate in the **ciliary ganglion.** Postganglionic parasympathetic axons originating in the ciliary ganglion travel along **short ciliary nerves** to reach the eye. The primary targets of parasympathetic innervation to the eyes are the **ciliary muscles,** which are responsible for changing the shape of the lenses during **accommodation,** and the **sphincter pupillae muscles,** which are responsible for **miosis** (pupillary constriction). In the **pupillary light reflex,** light entering the eye is conveyed by the optic nerve through the lateral geniculate nucleus (LGN) of the thalamus to the Edinger-Westphal nucleus in the midbrain. Reactive pupillary constriction is then mediated by the parasympathetic portion of CN III. The same type of reflex arc conveys information mediating the **accommodation reflex.**

The eye receives **sympathetic** autonomic innervation from the **superior cervical ganglion.** Postganglionic sympathetic axons originate in the paraspinous **sympathetic chain.** Sympathetic innervation also reaches the eyes via the **ciliary nerves.** The primary targets of sympathetic innervation to the eyes are the **dilator iridis muscles,** which contract to cause **mydriasis** (pupillary dilation). There is also a small amount of sympathetic innervation to the **ciliary muscles,** which counteracts the parasympathetic effect and opposes accommodation.

Neuroanatomy of the Visual System

Retina Visual processing begins in the retina, predominantly in the central portion, called the **macula.** The most sensitive part of the macula, the **fovea,** has the highest concentration of **cone photoreceptors.** They are responsible for **high-acuity central vision** and **color. Rod photoreceptors** are more prominent in the peripheral retina and mediate **low-acuity vision.** Energy from light is transduced to electrochemical energy by the photoreceptors, which are contained within the outer nuclear layer on the retina. Photoreceptors synapse onto **bipolar neurons** contained within the inner nuclear layer of the retina. These cells, in turn, synapse onto **ganglion cells** in the ganglion cell layer. Axons of the ganglion cells join to form the **optic nerve.** Numerous photoreceptors may converge on a single ganglion cell. The **receptive field** of a ganglion cell refers to the collective information from all the photoreceptors converging on that cell. However, there is minimal convergence within the fovea. This allows for higher acuity vision in this region.

Optic Chiasm The medial half of each optic nerve (coming from the medial half of each retina and carrying information from the lateral half of each visual field) crosses the midline at the **optic chiasm** to become part of the contralateral **optic tract.** The lateral half of each optic nerve continues on as part of the ipsilateral optic tract. This means that information from each half of the visual field (the sum of what both eyes see on one side) is carried by the contralateral optic tract (upside down and backward). This relationship is maintained throughout the remainder of the visual system, all the way to the level of the primary visual cortex.

Lesions that compress the optic chiasm cause loss of peripheral vision in the lateral half of the visual field of each eye (a bitemporal visual field deficit). Pituitary tumors can cause this visual deficit. This can also be seen in pregnancy, when the pituitary gland can become significantly enlarged.

Thalamus The optic tract ends in the **LGN** of the thalamus, where further processing of visual information occurs. The LGN has six layers. Axons from the ipsilateral retina project to layers 2, 3, and 5. Axons from the contralateral retina project to layers 1, 4, and 6. Layers 1 and 2 **(magnocellular layers)** respond to low contrast and are involved in the detection of motion. The remaining layers **(parvocellular layers)** respond to high contrast and color.

Optic Radiations From the LGN, the visual system projects to the **primary visual (calcarine) cortex** via the **optic radiations.** Information from the lower portion of the visual field is carried within the upper portion of the corresponding optic tract and along the **geniculocalcarine fibers** of the optic radiations. These fibers project straight back from the LGN to the superior portion of the visual cortex (the area above the calcarine sulcus). Information from the upper portion of the visual field is carried within the lower portion of the corresponding optic tract. Within the optic radiations, the fibers carrying this information follow a less direct route, looping somewhat anteriorly and superiorly through the temporal lobe **(Meyer loop),** before ending in the inferior portion of the visual cortex (the area below the

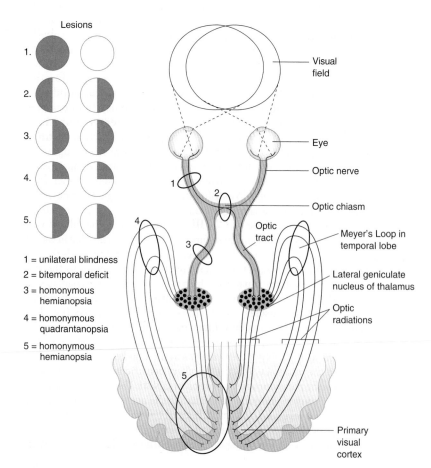

Lesions

1.

2.

3.

4.

5.

1 = unilateral blindness
2 = bitemporal deficit
3 = homonymous hemianopsia
4 = homonymous quadrantanopsia
5 = homonymous hemianopsia

Visual field

Eye

Optic nerve

Optic chiasm

Optic tract

Meyer's Loop in temporal lobe

Lateral geniculate nucleus of thalamus

Optic radiations

Primary visual cortex

• **Figure 10-5.** Visual system.

calcarine sulcus). The organization of the visual cortex is discussed in Case 10-3. Figure 10-5 summarizes the visual pathways leading to the occipital cortex.

Visual Field Deficits

A loss of vision in one half of the "visual field" (**homonymous hemianopia**) can be localized to a contralateral lesion involving the optic tract, LGN, or visual cortex. Clinicians refer to these deficits as "field cuts." As a general rule, cortical homonymous hemianopias tend to be more congruous (the shape of the visual defect is the same in both eyes) than lesions involving the optic tracts. Lesions in the optic radiations would not be expected to cause complete hemianopias because these fibers are spread too far apart anatomically. It is important to note that temporal lobe lesions can involve Meyer loop and thus lead to a loss of vision in the contralateral upper and outer quadrant of the visual field (**homonymous quadrantanopia**). Such "pie in the sky" lesions tend to spare central vision. These deficits are reviewed in Figure 10-5 and in the Thumbnail below.

Vision Loss

Sudden vision loss is a particularly disturbing symptom for patients and can be localized to lesions anywhere from the eye (globe) to the visual cortex. Ocular causes include corneal disease, refractive error, cataracts, and glaucoma. These often manifest as blurring, but vision loss can also be seen. Double vision is most commonly associated with disturbance of extraocular movement. Lesions affecting the retina or visual pathways generally are associated with visual field defects, called **scotomas**. Diseases affecting the retina, especially the macula, often present with a **positive scotoma** (a dark spot in the field of vision). Diseases affecting the optic nerve often present with a unilateral **negative scotoma** (a "blind spot"). Lesions affecting the optic chiasm, optic tract, or visual cortex affect vision in both eyes.

CASE CONCLUSION

Optic neuritis is generally self-limited, with peak disability within days to weeks. Most patients regain normal vision within the first 6 months. Subclinical demyelination may manifest as a decrease in visual acuity under certain stressors, such as fever (Uhthoff phenomenon). As a general rule, about half of patients who present with a single demyelinating event, like optic neuritis, will ultimately be diagnosed with MS. The risk is higher in the setting of supportive imaging or CSF laboratory data, and lower in the absence of such findings. The differential diagnosis in this case should include acute angle-closure glaucoma and amaurosis fugax (sudden, transient monocular loss of vision "like a curtain coming down," suggesting vascular compromise of the optic nerve and retina). Trauma, vitreous hemorrhage, retinal detachment, orbital infection, tumor, or pseudotumor and intracranial mass lesions would also have to be considered.

AF was admitted to the hospital and lumbar puncture was performed. MRI scan was ordered and revealed increased signal and contrast enhancement in the right optic nerve. CSF studies were normal. A 3-day course of IV methylprednisolone was initiated. After discharge, her vision gradually returned to normal over 8 weeks.

THUMBNAIL: Visual System Lesions

Location	Lesion	Clinical Features
Anterior to chiasm	Refractory error	Blurring
	Cataract	Blurring, dimming
	Glaucoma	Blurring, peripheral vision loss
	Orbital pseudotumor	Blurring, pain, proptosis
	Macular degeneration	Positive scotoma centrally
	Amaurosis fugax	Scotoma "like a curtain coming down"
	Optic neuritis	Negative scotoma centrally
Optic chiasm	Pituitary adenoma	Bitemporal peripheral vision loss
Posterior to chiasm	Optic tract/LGN lesions	Incongruous homonymous hemianopia
	Optic radiation lesions	Homonymous quadrantanopia
	Primary visual cortex lesions	Congruous homonymous hemianopia
	Associative visual cortex lesions	Higher-order visual defect (visual agnosia, alexia)

✓ KEY POINTS

■ A Marcus Gunn pupil "dilates paradoxically" in response to light (afferent pupillary defect)

■ Only the "superior muscles" are innervated contralaterally

■ Each superior oblique muscle is innervated by the contralateral trochlear nucleus

■ Each superior rectus muscle is innervated by the medial subnucleus of the contralateral oculomotor nuclear group

■ The remaining muscles mediating eye movement are innervated ipsilaterally

■ Parasympathetic and levator palpebrae innervation is bilateral

■ Lesions that compress the optic chiasm cause bitemporal visual field deficits

■ **Meyer loop** describes the optic radiations arising from the ventral portion of the optic tracts, which loop anteriorly in the temporal lobe

■ Lesions of Meyer loop cause homonymous quadrantanopsias

■ Lesions involving the optic tract, LGN, or visual cortex cause homonymous hemianopias

QUESTIONS

1. A 36-year-old man presents with difficulty reading for 1 day. Examination reveals a left centrocecal scotoma. Peripheral vision is relatively spared, as is vision in the right eye. He also is noted to have brisk reflexes and a positive Babinski sign on the left. Where is the lesion?

   A. Midbrain on the left, involving the oculomotor nerve and corticospinal tract
   B. Left optic nerve and right cervical spinal cord
   C. Left optic nerve and left cervical spinal cord
   D. Left optic nerve and left pons
   E. Optic chiasm and right internal capsule

2. An 18-year-old girl with intractable epilepsy and documented right mesial temporal sclerosis (MTS) by MRI undergoes an anterior temporal lobectomy. Postoperatively, she is seizure free but reports difficulty seeing the television. Where is the television located?

   A. Eye level and to the left
   B. Near the ceiling and to the right
   C. Centrally, beyond the foot of the bed
   D. Near the ceiling and to the left
   E. Eye level and to the right

3. A 23-year-old woman who is 15 weeks into her first pregnancy is referred to your office because of vision problems. She reports that at times she has been seeing things out of the corner of her eye. On further discussion, you discover that she also has been more prone to bump into things lately. Her examination is nonfocal. What is the most likely explanation?

   A. An electrical disturbance of the visual cortex related to migraine
   B. Substance abuse; check the urine drug screen
   C. An electrical disturbance of the visual cortex related to seizure
   D. Compression of the optic chiasm
   E. Demyelination in the optic tracts

4. A 63-year-old man with a history of diabetes, HTN, and intermittent AF has sudden onset of vision loss in his left eye. He says it was as though someone pulled down a curtain over his eye. His symptoms resolved after about 20 minutes. Which structure was most likely to have been affected?

   A. Optic nerve
   B. Retina
   C. Optic chiasm
   D. Optic tract
   E. Visual cortex

5. A 36-year-old man presents with sudden onset of the worst headache of his life. Examination reveals a dilated pupil on the left as compared with the right. Diplopia can be elicited with extreme right lateral gaze and he reports some difficulty reading. Where is the lesion?

   A. Compressive lesion, right sixth nerve
   B. Intrinsic lesion, left third nerve
   C. Compressive lesion, left third nerve
   D. Compressive lesion, right third nerve
   E. Intrinsic lesion, left sixth nerve

6. You evaluate a patient with unusual eye findings including restricted upward gaze. When he tries to look up, his eyes seem repeatedly to converge and retract deeper into his sockets (convergence-retraction nystagmus). His pupils do not constrict in response to light but do constrict when he focuses on near objects, like the tip of his nose. Which of the following structures is most likely being compressed?

   A. Ventral midbrain
   B. Dorsal midbrain
   C. Oculomotor nerve
   D. Optic nerve
   E. Pituitary gland

HPI: FP, a 52-year-old man, comes to your office for evaluation of headache. He reports that several times per day, he experiences sharp pain on the right side of the face and jaw. The pain lasts only a few seconds but is so severe that it cannot be ignored. The problem first developed several weeks ago, and his spells are getting more frequent. He has gone to his dentist, who found nothing wrong and referred him to you. Lately, he has noticed that his symptoms can be triggered by stimulation of a spot on his right jaw. He has since stopped shaving. He denies any other problems or illnesses. He has not had any rashes. His examination is unremarkable.

THOUGHT QUESTIONS

- Does this patient have a peripheral or central process?
- What is the most likely structure to be involved?
- What functions are mediated by this structure?

BASIC SCIENCE REVIEW AND DISCUSSION

FP presents with brief, episodic, lancinating pain involving the right side of the face. The upper face and eye are spared. There are no visible skin lesions. In this age group, the most likely diagnosis is **trigeminal neuralgia,** a clinical entity whose etiology is not clearly defined. The absence of other associated signs or symptoms makes the possibility of a central lesion less likely, especially in the setting of a spared first division of the trigeminal nerve. A mass lesion compressing the trigeminal nerve should be excluded. Migraine can present with unilateral head pain and belongs in the differential. Cluster headache can also present with unilateral head pain but is usually localized to the first branch of the trigeminal nerve rather than sparing it. As always, an understanding of the anatomy involved is important for the clinical evaluation.

Anatomy of the Trigeminal Nerve

CN V is the only cranial nerve to exit from the body of the **pons.** It does so from the midlateral surface, originating as two roots: a larger sensory root and a smaller motor root. The roots come together to form the nerve, which enters the **trigeminal ganglion.** The trigeminal ganglion has a purely sensory function, analogous to the dorsal root ganglia along the spinal cord. As its name implies, the trigeminal nerve has three main divisions that emerge from the trigeminal ganglion before exiting the skull. Some studies have implicated anatomic compression of the trigeminal ganglion or its main divisions as a possible cause for trigeminal neuralgia. Surgical decompression has been used in some cases but has not gained wide use. Chemical or radioablation is reserved for intractable cases not responsive to conservative medical management because of the resulting permanent sensory disturbance. These procedures are generally limited to the most affected of the three major divisions of the trigeminal nerve.

Divisions of Trigeminal Nerve The first division is the **ophthalmic nerve (V1),** which conveys purely sensory information. It passes through the **cavernous sinus** and exits the skull through the **superior orbital fissure.** It has several branches, including lacrimal, frontal, ciliary, and meningeal branches. The ophthalmic nerve conveys sensory information from the upper face, eye, cornea, and nose. The meningeal branch conveys sensory information from the tentorium cerebelli. Although the ophthalmic

division of the trigeminal nerve mediates purely sensory information, small sympathetic nerves that originate in the superior cervical ganglion and ascend along the internal carotid artery follow the ciliary branches to reach the eye. The patient in this case did not have any pain or abnormality associated with the ophthalmic division of the trigeminal nerve. However, there are a few clinical syndromes associated with this nerve. Herpes zoster ophthalmicus is one example. Although herpes zoster can affect any nerve and most commonly affects thoracic spinal nerves, herpes zoster ophthalmicus is an important entity to recognize because vesicular involvement of the cornea can lead to loss of vision.

The second division is the **maxillary nerve (V2),** also a pure sensory nerve. It generally passes through the cavernous sinus before exiting the skull through the **foramen rotundum.** It has several branches, including zygomatic, infraorbital, pterygopalatine, and meningeal branches. The maxillary nerve conveys sensory information from the middle face, nose, upper lip, and pharynx. The meningeal branch of the maxillary nerve conveys sensory information from the meninges of the anterior and middle cranial fossae. The maxillary nerve is often involved in trigeminal neuralgia (also called **tic douloureux** because the severe sudden pain can cause patients to wince).

The third division is the **mandibular nerve (V3).** The mandibular nerve has both a sensory and a motor component. It exits the skull through the **foramen ovale.** It has several branches, including buccal, lingual, auriculotemporal, inferior alveolar, and meningeal branches. The mandibular nerve conveys sensory information from the lower face, lower lip, buccal mucosa, and anterior two thirds of the tongue. Nerve fibers that convey taste information from the anterior two thirds of the tongue also are contained within the lingual nerve for a short distance. Rather than continuing to the trigeminal nucleus, these fibers leave the mandibular nerve as the **chorda tympani,** passing through the petrotympanic fissure and joining CN VII. The meningeal branch of the mandibular nerve also conveys sensory information from the meninges of the anterior and middle cranial fossae. The mandibular nerve also has several branches, which innervate each of the **muscles of mastication.** These represent the only motor function mediated by the trigeminal nerve.

Brainstem Trigeminal Nuclei The trigeminal nerve enters the brainstem on the midlateral surface of the pons. Within the pons, there are two **trigeminal nuclei:** a motor nucleus and a sensory nucleus. Both are located within the **pontine tegmentum** and are medial to the middle cerebellar peduncle, lateral to the medial longitudinal fasciculus (MLF), ventral to the superior cerebellar peduncle, and dorsal to the medial lemniscus. In keeping with the brainstem organizational principles previously discussed, the motor trigeminal nucleus is medial to the sensory nucleus.

The **motor trigeminal nucleus** is restricted to the pons. Its role is analogous to the anterior horn of the spinal cord. UMNs whose cell bodies are located within the primary motor cortex project to this nucleus where they synapse onto the LMNs. Each motor nucleus receives bilateral cortical input. Output from the motor nucleus projects out the ipsilateral trigeminal nerve, along the mandibular division, to reach the **muscles of mastication.** Because these nuclei **receive bilateral cortical input,** UMN lesions of the muscles of mastication are rarely seen.

The sensory trigeminal nucleus has three components. The rostral portion of the trigeminal sensory nucleus extends into the midbrain. This mesencephalic portion of the trigeminal nucleus is responsible for proprioceptive input from the muscles of mastication. The neurons of the **mesencephalic trigeminal nucleus** are unique in that they are the only primary sensory neurons known to exist within the CNS, rather than within sensory ganglia. Their peripheral processes come directly from the muscles of mastication without synapsing in the trigeminal ganglion. Their central processes project primarily onto the neurons of the motor trigeminal nucleus, forming a monosynaptic arc that mediates reflexes, such as the jaw jerk. The **principal sensory trigeminal nucleus is located within the pons** and is primarily responsible for tactile sensation from the face, analogous to the dorsal columns of the spinal cord. The **nucleus of the spinal tract of the trigeminal nerve extends caudally through the medulla and into the upper segments of the spinal cord.** It is primarily responsible for pain and temperature sensation from the face, analogous to the anterolateral sensory system of the spinal cord. Both the principal trigeminal nucleus and the nucleus of the spinal tract of the trigeminal nerve contain second-order sensory neurons. They receive input from primary sensory neurons in the trigeminal ganglion. The central projections from neurons within the trigeminal nuclei decussate within the pons to join the contralateral ascending spinothalamic pathways as the **trigeminal lemniscus.** Upon reaching the thalamus, nerve fibers from the trigeminal system synapse onto third-order sensory neurons in the **ventral posterior medial nucleus,** which then project to the primary sensory cortex.

Clinical Correlation

As mentioned previously, the constellation of symptoms in this patient is most consistent with trigeminal neuralgia. This clinical entity may be triggered by focal stimulation and is often responsive to carbamazepine. In younger patients, particularly in younger women, demyelinating disease should be considered as a cause for trigeminal neuralgia. Migraine can present with hemicranial pain, but attacks are more prolonged, pain is described as throbbing, and there are often other associated features (photophobia, phonophobia, nausea). Herpes zoster also can present with facial pain. In the acute phase, pain can precede vesicular eruption, but our patient is well into the subacute phase of his syndrome. In a patient with a history of herpes zoster, postherpetic neuralgia can present as severe facial pain that is generally more persistent. Trauma is another important potential cause for trigeminal nerve dysfunction. New-onset facial pain in an older individual should always raise the suspicion for tumor and an imaging study of the head should be performed.

CASE CONCLUSION

Routine laboratory studies were unremarkable. An MRI of the head with contrast was obtained and was also unremarkable. The patient was started on carbamazepine at the initial visit based on a presumptive diagnosis of trigeminal neuralgia. The dose was gradually increased with good response. Several months later the medication was weaned and the patient remained free of symptoms.

THUMBNAIL: Major Branches of the Trigeminal Nerve

Divisions	Main Branches
Ophthalmic (V1)	Lacrimal
	Frontal
	Nasociliary
	Meningeal
Maxillary (V2)	Zygomatic
	Infraorbital
	Pterygopalatine
	Meningeal
Mandibular (V3)	Buccal
	Auriculotemporal
	Lingual
	Inferior alveolar
	Meningeal
	Motor branches (to muscles of mastication)

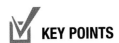

KEY POINTS

- Trigeminal nerve has predominantly sensory function
- The motor component of the trigeminal nerve innervates the muscles of mastication
- Proprioceptive information goes to the mesencephalic trigeminal nucleus
- Tactile sensation information goes to the principal trigeminal nucleus in the pons
- Pain and temperature information goes to the spinal trigeminal nucleus in the medulla and upper spinal cord

QUESTIONS

1. A 40-year-old woman presents with brief severe headaches over the right eye. They occur several times per day and are associated with runny nose, sweating, and reddening of the eye. What structure is involved?

   A. Maxillary sinus
   B. Ophthalmic nerve
   C. Trigeminal ganglion
   D. Ophthalmic artery
   E. Ciliary ganglion

2. A 72-year-old hypertensive man has been having brief spells that he describes as tingling on the right side of his face. They have generally lasted only minutes at a time. This morning he awoke to find a similar sensation involving his left arm and leg. The symptoms have persisted throughout the day and he is getting worried. Where is his lesion?

   A. Dorsal pontine tegmentum on the left
   B. Ventral pontine tegmentum on the left
   C. Dorsal pontine tegmentum on the right
   D. Ventral pontine tegmentum on the right
   E. Trigeminal ganglion on the right

3. A 34-year-old man presents with left facial droop and diminished sensation on the left side of the face. Both the upper and the lower face are affected. His ability to taste is also diminished on the left side of the tongue. Which structure is affected?

   A. Trigeminal nerve on the right
   B. Trigeminal nerve on the left
   C. Pons on the left
   D. Facial nerve on the left
   E. Cerebral cortex on the left

4. Another 34-year-old man presents with a left facial droop involving both the upper and lower face. Taste is diminished on the left side of the tongue. Which muscles are spared?

   A. Orbicularis oculi and frontalis
   B. Levator palpebrae and frontalis
   C. Masseter and levator palpebrae
   D. Orbicularis oculi and masseter
   E. Frontalis and masseter

CASE 10-13 Taste and Facial Nerve

HPI: A 35-year-old otherwise healthy woman presents to your office complaining of an inability to close her left eye. She had been in good health (other than a case of the flu several weeks ago) when she noticed upon waking the previous day that her left eye would not close all the way and was somewhat irritated. Her family notes that the left side of her face doesn't seem to move as much as the right, and the left corner of her mouth appears to droop. She also complains that she is not able to taste food on the left side of her tongue.

PE: Her exam is notable for a fairly noticeable left facial droop with a decreased left nasolabial fold, and slightly increased size of the palpebral fissure on the left versus the right. When asked to close her eyes, her left eye looks upward, but the lids are not able to completely close. She is unable to appreciate sweet taste on the left side of her tongue. Otherwise, her exam is completely benign.

THOUGHT QUESTIONS

- What area of the nervous system has been affected?
- How is motor innervation of the face controlled?
- How is taste appreciated?
- What is her prognosis?

BASIC SCIENCE REVIEW AND DISCUSSION

Control of Facial Muscles and CN VII

Motor function of the face is almost completely governed by CN VII (the facial nerve), with the exception of the levator palpebrae superioris, which is controlled by CN III. It is the lack of opposition to the levator palpebrae that resulted in this patient's inability to close her eye (normally closure is performed by the orbicularis oculi). In addition, CN VII also (at some points in its course) contains fibers for taste, sensation of the ear, and some of the autonomic fibers controlling salivation.

Facial motor function originates in the **motor cortex,** located in the precentral gyrus of the frontal lobe. Motor fibers projecting to the pons (also known as *corticobulbar fibers*) coalesce with all other motor fibers, forming the corona radiata and then the internal capsule, then passing through the cerebral peduncles. After entering the brainstem, the corticobulbar fibers (which control all motor function governed by cranial nerves) diverge to the various cranial nerve nuclei, crossing the midline in most cases. The **corticospinal** fibers progress onward to the spinal cord.

The pons contains the **facial nucleus,** in which the UMNs (in this case, the corticobulbar fibers to the facial nucleus) synapse to the LMNs, whose cell bodies essentially make up the facial nucleus. The facial nucleus is separated into two basic halves, one of which projects to the lower face and one of which projects to the upper face. Because these parts are innervated differently, they are discussed separately. The projections from the facial nucleus exit the brainstem to form the majority of the facial nerve, or **CN VII.**

The Facial Nucleus The facial nucleus is concerned only with motor function, namely that of the head and neck. The **lower half** of the facial nucleus receives axons solely from the contralateral motor cortex. These "singly innervated" LMNs project fibers (axons) that exit the brainstem to form part of the facial nerve. They innervate the lower half of the face and neck, generally at and below the level of the nose. Because the lower half of the face is innervated only by the contralateral cortex, it is susceptible to both UMN and LMN lesions, which includes stroke and Bell palsy (discussed subsequently).

The **upper half** of the facial nucleus receives bilateral projections from the motor cortex: Both the ipsilateral and contralateral cortex synapses with these LMN cell bodies. These "dual-innervated" LMNs then run to the muscles of the upper half of the face. As a result, processes that affect the UMN only (stroke) generally do not cause upper facial weakness, because the opposite cortex also projects to the upper half of the facial nucleus, and thus may compensate. As a result, only LMN processes (Bell palsy) affect strength in the upper portion of the face.

CN VII Fibers from both the upper and the lower half of the facial nucleus coalesce to form the facial tract, which loops around the abducent nucleus in the dorsal pons. This loop forms a dorsal bulge on the floor of the fourth ventricle known as the **facial colliculus.** These motor fibers then exit the ventral pons at the pontomedullary junction. These motor fibers have joined with other autonomic, taste, and sensory fibers before exiting the brainstem. CN VII comprises this complex collection of nerve fibers outside of the brain. Upon leaving the brainstem, CN VII enters the **internal auditory meatus** and the **facial canal** within the skull. The facial canal leaves little room for expansion in its tighter segments, resulting in the possibility of facial nerve compression if CN VII should become swollen or inflamed (to be discussed later).

Motor Fibers

The first motor branch diverges within the facial canal to the **stapedius** muscle of the inner ear. The stapedius dampens tympanic membrane vibration, which is helpful when excessively loud noises are encountered. Remaining motor fibers exit the skull via the **stylomastoid foramen.** Branches are sent to the **posterior digastric belly** and **stylohyoid** muscles. They then weave through the parotid gland and then divide into the five major motor branches of the facial nerve: **cervical, mandibular, buccal, zygomatic,** and **temporal.** These innervate the platysmas and muscles of facial expression.

Sensory Fibers

The sensation of the outer ear is governed by sensory fibers whose cell bodies are located in the **geniculate ganglion** (so named because it lies in the curve, or **genu,** of the facial canal) after joining the other facial nerve fibers in the facial canal. These sensory fibers enter the brainstem as part of CN VII, and then diverge to the **spinal trigeminal nucleus.** (General sensory fibers associated with cranial nerves generally project to the spinal trigeminal nucleus.)

Taste Fibers

Taste of the anterior two thirds of the tongue, in addition to taste of the hard and soft palates, is governed by fibers that also form part of CN VII. These gustatory fibers initially run or "hitchhike" with the lingual branch of the trigeminal nerve before diverging to form the **chorda tympani.** The **chorda tympani** is an important branch of CN VII, which enters the skull at the **petrotympanic fissure** and then runs through the middle ear, adjacent to the tympanic membrane (thus giving it its name) before joining the rest of CN VII in the facial canal. It synapses in the geniculate ganglion and then continues with CN VII into the brainstem, where the gustatory fibers run to the **nucleus solitarius,** which governs taste. The nucleus solitarius also projects onto the superior salivary nucleus, which governs salivation and lacrimation (discussed later in this case).

Autonomic Fibers (Secretory Function)

The autonomic fibers of CN VII essentially control all major salivary and mucous glands of the head, with the important exception of the parotid gland. This is accomplished by projections from the **superior salivary nucleus,** which join the facial tract as it exits the brainstem. These autonomic fibers form two branches that diverge from CN VII in the facial canal.

The first branch is the **greater superficial petrosal nerve**. It enters the pterygoid canal and then synapses in the pterygopalatine (or sphenopalatine) ganglion. Postganglionic nerve fibers leave the ganglion and follow a complicated course ("hitchhiking" on different branches of CN V) en route to the lacrimal glands of the orbit and mucous glands of the nose and pharynx. The second branch runs with the chorda tympani to synapse in the submandibular ganglion, which sends postganglionic fibers to the submandibular and sublingual salivary glands.

Clinical Presentations of Facial Weakness

Because of the anatomy described earlier in regards to the upper and lower halves of the facial nucleus, UMN lesions present differently from LMN lesions.

UMN Lesions Processes affecting the facial aspect of the motor strip are only evident in their exclusive projections to the lower half of the contralateral facial nucleus. As a result, they generally present with contralateral weakness of the lower half of the face, with relative preservation of periorbital and forehead muscles. Patients present with a droop of the mouth and diminished nasolabial fold on the affected side. Stroke (cerebrovascular accident [CVA]) is the most common cause of UMN dysfunction, but brain tumors, MS, and head trauma are other possibilities, to name a few.

LMN Lesions Lesions affecting the facial nerve itself, the final common pathway to the innervation of facial musculature, **affect motor function of the entire side of the face,** including the periorbital muscles and the forehead. They may also affect taste on the ipsilateral tongue due to compromise of the chorda tympani fibers, and theoretically salivation and sensation of the ear may be affected, although these are less obvious. The presence or absence of upper facial weakness often allow LMN versus UMN lesions to be distinguished clinically.

Bell Palsy

Bell palsy refers to an acute hemifacial palsy of unknown cause. It occurs in about 30 patients per 100,000 per year (rare) and is more likely in diabetics and pregnant patients (third trimester or 1 week postpartum). Patients will present with a partial or complete paralysis of both the upper and the lower half of one side of the face. This presentation can be caused only by LMN dysfunction, because UMN lesions spare the upper half of the face. There are other causes of hemifacial palsy, including trauma, severe otitis media, Lyme disease, tumor, sarcoidosis, and HIV. However, most patients with acute hemifacial palsy will not have any clear etiology, and aggressive diagnostic testing is generally unnecessary unless the problem persists for more than 2 weeks.

Although Bells palsy refers to unknown causes by definition, some evidence suggests that most cases are caused by a neuritis secondary to HSV-1 infection. HSV-1, when present, resides within CN ganglia and may periodically reactivate, often resulting in vesicular eruptions (cold sores) and possibly facial nerve inflammation. This inflammatory response causes swelling. The facial canal is constrictive and compression of CN VII may follow, resulting in dysfunction and hemifacial paralysis. It may also cause loss of taste and salivation on the affected side, although many patients will not notice this.

Most patients with Bell palsy (about 70%) will completely recover. A good rule of thumb is that patients with an incomplete palsy will recover (about 95%), whereas significantly fewer of those with a complete palsy (60%) recover. In severe cases, regeneration of the facial nerve may be inappropriate, leading to tearing of the eye when salivation should occur. This is known as **"crocodile tears."** Treatment is usually supportive, although medium-dose oral steroids and antiherpetic agents (acyclovir or valacyclovir) are sometimes used.

CASE CONCLUSION

Because both the upper and the lower portion of her face was clearly involved, it is clear that the LMN (the peripheral nerve) is the culprit. The patient was diagnosed with a Bell palsy in light of the lack of other cranial neuropathies or physical findings. She was given a 2-week regimen of oral prednisolone and valacyclovir and allowed to go home. She was also told to tape her eye closed at night and to use eyedrops to keep it moist, because she is unable to close it. Within 3 weeks, she reported return of eye closure and some use of her face, and she regained complete use of her face after 2 months.

THUMBNAIL: Facial Nerve and Selected Cranial Nerve Functions

Cranial Nerve	Motor Function	Sensory Function	Autonomic Function	Other
VII	Facial muscles; stapedius	External ear	Salivary, lacrimal; nasal glands	Taste, anterior two thirds of tongue
V	Mastication	Face, eyes, mouth	None	
IX	Stylopharyngeus	External ear, middle ear; pharynx	Parotid gland; carotid sinus	
X	Pharynx, larynx	External ear; pharynx, larynx	Parasympathetic; of internal viscera	

 KEY POINTS

- The facial nucleus receives bilateral projections to its upper half, such that central or UMN lesions affect only the lower contralateral facial quadrant; facial hemiplegia involving the upper and lower face results from lesions of the LMN, often within the facial canal
- CN VII is a complex nerve that controls almost all voluntary facial musculature, sensation of the ear, secretory function of the eye,

nasopharynx, and salivary glands (except the parotid), and taste of the anterior two thirds of the tongue
- Bell palsy refers to idiopathic acute facial hemiplegia; it is thought to often be caused by facial neuritis, leading to compression in the facial canal, generally due to HSV-1 reactivation; patients usually fully recover

QUESTIONS

1. You meet a patient in the hospital who has an isolated schwannoma of the left facial nerve, which has completely compromised all function of all the nerve fibers just as they exit the brainstem. What symptoms do you expect this patient to have?

    A. Left hemifacial palsy (upper and lower), decreased taste on anterior left tongue, hyperacusis in left ear, decreased sensation in external left ear, decreased secretion of left salivary and nasal glands
    B. Left lower facial palsy, decreased taste on anterior left tongue, hyperacusis in left ear, decreased sensation in external left ear, decreased secretion of left salivary and nasal glands
    C. Right hemifacial palsy (upper and lower), decreased taste on anterior right tongue, hyperacusis in right ear, decreased sensation in external left ear, decreased secretion of left salivary and nasal glands
    D. Asymptomatic
    E. Left hemifacial palsy (upper and lower) only

2. A 75-year-old man with a history of left lower facial droop due to stroke and recurrent left-sided otitis media is noted to have diminished taste on the anterior left tongue. Sensation is otherwise intact. What is the most likely explanation?

    A. Congenital absence of taste buds on the left tongue
    B. Infarction of cerebral taste pathways from stroke

    C. Benign changes related to aging
    D. Involvement of chorda tympani from otitis media
    E. New-onset Bell palsy

3. A 70-year-old male patient has a persistent left hemifacial droop secondary to a parotid gland tumor that was excised 5 years ago. What other deficiencies would he be expected to have?

    A. Lack of taste in left anterior tongue
    B. Lack of salivation in left salivary glands
    C. Lack of sensation in left face
    D. No other deficits
    E. Left hyperacusis

4. A 46-year-old woman developed an apparent Bell palsy several months ago with residual right hemifacial droop. Over time, the droop slowly improves, but she begins to note that her right eye tears when she eats or salivates. What is a possible explanation?

    A. Inappropriate regeneration of salivary autonomic fibers to lacrimal glands
    B. Recurrence of Bell palsy
    C. Conjunctivitis
    D. Hyperlacrimation syndrome
    E. Normal prodrome of recovery

HPI: HM, a 56-year-old right-handed man, comes to your office complaining of hearing loss and ringing in the right ear. He reports that his symptoms were initially subtle. In retrospect, he admits to diminished hearing over the past year. More recently, he becomes dizzy at times, although this is mild. He also reports that food just doesn't taste the same anymore. His health has been good in all other respects.

PE: His exam reveals asymmetry on the Weber test, with sound heard better on the left. Air conduction is louder than bone conduction bilaterally on the Rinne test. He has a subtle right lower facial droop and diminished taste sensation on the right side of the tongue. The remainder of the exam is unremarkable.

THOUGHT QUESTIONS

- Where is this patient's lesion?
- What are the structural implications of the exam findings?
- What other structures could be involved?
- Can you describe the auditory pathways involved?

BASIC SCIENCE REVIEW AND DISCUSSION

Hearing loss can be divided into central and peripheral causes. **Central hearing loss** is usually relatively mild unless the cochlear nuclei are involved. **Peripheral hearing loss** can be either **conductive** (sound not getting to the inner ear) or **sensorineural** (sound gets in but cannot be conveyed centrally). In the **Weber test**, a tuning fork is held at the midline on the skull. The sound is perceived asymmetrically if there is a deficit. Sound is louder in the affected ear with a conductive deficit but louder in the intact ear with a sensorineural deficit. In the **Rinne test**, conduction of sound waves in bone and air are compared. Bone conduction is louder only in the setting of a conductive deficit. This patient's complaint and exam findings suggest a sensorineural hearing loss on the right. The LMN facial weakness and loss of taste on the right implicate the right facial nerve. Given the absence of other associated symptoms, the lesion is more likely to be extra-axial and involving CN VII and VIII on the right.

A slow-growing mass lesion in the cerebellopontine angle could produce this clinical syndrome. The mass lesion most often associated with this location is an **acoustic neuroma.** These tumors usually begin on the vestibular portion of the eighth nerve but grow slowly enough that hearing loss is seen more often than vertigo as an initial manifestation. Acoustic neuromas can occur either sporadically or in association with **neurofibromatosis.** This is the most common of the neurocutaneous syndromes (associated with both neurologic deficits and characteristic skin lesions). Two types of neurofibromatosis are recognized. Both are inherited in a dominant pattern. Type 1 (von Recklinghausen disease) is primarily peripheral in its manifestation. Type 2 is more commonly associated with CNS manifestations. Bilateral acoustic neuromas are classically associated with neurofibromatosis type 2.

Sound Reception

The auricle of the ear concentrates sound toward the external acoustic meatus. These sound waves cause vibration of the **tympanic membrane,** which converts the sound wave energy into mechanical energy. Movement of the tympanic membrane sets the ossicles in motion. Within the tympanic cavity, two muscles exert control over the sensitivity of this system. The **tensor tympani muscle,** innervated by the trigeminal nerve, can reduce tympanic membrane flexibility. The **stapedius muscle,** innervated by the facial nerve, can reduce ossicle motion. The first of the **ossicles,** the **malleus,** is attached to the tympanic membrane. The **stapes** is attached to the membrane covering the oval window. The **incus** connects the malleus to the stapes. Movement of the stapes causes movement of the membrane covering the **oval window** of the cochlea.

Cochlea The **cochlea** is a coiled tube with three fluid-filled compartments (scalae) divided by two membranes (Fig. 10-6). The **Reissner membrane** separates the **scala vestibuli** from the **scala media.** The **basilar membrane** separates the **scala media** from the **scala tympani.** The scala media is completely isolated from the other two compartments and contains potassium-rich **endolymph.** The scala vestibuli and scala tympani are connected through an opening at the apex of the cochlea, called the **helicotrema.** The **oval window** is at the proximal end of the scala vestibuli. The **round window** is at the proximal end of the scala tympani. The flexible membrane covering the round window accommodates the piston-like movement of the stapes against the membrane of the oval window (as one moves in, the other moves out). The resulting fluid waves set the basilar membrane in motion. The **organ of Corti,** which transduces this motion into electrochemical energy, is located within the basilar membrane. The shape of the basilar membrane is such that it is stiffer near the base of the cochlea and more flexible at the apex. This allows for sound frequency differentiation. Higher frequencies are best detected at the cochlear base, and lower frequencies are best detected at the apex. This **tonotopic organization** starts in the cochlea and is maintained all the way up to the **primary auditory cortex.**

Organ of Corti The organ of Corti converts mechanical energy into electrochemical energy. It contains one row of inner **hair cells** and three rows of outer **hair cells.** The **cilia** of the hair cells are attached to an overlying **tectorial membrane** and are surrounded by potassium-rich endolymph. Movement of the basilar membrane and hair cells relative to the tectorial membrane cause bending of the cilia, which causes **potassium ion channels** within them to either open or close. Altered potassium conductance changes the membrane potential of the hair cells. The hair cells are direction sensitive. Movement in one direction causes relative hair cell depolarization, and movement in the opposite direction causes relative hyperpolarization. The hair cells are in

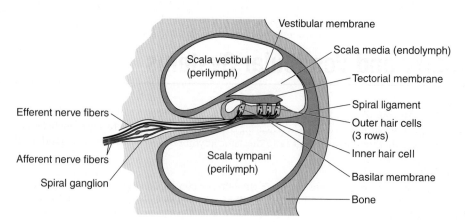

• **Figure 10-6.** Cochlea in cross-section.

synaptic contact with the peripheral processes of bipolar (primary) sensory neurons in the **spiral ganglion.** The hair cell membrane potential modulates neurotransmitter release from hair cells onto these dendrites.

Sensory Neurons The **primary auditory sensory neurons** are glutamatergic bipolar neurons in the **spiral ganglion** of the cochlea, which receive input from **cochlear hair cells.** The central projections from these neurons make up the cochlear portion of the eighth nerve. They enter the skull at the internal auditory meatus and enter the brainstem near the cerebellopontine angle, at the pontomedullary junction. They terminate on secondary sensory neurons in the **dorsal and ventral cochlear nuclei.** The cochlear nuclei are located in the dorsolateral pons, near the inferior cerebellar peduncle, and lateral to the vestibular nuclei.

Afferent Auditory Pathways The cochlear nuclei have bilateral central projections. Ipsilateral projections enter the **lateral lemniscus** on the same side. Three acoustic striae (the **dorsal, intermediate, and ventral striae**) project to the contralateral side of the brainstem. The dorsal and intermediate pathways decussate more dorsally in the pons and enter the lateral lemniscus directly. The ventral pathway (also called the **trapezoid body**) decussates more ventrally in the pons, terminating in the **superior olivary nuclear group** and reticular formation. Tertiary auditory neurons from these areas then project into the **lateral lemniscus.** The lateral lemniscus terminates in the **inferior colliculus.** Neurons in the inferior colliculus project to the **medial geniculate nucleus of the thalamus.** Neurons from this nucleus then project to the **primary auditory cortex.**

Organization of Sound Processing

Beginning at the level of the cochlear nuclei, **auditory pathways have bilateral representation.** This means that unilateral deafness can only be caused by a peripheral lesion (cochlea, eighth nerve) or a lesion involving the cochlear nuclei (which would likely involve other structures too). Any higher lesion in the auditory pathways may cause mild diminished hearing bilaterally but would not cause unilateral deafness. Auditory pathways are further complicated by feedback loops at every level of processing. Integration of auditory input from the two ears allows **localization of sounds in space.** Neurons in the auditory cortex either respond preferentially to sounds heard best in both ears (type EE neurons) or to sounds heard best in the contralateral ear (type EI neurons). Further processing of auditory input occurs within the auditory cortex and higher associative cortices.

Detection of Movement

The **vestibular apparatus** is a collective term for the fluid-filled labyrinthine structures involved in the detection of movement. It includes **three semicircular canals,** which are arranged perpendicular to each other, as well as the **utricle** and **saccule.** The semicircular canals are involved in the detection of **angular acceleration,** and the utricle and saccule are involved in the detection of **linear acceleration.**

Each semicircular canal responds maximally to movement in a specific plane. The lateral canal responds to head turning. The anterior canal responds to head nodding. The posterior canal responds to lateral head tilting. Movement that causes increased activity in one canal will generally cause decreased activity in the corresponding contralateral canal. For this reason, lesions on one side of the vestibular system result in a subjective sensation of motion, called **vertigo.**

The physiologic basis for the detection of motion is very similar to the system previously described for the cochlea. In fact, the endolymph of the cochlear duct (scala media) is continuous with the endolymph of the vestibular structures. Motion is detected by **ciliated hair cells** bathed in endolymph. The hair cells of the semicircular canals are located in the ampulla of each canal, in the **crista ampullaris.** Hair cells of the utricle and saccule are similarly arranged in structures called **maculae.** Hair cells in the macula of the utricle respond to linear acceleration along the long axis of the body, while hair cells in the macula of the saccule respond to linear acceleration along the dorsoventral axis of the body.

Causes of Vertigo

Ménière disease causes paroxysmal attacks of severe vertigo that usually last for minutes at a time, are not precipitated by any particular movement, and can be associated with hearing loss, nausea, and vomiting. Attacks of benign positional vertigo **(BPV)** often are shorter in duration (less than 1 minute) and usually are associated with a particular provocative head position. **Vestibular neuritis** and other peripheral inflammatory conditions are often associated with spells of longer duration (minutes to hours), may be provoked by movement, but generally are not associated with a specific head position. **Central vertigo** can last days to months, is less likely to be episodic, and is far more likely to be associated with other neurologic deficits.

Vestibulo-Ocular System

The vestibular nuclei receive input from the visual system and project to the nuclei, controlling eye movement through the **MLF.** This system helps to coordinate eye movement with head movement to maintain the image of an object of interest focused on the fovea in the retina. As previously described, damage to the vestibular system on one side causes disequilibrium of vestibular input, which is interpreted as motion by the nervous system (vertigo). This results in compensatory slow eye movement opposite to the direction of perceived motion followed by rapid (saccadic) correction. This repetitive process is called **nystagmus.** Nystagmus is named for the direction of the fast phase by convention.

Testing the **vestibulo-ocular reflex (VOR)** is important in the evaluation of the comatose patient. This can be done by oculocephalic testing (if there is no head or neck trauma) or by caloric testing. Passive head turning in an unconscious patient should elicit reflexive movement of the eyes toward the contralateral side such that the direction of gaze remains fixed, or the **doll's eyes response.** If intact, this reflex suggests that the brainstem is intact from the level of the vestibular nuclei at the pontomedullary junction up to the third and fourth nerve nuclei in the midbrain. When the VOR is absent, the eyes do not move as the head is turned and the direction of gaze changes. The VOR is normally suppressed in the awake patient, so the absence of the VOR either indicates an awake patient with an intact brainstem or a comatose patient with a brainstem lesion.

The VOR can also be evaluated by **caloric testing.** Cold water infusion into the ear creates a convection current within the semicircular canals on one side and the illusion of motion. The eyes will deviate toward the cold ear and a compensatory nystagmus will develop. The direction of the nystagmus (named for the fast phase) will be away from the cold ear. The opposite will occur with infusion of warm water. The mnemonic *COWS* (*c*old *o*pposite, *w*arm *s*ame) refers to the nystagmus, not to the direction of initial eye deviation.

CASE CONCLUSION

An MRI scan was ordered and revealed an enhancing mass near the cerebellopontine angle on the right. The patient was referred for neurosurgical evaluation and resection of the mass. The eighth nerve on the right could not be spared. Postoperatively, the patient was left with permanent unilateral deafness on the right. He was initially vertiginous, but this ultimately resolved with vestibular therapy. His facial nerve deficits also resolved.

THUMBNAIL: Peripheral Hearing Loss

	Conductive	Sensorineural
Structures involved	Outer or middle ear	Cochlear or retrocochlear
Frequencies affected	Same for all frequencies	High frequencies affected
Speech discrimination	Intact	Impaired
Tinnitus	May be present	Usually present
Causes	Usually acquired (structural, trauma, toxic, tumors)	Congenital or acquired (noise, aging, inflammation, infection, trauma, toxic, tumor)

KEY POINTS

- Unilateral deafness suggests a peripheral, neural, or nuclear lesion
- Conductive hearing loss is caused by lesions in the external or middle ear
- Sensorineural hearing loss is caused by lesions in the inner ear or nerve
- The auditory system is tonotopically organized
- In the Weber test, a tuning fork is held at the midline on the skull; sound is louder in the affected ear with a conductive deficit and louder in the intact ear with a sensorineural deficit
- In the Rinne test, conduction of sound waves in bone and air are compared; bone conduction is louder than air conduction in the setting of a conductive deficit

- Semicircular canals are involved in the detection of angular acceleration
- The utricle and saccule are involved in the detection of linear acceleration
- Peripheral vertigo has a relatively short duration and may be caused by Ménière disease, vestibular neuritis, BPV, or vestibular toxicity (e.g., aminoglycosides)
- Central vertigo has a longer duration and may be familial or caused by migraine, stroke, or tumors

QUESTIONS

1. A 30-year-old woman presents with sudden onset of hearing loss and tinnitus on the right. She asks if this could be a manifestation of her MS. Where might her lesion be located?

   A. Trapezoid body
   B. Left superior olivary nuclei
   C. Right cochlear nuclei
   D. Right lateral pons
   E. Left lateral lemniscus

2. A 63-year-old man comes to the ED complaining of gradual loss of hearing on the left. This is confirmed objectively. The Weber test reveals asymmetric findings with sound louder on the left. The Rinne test reveals bone conduction to be louder than air conduction on the left. What is the most likely explanation?

   A. Excessive cerumen buildup; his ears need to be cleaned
   B. Probable exposure to an aminoglycoside
   C. Tumor in the cerebellopontine angle on the left
   D. Too many rock concerts
   E. Increased endolymph pressure and distended semicircular canals

3. A 53-year-old man complains of attacks of vertigo associated with fullness in the ears and impaired hearing. This is worse on the right than on the left. These attacks can last hours and have been occurring on and off for several years. More recently, he has noticed trouble hearing between attacks too. What is the most likely explanation?

   A. Excessive cerumen buildup; his ears need to be cleaned
   B. Probable exposure to an aminoglycoside
   C. Tumor in the cerebellopontine angle on the left
   D. Too many rock concerts
   E. Increased endolymph pressure and distended semicircular canals

4. A 28-year-old man comes to the ED with sudden onset of a left facial droop. He complains that sounds are louder on the left than on the right. You determine that he has impaired taste sensation on the right side of the tongue. What is the explanation for his hearing problem?

   A. Impaired tensor tympani muscle function on the left
   B. Impaired stapedius muscle function on the right
   C. Impaired tensor tympani muscle function on the right
   D. Impaired stapedius muscle function on the left
   E. Tumor in the cerebellopontine angle on the left

5. A 25-year-old female patient with a known history of MS presents with sudden onset of vertigo and tinnitus in the right ear. Where might her lesion be located?

   A. Right dorsolateral pons
   B. Cerebellum
   C. Right vestibular nuclei
   D. Right MLF
   E. Left MLF

6. A 56-year-old man complains of sudden onset of severe dizziness, "like the room was spinning," which he first noted while checking his car tire pressure. His symptoms resolved quickly but recurred for several seconds when turning in bed this morning. He has no other symptoms and his hearing is normal. Where is the problem?

   A. Utricle
   B. Eighth nerve
   C. Vestibular nuclei
   D. Semicircular canal
   E. Saccule

CASE 10-15   Pons

HPI: A 32-year-old female school teacher comes to your office for evaluation. She has been having episodic double vision for several days. She first noticed it while writing on her chalkboard and trying to look over her right shoulder at her class. It also occurs when she tries to back up her car. It has never occurred with central gaze. She has never experienced anything like this before and is otherwise healthy. You ask if she has had difficulty reading and she denies it.

PE: Her exam is remarkable for impaired left eye adduction on right lateral gaze with associated diplopia. All other extraocular movements are intact in both eyes. Interestingly, when you ask her to watch your finger as you move it closer to her face (vergence testing), both eyes adduct equally and diplopia is denied. Pupillary responses are intact bilaterally and her exam is otherwise unremarkable.

THOUGHT QUESTIONS

- Does this patient have a peripheral or central lesion?
- What is the most likely structure to be involved?
- What functions are mediated by this structure?

BASIC SCIENCE REVIEW AND DISCUSSION

The patient presents with episodic diplopia in association with right lateral gaze. Although she is unable to adduct her left eye with right lateral gaze, the eye does adduct with vergence. This apparent paradox defines the deficit as an **internuclear ophthalmoplegia (INO)** and localizes the lesion to the left **MLF.** The MLF provides a functional connection between the pontine abducens nucleus on one side and the contralateral mesencephalic oculomotor nucleus, allowing for the coordination of conjugate eye movements.

Coordination of Horizontal Gaze

Remember that extraocular movement is mediated by three cranial nerves, two of which (third and fourth) are located in the midbrain and one of which (sixth) is located more caudally, in the pons. The **abducens nucleus** is located at the midpontine level and is relatively medial and dorsal within the pontine tegmentum. Its location beneath the floor of the fourth ventricle is anatomically analogous to the location of the third and fourth CN nuclei with respect to the cerebral aqueduct in the midbrain. Although these different CN nuclei have unique control over their respective muscles, their actions must be coordinated to maintain conjugate gaze. The pathway connecting these three CN nuclei, the **MLF,** allows for this coordination to take place. Brainstem regulatory fibers projecting down to the medulla and spinal cord are contained within a caudal extension of the MLF.

Whereas the **MLF** is needed for **coordination of lateral gaze,** it is not needed for vergence (bilateral medial rectus activation). Vergence is mediated within the midbrain and would not be affected by a pontine MLF lesion. This explains why this patient has impaired left eye adduction only on right lateral gaze. The MLF runs along the dorsomedial aspect of the pontine and mesencephalic tegmentum and is so close to the midline that central lesions can sometimes cause a bilateral INO. Another important clinical syndrome to recognize is the **one-and-a-half syndrome.** This occurs when a single lesion affects both the abducens nucleus and the MLF on the same side. The result is a loss of ipsilateral abduction and an ipsilateral INO. Thus, the only horizontal gaze movement to remain intact is abduction in the contralateral eye. Think of the one-and-a-half syndrome as one

in which three fourths of the horizontal gaze movements are lost and in which the lesion is on the same side as the most affected eye. Coordination of horizontal gaze is also facilitated by the **horizontal gaze center,** located adjacent to the abducens nucleus in the **para-pontine reticular formation (PPRF).** The PPRF also can be involved in the one-and-a-half syndrome. Although it is important to recognize these clinical scenarios, the location of the lesions can also be determined by understanding the anatomy of the pons.

Pontine Anatomy

External Features and Cranial Nerves The **basilar pons** makes up the central portion of the brainstem. It is bounded rostrally by the mesencephalon, caudally by the medulla, and dorsally by the fourth ventricle and cerebellum. It contains the continuation of both ascending and descending pathways. The major sensory and motor systems are discussed separately. Their location in the pons remains relatively similar to their location in other parts of the brainstem and spinal cord. One exception to this is the medial lemniscus. As it ascends through the pons, it shifts gradually from its medial location in the medulla to a more dorsolateral position, twisting like a ribbon. The pons also contains the nuclei of the fifth, sixth, seventh, and eight cranial nerves, portions of the reticular formation, and the ventral pontine nuclei. Figure 10-7 illustrates the location of some of the major structures one should be able to recognize.

The **fifth cranial nerve** is the only one to emerge from the surface of the basilar pons. Its sensory nucleus extends rostrally into the midbrain and caudally into the cervical spinal cord. Nerve fibers exiting the **sixth nerve nucleus** travel caudally and ventrally to traverse the pontine tegmentum and exit the brainstem near the midline. Because they loop caudally before exiting the brainstem, these CN fibers are thought to have the longest intracranial course. The **seventh and eight cranial nerves** also exit from the border of the pons and the medulla. The sixth nerve (motor function) exits most medially, and the eighth nerve (sensory function) exits most laterally. The seventh nerve has both motor and sensory functions and exits between the other two. These cranial nerves, their nuclei, and their associated systems have already been discussed in other cases. However, the present case uses conjugate eye movement as an example to emphasizes how different brainstem structures need to work in a coordinated manner.

Cerebellar Connections The pons is a bulbous structure extending from the ventral surface of the midbrain. This bulge is caused by many small **pontine nuclei,** which are interspersed among the fascicles of the corticospinal and corticobulbar tracts. The primary function of the pons is as a relay station between the cerebrum

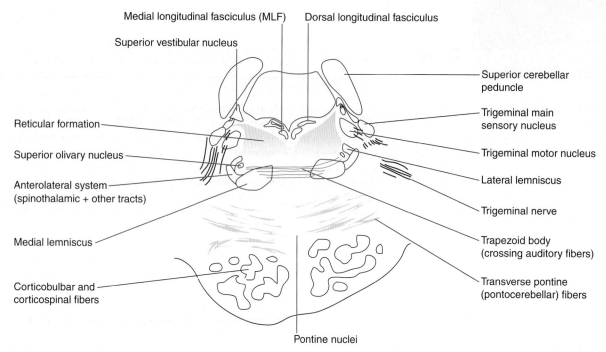

Medial longitudinal fasciculus (MLF)   Dorsal longitudinal fasciculus

Superior vestibular nucleus

Superior cerebellar peduncle

Trigeminal main sensory nucleus

Reticular formation

Trigeminal motor nucleus

Superior olivary nucleus

Lateral lemniscus

Anterolateral system (spinothalamic + other tracts)

Trigeminal nerve

Medial lemniscus

Trapezoid body (crossing auditory fibers)

Corticobulbar and corticospinal fibers

Transverse pontine (pontocerebellar) fibers

Pontine nuclei

• **Figure 10-7.** Mid-pons in cross-section.

and the cerebellum. Descending corticopontine fibers terminate onto the pontine nuclei. These nuclei then give off transverse fibers that decussate before ascending dorsally into the cerebellum through the **middle cerebellar peduncle,** the main cerebellar afferent pathway. Reciprocal cerebellar output exits primarily through the **superior cerebellar peduncle,** which decussates at the border between the pons and midbrain and represents the main cerebellar efferent pathway. **The inferior cerebellar peduncle (restiform body)** is also predominantly an afferent cerebellar pathway. It conveys information from the spinal cord and medulla. A small component of the inferior cerebellar peduncle **(juxtarestiform body)** conveys cerebellar fastigial efferents, which project to brainstem nuclei. Cerebellar systems are discussed in more detail separately. However, the cerebellar peduncles and pontine nuclei are important to consider here because their injury in disorders of the pons manifests as ataxia.

Vascular Supply of the Pons Like other parts of the brainstem, the vascular supply to the pons can be divided broadly into **paramedian branches of the basilar artery, short circumferential branches,** and **long circumferential branches.** Different clinical syndromes

are associated with disruption of these vessels. As a general rule, paramedian and short circumferential branches are implicated when weakness is present because motor systems tend to be concentrated ventromedially. Sensory disturbance with sparing of motor function, on the other hand, implicates longer circumferential branches. Involvement of facial sensation often implicates a more rostral level of dysfunction, whereas involvement of the sixth, seventh, or eighth nerves implicates a more caudal pontine process.

Internuclear Ophthalmoplegia As previously mentioned, INO is caused by disruption of the MLF. The MLF provides a functional connection between the sixth CN nucleus on one side and the contralateral third CN nucleus. This communication allows for conjugate eye movement in the horizontal plane. The two most likely causes for small pontine lesions like this would be small-vessel ischemia and demyelinating disease. Mass lesions such as tumors or vascular malformations would be less likely. In our young female patient, demyelinating disease is most likely. A vascular etiology also would have to be considered, particularly if the patient had a history consistent with coagulopathy or connective tissue disease.

CASE CONCLUSION

Routine laboratory studies were unremarkable. A hypercoagulability work-up also turned out to be unrevealing. An MRI of the head was obtained and revealed multiple brainstem and periventricular white matter lesions. The patient was admitted to the hospital for a course of IV methylprednisolone. A lumbar puncture was performed and CSF studies were consistent with a demyelinating process. The patient reported that she had had episodes of transient sensory and motor deficits over the past few years but was afraid to seek medical attention. The diagnosis of MS was made. An immunomodulatory agent was started in the outpatient setting.

THUMBNAIL: Midbrain and Pontine Syndromes

Midbrain Syndromes	Structures	Deficits
Weber	Third nerve; cerebral peduncle	Ipsilateral third nerve palsy; contralateral hemiparesis
Parinaud	Superior colliculi; periaqueductal gray	Light-near pupillary dissociation; paralysis of upgaze
Medial (paramedian basilar artery branches)	Fascicles of pyramidal tract; cerebellar pathways; MLF; PPRF	Contralateral hemiparesis; ipsilateral ataxia; ipsilateral INO; horizontal gaze paresis
Lateral (anteroinferior cerebellar artery [AICA] and long circumferential arteries)	Medial lemniscus; descending autonomic fibers; trigeminal nucleus; cerebellar pathways	Contralateral hemianesthesia; ipsilateral Horner syndrome; ipsilateral facial hemianesthesia; ataxia
Caudal (short and long circumferential arteries)	Seventh nerve; sixth nerve; eighth nerve	Ipsilateral LMN facial palsy; ipsilateral lateral rectus palsy; ipsilateral deafness; vertigo
INO (small vessel lacuna)	MLF	Ipsilateral adduction palsy on contralateral gaze
One-and-a-half syndrome (small vessel lacuna)	Sixth nerve nucleus; MLF; PPRF	Ipsilateral lateral rectus palsy; ipsilateral INO; functionally, contralateral INO
Dysarthria, clumsy hand, and other small vessel lacunae	Fascicles of pyramidal tract; pontocerebellar fibers	Partial corticospinal disorders occurring because pyramidal fascicles are separated by pontine nuclei, so only some affected
Locked-in syndrome	All motor systems; below pontine lesion	Retained awareness; retained eye movements; unable to speak or move

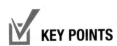

KEY POINTS

- Crossed findings implicate the brainstem
- Crossed findings involving the fifth, sixth, seventh, or eighth cranial nerve implicate the pons
- Coordination of conjugate horizontal gaze is mediated by the MLF and PPRF
- Vertigo and ataxia implicate the cerebellum, its peduncles, and/or the vestibular system
- Pontine syndromes most commonly present with mixed long-tract, cerebellar, and cranial nerve findings

QUESTIONS

1. A 73-year-old woman presents to the ED with sudden onset of left face and right extremity numbness. She is noted to be profoundly ataxic on exam. What other finding might one expect to find?

   A. Tongue deviation to the left
   B. Right eye deviated down and out
   C. Smaller pupil on the left
   D. Left eye deviated down and out
   E. Smaller pupil on the right

2. A 66-year-old man presents complaining of vision problems manifesting as double vision when he looks to the left. This has been going on for several hours. On exam, he fails to adduct the right eye on left lateral gaze. On right lateral gaze, his eyes do not cross the midline. His reading ability is relatively spared. What structures are involved?

   A. Left sixth nerve nucleus and right PPRF
   B. Right sixth nerve nucleus and left MLF

   C. Left sixth nerve nucleus and left MLF
   D. Right sixth nerve nucleus and right MLF
   E. Right sixth nerve nucleus and left PPRF

3. Branches from which of the following vessels would be affected in a patient with a pontine lacunar infarction?

   A. Basilar artery
   B. Posteroinferior cerebellar artery (PICA)
   C. AICA
   D. Vertebral artery
   E. Superior cerebellar artery (SCA)

4. Which of the following cranial nerves would be least affected by a large lateral pontine demyelinating plaque?

   A. Facial nerve
   B. Abducens nerve
   C. Trigeminal nerve
   D. Trochlear nerve
   E. Vestibulocochlear nerve

HPI: A 75-year-old woman who has not been able to speak or use her right side for the past hour is seen in the ED. She was at home with her family around 8 p.m. when she developed a droop on the lower right side of her face, then dropped a pen from her writing (right) hand. She slumped over to her right side and appeared unable to speak, although she retained consciousness. Her eyes were deviated to the left.

PE: T 98.3°F; HR 92 beats/min; BP 165/85 mm Hg; RR 15 breaths/min; SaO$_2$ 95% at room air

History is notable for HTN and hypercholesterolemia. She is a bewildered elderly woman with a right lower facial droop and plegic right arm. She does not phonate or follow commands. She winces but does not move the right arm in response to painful stimuli, but abruptly and purposefully moves her right leg. Movement on the left side and the rest of her other cranial nerves are unaffected.

THOUGHT QUESTIONS

- Where is the lesion?
- What is the diagnosis?
- Why is her leg relatively spared?

BASIC SCIENCE REVIEW AND DISCUSSION

The Anterior Cerebral Circulation

The anterior or **carotid** circulation is composed of the internal carotid arteries (ICAs), the circle of Willis, and the MCAs and ACAs.

The **ICAs** are relatively straightforward and do not have the multiple branches for which the external carotid arteries are well known. The important branch derived from the ICA is the **ophthalmic artery,** which supplies the optic nerve and retina. Internal carotid disease may thus cause inadequate blood flow to the retina, which may result in **amaurosis fugax** (transient monocular blindness). After giving off the ophthalmic branch, the ICA rises superiorly to join the circle of Willis, and metamorphoses into the MCA.

The **circle of Willis** is a circular ring of adjoining arteries ultimately supplied by the ICAs and the basilar artery (Fig. 10-8). This circular connection allows compensation for vascular insufficiency on one side by allowing the other side's blood flow to cross over the midline. This is accomplished via the anterior and posterior communicating arteries (ACom and PCom). The **MCA,** originating from the circle of Willis, then forms multiple branches supplying the temporal lobe, the parietal lobe, and the superior and lateral aspects of the frontal lobe (Fig. 10-9). Both the cortex and subcortical white matter are supplied by the MCA. The MCA also gives off perforating arteries, which supply the corona radiata, internal capsule, and much of the basal ganglia. The **ACA** runs anteriorly from the circle of Willis to supply the medial aspect of the frontal lobe, curving superiorly and posteriorly as it does so. It often runs posteriorly enough to supply the medial parietal lobe as well.

The PCAs also originate from the circle of Willis, and are discussed in Case 10-17.

Organization of the Cortex by Vascular Territory

It is worthwhile to recognize which areas of the brain are supplied by which vessels, to recognize different types of strokes.

The **MCA** supplies the motor strip (precentral gyrus) pertaining to the face, trunk, and upper extremity, but not the leg. It also supplies the postcentral gyrus, which controls sensation in the same areas. The MCA supplies the **frontal eye fields,** which control conjugate horizontal eye movement. Injuries to the frontal eye field result in a gaze preference **toward the side of the lesion;** for example, left MCA strokes cause patients to look toward the left. Perforating arteries from the MCA supply the basal ganglia and the anterior thalamus. The MCA also supplies the language centers: **Broca area** in the posterolateral frontal lobe and **Wernicke area** in the adjacent anterior temporal lobe.

The **ACA** supplies the medial aspect of the motor strip and the medial aspect of the sensory strip in the parietal lobe. These areas control motor function and sensation of the lower extremity, respectively.

Of note, the **PCA** supplies the occipital lobes, which govern the contralateral hemifield of vision, as well as association visual cortex.

Clinical Discussion

This patient has had a **left MCA stroke** until proven otherwise. Her constellation of symptoms fits the areas of the cerebrum supplied by the left MCA: the motor cortex involving the face and arm (located laterally and superiorly, respectively) and Broca and Wernicke areas, resulting in a **global aphasia.**

The **language centers** of the cortex are located on the **left side** of the brain in more than 99% of right-handed patients (note that she was using her right hand to write). The sparing of her leg also suggests an MCA stroke. The motor cortex projecting to the leg is located on the medial aspect of the motor strip, which is supplied by the ACA and thus spared by MCA infarcts. Figure 10-10 depicts Brodmann areas, or areas of the brain with different cellular structure and functional roles.

Differential Diagnosis

Other considerations should involve the motor system as well. A stroke of the left internal capsule or corona radiata will cause right-sided face and arm weakness but will often involve the leg because all the motor fibers of the internal capsule coalesce into a small area sharing the same vascular supply. Language involvement would also be less likely. A seizure that involved primarily

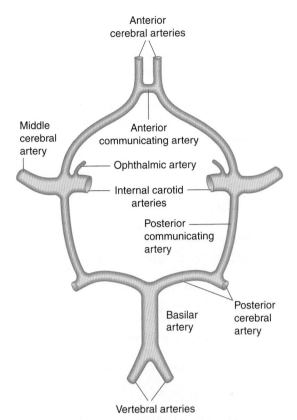

• **Figure 10-8.** Circle of Willis (simplified).

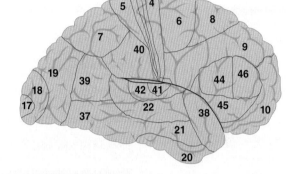

• **Figure 10-10.** Brodmann areas.

the left frontal cortex, which was not witnessed, could result in plegia as a result of the postictal hypofunction of the cortex. This phenomenon has been described as **Todd paralysis, and it usually resolves within 24 hours.** Hemorrhage of the left frontal lobe, as well as a subdural or epidural hematoma compressing primarily the left frontal lobe, might appear in similar fashion. A mass or tumor might compress or impinge on the frontal lobe, but this usually presents gradually rather than abruptly.

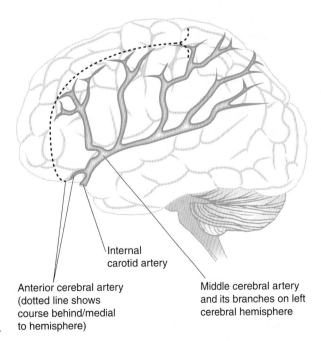

• **Figure 10-9.** Middle cerebral artery.

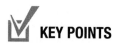

CASE CONCLUSION

Thankfully, head CT showed no hemorrhage, and the patient was given IV tissue plasminogen activator (tPA). IV tPA may be given up to 3 hours after the onset of symptoms in stroke patients without evidence of hemorrhage. She began to regain some use of her right arm and began to follow commands. Head MRI demonstrated infarct in the left frontal, temporal, and parietal cortices, with sparing of the medial frontal lobe and occipital lobe (ACA and PCA territories, respectively).

THUMBNAIL: Anterior Circulation

Vessel	Territory Supplied	Ischemic Syndrome
ICA/ophthalmic artery	Retina	Amaurosis fugax (transient monocular blindness)
MCA	Lateral motor strip	Contralateral face and arm weakness
	Lateral sensory strip	Contralateral face and arm anesthesia
	Internal capsule	Contralateral face, arm, and leg weakness
	Frontal eye fields (frontal lobe)	Gaze preference toward affected side
	Broca area (frontal lobe)	Expressive (motor) aphasia
	Wernicke area (temporal lobe)	Receptive (sensory) aphasia
ACA	Medial motor and sensory strips	Contralateral leg weakness and anesthesia

KEY POINTS

- The anterior circulation (internal carotid system) serves the retina, frontal lobe, parietal lobe, temporal lobe, internal capsule, and basal ganglia via the MCA and the ACA
- Anterior circulation stroke syndromes may be discerned by involvement of the leg (ACA territory) and the development of aphasias (suggests cortical involvement)
- The circle of Willis allows blood supply from any of its supply vessels to run to any of its outflow vessels

QUESTIONS

1. A 72-year-old man is brought in by his family for "not speaking right." Starting 2 days ago, his children noticed that he tends to put inappropriate words together or makes up words that do not exist (paraphasias). He also does not seem to understand everything that they tell him. Upon exam, you notice a subtle right lower facial droop and weakness of the right arm. He has no difficulty walking. What is a head CT most likely to show?

   A. Infarction of Wernicke area (left anterior temporal lobe) and the left motor cortex
   B. Brainstem infarct involving the left facial nucleus and hypoglossal nucleus
   C. Infarction of Broca area (left lateral frontal lobe) and left motor cortex
   D. Left ACA infarct
   E. Right posterior frontal lobe infarct with some involvement of parietal and temporal lobes

2. A 36-year-old right-handed healthy woman develops abrupt difficulty in producing words, essentially becoming completely mute over the course of a few minutes. Motor function and comprehension are retained. She takes oral contraceptives and is an avid smoker. Her medical history is notable only for a patent foramen ovale. What is the most likely cause?

   A. Paradoxical fat embolism to the left temporal lobe, causing embolic infarct
   B. Thromboembolism to the left posterior frontal lobe, causing embolic infarct
   C. Right frontal lobe hemorrhage
   D. Acute right internal carotid occlusion
   E. Septic emboli to the left parietal lobe, causing hemorrhagic infarct

3. An 85-year-old man complains of the complete inability to see out of the left eye for the past 15 minutes. He describes a "shade" or "blind" that appeared to abruptly cover his vision. Vision of the right eye is relatively unaffected. Physical exam shows a pale retina on the left side. What is the most likely explanation?

   A. Ocular migraine
   B. Acute left ophthalmic artery occlusion
   C. Acute right occipital lobe infarct
   D. Acute left occipital lobe infarct
   E. Elevated intracranial pressure (ICP)

4. A 79-year-old woman is noticed in the nursing home to have difficulty using her right leg over the past several days. She does not complain of any pain. The leg's appearance has not changed. She has diffuse weakness affecting both flexors and extensors in both the thigh and the leg, as well as the foot. What is the most likely diagnosis?

   A. Left ACA occlusion
   B. Pelvic mass impinging on the right sciatic and femoral nerves
   C. Left MCA occlusion
   D. ACom occlusion
   E. Left deep femoral venous thrombosis

HPI: RS is a 63-year-old right-handed man with a history of tobacco use, diabetes, and AF. He has had two MIs. He is brought to the ED because his wife can no longer control his behavior. Over the past 2 days, he has become progressively more argumentative. He insists that his wife must stop contradicting his mother. However, the wife reports that his mother passed away many years ago. He states that he does not want to be evaluated because "you can't trust those doctors," but she has talked him into this visit. Since this morning, he has been more confused. He has been falling and has been unable to get up on his own power. He reports that he has been seeing double all day.

PE: His BP is 189/100 mm Hg. His exam is remarkable for a homonymous left visual field deficit when each eye is tested separately. He has ptosis in the right. His right pupil is deviated downward and laterally. He has bilateral impairment of upward gaze. His reflexes are symmetric and his toes are up-going bilaterally.

THOUGHT QUESTIONS

- What structures are responsible for each of the symptoms?
- How are they anatomically related?
- What is their vascular supply?
- Could a single lesion cause all of these deficits?

BASIC SCIENCE REVIEW AND DISCUSSION

The posterior circulation of the brain and brainstem covers a large territory containing varied structures and pathways. However, a systematic approach to the vascular territories and functional systems can help to localize lesions and define clinical syndromes. This patient has a right homonymous hemianopsia, implicating the left visual cortex or optic tract. He has a right third nerve palsy but also has bilateral impairment of upward gaze. He has bilateral long tract signs. He is also confused, agitated, and delusional. This combination of findings can initially appear confusing. However, a systematic review can identify a single lesion at the top of the basilar artery. This case focuses on the posterior circulation of the brain and brainstem, which is derived from the vertebral arteries, the basilar artery, and their branches. The posterior circulation is connected to the anterior circulation through the circle of Willis. The anterior circulation is discussed in Case 10-16.

Vertebral Arteries

Cervical Portion Each **vertebral artery** originates from the proximal portion of the corresponding **subclavian artery.** They ascend and move posteriorly, entering the cervical vertebrae for which they are named in the midcervical region. From this point, they continue to ascend through the transverse foramina of each of the upper cervical vertebrae. The vertebral arteries are particularly susceptible to damage resulting from neck injury because of their proximity to the cervical vertebrae. Abrupt turning movements of the neck, as may be seen even with mild trauma or chiropractic cervical manipulation, can sometimes lead to **vertebral artery dissection** (tearing of the intimal layer of the arterial wall, leading to obstruction and/or formation of emboli) and **posterior circulation infarctions.** Throughout the neck, the vertebral arteries give off **spinal branches** to the spinal cord, as well as branches to the soft tissues of the neck. At the atlanto-occipital junction, they turn medially across the superior surface of the atlas and then enter the skull and penetrate the dura mater through the foramen magnum. Each gives off a **posterior meningeal branch** in this area.

Cranial Portion The vertebral arteries enter the posterior fossa through the foramen magnum and course along the ventrolateral aspects of the medulla oblongata. Although many branches come off of the vertebral arteries, they can be divided broadly into three categories. First, medial branches provide blood supply to the most ventral and medial aspects of the neuraxis. The largest of these are the two branches (one from each vertebral artery) that come together to form the **anterior spinal artery.** It courses caudally in the midline, along the ventral aspect of the spinal cord. Small **paramedian branches** of the vertebral arteries and anterior spinal artery represent the primary vascular supply to the pyramidal tracts and overlying paramedian portions of the medulla (medial lemniscus, MLF, hypoglossal nucleus). Lateral branches from the vertebral arteries can be further divided into short circumferential branches and long circumferential branches. Second, the (unnamed) **short circumferential branches** provide the vascular supply to the ventrolateral aspects of the medulla. Third, the **long circumferential branches** provide the vascular supply to the dorsal and dorsolateral aspects of the medulla, the dorsal spinal cord, and the ventrocaudal cerebellum. The two most important lateral branches of the vertebral arteries are the **posterior spinal artery** and the **PICA.** In addition to supplying the dorsal spinal cord and posterior inferior cerebellum, respectively, small branches from these important arteries supply the dorsal and dorsolateral medulla. One of the most important eponymous brainstem syndromes, the **lateral medullary syndrome of Wallenberg,** is classically attributed to occlusion of the PICA on one side. This syndrome is described separately in detail. In practice, a vertebral artery occlusion is more likely to be seen in the context of Wallenberg syndrome.

Basilar Artery

The two vertebral arteries join at the pontomedullary junction, near the midline, to form the **basilar artery.** The basilar artery continues along the ventral aspect of the pons, up to the level of the midbrain. Branches from the basilar artery supply the pons, the midbrain, the remainder of the cerebellum, and the posterior and inferior portions of the diencephalon (thalamus, hypothalamus) and cerebral hemispheres. As was the case with branches from the vertebral arteries, branches of the basilar artery can be divided broadly into *(a)* **paramedian,** *(b)* **short circumferential,** and *(c)* **long circumferential branches.** As a general rule, paramedian branches supply predominantly motor structures, which are more medial. Circumferential branches, on the other hand, supply predominantly sensory structures, which tend to be located dorsolaterally. These vascular territories help define the symptoms associated with brainstem stroke syndromes. Rather than trying to remember a long list of symptoms for each syndrome, ask yourself what the involved vascular territory might be. Then consider the cranial nerves and long tracts that are likely to be involved.

Lower and Middle Branches **Paramedian branches** of the basilar artery supply the corticospinal and corticobulbar fibers of the ventral pons, as well as the pontine nuclei interspersed among them. **Short circumferential branches** of the basilar artery supply more lateral aspects of the ventral pons, including pontocerebellar fibers, ascending sensory pathways, and descending sympathetic fibers that project from the hypothalamus to preganglionic autonomic neurons in the spinal cord. **Long circumferential branches** of the basilar artery supply dorsal and dorsolateral portions of the pons, including structures in and near the floor of the fourth ventricle. These structures include nuclei of the pontine cranial nerves, portions of the cerebellar peduncles, and portions of the ascending sensory pathways. As in the medulla, one can predict the clinical manifestations associated with disruption of each of the pontine vascular territories based on the affected structures.

The basilar artery also gives off several important large paired branches. Beginning at the caudal end, the first branch is the **AICA.** The AICA supplies portions of the inferior aspect of the cerebellum and portions of the cerebellar peduncles and contributes to the supply of the dorsolateral pons. The **labyrinthine artery** originates immediately rostral to the AICA and supplies the structures of the inner ear. Small and unnamed pontine branches dominate the midbasilar region. The basilar artery ends at the level of the midbrain.

Terminal Branches The basilar artery gives off another pair of large, important branches, the **SCAs,** at the level of the midbrain. The SCA supplies the remainder of the cerebellum. The basilar artery then bifurcates into the right and left **PCAs.** The PCA supplies the posterior and inferior aspects of the cerebral hemispheres, including the ventral temporal lobe and most of the visual cortex in the occipital lobe. Each PCA also receives flow from the anterior circulation via its corresponding PCom. It is important to note that the third cranial nerve passes between these two vessels as it exits the midbrain. Mass lesions in this area, such as an aneurysm involving either of these arteries (or more likely the PCom), can compress the third nerve and cause an isolated **third nerve palsy.** Penetrating branches from these large vessels supply most of the diencephalon, including the hypothalamus, the subthalamus, and the thalamus. The most prominent branch of the PCA is the **posterior choroidal artery,** which supplies the posterior aspect of the thalamus, the pineal gland, and the choroids plexus of the third ventricle and inferior portions of the lateral ventricles.

As was the case for the medulla and the pons, the vascular supply of the midbrain itself can be divided broadly into *(a)* **paramedian,** *(b)* **short circumferential,** and *(c)* **long circumferential branches.** These penetrating branches are derived from all of the large vessels discussed earlier (basilar artery, SCA, PCA, PCom). The paramedian branches supply the most medial portions of the cerebral peduncles, the occulomotor nuclear group, and portions of the red nucleus and substantia nigra. Infarction in this territory results in another important brainstem syndrome. **Weber syndrome** is characterized by unilateral third nerve palsy with associated contralateral hemiplegia. Short circumferential branches supply more lateral aspects of these same structures. Long circumferential branches supply the midbrain tectum. Infarction in this territory can lead to Parinaud syndrome and restricted upgaze, as seen with the patient in the present case.

Top-of-the-Basilar Syndrome RS had findings that were localized to many areas, including the visual cortex, midbrain, and diencephalon. Although relatively nonspecific, the altered mentation was most likely related to thalamic involvement. Several of the thalamic subnuclei are interconnected with the limbic system and prefrontal cortex. They are involved in the modulation of emotional behavior and the coordination of that behavior with sensory experience. The term **peduncular hallucinosis** is used to describe the confusion often associated with the top-of-the-basilar syndrome. The clinical manifestations of this syndrome can vary dramatically, depending on the location and extent of the lesion and on the presence of collateral vascular supply to critical areas.

CASE CONCLUSION

Shortly after presentation, the patient became comatose and required intubation. CT angiography confirmed occlusion of the distal basilar artery. Although the exact time of symptom onset could not be defined, the prognosis in the absence of intervention was felt to be poor. The endovascular team was activated and intra-arterial thrombolysis was performed. Blood flow was restored. Follow-up MRI scans confirmed a large region of infarction involving the midbrain, thalami, and left visual cortex. The patient remained comatose, requiring extensive supportive care. The prognosis remained grim and the family decided to withdraw supportive measures.

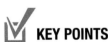

THUMBNAIL: Posterior Circulation

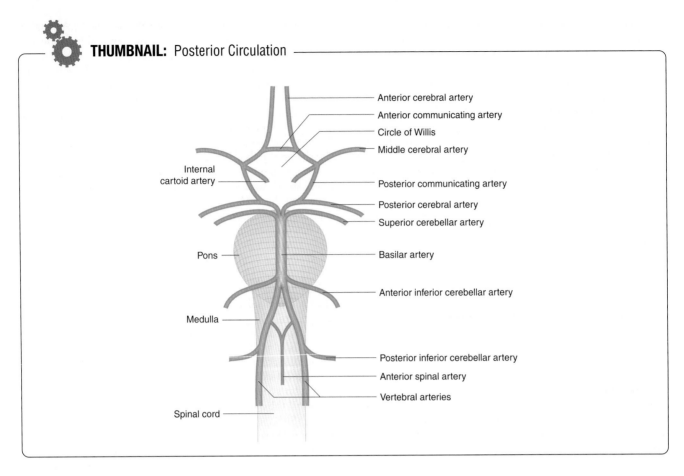

Anterior cerebral artery
Anterior communicating artery
Circle of Willis
Middle cerebral artery
Internal cartoid artery
Posterior communicating artery
Posterior cerebral artery
Superior cerebellar artery
Pons
Basilar artery
Anterior inferior cerebellar artery
Medulla
Posterior inferior cerebellar artery
Anterior spinal artery
Vertebral arteries
Spinal cord

KEY POINTS

■ Within the posterior circulation, vascular territories can be broadly defined on the basis of paramedian, short circumferential, and long circumferential branches

■ Paramedian branches supply predominantly motor structures

■ Short circumferential branches supply predominantly ventrolateral tracts and intrinsic nuclei

■ Long circumferential branches supply dorsal and dorsolateral structures

■ Large, named branches contribute to these territories

QUESTIONS

1. A 60-year-old man has a right vertebral artery occlusion. Which of the following symptoms is he most likely to have?

   A. Right-sided weakness
   B. Loss of pain and temperature on the left
   C. Left-sided Horner syndrome
   D. Left-sided weakness
   E. Loss of pain and temperature on the right

2. A 73-year-old woman has complete loss of sensation on the left (hemianesthesia) involving the face, arm, trunk, and leg equally. She has full strength. Which artery is most likely involved?

   A. Left vertebral artery
   B. Right PCA
   C. Right vertebral artery
   D. Left PCA
   E. Basilar artery

3. A 67-year-old man has had sudden loss of vision in his right visual field. Which arterial distribution is most likely involved?

   A. Left vertebral artery
   B. Right PCA
   C. Right vertebral artery
   D. Left PCA
   E. Basilar artery

4. A 45-year-old man presents with right-sided weakness. His symptoms quickly resolve to the point at which his only objective neurologic deficit is a mild degree of finger-to-nose dysmetria on the right. His MRI scan reveals a rather large new infarction. Which vascular territory is most likely affected?

   A. Left vertebral artery
   B. Right PICA
   C. Right vertebral artery
   D. Left MCA
   E. Left PICA

CASE 10-18 | Dural Venous Sinuses

HPI: BM is a 45-year-old right-handed man who collapsed while jogging in the desert today. He normally runs 15 miles every other day. Today was a particularly hot day. He has been stabilized in the ED. Rehydration has been initiated, but he remains unresponsive. When he was found, he complained of severe headache.

PE: He does not respond to voice, he withdraws to noxious stimulation but does so more briskly on the right, his CN reflexes are intact, and he has bilateral Babinski signs.

THOUGHT QUESTIONS

- What structures are responsible of each of the symptoms?
- How are they anatomically related?
- What is their vascular supply?
- Could a single lesion cause all of these deficits?

BASIC SCIENCE REVIEW AND DISCUSSION

The presence of lateralized findings on the neurologic exam implicates the CNS. The level of consciousness suggests that both cerebral hemispheres may be affected, although the left hemisphere seems more involved. In cases with such acute presentation, a vascular cause must be considered first. Given the apparent dehydration, one would suspect the possibility of a **dural venous sinus thrombosis.** Venous drainage of the brain and brainstem can be broadly divided into the dural venous sinuses and the veins that drain into them. This case focuses on the dural venous sinuses themselves.

Dural Sinus System

The vessels and sinuses that mediate venous drainage of the brain can be divided into those vessels draining superficial cortical regions and those draining deep regions. As a general rule, superficial regions of the cerebrum are drained by the superior sagittal sinus and the cavernous sinuses. The deeper regions of the cerebrum are drained by a system of lesser known veins and sinuses. The fundamental difference between the dural sinuses and the cerebral veins is that the veins drain the brain parenchyma and travel through the subarachnoid and subdural spaces, whereas the venous sinuses are all intradural. Dural sinuses are contained between the **periosteal and meningeal layers** of the **dura mater.** The dural venous sinuses are firm structures. They are lined with endothelium and, unlike systemic veins, they lack valves. They are located along the large fissures of the brain. Most of the dural sinuses drain posteriorly toward the **confluence of the sinuses** near the occipital pole or inferiorly toward the **jugular veins.** The dural sinuses are a **low-pressure system** with slow-moving blood. They are susceptible to congestion and thrombosis during hypercoagulable states. Sinus thrombosis should always be considered in the setting of headache in such patients. **Dehydration, pregnancy**, **oral contraceptives,** and **tobacco** are all associated with hypercoagulability and are often favored in test questions.

Superficial Drainage The largest of the dural venous sinuses, the **superior sagittal sinus,** is located within the **falx cerebri** along the superior aspect of the interhemispheric fissure. It is the most likely sinus to be affected by thrombosis in the clinical setting. The superior sagittal sinus receives blood from the superficial cerebral veins. It also receives venous blood from the scalp through **emissary veins** that penetrate the skull. Along its course, the superior sagittal sinus also receives CSF from the subarachnoid space via **arachnoid granulations** that penetrate the meningeal layer of the dura mater. The function of the arachnoid granulations is discussed in further detail within the context of CSF flow and the ventricular system. The superior sagittal sinus is smaller anteriorly, in the area of the prefrontal cortex, and gets larger posteriorly. It terminates posteriorly at the **confluence of the sinuses,** in the **tentorium cerebelli** near the occipital pole.

Deep Drainage The **inferior sagittal sinus** is parallel to its superior counterpart but drains deeper cerebral tissue. It also is contained within the **falx cerebri** but is located more deeply within the interhemispheric fissure and is situated along the superior surface of the corpus callosum. The **great cerebral vein of Galen** drains even deeper tissue. The inferior sagittal sinus and the vein of Galen come together to form the **straight sinus** at the anterior boundary of the **tentorium cerebelli.** The straight sinus continues posteriorly, through the tentorium cerebelli, to the confluence of the sinuses. Thus, all venous drainage from superior aspects of the cerebrum arrives at the confluence of the sinuses via the superior sagittal sinus and the straight sinus.

The **transverse sinuses,** one on each side, drain blood laterally from the confluence of the sinuses toward the jugular veins. They are the second most likely sinuses to be affected by thrombosis. They are usually asymmetric, and in most people, the right one is larger. The transverse sinuses follow the contour of the skull, along the tentorium cerebelli, between the cerebral and cerebellar hemispheres. At the boundary between the occipital and petrosal bones, the transverse sinus is joined by the **superior petrosal sinus** to form the sigmoid sinus. The **sigmoid sinus** curves inferiorly, medially, then inferiorly again and is joined by the **inferior petrosal sinus** at the jugular foramen to form the **jugular vein.**

Clinical Correlation

Dural venous sinus thrombosis is most commonly associated with hypercoagulability related to either intrinsic or acquired processes. Some of the more commonly encountered clinical situations include dehydration, pregnancy, oral contraceptive use, and tobacco use. Thrombosis can also occur in association with infections and direct infection spread. Frontal sinusitis can lead to superior sagittal sinus thrombosis. Sphenoid sinusitis can lead to **cavernous sinus thrombosis.** The most common presenting symptom is headache. Altered mentation and nausea are also seen often. Other symptoms vary, depending on the sinus involved and the extent to which the adjacent brain parenchyma is affected. Diagnosis is on a clinical basis and is supported by venography. The most important differential considerations are cerebral infarction or hemorrhage on an arterial basis. Dural sinus thrombosis can cause ischemia and infarction of adjacent tissue. Hemorrhage can also occur in these areas. Treatment is primarily with heparin anticoagulation and rehydration, although the use of anticoagulation in the setting of hemorrhage is somewhat controversial. If there is no hemorrhage, endovascular thrombolysis may be beneficial.

CASE CONCLUSION

An emergent CT scan of the head was performed and revealed no evidence of hemorrhage. A magnetic resonance venogram was performed and confirmed thrombosis of the superior sagittal sinus. Heparin therapy and rehydration were initiated. The patient was seen by the endovascular service and endovascular thrombolysis was performed. Venous flow was restored. The patient gradually recovered full function, after a prolonged period of rehabilitation.

THUMBNAIL: Dural Venous Sinuses

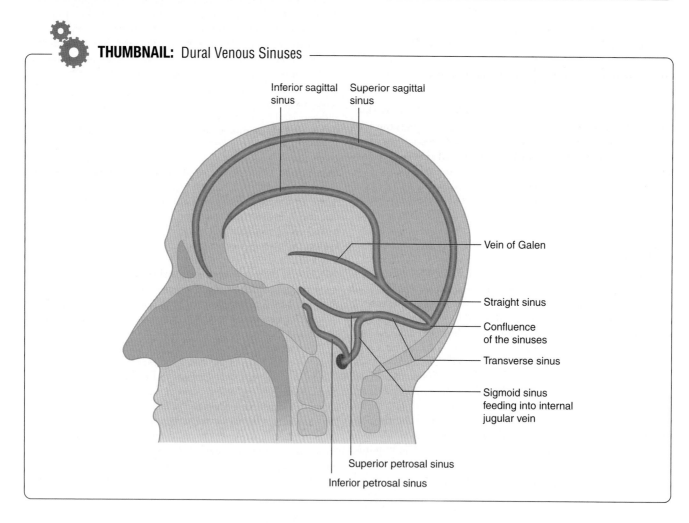

KEY POINTS

- Cerebral veins and dural venous sinuses mediate venous drainage of the cerebrum
- Venous drainage of the cerebrum can be divided broadly into superficial and deep regions
- Dural sinus thrombosis occurs in the setting of hypercoagulability
- The most common presenting symptom of sinus thrombosis is headache
- The sinuses most likely to be affected by thrombosis are the superior sagittal and the transverse sinuses

QUESTIONS

1. A 58-year-old woman presents to your office complaining of a severe headache that has been troubling her for the past week. Over the past 24 hours she has developed ringing in the right ear and severe positional vertigo. Which structure might be involved?

   A. Superior sagittal sinus
   B. Inferior sagittal sinus
   C. Transverse sinus
   D. Cavernous sinus
   E. Vein of Galen

2. A 23-year-old woman presents for evaluation of a severe headache that developed gradually over 5 days. She reports that this morning she found she is unable to walk because of weakness in both legs. What is the most likely vessel to be involved?

   A. Sigmoid sinus
   B. Transverse sinus
   C. Middle cerebral vein
   D. Superior sagittal sinus
   E. Vein of Rosenthal

3. A 68-year-old diabetic man presents to your office complaining of a severe head and eye pain on the right. He is proptotic on the right. Which structure might be involved?

   A. Superior sagittal sinus
   B. Inferior sagittal sinus
   C. Transverse sinus
   D. Cavernous sinus
   E. Vein of Galen

4. A 32-year-old female smoker who is taking oral contraceptives collapsed after the sudden onset of a headache. Her exam reveals UMN findings on the left. A CT scan of the head confirms hemorrhage on the right. A venous occlusion is suspected. In which space has the blood collected?

   A. Intraparenchymal
   B. Subarachnoid
   C. Subdural
   D. Epidural
   E. Intradural

HPI: An 18-year-old male is brought to the ED by his college roommate after having a witnessed seizure. He is becoming arousable again but remains confused and combative. His speech is slurred and he spits at the paramedics as he is brought in. His roommate explains that he has had a sore throat for several days but was otherwise completely normal yesterday.

PE: T 102.6°F; HR 136 beats/min; BP 185/90 mm Hg; RR 28 breaths/min; SaO$_2$ 94% on room air

PmHx: Broken right clavicle as a child; otherwise negative.

He did not take any medications before this incident and his toxicology screen is negative for alcohol or illicit drugs. He responds to pain in all four extremities with what appears to be normal strength; reflexes are intact. He is uncooperative and does not follow commands, and his consciousness is diminished with the exception of combativeness when stimulated. His neck is rigid. He reflexively flexes his knees when his hips are flexed and claims that his neck hurts when the knee is extended.

THOUGHT QUESTIONS

- What is the likely diagnosis?
- How are his symptoms explained by the process involved?
- What preventive measures should be taken at this point?

BASIC SCIENCE REVIEW AND DISCUSSION

The Meninges

The meninges are the three supportive and protective soft tissue layers that surround the CNS, which includes the brain and spinal cord. The relatively soft, gelatinous brain and spinal cord need a cushion to protect them from abrasion and shear forces with the activities of daily life. The surrounding skull and spine provide the first line of defense against compressive injury. Further shock absorption, support, and protection are provided by surrounding and suspending the brain and spinal cord in the meninges and CSF.

Three Layers of the Meninges

The meninges are divided into three layers: two light layers collectively called the **leptomeninges,** which includes the **pia mater** ("soft mother") and the *arachnoid* layer, and an outer fibrous layer called the **dura mater** ("hard mother").

The **pia mater** forms the innermost thin layer and is directly attached to the entire exterior of the brain and spinal cord. It acts to minimize abrasions or tearing of the CNS when subjected to trauma. It anchors the spinal cord in place via numerous **dentate ligaments,** which are attached to the arachnoid layer along the spinal cord. The pia also runs inferiorly beyond the conus medullaris to form the **filum terminale,** which is anchored to the outer meninges as they converge at spinal level S2.

The **arachnoid** forms the middle layer, which envelops the CSF. The space between the pia and arachnoid in which the CSF circulates is accordingly called the **subarachnoid space.** CSF is reabsorbed in the **arachnoid granulations** of the arachnoid layer, which are evaginations of the arachnoid membrane through which CSF may flow into the superior sagittal venous sinus via a pressure gradient. Cerebral arteries and bridging veins are also located within the subarachnoid space. **Arachnoid trabeculations,** running from the pia to the arachnoid throughout the subarachnoid space, gently tether the brain in place.

The **dura mater** is the tough, fibrous outermost layer that anchors the meninges to the skull or paraspinal tissue and is closely apposed to the arachnoid. It is composed in part of the actual periosteum of the skull and forms a supportive scaffolding for the brain, which is discussed in the subsequent "Structure" section. The space between the skull and dura, usually nonexistent, is called the **epidural space,** which becomes important when the dura is separated from the skull (usually from trauma). The space between the dura and arachnoid, which is also usually closed, is called the **subdural space,** which readily expands when blood or other fluid enters (also usually from trauma). The intracranial dura is innervated by CN V and spinal nerves C1–C3 and may be exquisitely sensitive to inflammation.

Peripheral Nerves

As cranial nerves or spinal nerves exit the CNS, they are "coated" by the subarachnoid and dural layers, which form the perineurium or sheath of the peripheral nerve.

Structure

The fibrous dura forms several "shelves" to hold the cerebellar and cerebral hemispheres in place. These supportive dividers prevent excessive movement of the brain but also cause compression and potentially herniation should expansion of the brain occur. They also contain the venous sinuses.

The dura eventrates into the medial longitudinal fissure of the brain, forming a midsagittal divider running anteroposterior within the skull called the **falx cerebri,** or "falx." The falx separates the cerebral hemispheres and contains the **superior sagittal venous sinus** (adjacent to the skull) and **inferior sagittal sinus** (along the deep aspect of the falx). Expansion of one of the cerebral hemispheres may force it to cross the midline under the falx, that is, **subfalcine herniation.**

A horizontal shelf of dura extends in the axial plane just inferior to the cerebrum, separating the occipital lobes from the cerebellum, called the **tentorium cerebellum.** The **transverse venous sinuses** run within the tentorium to the midsagittal **straight sinus,** where the falx and tentorium intersect. The presence of the tentorium creates a rigid "ceiling" in the posterior fossa, so small changes in cerebellar size may displace it inferiorly, causing cerebellar **tonsillar herniation** into the foramen magnum. The anterior aspects of the tentorium run under the uncus of the temporal lobe. Temporal lobe displacement secondary to mass effect may force it under the tentorium, causing **uncal herniation.**

The midsagittal plane of dura, which makes up the falx cerebri, extends inferior to the tentorium, at which point it is called the **falx cerebellum.**

Disease Processes of the Meninges

The most lethal and fulminant disease specific to the meninges is infectious meningitis. Meningitis refers to meningeal inflammation, which may arise from viral ("aseptic"), bacterial, fungal, parasitic, malignant, or autoimmune causes. Meningitis generally involves seeding of the CSF with the pathogen from either **bloodborne spread** or direct spread, in the case of meningeal injury or sinusitis. The CSF serves as an ideal culture medium with only limited immune response available from adjacent blood vessels. As an infection takes hold, an inflammatory response follows with exudate of leukocytes (and RBCs) into the CSF and meningeal irritation, causing neck pain and stiffness. Patients' necks may become entirely rigid **(meningismus)** to guard against movement, as movement places tension on the already inflamed meninges. They may develop photophobia, headache, seizures, mental status changes and coma, fever, and sepsis, among other conditions. Two other physical findings are worth noting:

- **Kernig sign:** pain with flexing hip and extending knee (places traction on lumbar roots, which is transmitted to the meninges)
- **Brudzinski sign:** flexing the hip and knees with neck flexion (to relieve traction on meninges)

Bacterial Meningitis Bacterial meningitis is among the most lethal of all known infections, although it is generally completely curable if treatment is started early. It is caused by three major organisms in the adult: *Haemophilus influenzae, Streptococcus pneumoniae,* and *Neisseria meningitidis. Listeria monocytogenes* may infect children younger than 5 years of age or elderly patients, and *Escherichia coli* may infect immunocompromised patients.

Patients may present with a **prodrome** of sinusitis, respiratory tract infection, or otitis media with backache. Severe meningismus and photophobia usually follow. Acute bacterial meningitis should lead to deposition of a purulent PMN exudate within the subarachnoid space, usually most concentrated around the brainstem, which leads to edema and inflammation of the external brain, cranial nerves, and penetrating arteries and veins, which can cause vasculitis and thrombosis. Ischemia, infarct, and seizures may develop.

CSF analysis correspondingly shows a **PMN pleocytosis with elevated protein** and **low glucose** levels because of the metabolic demands of the PMN cells. Gram stain and culture may reveal the bacteria and give further information about treatment, which must be started immediately. Untreated bacterial meningitis is lethal within hours to days.

Viral (aseptic) Meningitis Viral or "aseptic" meningitis is named for the inability to grow a pathogen out of CSF culture, which otherwise shows elevated leukocytes consistent with meningitis. **Enterovirus** causes the majority of viral meningitis cases, with a seasonal peak in late summer. Other viruses include *EBV,* mumps virus, *HSV-2* (HSV-1 tends to cause encephalitis), *lymphocytic choriomeningitis* (LCV, from rodent droppings), and *HIV.* Patients may present with meningismus and photophobia but otherwise appear much more stable than those with bacterial meningitis.

CSF analysis generally shows a **lymphocytic pleocytosis with normal or high protein and normal glucose levels.** Viral culture or polymerase chain reaction (PCR) may recover the infecting virus, but bacterial cultures remain bland. Patients generally do not require treatment and recover over several days.

Tuberculous Meningitis Tuberculous meningitis has a more vasculitic component, causing ischemia and stroke of the brain and spinal cord. *Mycobacterium tuberculosis* and *Mycobacterium bovis* are the causative organisms.

Presentation may be indistinguishable from bacterial meningitis, although hemiparesis from stroke is more common in tuberculous meningitis. It is seen mostly in adults, often years after primary TB infection. Onset may be acute or indolent over months.

CSF analysis generally shows **lymphocytic pleocytosis with elevated protein and low glucose levels.** *Acid-fast bacilli* may be seen on the CSF smear. Treatment is standard triple/quadruple antimycobacterial therapy in accordance with resistance patterns.

Syphilitic Meningitis Neurosyphilis usually causes asymptomatic meningitis, detectable only on lumbar puncture. In a minority of cases, meningismus and CN abnormalities will follow. This may resolve without treatment, allowing the later complications of neurosyphilis to ensue: meningovascular syphilis, optic atrophy, and tabes dorsalis.

CSF analysis shows **lymphocytic pleocytosis with elevated protein and low glucose levels.** CSF rapid plasma reagent (RPR) titer or dark field microscopy may be used to demonstrate neurosyphilis. **Penicillin** remains the treatment of choice, preventing later complications of syphilis.

Fungal Meningitis Fungal meningitis usually presents indolently in **immunocompromised** patients. **Cryptococcal meningitis** is the most common entity, although *Candida, Nocardia,* and *Aspergillus* may cause meningitis. CSF generally **shows lymphocytic pleocytosis with elevated protein and low glucose levels.** Gram stain or culture may show the causative organism, with **India ink stain** confirming *Cryptococcus.* **Amphotericin B** is usually the treatment for fungal meningitis.

Carcinomatous Meningitis Infiltration of the CSF with malignant cells (usually lung, breast, and GI tract cancers) may cause meningitis. Back pain and radiculopathy are common. CSF shows an abundance of **abnormal cells,** which may be used to diagnose the primary tumor. Treatment relies on chemotherapy and radiation, although carcinomatous meningitis usually portends a grave prognosis.

Autoimmune Meningitis Sarcoid or SLE may involve the meninges, causing possible CN abnormalities and CSF lymphocytic pleocytosis.

Parameningeal Infection Infection abutting the meninges, such as mastoiditis or epidural abscess, may give a lymphocytic pleocytosis. Organisms may not be present in the CSF, and protein and glucose levels may be normal.

Other Disease Processes of the Meninges

Epidural Hematoma Invasion of blood into the epidural space occurs after rupture of a meningeal artery, usually in the setting of trauma. The **middle meningeal artery** is particularly susceptible to shearing because it lies deep to the thin temporal bone, which is fractured relatively easily. Generally only arterial pressure may separate the fibrous dura to open the epidural space, causing epidural hematomas to be **"football shaped"** as the edges are slowly pried apart. If the epidural hematoma continues to expand, mass effect leading to cerebral herniation and death may occur if surgical decompression is not performed. Patients may be initially unconscious from a traumatic injury, wake up, and appear normal during the **"lucid interval,"** during which the epidural hematoma continues to expand. Once it causes adequate mass effect, consciousness is again impaired and the patient may become comatose.

Subdural Hematoma The subdural space, by contrast, is easily formed, and **bridging veins** penetrating the meninges may bleed into this space after blunt head trauma. This is most common in **elderly** patients with a history of **alcohol abuse** (bridging

veins are more likely to tear, as cerebral atrophy increases their "tethering"). Subdural hematomas are **crescentic** because arachnoid and dura come apart easily, spreading the subdural blood along the arc of the crescent. They may also cause mass effect, which may require surgical decompression.

Meningioma The arachnoid (particularly the granulations) may give rise to benign calcified tumors called **meningiomas.** They very rarely invade adjacent tissues but may cause symptoms resulting from local mass effect. Nearly half involve the falx or frontal convexities. Pathology shows characteristic "whorls" of fibrous tissue and calcified **psammoma bodies.** Surgical removal is performed to eliminate unacceptable symptoms.

CASE CONCLUSION

This patient was immediately treated with IV antibiotics empirically for suspected bacterial meningitis. Often vancomycin will be chosen to cover *S. pneumoniae*, with third- or fourth-generation cephalosporin added for coverage of *N. meningitidis* and *H. influenzae*. Ampicillin should be added if *Listeria* is suspected. After obtaining a normal head CT scan, a lumbar puncture was performed, which registered an elevated opening pressure. CSF Gram stain showed a significantly elevated WBC count with 98% PMN leukocytes and gram-negative coccobacilli consistent with *N. meningitidis* infection. The patient became afebrile with a normal neurologic exam 3 days after initiation of treatment; he was given 10 days of IV antibiotic therapy. Preventive single-dose ciprofloxacin was given to the patient's roommate, close contacts, and healthcare workers who were exposed to the patient's respiratory secretions.

THUMBNAIL: Meningitis

Type	Symptoms	CSF Studies		Treatment
Bacterial	Fever/meningismus, confusion, seizures, coma	High polys, high protein, low glucose, Gram stain		Vancomycin + third-generation cephalosporin (ampicillin (*Listeria*)
Viral	Meningismus, more benign	High lymphocytes, normal protein/glucose		Supportive
Tuberculous	More cranial neuropathies, strokes	Acid-fast smear		Antitubercular antibiotic therapy
Syphilitic	Often asymptomatic	CSF RPR		Penicillin
Fungal	More indolent, immunocompromised patients	India ink (Crypto)	Lymphocytic pleocytosis, elevated protein, low glucose	Amphotericin B
Carcinomatous	Back pain, radiculopathy	Cytology		Radiation/chemotherapy
Autoimmune	Cranial neuropathies			Immunosuppression

KEY POINTS

■ The three layers of meninges—pia mater, arachnoid, and dura mater—support and protect the brain and the venous sinuses within the bony skull

■ Infectious meningitis is caused by a variety of organisms and must be diagnosed and treated rapidly in most cases; CSF analysis is usually sufficient to make the diagnosis

■ Other complications involving the meninges include epidural hematoma, subdural hematoma, and meningioma, all of which may require surgery if they cause mass effect

QUESTIONS

1. An elderly patient is brought in for confusion by a stranger. You notice that the patient's neck is stiff and a fever of 101°F. Kernig and Brudzinski signs are present. What is the most appropriate next course of action?

   A. Start IV vancomycin/cefotaxime

   B. Obtain head CT scan

   C. Start IV vancomycin-cefotaxime-ampicillin

   D. Perform lumbar puncture

   E. Obtain plain neck films

2. A 68-year-old man is brought to the attention of his doctor because his wife says that his memory is poor and he has appeared vague and inattentive for the past 3 months. He is a retired physician but has difficulty giving his previous medical history when asked (it is notable for HTN and BPH). His wife mentions that he had a fall in the shower preceding this change, and he was able to recite esoteric medical facts in great detail before the fall occurred. What is the most likely cause of his mental status change?

   A. Meningioma

   B. Subdural hematoma

   C. Fungal meningitis

   D. Alzheimer dementia

   E. Viral meningitis

3. A 16-year-old girl is attending a hockey game when she is struck on the head by a stray puck. Although she is initially arousable and complains of pain over her left temple where she was struck, she becomes progressively more somnolent and is rushed to the hospital. Upon arrival an hour later, she has become comatose. What would the head CT be expected to show?

   A. Left temporal skull fracture with cerebral contusion

   B. Left temporal skull fracture with a crescentic mass adjacent to the brain with mass effect

   C. Left temporal skull fracture with a football-shaped mass adjacent to the brain with mass effect

   D. Left temporal skull fracture with a calcified mass adjacent to the brain with mass effect

   E. Intact skull with cerebral edema and mass effect

4. A 34-year-old patient with no previous medical history presents to his doctor's office with a complaint of stiff neck. He states that this began 5 days ago with headache and neck stiffness so bad that he could not move it, with fevers and chills. He says that this began to improve 2 days ago and he now has some residual neck stiffness and photophobia, but otherwise feels well. His exam is otherwise unremarkable and mental status is intact. He has no fever, has stable vital signs, and results of laboratory tests show no electrolyte or blood count abnormalities. What is the most appropriate course of action?

   A. Immediate IV vancomycin-cefotaxime

   B. Lumbar puncture for culture and cell count

   C. Head CT

   D. Observation

   E. Head MRI

Membrane Properties

HPI: A 32-year-old waitress presents to the ED complaining of double vision since the morning. She also reports on and off numbness of her foot this summer and is concerned she "might be having some kind of stroke." She cannot recall any specific event precipitating these symptoms, although she has been under more stress at work since she has been "more tired and clumsy lately." Three years ago, she had an episode of numbness of her other foot, but this spontaneously resolved after 1 week.

PE: You observe nystagmus and elicit heightened DTRs in her left leg. She has slightly decreased strength in her left lower extremity, but no diminished sensation.

THOUGHT QUESTIONS

- What is this woman's most likely diagnosis?
- How does axonal conduction normally occur?
- What properties affect the velocity of axonal conduction?
- What is the role of myelin in the CNS and peripheral nervous system (PNS)?
- What signs and symptoms would present if axonal conduction is impaired?

BASIC SCIENCE REVIEW AND DISCUSSION

This young woman with a variety of seemingly unrelated neurologic findings in her extremities and vision most likely has MS. The pathophysiology of MS is related to the transmission of the electrical signals along neurons; understanding of neuron and membrane function is critical to understanding this disease.

Action Potentials and Neuronal Function

Nerves transmit electrical signals from one point in the body to another. Action potentials are generated at the **axon hillock,** where the cell body meets the **axon,** a tubular elongated process. The signal must travel the full length of the axon, from hillock to the synaptic terminal, without degeneration. Although axons within the brain can be miniscule, those of spinal neurons are several feet long, transmitting impulses to the most distal points of our extremities.

The axonal membrane is a phospholipid bilayer containing voltage-gated ion channels that conduct impulses both passively and actively. Action potentials arise at the axon hillock and cause a depolarization of the surrounding membrane. This depolarization spreads to the portion of axon immediately downstream, which has a more negative charge. This spread is **passive;** it is due to the imbalance of charge and occurs without any facilitation by the axon. Once slightly downstream, the arriving depolarization causes voltage-gated ion channels to open and the action potential is regenerated. This is the **active propagation** of the signal; the action potential is regenerated by the flux of ions through membrane channels. The new action potential then passively spreads further downstream. The signal cannot return to the axon hillock because the ion channels upstream are immediately closed, in a refractory stage that prevents backward propagation. The entire process repeats until the action potential moves down the length of the axon (Fig. 10-13).

The velocity of an action potential is limited by the need to regenerate as it travels down the axon. Passive conduction alone is not sufficient for transmission. The axon membrane has inherent resistance, which wears down the charge of the impulse as it travels. Just as electricity flowing across uninsulated wire leaks out over distance, the magnitude of the depolarization "leaks" as it travels down stretches of axon. Furthermore, passive conduction is impeded by the bilayer structure of the axonal membrane. The space between the two conductive layers forms a capacitor; that is, for an action potential to move down the membrane, some voltage must serve to fully charge the space within the bilayer. This requirement also slows membrane conduction. (For the electrically inclined, the axon may be thought of as a resistor and a capacitor in parallel.) The result of these factors is that passive conduction cannot transmit an action potential down an entire axon. Therefore, the action potential must be actively regenerated as it moves. The cost of regeneration is conduction speed. The signal must "wait" to be regenerated at various points on the axon.

Because speed is essential in signal transmission, nerves have a few adaptations to recover the velocity of active propagation. First, increasing the numbers of ion channels ensures that action potentials will be regenerated quickly. Faster axons have greater **ion channel densities.** Second, increasing the **diameter** of the axon allows the charge to travel further without regeneration. (This increases the volume inside the axon, which transmits the impulse, relative to the membrane that impedes it.) Axons that have longer lengths are often thicker than their shorter counterparts. Finally, the best way to improve axonal conduction is to provide insulation to prevent charge from "leaking" out.

Myelin is a lipid-rich substance formed by **oligodendrocytes** in the CNS and **Schwann cells** in the PNS. It acts as an excellent insulator for axons, increasing the distance and speed with which an action potential may passively travel by minimizing the leak of charge. In the CNS, oligodendrocytes extend thin processes that wrap around axons, surrounding them in many layers of myelin. In the CNS, one oligodendrocyte can myelinate many different axons. One Schwann cell in the PNS also creates a myelin sheath, but for just one axon. Myelinated axons conduct charge quickly down their length to gaps in the myelin called **nodes of Ranvier.** At these unmyelinated nodes, clusters of ion channels regenerate the action potential, which in turn is conducted down the next segment of myelinated axon. The interspersed jumping of charges down myelinated segments with halting at regenerating nodes is called **saltatory conduction.** Myelin insulation greatly decreases the frequency with which the action potential must be regenerated, increasing its speed down the axon. Myelin greatly increases conduction velocity; although unmyelinated axons have a conduction velocity of about 2 m/second, myelinated axons can have a conduction

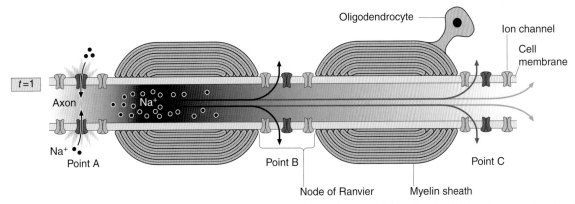

• **Figure 10-13.** Action potential propagation across neuronal membrane. The action potential begins at point A, where massive depolarization occurs. This charge travels passively down the membrane, which is insulated by a myelin sheath. At the node of Ranvier, where there is a gap in the myelin, the charge is regenerated as voltage-gated ion channels open and propagate the depolarization.

velocity of up to 100 m/second. By far, myelination is the most important enhancement that allows signals to be conducted down nerve fibers.

Clinical Correlates

MS is progressive demyelination throughout the CNS that is thought to be autoimmune in origin. It is a relatively common disease, usually affecting young adults (ages 20–50 years) and occurring in women more often than in men. Myelin insulation provided by oligodendrocytes is slowly destroyed and then is replaced by a glial scar. Conduction is impaired in affected axons; scarring can eventually block axonal conduction completely. The hallmark of MS is neurologic deficits that are **transitory and scattered** in location. In fact, the diagnosis of MS requires evidence of multiple lesions and more than one attack over time. Symptoms can appear after periods of infection or stress and tend to worsen with elevated body temperature. The most common complaints at presentation include paresthesia, weakness, abnormal gait, and visual loss. As demyelination periodically worsens and then remits, symptoms wax and wane. Most patients have

relapses every few years. Although there is no fixed pattern to the demyelination, MRI often shows plaque formation in the periventricular white matter. In addition to MRI evidence, the diagnosis can be supported by CSF analysis; most affected patients have increased IgG levels in the CSF with oligoclonal bands on electrophoresis. (This fact also supports the proposed autoimmune basis for the disorder.) MS always follows a progressive course. The rate of decline varies from patient to patient though. Deterioration cannot be reversed, but worsening of disease can be slowed by regular interferon-β (IFN-β) injections.

In addition to MS, **Guillain-Barré syndrome** is a well-understood example of a demyelinating disease. Guillain-Barré is an acute, idiopathic demyelination of the PNS. Symptoms of weakness and eventual paralysis usually occur after resolution of an infectious illness, inoculation, or surgery. Weakness begins in the distal lower extremities and spreads upward. Immediate medical care is essential, as weakness can progress to paralysis of the muscles of respiration. If ventilation is maintained, the illness is self-limited. It generally resolves with no permanent sequelae.

CASE CONCLUSION

CSF analysis demonstrates oligoclonal IgG bands on electrophoresis. MRI reveals multiple periventricular white matter plaques. You refer the patient to a neurologist, who confirms the diagnosis of MS. The neurologist gives the patient a guarded prognosis: Although her immediate symptoms will probably resolve, most patients develop some degree of disability within 10 years of diagnosis. Her young age and relatively mild symptoms are good prognostic signs. A course of weekly IM IFN-β injections is begun in hopes of lengthening the interval before the next relapse. The patient also joins a support group, where she can learn more about MS and the experiences of others who share her illness.

THUMBNAIL: Membrane Properties

Property	Effect on Conduction Velocity
Density of ion channels	Increases
Diameter	Increases
Myelination	Increases

☑ KEY POINTS

- Axons actively propagate action potentials as they travel down nerves
- Conduction velocity increases with increased membrane channel density and diameter
- Myelin serves as an insulator for axons; in the CNS, myelin is supplied by oligodendrocytes; in the PNS, it is supplied by Schwann cells
- In myelinated axons, action potentials travel passively through myelinated segments and are regenerated at the nodes of Ranvier
- One oligodendrocyte can insulate many neurons in the CNS, but one Schwann cell insulates only one axon in the PNS

QUESTIONS

1. Which of the following would most likely remain unaffected in a patient with MS?

   A. Oligodendrocyte structure
   B. Muscle strength
   C. DTRs
   D. Optic nerve function
   E. Schwann cell function

2. Which of the following nerves would be expected to have the greatest conduction velocity?

   A. An unmyelinated pain fiber, 30 cm long, 1 µm in diameter
   B. An unmyelinated interneuron, 5 mm long, 0.8 µm in diameter
   C. An unmyelinated interneuron, 1 mm long, 0.2 µm in diameter
   D. A myelinated motor fiber, 20 cm long, 0.9 µm in diameter
   E. A myelinated sensory fiber, 10 cm long, 0.8 µm in diameter

3. Gliosis at the cell membrane would have which of the following effects?

   A. Enhance action potential propagation by insulating axonal membrane
   B. Slow action potential propagation by blocking passive movement of depolarization
   C. Enhance action potential propagation by increasing the diameter of the axon
   D. Slow action potential propagation by increasing the depositions of oligodendrocytes
   E. Enhance action potential propagation by increasing the density of ion channels

4. A 26-year-old kindergarten teacher comes to the ED with rapidly increasing weakness. She notes that a few weeks ago, she felt "run down" with a flu, but over the past 2 days she has become very weak; what began as tripping over her feet evolved to trouble with stairs and now she has difficulty with any walking. Her exam is notable for areflexia of the lower extremities. Which of the following structures is impaired in this patient?

   A. Axon hillock
   B. Nodes of Ranvier
   C. Axonal ion channels
   D. Oligodendrocytes
   E. Schwann cells

HPI: A 44-year-old office manager is referred to your neurology clinic by her primary care physician, who observed ptosis and mild nystagmus at her last visit. The patient reports increasing fatigue over the last few months and has considered switching to part-time work because she "can never make it through the day anymore." Even though her only flu this year was several months ago, she describes persistently "getting tired more easily: By 3 p.m., I can't stand looking at my computer screen for another minute."

PE: You elicit mild nystagmus and note ptosis, greater in the left eye than in the right. When you ask the patient to maintain an upward gaze, this ptosis worsens notably. Facial sensation is normal, but you observe mild facial muscle weakness. DTRs are normal, and strength and sensation of the extremities are within normal limits.

THOUGHT QUESTIONS

- What is this patient's most likely diagnosis?
- What effect does ACh normally have at the neuromuscular junction (NMJ)?
- How does neurotransmitter release usually lead to postsynaptic action potentials?
- How can the events at the synapse be altered by drugs to change postsynaptic effects?

BASIC SCIENCE REVIEW AND DISCUSSION

In this patient with increasing fatigue over the past few months and neurologic findings of nystagmus and ptosis, particularly with worsening of ptosis upon maintained gaze, myasthenia gravis should be considered. The pathophysiology of myasthenia gravis is related to ACh and its function.

Acetylcholine

A neurotransmitter released into the synaptic cleft is a chemical signal that can diffuse toward the postsynaptic neuron. However, for transmission to be complete, this chemical signal must be converted back into an electrical signal. The classic illustration of this process includes the events at the NMJ. After ACh is released from the presynaptic membrane into the synaptic cleft, it diffuses toward the postsynaptic membrane of the muscle fiber. There, ACh receptors bind the transmitter. These receptors are attached to ion channels; the entire unit at the NMJ is called a **nicotinic ACh receptor.** This is an example of a **ligand-gated ion channel.** When ACh binds to its receptor, the protein changes conformation and directly opens the ion channel, allowing an influx of Na^+ and an efflux of K^+. The net result is depolarization at the postsynaptic membrane, an area called the **endplate** of the muscle fiber. Each molecule of ACh that binds with a receptor opens an ion channel, producing a **miniature endplate potential (MEPP).** If enough ACh binds to enough receptors, the potentials from many MEPPs are summed into one larger depolarization, an **endplate potential (EPP).** This depolarization, in turn, is large enough to open voltage-gated ion channels, which generate an action potential. The action potential travels across the muscle fiber, triggering calcium release and resulting in muscle contraction. The chemical signal of ACh has been converted to an electrical signal at the postsynaptic membrane. The unit then "resets" by clearing out ACh from the synaptic cleft. Acetylcholinesterase is an enzyme in the synaptic cleft that degrades ACh to acetate and choline. These breakdown products re-enter the presynaptic cell, where they are recycled into ACh. The presence of acetylcholinesterase ensures that the effect at the NMJ is limited; synaptic activity is transitory rather than permanent (Fig. 10-14).

Postsynaptic Membrane

Although the example of the NMJ is well understood, the exact events at the postsynaptic membrane vary throughout the nervous system. Postsynaptic receptors vary in structure and in their effects on neurons. For example, not all cholinergic synapses work through ligand-gated ion channels. Muscarinic ACh receptors instead are bound to G proteins, which activate second messengers. When ACh in the synaptic cleft binds with a muscarinic receptor, an enzyme cascade is triggered, with varying final results depending on the specific type of cascade triggered. These second-messenger receptors are sometimes called **metabotropic** receptors (as opposed to directly **ionotropic** receptors). In some cases, the second messengers cause the opening of Na^+ channels or closing of K^+ channels, resulting in a depolarization much like that at the endplate. This brings the postsynaptic neuron closer to threshold; it is now in an "excited" state where action potential generation is facilitated. The general term for a potential of this type is **EPSP.** A series of EPSPs (either repeatedly from the same presynaptic input or at once from several presynaptic synapses) can sum to push the neuron past threshold and fire an action potential. In other instances, the second messenger leads to the opening of K^+ or Cl^- channels or the closing of Na^+ channels. In this case, the result at the postsynaptic membrane is a hyperpolarization, moving the cell further from threshold. Because the cell is now further from the threshold required to generate an action potential, these potentials are called **IPSPs.** Various combinations exist in which a given transmitter activates either a metabotropic or ionotropic receptor, eliciting either an EPSP or an IPSP. Any neurotransmitter can have either excitatory or inhibitory effects depending on the structure of its receptor. Nonetheless, certain receptors predominate in the nervous system, and so neurotransmitters can have a generally excitatory or inhibitory effect. (For example, glutamate is largely excitatory, whereas GABA is usually inhibitory.)

These effects can occur simultaneously at one postsynaptic neuron, which allows integration of multiple incoming signals. If the EPSPs outweigh the IPSPs at a postsynaptic membrane, an action potential results. Likewise, IPSPs can counteract excitatory input from upstream neurons. In this way, multiple synapses on one neuron can be processed to result in one event, the firing (or nonfiring) of an action potential.

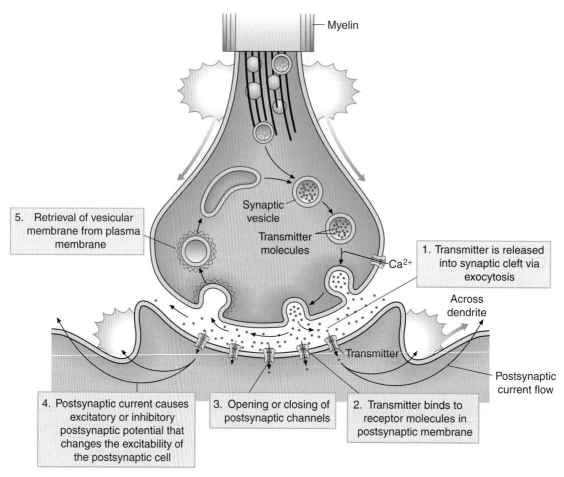

5. Retrieval of vesicular membrane from plasma membrane

Synaptic vesicle

Transmitter molecules

Myelin

1. Transmitter is released into synaptic cleft via exocytosis

Ca²⁺

Across dendrite

Transmitter

Postsynaptic current flow

4. Postsynaptic current causes excitatory or inhibitory postsynaptic potential that changes the excitability of the postsynaptic cell

3. Opening or closing of postsynaptic channels

2. Transmitter binds to receptor molecules in postsynaptic membrane

• **Figure 10-14.** Steps of synaptic transmission at the postsynaptic membrane.

Just as there are many different receptor types, there are various methods by which the neurotransmitter is cleared from the synaptic cleft. Some synapses employ enzymatic degradation, like **acetylcholinesterase,** to break down the neurotransmitter. Others use transporter pumps to bring the neurotransmitter back into the presynaptic terminal or into surrounding glial cells. All rely on simple diffusion to some degree. These mechanisms are popular targets for pharmaceutical therapy; by prolonging neurotransmitter release in the synaptic cleft, they increase its activity. Examples of such drugs are selective serotonin reuptake inhibitors (SSRIs) (e.g., fluoxetine), which block reuptake pumps, or monoamine oxidase inhibitors (MAOIs) (e.g., phenelzine), which prevent degradation of catecholamines. Eventually, though, the neurotransmitter is removed from the synaptic cleft and the signaling process can start over.

Clinical Correlates

Myasthenia gravis is an autoimmune disorder that attacks the NMJ. Autoantibodies to nicotinic ACh receptors block signaling; ACh release in the synaptic cleft thus has less effect on the postsynaptic membrane. The disease most often affects cranial muscles, such as the extraocular muscles and those innervated by CN VII. The resulting symptom is fatigable weakness, that is, muscle weakness that worsens with sustained contraction and improves after rest. The diagnosis is classically confirmed by a **Tensilon (or edrophonium) test.** Tensilon is an acetylcholinesterase inhibitor; it counters the enzyme that normally degrades ACh in the synaptic cleft. In a patient with myasthenia gravis, Tensilon administration lengthens the life of ACh in the synapse, which allows increased effect at the postsynaptic membrane and thus improved strength and immediate relief from symptoms. Likewise, long-term treatment usually involves regular administration of an anticholinesterase drug. The origin of the autoantibodies in myasthenia gravis is unclear, but there is a high incidence of comorbidity in the thymus. Therefore, each patient should be evaluated for thymoma, and thymectomy may be performed in an effort to lessen symptoms. Likewise, because symptoms are mediated through autoantibodies, steroid treatment to inhibit immune function can alleviate symptoms of myasthenia gravis. Generally, myasthenia gravis is progressive, although the course may involve lengthy periods of maintenance without remission of symptoms.

CASE CONCLUSION

A Tensilon test in the office produces dramatic improvement in the ptosis, as well as complete cessation of nystagmus. Facial musculature shows increased strength. The patient is begun on a regular schedule of anticholinesterase drugs, which allow her to resume her prior activities. Although a CT shows no thymic mass, the patient elects thymectomy, which leads to an almost total remission of her symptoms. She understands she is not "cured" of her disease, but her symptoms remain minimal after surgery and with her new drug regimen.

THUMBNAIL: Postsynaptic Receptors

Receptor Type	Ionotropic	Metabotropic
Works via . . .	Ligand-gated ion channels	G proteins and second messengers
Speed	Faster	Slower
Example of excitatory receptor	Nicotinic ACh receptor at NMJ	M_1 muscarinic ACh receptors in the ANS
Example of inhibitory receptor	$GABA_A$ receptors in the brain	$GABA_B$ receptors in the brain

KEY POINTS

- ACh in the NMJ directly opens ligand-gated ion channels, causing a depolarization of the endplate (EPP)
- A sufficient number of depolarizations at the postsynaptic membrane (EPSPs) can drive a neuronal membrane past threshold and generate an action potential
- Hyperpolarizations (IPSPs) drive the cell further from threshold, preventing action potential generation

- Postsynaptic receptors either can be ligand-gated ion channels (ionotropic) or affect channels via a second messenger (metabotropic)
- The effects of a neurotransmitter on the postsynaptic membrane are determined by the properties of the specific receptor on that membrane, not by the neurotransmitter itself
- Neurotransmitter effects can be enhanced by drugs that prolong their time in the synaptic cleft

QUESTIONS

1. Dopamine is an example of a neurotransmitter that has both excitatory and inhibitory effects in the CNS. Dopamine can have an excitatory effect on a given postsynaptic neuron in the striatum, but an inhibitory effect on a postsynaptic neuron in the cortex. The best explanation for this is which of the following?

   A. More dopaminergic vesicles are released at the striatal synapse than at the cortical synapse.
   B. The receptors on the striatal neuron are ionotropic, and the cortical receptors are metabotropic.
   C. The receptors on the striatal neuron have a higher affinity for dopamine than those of the cortical neuron.
   D. The ion channels affected in the striatal postsynaptic neuron are different from those in the cortical cell.
   E. The receptors at the striatal membrane have greater dopaminergic activation because of lower levels of enzymatic degradation.

2. A spinal interneuron integrates signals from two presynaptic inputs. One input has an excitatory effect via glutamate

release, and the other has an inhibitory effect via glycine release. When the excitatory presynaptic neuron fires alone, glutamate release leads to an action potential in the postsynaptic neuron. When both presynaptic neurons are fired simultaneously, the postsynaptic membrane is inhibited; it does not fire an action potential. How does glycine negate the otherwise excitatory effect of glutamate on this cell?

   A. Glycine blocks glutamate release at the presynaptic membrane.
   B. Glycine binds to glutamate, rendering it unable to bind to postsynaptic receptors.
   C. Glycine competes with glutamate for the same receptors on the postsynaptic membrane.
   D. Glycine binds to different receptors on the postsynaptic membrane, affecting ion channels.
   E. Glycine activates the pump on the presynaptic membrane, which removes glutamate from the synaptic cleft.

3. Some nerve gases are potent acetylcholinesterase inhibitors. Through what mechanism do they have their effect?

    A. Inhibiting the release of ACh, thus blocking signaling
    B. Acting as antagonists at postsynaptic ACh receptors, thus blocking signaling
    C. Inhibiting postsynaptic G protein signaling pathways
    D. Inhibiting the synthesis of signaling neurotransmitter
    E. Increasing ACh available in the synaptic cleft

4. Fluoxetine, sertraline, and paroxetine are all examples of SSRIs. How do these drugs increase activity at the synapse?

    A. Acting as agonists at the postsynaptic membrane
    B. Increasing vesicle fusion at the presynaptic membrane
    C. Inhibiting transporters on the postsynaptic membrane
    D. Directly depolarizing the postsynaptic membrane
    E. Inhibiting transporters on the presynaptic membrane

CASE 10-22 Dopamine and Substantia Nigra

HPI: A 65-year-old retired professor comes to your practice complaining of difficulty "getting around," gradually increasing for more than 1 year. On observation, you see he has difficulty standing and is slow to begin walking. He walks slowly, taking very small short steps.

PE: You note rigidity with intermittent bursts of movement on attempting to extend the arms. The patient sits quietly throughout the exam, continually making small, repetitive movements of his hands and fingers. Although he states he is very distressed by his symptoms, he remains almost completely without facial expression during his visit.

THOUGHT QUESTIONS

- What is the most likely diagnosis of this patient?
- What is the possible cause of and which areas of the CNS are affected by this disorder?
- How is dopamine synthesized?
- Where else in the body does dopamine act?

BASIC SCIENCE REVIEW AND DISCUSSION

This gentleman's most likely diagnosis is Parkinson disease (PD). His gait, with small, short steps, diminished extremity movements, and limited facial expression are all classic findings. The physiology of the neurotransmitter dopamine is intimately involved in this disease, so understanding its biochemistry, receptors, and actions is important in understanding and treating **PD.**

Dopamine

Dopamine is a catecholamine neurotransmitter that acts both in the brain and outside the CNS. All the catecholamines (dopamine, NE, epinephrine) are synthesized via a common pathway from the amino acid phenylalanine, which is also the precursor to melanin and T_4 synthesis. The dopamine synthesis pathway is important both as a frequent topic in Step 1 questions and as a target for drug therapy in PD, in which there is a deficit of dopamine (Fig. 10-15).

Dopamine acts primarily on five types of receptors, D_1 to D_5. All are seven-transmembrane segment G-protein receptors. These receptors are found on tissues throughout the body, including the renal vasculature, anterior pituitary, and the GI tract. In the brain, dopamine acts in the basal ganglia, limbic system, and cortex, affecting mood, reward pathways, cognition, and movement. Drugs such as amphetamine and cocaine produce euphoria and motor agitation by increasing dopaminergic activity in the brain. In the basal ganglia, D_1 has an excitatory effect on adenylate cyclase postsynaptically, whereas D_2 has an inhibitory effect on adenylate cyclase both presynaptically and postsynaptically. Although dopamine is found throughout, 80% of the brain's dopamine is found in the substantia nigra.

The **substantia nigra** is a nucleus at the base of the midbrain composed of two parts, the **substantia nigra pars compacta** and the **substantia nigra pars reticulata.** The cells of the nucleus have high concentrations of melanin and thus have a dark appearance to the naked eye. (Hence the name, which is Latin for "dark substance.") The substantia nigra compacta projects dopaminergic axons to the striatum, where dopamine acts on both D_1 and D_2 receptors in the caudate and putamen. The overall effect of increased dopamine from the substantia nigra is increased motor activity.

In the normal brain, the dopaminergic axons from the substantia nigra have a net excitatory effect on the striatum, which in turn inhibits the internal segment of the globus pallidus via the direct pathway. This dampens the effect of the internal segment of the globus pallidus, which otherwise acts to inhibit the excitatory stimulation of the ventrolateral thalamus, on the motor cortex. If the substantia nigra is not functioning, there is less excitement to the striatum, and thus less inhibition of the internal segment of the **globus pallidus.** The globus pallidus is then free to inhibit the ventrolateral thalamus, and end motor activity is decreased as a result of excessive indirect pathway activity (Fig. 10-16). "Short-circuiting" the indirect pathway by deep brain stimulation of the subthalamic nucleus has proven to be a good symptomatic treatment for PD.

Clinical Correlates

Parkinsonism is a syndrome defined by a collection of motor deficits such as "cogwheel" **rigidity,** resting "pill-rolling" or "head-nodding" **tremor, bradykinesia,** difficulty initiating movement, stooped posture, diminished facial expression ("Parkinson mask"), and festinating gait. This syndrome is found after damage to the substantia nigra or its connections to the striatum. The substantia nigra may be damaged after exposure to certain drugs or toxins, such as dopamine antagonists, 1-methyl-4-phenyl-1,2,5,6-tetrahydropyridine (MPTP), or manganese; during an acute viral encephalitis, although this has become exceedingly rare; or due to ischemia in atherosclerotic disease. In each of these cases, parkinsonism may occur (Fig. 10-17).

Although parkinsonism is a clinical syndrome with a number of possible causes, **PD** is the most common. Idiopathic PD occurs later in life, when degeneration of the dopaminergic cells of the substantia nigra causes an overall deficit of dopamine in the basal ganglia. For symptoms to be present, there must be a loss of at least 80% of the cells of the substantia nigra. On microscopic exam, the remaining neurons can show Lewy bodies, which are dense deposits of filament inside the neuronal body. The cause of these deposits and of neuronal degeneration is unclear. Untreated, PD will progress, with symptoms worsening until death. About 15 to 30% of patients also develop dementia, usually attributed to Lewy body deposits in the cortex. Although there is no cure for PD, a number of therapies attempt to correct the dopamine deficiency and relieve symptoms. Action on D_2 receptors has been shown to be particularly important, although some benefit can be gained by action on

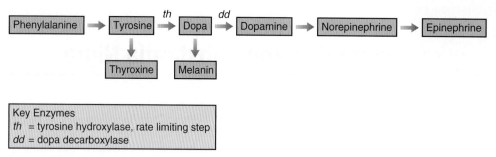

• **Figure 10-15.** Dopamine and catecholamine synthesis.

D_1 receptors as well. Drug therapy includes **levodopa (L-dopa)**, a form of dopa that can cross the blood–brain barrier and be converted to dopamine. Other useful drugs are dopamine agonists and MAOIs. Although these may allow dramatic improvement when initiated, there is often a "wearing off" of the drug's effect and responsiveness may be lost completely. In severe cases, surgery may also be employed, as described above.

CASE CONCLUSION

The patient underwent neuropsychiatric testing and was found to have no signs of dementia. Drug therapy was initiated, consisting of oral L-dopa daily. The patient began physical therapy to maximize his mobility. This resulted in significant improvement, and after 1 month the patient was able to walk relatively well with a cane. The patient was advised that this gain may be temporary and was informed that future options may include addition of other drugs to his regimen or possibly surgical intervention.

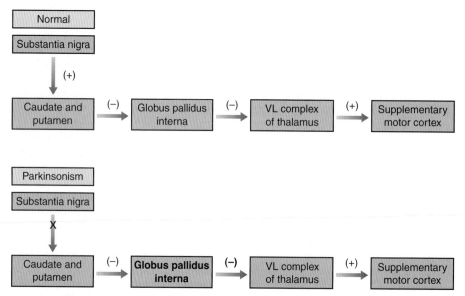

• **Figure 10-16.** Normal motor pathways are altered in PD by a lack of dopaminergic input from the substantia nigra; the result is increased inhibition by the globus pallidus and decreased motor output. For simplicity, only the direct pathway is depicted.

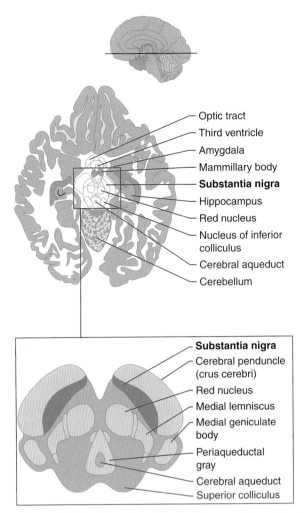

THUMBNAIL: Dopamine Receptors

Type of Receptor	Primary Location	Effect on cAMP
D$_1$	Striatum, vascular tissue	↑
D$_2$	Throughout brain, smooth muscle, presynaptic nerve terminals	↓
D$_3$	Limbic system, cortex	↓
D$_4$	Limbic system, cortex, cardiovascular muscle	↓
D$_5$	Cortex, hippocampus, renal vasculature	↑

KEY POINTS

■ Dopamine is a catecholamine; its synthesis is limited by the conversion of tyrosine to dopa, dopamine's immediate precursor

■ In the basal ganglia, the net effect of dopamine is to promote movement

■ The substantia nigra is located in the midbrain; although the dark pigment distinguishes the nucleus in normal specimens, the region can be completely pale in cases of PD with severe neuronal loss. Thus, to identify the substantia nigra, know the characteristic color *and* the relative location of the nucleus in the midbrain.

■ Parkinsonism is a syndrome characterized by rigidity, difficulty initiating movements, resting tremor, slow movement, diminished facial expression, and shuffling gait; it may occur after any type of damage to the substantia nigra

■ Idiopathic PD is the most common cause of parkinsonism

• **Figure 10-17.** Axial section of brain at the level of the midbrain. Note the location of the substantia nigra in relation to the cerebral peduncles, red nucleus, and tegmentum of the midbrain.

QUESTIONS

1. A 26-year-old chef with schizophrenia has been admitted to the inpatient psychiatry service after her second florid episode in a year. Her physician prescribes chlorpromazine and alprazolam to be taken immediately. At the urging of her family, the patient also resumes taking the haloperidol she was prescribed by another doctor after her earlier episodes. After a week in the hospital, her nurses notice a resting "head-nod" tremor, as well as slowness in movements. Her facial expression is also markedly diminished. A review of medication reveals she is taking high doses of two antipsychotics, which are considered the cause of her parkinsonism. The haloperidol is discontinued and L-dopa begun to alleviate symptoms. Which of the following enzymes catalyzes the rate-limiting step required for L-dopa to be converted to dopamine in the brain?

A. Phenylalanine hydroxylase
B. Tyrosine hydroxylase
C. Dopa decarboxylase
D. Monoamine oxidase A
E. Monoamine oxidase B

2. MPTP is a toxin that can be unintentionally synthesized in the illicit manufacturing of opioid drugs. MPTP is selectively taken up by the dopaminergic neurons of the substantia nigra, where its active form causes neuronal death. Cases have been reported of opioid users self-administering MPTP contaminate and developing a severe acute-onset PD. A patient developing this type of toxin-mediated PD will have symptoms resulting from altered activity in which set of brain areas?

A. Substantia nigra reticulata, caudate, putamen, cerebellum
B. Substantia nigra reticulata, striatum, internal segment of the globus pallidus, motor cortex
C. Substantia nigra reticulata, putamen, ventrolateral thalamus, motor cortex
D. Substantia nigra compacta, striatum, internal segment of the globus pallidus, ventrolateral thalamus
E. Substantia nigra compacta, striatum, internal segment of the globus pallidus, cerebellum

3. Which of the following is an identified cause of parkinsonism?

A. Viral encephalitis
B. Head trauma
C. Ischemia
D. All of the above
E. None of the above

4. Which structures lie directly adjacent to the substantia nigra?

A. Cerebral peduncle
B. Red nucleus
C. Cerebral aqueduct
D. A and C
E. All of the above

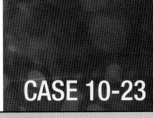

CASE 10-23 Serotonin and Nucleus Raphe

HPI: A 25-year-old paralegal comes to your family practice office complaining of months of fatigue. She is also bothered by occasional headaches and sporadic stomach and back pain. She reports difficulty sleeping: She wakes early every morning and is unable to fall back asleep. On questioning, the patient reports she has also lost about 20 pounds over the past 8 months, since moving across the country to begin her new job. She looks at the floor throughout the conversation, maintaining a flat affect with little positive expression. She does not have friends or family in the area and finds it difficult to come up with any interests or activities she enjoys as recreation.

PE: Normal, not revealing any obvious pathology.

THOUGHT QUESTIONS

- How can major depression present?
- Which neurotransmitters have been implicated in depression?
- How is serotonin formed?
- Where does serotonin act?

BASIC SCIENCE REVIEW AND DISCUSSION

This patient comes to her physician with multiple vague physical complaints, including fatigue and insomnia. Such a presentation is very common in cases of major depression. Because understanding the action of serotonin is useful in the diagnosis and treatment of depression, we begin with a discussion of its biochemistry and physiology.

Serotonin

Serotonin, or 5-hydroxytryptamine **(5-HT),** is an indolamine neurotransmitter. Serotonin is synthesized from the amino acid tryptophan (also the precursor of niacin and melatonin). Its major metabolite is 5-hydroxyindole acetic acid (5-HIAA) (Fig. 10-18).

Serotonin receptors are found throughout the body; there are more than 12 receptor subtypes. Some play important roles in pain and local inflammation after tissue damage. Others are important in local signaling in the GI tract. In fact, more than 80% of the body's serotonin is in the enterochromaffin cells of the intestine. In the brain, serotonergic neurons are mainly located in the **nucleus raphe.** This is a vertical cluster of neurons in the pons and upper midbrain that sends projections both up throughout the brain and downward into the spinal cord. Serotonin acts primarily on the 5-HT_1, 5-HT_2, and 5-HT_3 subsets of receptors in the CNS.

The projections of the nucleus raphe have been implicated in control of pain, nausea, sleep, and mood. The **descending analgesia circuit** of the midbrain and spinal cord is a hierarchic system that can suppress ascending pain signals. The circuit begins in the midbrain, where the periaqueductal gray is activated by endorphin release. When activated, projections from the periaqueductal gray stimulate the nucleus raphe. In turn, the projections of the nucleus raphe release more serotonin in the dorsolateral spinal cord. There, serotonin inhibits pain signals and mediates release of enkephalins. This decreases the transmission of pain signaling before it can reach the brain. This circuit is

thought to be one mechanism by which extreme emotion or physical stress can modulate the sensation of pain.

Other circuits that require serotonin are not as well understood. For example, the nucleus raphe is known to be a part of the **reticular formation,** a dispersed mesh of neurons that control sleep patterns via inputs to the thalamus. It has been observed that increased serotonin activity in the reticular formation is correlated with slow-wave (non-REM) sleep. Furthermore, decreased serotonin activity is required to "turn on" REM sleep. The exact mechanism, though, is unclear. Likewise, serotonin is known to be important in controls of nausea through 5-HT_3 receptors on the gut and in the brainstem. Particularly, serotonin acting at specific areas of the medulla is thought to underlie nausea and vomiting in response to noxious stimuli. The interplay between signals from the GI tract and the **medullary vomiting center,** though, is unclear. Finally, serotonin levels are known to have a profound effect on mood. However, much remains unknown about how exactly mood is controlled.

Clinical Correlates

Major depressive disorder is very common; it affects 10 to 20% of individuals at some point during their life. Patients experience fatigue, anhedonia, and a loss of interest in formerly motivating activities. A sense of hopelessness is a common feature, and suicidal ideation may result. Although some spend more time eating or sleeping, most depressed persons experience a loss of appetite and insomnia. Classically, depressed individuals sleep less, have less slow-wave sleep, and wake early in the morning. The exact pathophysiology of depression is unclear, but a number of theories have been suggested. The **amine hypothesis** is based on the known effects of drugs that act at amine synapses. Drugs that block the release of NE and serotonin have been found to induce depression in some patients. Likewise, drugs that inhibit monoamine degradation or reuptake have been found to ameliorate symptoms of depression. In normal persons, drugs that increase amine transmitter activity cause a sense of euphoria or symptoms of mania. This evidence has been proposed to suggest that decreased levels of NE and serotonin in the brain cause depression and insomnia, whereas increased levels cause mania. A variation of the amine hypothesis is based on more recent findings that drugs that affect only serotonin, such as SSRIs, can also give relief from depression with a much lower incidence of side effects. The **permissive serotonin hypothesis** proposes that dysfunction of serotonin allows altered catecholamine levels to

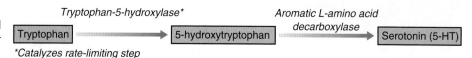

Figure 10-18. Serotonin is synthesized in a series of steps from its precursor tryptophan.

cause changes in mood. That is, alterations in serotonin levels are required for abnormal catecholamine levels to affect on mood. Current research aims at elucidating the exact relationship between serotonin, catecholamines, and mood disorders.

Pharmaceutical agents that increase functional serotonin levels have been proven effective in many cases of depression. In addition to SSRIs, MAOIs and tricyclic antidepressants (TCAs) increase the time serotonin lasts in the synaptic cleft. Drugs that act directly on 5-HT receptors have not been widely employed in depression but

have found other applications. Sumatriptan is a 5-HT$_{1D}$ agonist that acts at receptors on the cerebral and meningeal vasculature. By directly stimulating these receptors, it provides immediate relief from migraine headaches for many patients. Ondansetron is a 5-HT$_3$ antagonist that is a powerful antinauseant and antiemetic. Its effects at the medullary vomiting center have been extremely helpful to patients undergoing chemotherapy. Although the primary application of serotonin-affecting drugs is in mood disorders, other applications are of significant importance as well.

CASE CONCLUSION

With further discussion, the patient admits she has been feeling sad and even hopeless lately. At times she feels guilty or worthless for no particular reason, but she denies contemplating suicide. You suggest that her symptoms could be a part of a larger case of depression. She reluctantly agrees and accepts your recommendation to visit a psychologist for a trial of cognitive behavioral therapy with antidepressant medication. With this combination of treatment, more than two thirds of patients can expect significant remission of symptoms.

THUMBNAIL: Important 5-HT Receptors in the CNS

Receptor Subtype	Location	Receptor Type	Effect
5-HT$_{1A}$	Nucleus raphe, hippocampus	Metabotropic	Inhibition
5-HT$_{1D}$	Cerebral and meningeal vessels	Metabotropic	Vasoconstriction
5-HT$_2$	Cortex, striatum	Metabotropic	Excitation
5-HT$_3$	Medullary vomiting center (aka, area postrema)	Ionotropic	Excitation

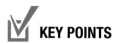

KEY POINTS

- Serotonin is an amine neurotransmitter synthesized from tryptophan
- Serotonin acts throughout the body in pain, inflammation, and GI tract function

- In the brain, serotonin-containing neurons are found mainly in the nucleus raphe and send projections throughout the CNS
- Serotonin is active in descending inhibition of pain in the spinal cord, sleep and wakefulness, and mood

QUESTIONS

1. Serotonergic projections from the nucleus raphe act on neurons in the spinal cord and dorsal root ganglia as part of the descending analgesia circuit. This activation of 5-HT receptors in the spinal cord has which of the following effects on ion channels?

A. Increase postsynaptic K$^+$ conduction
B. Decrease postsynaptic K$^+$ conduction
C. Increase postsynaptic Na$^+$ conduction
D. Decrease postsynaptic Cl$^+$ conduction
E. Increase presynaptic Ca^{2+} conduction

2. Which of the following receive serotonergic projections from the nucleus raphe?

   A. Reticular formation
   B. Enterochromaffin cells
   C. Descending analgesia circuit
   D. A and C
   E. All of the above

3. A strong serotonin agonist that acts in the area postrema of the medulla would most likely have which of the following effects?

   A. Elevate mood
   B. Cause vasodilation
   C. Cause headache
   D. Promote vomiting
   E. Descending analgesia

4. The pontine reticular formation regulates sleep patterns mainly through direct inputs to which brain region?

   A. Periaqueductal gray
   B. Thalamus
   C. Nucleus raphe
   D. Hippocampus
   E. Cerebral cortex

ANSWERS

PART I: CARDIOVASCULAR

CASE 1-1

1. C. Concentric hypertrophy is the result of pressure overload, which is usually the result of AS or uncontrolled, long-term hypertension. Eccentric hypertrophy and subsequent chamber dilatation are secondary to long-term volume overload. Severe aortic and mitral regurgitation impose a volume overload on the LV. A VSD or ASD with a large left-to-right shunt would also result in volume overload and eccentric hypertrophy.

2. D. Nitrates result in vascular smooth muscle relaxation and produce greater dilatation of the veins than do the arterioles. The resulting venodilation induces venous pooling and decreased preload because of diminished venous return. At higher doses, nitrates can also cause increased arteriolar dilatation and afterload reduction. Choices (A), (B), (C), and (E) are all effective treatments for CHF, but all four choices are pure afterload reducing agents.

3. B. Treatment of heart failure secondary to diastolic dysfunction is similar to that for heart failure secondary to systolic dysfunction, except for the use of positive inotropic drugs (digoxin, dobutamine, dopamine, milrinone). Positive inotropic drugs can worsen diastolic dysfunction by (*a*) promoting tachycardia: (*b*) decreasing diastolic filling time: (*c*) increasing myocardial oxygen requirements: and (*d*) worsening underlying myocardial ischemia.

4. E. Beta-blockers improve diastolic filling via choices (A) through (D). Choice (E) is incorrect because beta-blockers decrease the LV outflow gradient.

In addition to diastolic dysfunction, beta-blockers are also used to treat patients with elevated subaortic valve gradients secondary to LV hypertrophy (asymmetric septal hypertrophy/hypertrophic obstructive cardiomyopathy). With severe septal or LV hypertrophy, the LV outflow tract is narrowed. With increased contractility (as seen with increased physical activity) the LV outflow tract narrowing and obstruction increases further. This dynamic narrowing (or dynamic outflow obstruction) increases the LV outflow gradient and LV end-diastolic pressure with resultant pulmonary edema. Beta-blockers therefore can decrease this narrowing, decrease the LV outflow gradient, improve LV outflow, and decrease pulmonary edema.

CASE 1-2

1. C. All five of these biochemical markers increase in MI, but troponin is the most specific and has the longest duration of elevation. Myoglobin and creatinine kinase decrease to baseline within 24–36 hours. SGOT peaks in 2 days but returns to baseline within 5 days. LDH can remain elevated for up to 6 days but is a relatively nonspecific marker. Troponin I can remain elevated for up to 10 days and is very specific for myocardial necrosis.

2. D. Approximately one third of patients with inferior MI develop RV necrosis because the right coronary artery (RCA) supplies both the LV inferior wall and the RV. Patients with RCA occlusion often present with severe bradycardia and heart block because the AV node receives its blood supply from the RCA. Occlusion of the RCA results in poor RV contractile function, but LV systolic function remains relatively unimpaired. As a result, signs of right-sided heart failure (elevated JVP, pulsatile liver) are out of proportion to signs of left-sided heart failure (lack of CHF and clear lungs). The impairment of LV filling due to poor RV contractile function is the main cause for the hypotension, and the treatment of choice is IV fluid resuscitation.

CASE 1-3

1. B. This patient presents with syncope secondary to critical AS. The median survival for severe AS patients is 5 years for angina, 3 years for syncope, and 2 years for CHF. His exam is notable for the prototypical systolic murmur radiating upward. The apical component of the murmur is the Gallavardin phenomenon. The second heart sound (composed of an aortic and pulmonic component) is paradoxically split (P_2 occurs before A_2) because LV ejection is prolonged in severe AS. Unlike in MR, handgrip does not change the AS murmur. The cardiac catheterization tracing consistent with AS is that shown in (B), with the solid line representing the LV pressure and the dotted line representing the aortic pressure. The difference between the two lines at mid-systole is the peak-to-peak gradient generated by the stenotic valve. Choice (A) is the pressure tracing for a normal aortic valve. Choice (C) is the pressure tracing for severe aortic insufficiency when there is a rapid decrease in aortic pressure during diastole and a concomitant rise in LV pressure from the regurgitant volume.

2. E. This patient presents with chronic decompensated aortic insufficiency and CHF secondary to increased LVEDP and pulmonary congestion. The primary treatment for decompensated aortic insufficiency is afterload reduction (with ACE inhibitors, angiotensin receptor blockers, or hydralazine) to improve forward cardiac output, diuresis to decrease the LVEDP, and increased inotropy with digoxin. Although the patient presents with angina, it is unlikely secondary to coronary artery disease, and beta-blockers are therefore unlikely to improve his angina. With aortic insufficiency, relative bradycardia actually worsens the clinical symptoms and can precipitate angina. Bradycardia causes an increase in the diastolic filling period and regurgitant volume with a resultant increase in LVEDP and a decrease in diastolic coronary perfusion.

3. C. This patient presents with MS secondary to rheumatic heart fever. As a result of her MS, she has LA hypertension, which induces LA enlargement, atrial fibrillation, and pulmonary congestions. The elevated left-sided pressures are then transmitted to the right-sided chambers, resulting in RV dilatation and hypertrophy and peripheral edema. She also presents with the prototypical malar erythema and OS secondary to the sudden tensing of the chordae upon opening. The cardiac catheterization tracing for MS is choice (C), with the solid line representing the LV pressure and the dotted line representing the LA pressure. A pressure gradient is present throughout diastole.

4. D. After mitral valvuloplasty, one of the most common complications is acute MR. The hemodynamic profile of MR is best characterized by choice (D), with a large C-V wave noted in the

LA tracing, corresponding to the large regurgitant pressure wave transmitted retrograde from the LV to the LA through the incompetent mitral valve.

CASE 1-4

1. C. *S. bovis* is almost always associated with GI tumors, interventions on the GI tract, or digestive infectious diseases. Genitourinary tumors such as transitional cell carcinoma of the bladder would be more commonly associated with enterococci, gram-negative bacilli, or *S. aureus*. Endocarditis associated with infections of the respiratory tract would include penicillin-sensitive streptococci.

2. C. Mitral valve prolapse without MR is associated with no risk of IE and does not require antibiotic prophylaxis. However, mitral valve prolapse with mitral valve regurgitation is associated with a risk of IE 6–14 times greater than normal and does require antibiotic prophylaxis. Bicuspid aortic valve also requires antibiotic prophylaxis and is found in up to 25% of cases of aortic endocarditis. A PDA also requires antibiotic prophylaxis, but risk is greatly decreased with correction. Prosthetic heart valves carry a risk 5–10 times greater for IE than patients with native valves and therefore require antibiotic prophylaxis.

CASE 1-5

1. E. The patient's postoperative state increases his risk for all SVTs. However, the prompt resolution of the tachycardia with IV adenosine suggest that the tachycardia circuit involves the AV node and is most likely to be either AVNRT or AVRT. Although adenosine decreases the rate of conduction through the AV node and can slow the ventricular rate of non-AV node-dependent tachycardia circuits (sinus tachycardia, atrial flutter, AF, multifocal atrial tachycardia), the inhibition of the AV node usually does not terminate the tachycardia.

2. C. The most straightforward arrhythmia for ablation is typical flutter. In typical flutter, the re-entrant circuit is usually located in a defined anatomic location within the RA (the circuit passes along a narrow isthmus of tissue between the tricuspid valve annulus and entrance of the inferior vena cava) and is easily interrupted. Atypical atrial flutter is much more difficult to locate because the flutter circuit can exist anywhere within the RA or LA. Although experimental protocols are now available, multifocal atrial tachycardia and AF are not typically amenable to ablation because of their multiple foci. Sinus tachycardia is a physiologic response to a stressor, and the treatment is correction of the underlying stressor (pain, dehydration, fever, etc.), not ablation.

3. E. Polymorphic VT suggest that the underlying etiology for the recurrent arrhythmia is ongoing ischemia. Although IV magnesium replacement and IV antiarrhythmics may temporize the situation, these steps will not address the underlying ischemia. An activation-induced cell death (AICD) will correct the VT but will defibrillate incessantly for recurrent VT until the underlying ischemia is corrected. Thrombolysis could potentially address the occluded coronary artery, but given the patient's presumed cardiogenic shock, cardiac catheterization and angioplasty would be the most reasonable option.

4. D. Patients with MI secondary to proximal RCA occlusion are most likely to present with severe bradycardia. Although the SA node receives its blood supply only 60% of the time from the

RCA, the AV node receives blood from the RCA 90% of the time. Patients with severe right coronary infarcts often require temporary electronic pacing.

CASE 1-6

1. D. With TGA, it is imperative to maintain ductus arteriosus (DA) patency to allow for right-to-left shunting of oxygenated blood. Prostaglandin infusion allows for the DA to remain patent until a definitive surgical procedure is performed. Balloon atrial septostomy is another palliative procedure to establish shunting at the interatrial level. Supplemental oxygen would have little effect since the increasingly oxygenated blood would remain isolated within the LV circuit. Inotropic support would not increase oxygenation due to persistent shunting. Indomethacin would actually hasten DA closure. Finally, TGA patients are already polycythemic from hypoxia, and additional blood transfusion can exacerbate symptoms.

2. E. In TOF, deoxygenated blood is routed from the RV, through a VSD, and into the systemic circulation. Therefore, any condition causing (*a*) lower SVR, (*b*) increased venous return, or (*c*) worsened pulmonic stenosis can exacerbate the baseline hypoxemia. Although hydralazine is an afterload-reducing agent often used in systolic heart failure, this medication could potentially worsen the clinical situation because right-to-left shunting would increase, resulting in increased hypoxia. TOF patients are at risk for endocarditis, and prophylactic antibiotics are appropriate. Supplemental oxygen would improve their baseline hypoxia. Supplemental iron will prevent anemia by providing the iron reserves for the adaptive polycythemia. Beta-blockers are also considered standard of care for TOF because they decrease the degree of dynamic RV outflow obstruction/pulmonic stenosis during ventricular systole.

PART II: PULMONARY

CASE 2-1

1. D. The internal intercostal muscles point backward as they are followed from the upper rib to the lower rib, such that contraction pulls the rib cage down and inward. This acts to decrease thoracic volume and facilitate forced expiration. The external intercostal muscles point forward, and contraction pulls the rib cage up and outward. The diaphragm in contraction acts to compress the abdominal contents and pull up the lower ribs. Scalene and sternocleidomastoid muscles are attached to the first two ribs and sternum; thus, contraction pulls up the anterior rib cage. Any upward force on the anterior rib cage allows the entire rib cage to pivot up and out until its posterior hinge points on the thoracic vertebrae. Muscles that perform this action are accessory muscles of inspiration, and include the diaphragm, external intercostals, scalenes, and sternocleidomastoids. Accessory muscles of expiration pull down on the anterior rib cage and include abdominal muscles and the internal intercostals.

2. D. Diffusion of oxygen across the alveolar capillary membrane is a rapid process in the normal lung, taking approximately 0.25 seconds for oxygen partial pressures to equilibrate on both sides. The transit time of pulmonary blood through capillary beds is about 0.75 seconds at rest, which allows ample time for oxygen diffusion to take place. The equation that governs diffusion of a gas across a membrane is the Fick equation: $v = \{A/T\} \times D \times (Pa - Pc)$, where

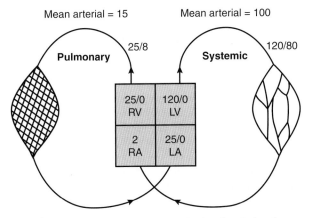

Mean arterial = 15   Mean arterial = 100

• **Figure A-1.** Vascular pressure found in the four heart chambers, and systemic and pulmonary circulation.

A = area, T = thickness, Pa = partial pressure of gas in the alveolus, and Pc = partial pressure of gas in the capillary. D is a diffusion constant proportional to $Sol/(MW)^{1/2}$.

3. D. It is important to have a general idea of vascular pressures and to know the differences between the pulmonary and systemic systems (Fig. A-1). The pulmonary circulation is a low-pressure system. The right ventricle is much smaller than the left ventricle and produces only about 25 mm Hg of pressure during systole. Pulmonary arteries are very thin-walled and do not provide diastolic recoil or much resistance to flow before it reaches the pulmonary capillary beds. The mean pressure in the pulmonary arterial system is about 15 mm Hg and about 12 mm Hg at the origin of the capillary beds. The majority of flow resistance in the pulmonary system occurs at the level of the capillaries, where the pressure drops from 12 to about 8 mm Hg, and the pressure in the left atrium is about 5 mm Hg. In contrast, the left ventricle produces a high pressure (120 mm Hg) during systole. The systemic arterial system consists of thick-walled elastic vessels that recoil during diastole and act to maintain a higher diastolic pressure (80 mm Hg) and a higher overall mean pressure (100 mm Hg). The majority of flow resistance in the systemic vasculature occurs in the small arterioles that contract and expand to regulate flow to certain vascular capillary beds during different physiologic needs. On average, the mean pressure drops from 100 to about 30 mm Hg across these arterioles. Pressure across the systemic capillary beds drops to about 10 mm Hg, and pressure in the systemic venous system drops to about 2 mm Hg by the time blood reaches the right atrium.

4. D. Inspired air pressure is equal to ambient air pressure when there is no flow through the airways. Ambient air pressure at sea level is 760 mm Hg, and thus inspired air pressure is 760 mm Hg during full inspiration. The fraction of air composed of oxygen is 0.21; therefore, the partial pressure of oxygen is 0.21×760 mm Hg, or 160 mm Hg. However, this assumes that inspired air is dry, when in fact it picks up water vapor as it is inhaled through the respiratory airways. Water vapor consists of about 47 mm Hg in inspired air, which means that the total dry gas pressure is about 760 to 47 mm Hg, or 713 mm Hg. The ratio of oxygen to total dry gas remains 0.21, and the partial pressure of inspired oxygen is 0.21×713 mm Hg, or 150 mm Hg. Once inspired air reaches the alveoli, it is further diluted by the presence of CO_2, which is discussed in Case 2-2.

CASE 2-2

1. A. Peripheral chemoreceptors in the carotid bodies respond to decreases in arterial Pa_{O_2}, decreases in pH, and increases in arterial Pa_{CO_2}. Their response to hypoxemia is profound below oxygen tension levels of 70 mm Hg, although smaller responses are present at oxygen levels slightly below normal. Even though the peripheral chemoreceptors respond to changes in pH and Pa_{CO_2}, the central chemoreceptors play a larger role in regulating CO_2 levels.

2. C. At high altitude, hyperventilation is triggered by the peripheral chemoreceptors in the carotid bodies as a response to hypoxemia. In the alveoli, the partial pressure of CO_2 (PA_{CO_2}) is governed by the alveolar ventilation equation: $PA_{CO_2} = V_{CO_2}/V_A \times K$, where V_{CO_2} is the production of CO_2 by peripheral tissues, V_A is alveolar ventilation, and K is a constant. At rest, V_{CO_2} remains constant and PA_{CO_2} is inversely proportional to V_A. Therefore, doubling the respiratory rate decreases the PA_{CO_2} twofold, or from the normal 40 mm Hg to 20 mm Hg. This accommodates a greater alveolar PA_{O_2}, which is important in order to maintain the PA_{O_2} as close to the normal 100 mm Hg as possible.

3. B. The first step to analyzing a blood gas is to look at the pH. If the pH <7.4, then the primary disturbance is acidosis; if the pH >7.4, then the primary disturbance is alkalosis. Next look at the Pa_{CO_2} and $[HCO_3^-]$ to determine whether the process is respiratory or metabolic. If the primary disturbance is acidosis, then $Pa_{CO_2} >40$ means there is a respiratory acidosis (hypoventilation), and an $[HCO_3^-] <24$ means there is a metabolic acidosis (excess organic acid). If the primary disturbance is alkalosis, then $Pa_{CO_2} <40$ means there is a respiratory alkalosis (hyperventilation), and an $[HCO_3^-] >24$ means there is a metabolic alkalosis (loss of organic acid). Once the primary disturbance is determined, the compensatory mechanism can be predicted by the ratio $[HCO_3^-]/[CO_2]$. In this instance, since the pH <7.4 and the $[HCO_3^-] <24$, the primary disturbance is metabolic acidosis. One can therefore predict that the compensation will be a decrease in $[CO_2]$. This is accomplished by hyperventilation, a common presenting symptom in patients with metabolic acidosis. In metabolic acidosis, the Winter equation predicts the level of Pa_{CO_2} when compensation is complete: $Pa_{CO_2} = 1.5 \times HCO_3^- + 8$, or in this case, $1.5 \times (12) + 8 = 26$ mm Hg, which is the measured value for Pa_{CO_2}. This means that the compensatory respiratory alkalosis is complete. A quick rule of thumb for the Winter equation is that the measured Pa_{CO_2} should be equal to the last two digits of the pH for compensatory respiratory alkalosis to be complete (26 in this case).

4. A. Again, the pH <7.4 indicates the primary disturbance is acidosis, and the $Pa_{CO_2} >40$ mm Hg indicates that it is a respiratory acidosis (e.g., effective hypoventilation or CO_2 retention that is typical of COPD). The ratio $[HCO_3^-]/[CO_2]$ dictates that the compensation will be an increase in $[HCO_3^-]$ that takes place at the level of the kidneys. This is a compensatory metabolic alkalosis and it takes at least 2–3 days to occur. Most patients with COPD have chronic respiratory acidosis and are referred to as CO_2 retainers because they have a chronically elevated arterial Pa_{CO_2}. Their compensation is also therefore chronic, meaning that the serum $[HCO_3^-]$ is always elevated. As a rule of thumb, in chronic compensation for respiratory acidosis, the $[HCO_3^-]$ is elevated 2 mEq/L and the pH is decreased by 0.03 for every 10 mm Hg elevation of Pa_{CO_2} above the normal 40 mm Hg. In this patient, the Pa_{CO_2} of 60 mm Hg is 20 mm Hg above the normal value. Expected chronic compensation would be an increase in $[HCO_3^-]$ of 4 mEq/L (or 28 mEq/L) and a decrease in pH of 0.06 (or 7.34). This means that this patient's respiratory acidosis is fully compensated with a metabolic alkalosis.

CASE 2-3

1. A. The Henry law dictates how much of a gas can be dissolved into a liquid depending on the partial pressure imparted on the liquid by the surrounding gas: $C_x = K \times P_x$, where C_x is gas concentration (mL/dL), K is a constant specific to the type of gas, and P_x is the partial pressure of the gas. For oxygen, K is 0.003 mL/dL/mm Hg; therefore, the oxygen concentration of oxygenated blood is $C_x = 0.003 \times 100 = 0.3$ mL/dL. This is only about 1.5% of the total oxygen content of oxygenated blood (about 20 mL/dL). The remaining oxygen is bound to hemoglobin. Keep in mind that partial pressures (referred to as O_2 or CO_2 tension) are often used instead of actual concentrations when describing dissolved gas contents in blood. For example, the oxygen content of pulmonary venous blood is described as 100 mm Hg, meaning that it contains the amount of oxygen (both dissolved and bound to hemoglobin) that an equal volume of blood would if in contact with oxygen at a partial pressure of 100 mm Hg. This number does not correlate with the actual pressure exerted on the fluid, which is only about 5–10 mm Hg in the pulmonary venous system. Similarly, the CO_2 content of mixed venous blood (P_{VCO_2}) is reported as 40 mm Hg, which means that when venous blood comes in contact with the alveolar membranes it will result in an alveolar partial pressure of CO_2 (PA_{CO_2}) of 40 mm Hg.

2. D. As explained in Case 2-1, diffusion across the alveolar membrane is governed by the Fick equation: $v = \{A/T\} \times D \times (Pa - Pc)$, where A = area, T = thickness, Pa = partial pressure of gas in the alveolus, and Pc = partial pressure of gas in the capillary. D is a diffusion constant proportional to $Sol/(MW)^{1/2}$. The solubility of carbon dioxide is about twenty-fold greater than that of oxygen, which accounts for its more rapid diffusion across the alveolar capillary membrane. Carbon dioxide therefore reaches equilibrium much quicker than does oxygen.

3. D. The oxygen tension is the partial pressure of oxygen if the blood were placed in a closed container and allowed to equilibrate. Based on the Henry law, it is proportional to the amount of oxygen dissolved in the blood. Physiologically, the container represents the alveoli, and the partial pressure of oxygen is dictated by the partial pressure of oxygen in inspired air. At higher altitudes the barometric pressure (air pressure, 760 mm Hg at sea level) decreases, yet the ratio of oxygen to total air molecules remains 0.21. Therefore, the partial pressure of oxygen decreases in the alveoli, which translates into a lower oxygen tension in arterial blood. Even though hemoglobin is the primary oxygen carrier in the blood, oxygen tension is independent of hemoglobin; therefore, anemia and CO poisoning have no effect on oxygen tension. They do, however, have a great effect on the oxygen-carrying capacity. Each gram of hemoglobin is capable of carrying 1.39 mL of oxygen. The normal hemoglobin concentration is about 15 g/dL; therefore, the normal carrying capacity of blood is about 20.8 mL/dL assuming a saturation of 100%. Again, compare this with the 0.3 mL/dL oxygen dissolved in blood that was calculated in question 1, Case 2-3. All of the factors listed in this question decrease oxygen delivery to peripheral tissues.

4. C. A shift to the right of the oxygen-hemoglobin dissociation curve occurs in conditions of increased temperature, acidity, P_{CO_2}, and 2,3-DPG; all conditions that exist in exercising muscles. Shifting the curve to the right has the effect of decreasing the size of the plateau and moving the steep portion of the curve toward higher oxygen tensions. Therefore, for a given oxygen tension, the saturation of hemoglobin will be less. This means that hemoglobin binds less avidly to oxygen and off-loading is facilitated. In the pulmonary capillary beds the opposite conditions exist, shifting the curve back to the left and making the plateau larger. This represents the greater avidity of hemoglobin for oxygen in the pulmonary capillaries. CO poisoning causes hemoglobin to adhere strongly to oxygen molecules and prevents off-loading in peripheral tissues. This is represented by an extreme shift to the left of the oxygen-hemoglobin dissociation curve. The normal P_{50} (O_2 tension at which hemoglobin is 50% saturated) is about 27 mm Hg. The P_{50} increases when the curve is shifted to the right. Of note, the oxygen tension of mixed venous blood is about 40 mm Hg, corresponding to about 60% saturation, which is still above the P_{50} level.

CASE 2-4

1. A. Emphysema is the result of alveolar wall destruction and its associated elastic properties. Alveolar wall destruction results in increased dead space where gas exchange cannot occur. Loss of elasticity results in greater lung compliance, or distensibility. This hinders the ability for normal passive exhalation to occur, resulting in increased FRC and RV. Without the normal recoil mechanism, the thoracic cage expands, which increases TLC and results in the characteristic barrel chest. This results in decreased VC.

2. B. In COPD, air trapping occurs mostly at the bases, which results in shunting of ventilation to the apices where little perfusion occurs. This results in a ventilation/perfusion mismatch, which has a deleterious effect on gas exchange. The lung tissue is more "relaxed" at the bases due to the settling effect of gravity. This increased compliance at the bases, along with the loss of alveolar integrity, causes respiratory bronchioles to collapse when intrathoracic pressure is applied during exhalation.

3. C. Respiratory acidosis is the result of poor alveolar ventilation, which causes the inadequate elimination of carbon dioxide. It is the characteristic metabolic disorder in those who have lost their respiratory drive due to CNS lesions, sedative overdose, or muscular disorders (e.g., kyphoscoliosis, rib fractures). It is also the primary metabolic disorder seen in obstructive lung disease. Acute CO_2 retention results in an increase in PA_{CO_2} and a decrease in pH. As a rule of thumb, the pH decreases by 0.08 for every increase of 10 mm Hg in PA_{CO_2}. Over the course of several days, renal compensation occurs with retention of HCO_3^- and an increase in the pH. However, the pH will not fully return to 7.40 until serum PA_{CO_2} has normalized. The rule of thumb for chronic CO_2 retention is that for every 10 mm Hg increase in PA_{CO_2} over 40, the pH will be decreased by 0.03 and the $[HCO_3^-]$ increased by 4 mEq.

4. B. Increasing lung volume results in stretching of alveoli and interstitial elastin, causing greater stiffness and recoil; therefore, compliance diminishes as lung volume increases. As mentioned previously, lung volumes are increased in those with COPD, which means that they function at a point on the pressure-volume curve where compliance is significantly lower. Thus, more work is required to generate a sufficient amount of negative intrapleural pressure to draw in the same volume of air.

CASE 2-5

1. D. This patient presents with symptoms and signs of classical pneumonia, which is typically caused by bacterial pathogens such as *S. pneumoniae*, *H. influenzae*, *M. catarrhalis*, or *S. aureus*. *M. pneumoniae* is the most common causative organism for atypical pneumonia in young, healthy adults.

2. C. The illness described is *Legionella* pneumonia, caused by the organism *L. pneumophila*. This organism is ubiquitous in moist environments. Outbreaks have been linked to a variety of sources, including cooling towers, air conditioning systems, whirlpools, respiratory nebulizers, and other man-made water-containing units. *Legionella* is thought to consist of 10% of both community- and hospital-acquired pneumonias. *Legionella* pneumonia is usually preceded by a prodrome of malaise, headache, myalgia, and weakness. Later, the onset of high fevers and rigors is not uncommon. Patients usually have a nonproductive cough and may have pleuritic chest pain. The radiographic findings include a patchy, diffuse infiltrate, but they may also include focal consolidation. GI symptoms are a hallmark of *Legionella* infection and include diarrhea, vomiting, and abdominal pain. Relative bradycardia is also common. The treatment of choice for *Legionella* is erythromycin, a macrolide. Other macrolides (e.g., azithromycin, clarithromycin), sulfamethoxazole/trimethoprim (Bactrim), and fluoroquinolones are effective as well.

3. A. This patient most likely has *M. pneumonia*, which is the most common bacterial atypical pneumonia. Other likely etiologies for a young healthy patient would be *C. pneumoniae* or a viral pneumonia. First-line treatment would be a macrolide (e.g., azithromycin, clarithromycin, erythromycin). A fluoroquinolone is a good alternative. Amoxicillin/clavulanate and cephalosporins are not active against *Mycoplasma* because of its lack of a true cell wall.

4. B. This patient presents with a syndrome typical for *P. carinii* pneumonia. Common presenting symptoms include fever, dyspnea, and nonproductive cough. Physical exam usually reveals tachypnea, tachycardia, hypoxia, and ill appearance. Pulmonary exam is often unrevealing. The chest x-ray findings show bilateral, diffuse, interstitial infiltrates that tend to be perihilar. Lab abnormalities often include an elevated serum LDH, which likely reflects parenchymal lung damage. The two mainstays of therapy for *Pneumocystis* include trimethoprim-sulfamethoxazole and pentamidine, both of which are administered intravenously. Other drugs used include dapsone, clindamycin, and primaquine. Studies have shown that administration of glucocorticoids is beneficial for patients with a Pa_{O_2} <70 mm Hg or an A-a gradient >35 mm Hg. *Pneumocystis* prophylaxis is indicated for AIDS patients with a CD4 count <200 because these patients are at high risk for contracting *Pneumocystis*. Prophylaxis consists of either trimethoprim-sulfamethoxazole one double-strength tablet daily or aerosolized pentamidine administered in an inhaler.

CASE 2-6

1. D. Primary infection with TB occurs by inhaling bacilli into the lungs where these are phagocytized by alveolar macrophages and carried to regional lymph nodes. During the first few weeks after primary infection, the bacilli replicate locally and T cell-mediated cellular immunity develops. Lymphocytes and monocytes migrate to the area of infection and form histiocytic cells that organize into a granuloma. These granulomas most often contain the infection and eventually become calcified. TB bacilli remain viable within macrophages in the granuloma for years and often never reactivate. Primary infection is usually asymptomatic; however, a small percentage of patients develop active TB after primary infection. Once infected, patients develop lifelong immunity to re-infection as is manifested by a positive response to PPD antigen. Patients with primary infection are not contagious as long as the infection is contained within a granuloma.

2. C. Secondary TB, or reactivation TB, usually occurs many years after the primary infection. Reactivation is more prevalent in the elderly, the debilitated, and the immunocompromised. It occurs when contained bacilli begin to multiply and proliferate. As pulmonary lesions progress, they necrotize and become caseating granulomas. These can necrotize into adjacent bronchi and become cavitary lesions. Secondary TB can also manifest as lobar infiltrates. It is during this phase that patients are contagious. The PPD typically remains *positive* during secondary TB. Anergy, or a false-negative PPD test, often occurs in end-stage AIDS and in miliary TB, which is a widespread hematogenous spread of bacilli.

3. B. The size of the PPD reaction considered positive depends on the likelihood of disease in that particular patient. This is done because there is some degree of cross-reactivity with other antigens and subsequent false-positive reactions in some patients. Therefore, the threshold of positivity is set higher for patients with relatively low risk to avoid overtreating false-positive reactions. For immunocompromised patients, any reaction is considered positive because of the high prevalence of anergy. Persons who are exposed to active TB are considered positive with reactions of 5 mm or greater. For individuals at elevated risk for TB (e.g., homeless, urban dwellers, highly endemic region), reactions of 10 mm or greater are considered positive.

4. A. The most common side effect of treatment for TB is hepatitis. Isoniazid, rifampin, and pyrazinamide can all cause hepatitis. Isoniazid is also known to cause peripheral neuropathy. Rifampin causes orange urine and flu-like symptoms; it can also cause thrombocytopenia. Pyrazinamide can cause hyperuricemia. Patients who are started on isoniazid or rifampin must have liver function tests done at 2 weeks and followed up every several months thereafter.

CASE 2-7

1. A. Squamous cell carcinoma, which accounts for about 40% of bronchogenic carcinomas, tends to occur more centrally. It is locally invasive and has a tendency to cavitate into surrounding bronchi, which leads to hemoptysis. Massive hemoptysis results from tumor invasion through the wall of a bronchiolar vessel. Because of its undifferentiated and invasive nature, large cell carcinoma also tends to cavitate; however, the tumors tend to be more peripherally located and thus hemoptysis is less common. Adenocarcinoma is also a peripheral tumor with less likelihood to cavitate. Small cell carcinoma is centrally located but not locally invasive and does not cavitate. It does, however, metastasize rapidly by hematogenous spread.

2. B. Adenocarcinoma, which also accounts for about 40% of bronchogenic carcinomas, has a variation referred to as *bronchioloalveolar* carcinoma because of its more diffuse involvement of bronchioles and alveoli. This type of carcinoma can appear on chest x-ray as diffuse, peripheral, multinodular, or fluffy infiltrates. Diagnosis is usually made via cytologic exam of bronchoalveolar lavage fluid. Adenocarcinoma and squamous cell carcinoma metastasize more slowly than do large or small cell carcinomas; therefore, lesions are often amenable to surgical resection. The 5-year survival rate for solitary tumors less than 4 cm in diameter is 40% and 30% for squamous cell carcinoma and adenocarcinoma, respectively. In general, adenocarcinoma tends to be more common in women and in nonsmokers. About 90% of patients who develop bronchogenic carcinoma have a strong history of tobacco use. Tobacco is very strongly associated with both squamous cell and small cell carcinoma.

3. C. This patient likely has a postobstructive pneumonia as a result of a bronchial tumor. This must be suspected in patients with pneumonia that does not resolve with appropriate therapy, especially in elderly patients with risk factors for bronchogenic carcinoma. In some hospitals, the next step in the work-up for this patient would be further imaging of the chest in an attempt to identify an obstructing mass and to identify mediastinal metastases. CT scan is the quickest and most cost-effective imaging study that will provide enough detail regarding pulmonary parenchyma and mediastinal structures. Whether or not a mass is identified by CT scan, this patient would likely undergo bronchoscopy to directly visualize the bronchi and obtain washings for culture and cytology. This test has the highest likelihood of arriving at a specific diagnosis.

4. E. Bronchogenic carcinoma can lead to a number of physical exam findings that are related to both tumor invasion of local thoracic structures and systemic neuroendocrine effects of factors released by the tumor. Eyelid drooping is one feature of Horner syndrome (ptosis, myosis, anhydrosis) that can occur as result of tumor invasion of the cervical sympathetic chain that originates anterior to the thoracic vertebrae in the posterior mediastinum. Hoarseness can result from invasion of the recurrent laryngeal nerve near the lung apices. Facial swelling can be the result of superior vena cava syndrome, which is caused most frequently by small cell carcinomas that obstruct the thoracic outlet and compress the superior vena cava. This results in decreased venous return from the head and upper extremities. Leg swelling is an indication of a lower extremity deep venous thrombosis, which occurs frequently in patients with cancer. The specific etiology of cancer-related hypercoagulability is not understood, although it is thought to be an alteration of normal clotting factor function.

PART III: RENAL

CASE 3-1

1 D. $C_1V_1 = C_2V_2$; so $250 * 500 = 25 * X$; so $X = 5000$. Plasma volumes may be calculated under experimental conditions but are not used clinically.

2. A. Our patient is suffering from iso-osmotic volume contraction, and 0.9% saline is the replacement fluid of choice to rapidly replete the intravascular volume and restore his BP. Over time, the water infused into the intravascular space also distributes to the interstitial space and more fluids may be needed. The 0.45%

saline, a hypotonic fluid (as compared with plasma), more rapidly distributes from the vascular space to the interstitial space, making it a poor choice for fluid resuscitation. A 5% dextrose solution is the equivalent of giving water only, since dextrose readily diffuses into cells and is thus unable to exert any osmotic activity in the intravascular space. The 3% saline is used almost exclusively to correct life-threatening hyponatremia and is rarely used for volume contraction. Oral chicken soup with its high salt concentration is not a bad choice for fluid replacement in a volume-contracted patient. Oral replacement fluid is not appropriate in patients unable to tolerate oral intake or in patients with orthostatic hypotension. **Orthostatic hypotension,** also called postural hypotension, is an increase in pulse of 20 beats per minute and/or a drop in BP of 20 mm Hg upon assuming an erect position. Our patient's complaint of dizziness stems from the drop in his BP and decreased perfusion to his brain upon standing.

CASE 3-2

1. B. The patient has had a rapid onset of hyponatremia and is symptomatic. Care must be taken not to "volume overload" the patient. The patient's sodium deficit can be calculated as follows:

$$Na^+ \text{ deficit} = (TBW)(Na^+ \text{ desired} - Na^+ \text{ measured})$$
$$Na^+ \text{ deficit} = (0.60 \times 70 \text{ kg})(130 \text{ mEq/L} - 122 \text{ mEq/L})$$
$$= (42 \text{ L} \times 8 \text{ mEq/L})$$
$$Na^+ \text{ deficit} = 336 \text{ mEq}$$

The volume of 3% saline required to replace 336 mEq of sodium can be calculated as follows:

$$\text{Volume of 3\% saline} = 336 \text{ mEq/513 mEq/L}$$
$$= 0.650 \text{ L} = 650 \text{ mL}$$

The rate of sodium correction is 0.5 mEq/L/h; 8 mEq/L should be replaced over 16 hours.

2. B. DI is the best choice given the clinical setting and the abrupt onset of polyuria, which is characteristic of central DI. The differential diagnosis for polyuria includes four of the five choices: DI, postobstructive diuresis, osmotic diuresis due to hyperglycemia, and inadvertent administration of diuretics. SIADH does not present with polyuria. Both DI and SIADH can occur, although not commonly, after subarachnoid hemorrhage.

3. E. SIADH presents with variable degrees of hyponatremia, and most patients are asymptomatic. A search for the cause of SIADH must be carried out. A mild weight gain is characteristic of mild water retention. Hyponatremia and weight gain could be characteristic of hypothyroidism, not hyperthyroidism, and must be ruled out as a cause of hyponatremia. Both advanced hyperglycemia and hyperlipidemia cause factitious hyponatremia, but there is no information to support those diagnoses. Surreptitious use of diuretics must be considered, but in light of a normal serum potassium, SIADH is the best answer.

CASE 3-3

1. E. We treat hyperkalemia by antagonizing the effects of potassium, increasing the movement of potassium into cells, and removing excess potassium. Our patient was given calcium chloride intravenously to antagonize the effects of potassium at the cardiac conduction system. Calcium is cardioprotective but does not change the serum potassium concentration. IV insulin preceded by IV glucose helps to shift potassium into the cells as does sodium bicarbonate. We also use β_2-agonists such as albuterol (a catecholamine agonist) to this effect. Sodium polystyrene sulfonate, not used in the urgent setting as it is slow acting, is an ion exchange resin that acts in the GI lumen to absorb potassium in exchange for sodium, thereby removing potassium from the body. Dialysis is the proper treatment for this patient's severe hyperkalemia.

2. B. Loop diuretics cause an increased flow of sodium and water to the distal nephron and cause potassium loss by disrupting the normal mechanisms for potassium balance. Increased sodium delivery to the distal tubules increases the action of the Na^+/K^+ exchange pump there, increasing potassium loss in the urine. Aldosterone acts on the cortical collecting tubule to increase potassium secretion, and an excess, not a deficiency, of aldosterone would cause hypokalemia. Spironolactone is a potassium-sparing diuretic that can cause hyperkalemia. Metabolic alkalosis is associated with a shift of potassium into the cells and a lowered serum potassium. Hyperthyroidism does not affect serum potassium levels. Dietary deficiency is the most common cause for a decreased serum potassium. The ability of the kidney to conserve potassium is limited by the obligatory excretion of approximately 10 mEq/L in the urine even in the presence of hypokalemia.

3. E. All of the above ECG changes happen with hyperkalemia, and in general occur in the order listed. The final ECG in hyperkalemia looks like a sine wave. The increased serum potassium causes changes in the cardiac conduction system and can lead to supraventricular tachycardia, sinus arrest, AV dissociation, ventricular fibrillation, and cardiac arrest.

CASE 3-4

1. C. Metabolic acidosis is one of the hallmarks of long-standing renal disease due to the accumulation of organic acids. This patient's renal disease is likely a result of hypertension and type 2 diabetes. He has a mild metabolic gap acidosis of 14. His elevated potassium is also likely caused by his renal insufficiency. **Hypertension** alone cannot cause decreased bicarbonate. **Diabetic ketoacidosis** is an emergent medical condition and often presents with a larger anion gap acidosis, obtundation, vomiting, and abdominal pain. **Diarrhea** causes a loss of bicarbonate and is a cause of a non-gap or hyperchloremic acidosis. COPD causes a respiratory acidosis secondary to retained CO_2 and is usually accompanied by elevated serum bicarbonate as metabolic or renal compensation for a respiratory acidosis.

2. C. Hyperventilation is the appropriate response to a metabolic acidosis, allowing rapid diffusion of the volatile acid CO_2. Hyperventilation secondary to acidosis is often termed Kussmaul breathing, and is characterized by deep breaths. It is a prominent clinical sign of an acidemic patient. Severe acidosis may result in depression of cardiac contractility, hyperkalemia, and altered mental status. We can see from the blood gas that our patient is not **hypoxic**. **Diarrhea** causes a loss of bicarbonate and a hyperchloremic acidosis rather than an anion gap acidosis. **Vomiting** causes a metabolic alkalosis due to a loss of hydrochloric acid from the stomach. COPD results in retention of carbon dioxide and compensatory elevation of bicarbonate by the kidney.

3. C. Acetylsalicylic acid, more commonly known as aspirin, causes a metabolic acidosis (decreased bicarbonate) due to ingestion of the acid and increased production or decreased removal of lactate by the liver. A concomitant respiratory alkalosis occurs due to direct stimulation of central respiratory centers, leading to hyperventilation and the "blowing off" of the volatile acid CO_2. Acute ingestion leads to nausea, vomiting, tachycardia, and tinnitus, and may result in coma, cardiovascular shock, and death.

4. D. Vomiting results in a loss of potassium and hydrochloric acid from the stomach. Surreptitious diuretic use for weight loss can also deplete chloride; as a result, sodium must be reabsorbed with bicarbonate instead of chloride, causing alkalosis. The dehydrated alkalemic patient suffers from a (volume) "contraction" alkalosis. Consumption of antacids such as *calcium carbonate* with milk is a cause of milk alkali syndrome, but would not explain our patient's physical findings or hypokalemia. Milk alkali syndrome was seen more frequently when calcium-based antacids were used to treat PUD; alkalosis and hypercalcemia occurred in those patients with underlying renal insufficiency. *Renal failure* commonly causes acidosis, not alkalosis. **Polydipsia** can cause mild hyponatremia but would not cause alkalosis.

CASE 3-5

1. C. Hyperparathyroidism is the most common cause of hypercalcemia due to an overgrowth of a single parathyroid gland, an adenoma. It is more common in women than in men. In addition to hypercalcemia, an important clue to an excess of PTH is the low serum phosphorus level due to the increased renal excretion of phosphorus. Long-standing renal insufficiency is more apt to cause hypocalcemia and hyperphosphatemia. Familial hypocalciuric hypercalcemia is a rare autosomal dominant disease due to decreased urinary excretion of calcium. Diagnosis is confirmed by low levels of urinary calcium and corroborated with a family history of hypercalcemia. Pseudohypoparathyroidism is an inherited disorder of end organ resistance to PTH, resulting in elevated levels of PTH, hypocalcemia, and hyperphosphatemia. It is a component of Albright hereditary osteodystrophy, and patients usually have somatic features, which include short stature, round face, short metacarpals and metatarsals, obesity, mental retardation, and basal ganglia calcifications. Excessive vitamin D results in elevated serum calcium and phosphorus due to increased absorption from the gut.

2. D. Chronic renal insufficiency that occurs with long-standing hypertension is characterized by small, scarred kidneys. With decreased nephron mass, less tissue is available for the hydroxylation of vitamin D and hypocalcemia results. A decreased GFR also occurs in long-standing renal disease, and as a result hyperphosphatemia is likely to be present. Other abnormalities such as hyperkalemia, acidosis, and anemia are also characteristic of kidney failure. Neither ACEIs nor beta-blockers have significant effects on renal excretion of phosphate or calcium.

3. B. This question is intended to remind us of what happens to serum-ionized calcium levels in the presence of alkalemia. Our anxious medical student hyperventilated, inducing a respiratory alkalosis, leading to an increase of calcium bound to protein and ionized hypocalcemia. As discussed above, hypocalcemia may cause acral and perioral paresthesias. Both metabolic and respiratory alkalosis cause an increased binding of calcium to protein, and in the presence of low serum calcium may lower the threshold for tetany. Acidosis causes a decreased binding of calcium to protein and increased levels of ionized serum calcium. Long-standing acidosis leeches calcium from bone and may contribute to renal osteodystrophy.

CASE 3-6

1. E. ACEIs reversibly inhibit the conversion of angiotensin I to angiotensin II, a potent vasoconstrictor. Inhibiting systemic vaso-constriction results in vasodilatation and lowering of BP. Reduced levels of aldosterone, causing less sodium and water reabsorption, also aid in reducing BP. Angiotensin II aids in maintaining the GFR by causing vasoconstriction of the efferent arteriole. The loss of this mechanism may precipitate a usually reversible renal failure, especially in those with impaired renal function at baseline. There is often a mild rise in serum creatinine upon institution of ACEIs, even in those with normal renal function. They may also result in hyperkalemia due to the decrease in aldosterone. Hyperkalemia occurs in approximately 5% of patients started on ACEIs, so serum levels of potassium must be monitored. There is a risk of hypotension with any antihypertensive medication. Angioedema is a common allergic reaction with any ACEI. A persistent dry cough is also a side effect of this class of drugs (the "captopril cough").

2. C. Causes of secondary hypertension are important to detect, as many are treatable. Our patient has many of the physical signs of long-standing hypertension, plus a carotid bruit indicative of fibromuscular dysplasia. Her young age, severe hypertension, and lack of family history should lead us to investigate causes of secondary hypertension. Hyperaldosteronism usually is due to an adrenal adenoma and leads to hypertension and hypokalemia. Cushing syndrome is due to adrenal hyperplasia causing an excess of glucocorticoids and hormones that, like aldosterone, may have mineralocorticoid activity (aldosterone levels are usually normal). Findings associated with Cushing syndrome include centripetal obesity, moon face and buffalo hump, peripheral muscle wasting, striae, and hypokalemia. Pheochromocytoma is usually an adrenal tumor but can be found extra-adrenally and presents with episodic hypertension, palpitations, diaphoresis, and throbbing headaches. Atherosclerosis in a 29-year-old patient is unlikely. Drugs such as birth control pills, cocaine, and amphetamines may also cause hypertension.

3. E. Patients with inadequately controlled BP are at risk for renal failure, retinopathy, left ventricular failure, and stroke. Long-standing hypertension increases the rate of decline in GFR. Eventually, glomerular damage leads to proteinuria and microscopic hematuria. This process is retarded by ACEIs. Retinal changes can be seen early in hypertensive disease. On the fundal exam, one sees progressive narrowing of retinal arteries, retinal hemorrhages, and exudates, which can obscure vision, and nicking of the retinal veins by fibrotic retinal arteries that impede retinal venous flow. Increased systemic BP increases afterload on the heart, leading to left ventricular hypertrophy and, eventually, ventricular dilation and CHF. Hypertension is the main risk factor predisposing to stroke. Elevations in systolic BP correlate well with increased risk of stroke, and even small reductions in BP can diminish that risk.

CASE 3-7

1. E. IgA nephropathy (Berger disease) is the most common form of acute GN worldwide, especially in Asia. It is most commonly seen in children, with boys outnumbering girls two to three times.

It presents with gross hematuria 2–3 days after pharyngitis or a GI infection. Fifty percent progress to renal insufficiency. **Poststreptococcal GN** is also postinfectious, but presents 10 days to 2 weeks after streptococcal pharyngitis or skin infection and is associated with elevated ASO titers and IgG deposition. **Henoch-Schönlein purpura** is indistinguishable from IgA nephropathy on microscopy and immunofluorescence but is associated with palpable purpura, arthralgias, and abdominal pain. **Alport syndrome** is an X-linked mutation in the collagen IV gene that is associated with nerve deafness and eye problems. **Benign familial hematuria (thin basement membrane disease)** also results from hereditary defects in type IV collagen but is asymptomatic, requires no treatment, and has no serious sequelae.

2. D. This patient has **Goodpasture syndrome,** in which circulating autoantibodies bind to the NC1 domain of the α3-chain of type IV collagen ("Goodpasture antigen"), a normal component of the GBM. Since the GBM is a linear structure, the IgG autoantibodies form a linear pattern on IF. The lung endothelium also contains the same locus on type IV collagen. The binding of Ab to Ag starts the complement cascade leading to endothelial injury and hemoptysis and hematuria. (A) is not correct, as there are no circulating antigens in Goodpasture. (B) is not correct because there is no mutation present. (C) is not correct because there are no exogenous antigens and antibodies tend not to be stationary. (E) is not correct because the pathophysiology is understood (at least in part).

3. B. **Churg-Strauss,** like Wegener granulomatosis, is a small vessel vasculitis that often affects the renal vasculature. Both involve hematuria presenting in the context of systemic involvement. However, Churg-Strauss tends to occur in patients with a history of asthma or atopy (thus the connection with eosinophilic infiltration), whereas **Wegener granulomatosis** is more commonly diagnosed in patients with upper respiratory (especially sinus) involvement. **Amyloidosis** also has systemic involvement but presents with nephrotic syndrome and Congo red staining of the mesangium due to light chains deposition. **Minimal change disease** and **thin basement membrane disease** also have no deposits seen on IF, but the former presents with nephrotic syndrome in *children* and the latter is a familial nephritic disease with no symptoms or sequelae.

4. B. **Alport syndrome** is classically described as an X-linked dominant mutation in components of type IV collagen (though there are other non–X-linked variants). It is associated with sensorineural hearing loss and abnormalities in the shape of the ocular lens. Hematuria can progress to serious nephritis and can cause renal failure in adolescence or young adulthood. None of the other syndromes are X-linked or associated with hearing or eye problems. **Goodpasture syndrome** is also seen in young men, but is associated with hemoptysis. **Berger syndrome (IgA nephropathy)** has IgA deposits in the mesangium. **Type IV lupus GN** is found more often in women and has IgG in a "wire-loop" pattern on IF. **Type I membranoproliferative GN** is also characterized by a split GBM on EM, giving the characteristic "train track" appearance, but it presents with nephrotic syndrome.

CASE 3-8

1. B. **FSGS** and **minimal change disease** are both nephrotic syndromes characterized by normal findings on LM and no immunoglobulin deposition on IF. The only way to confirm these diagnoses is by visualizing effacement of foot processes on EM. As this requires an invasive renal biopsy, this is rarely done in practice. In this case, FSGS would be the more likely diagnosis for this older patient with multiple comorbidities, since minimal change disease is seen primarily in children 2–6 years old. **Membranous GN** demonstrates mesangial proliferation on LM and significant IF findings, and thus does not require EM for definitive diagnosis, although splitting of the GBM is seen on EM. **Lupus GN** and **diabetic nephropathy** also present with nephrotic syndrome, but are seen in the context of a systemic illness and have significant LM and IF findings (wire-loop and Kimmelstiel-Wilson nodules, respectively).

2. E. Renal biopsy of a patient with **amyloidosis** will reveal deposits that stain Congo red under normal LM and show apple green birefringence with polarized LM. **Lesch-Nyhan syndrome** is a rare genetic syndrome characterized by spastic behavior, self-mutilation, and mental retardation. It results from a deficiency of the enzyme that catalyzes the central reaction in purines metabolism, resulting in hyperuricemia. This causes strongly birefringent uric acid crystals to precipitate, leading to uric acid kidney stones. **Diabetes mellitus** and **systemic lupus erythematosus** can lead to renal failure and nephrotic syndrome, but they have very different microscopic findings. *Diabetes insipidus* creates a water diuresis due to insensitivity to or inadequate production of antidiuretic hormone/vasopressin and does not lead to nephrotic syndrome.

CASE 3-9

1. D. Although the correct answer is <1%, FE_{Na^+} is useful only in oliguric patients. The calculation is as follows:

$$FE_{Na^+}\,[\%] = \frac{U_{Na^+}/P_{Na^+}}{U_{Cr}/P_{Cr}} \times 100$$
$$= \frac{5/140 \times 100}{25/3.5}$$
$$= 0.5\%$$

2. C. This patient's age and sex makes BPH likely, and BPH leads to postrenal obstructive failure. Kidney **stones** do cause postrenal failure; however, they are usually very painful, and one might expect an elevated BP or tachycardia. In patients with both kidneys, stones cause ARF only if they are lodged in the urethra or the bladder-urethral junction, not in one of two ureters. **Diabetes mellitus** is common in this age group, but most often leads to chronic renal insufficiency rather than ARF. **Sepsis** is a common cause of prerenal ARF in elderly men, but this patient has no other signs or symptoms of systemic illness. **Goodpasture syndrome** is a vasculitis that can cause GN and intrinsic ARF, but occurs in young men with hemoptysis.

PART IV: GASTROINTESTINAL

CASE 4-1

1. B. GERD develops when acidic gastric contents splash into the distal portion of the esophagus, irritating the tissues. It is true that GERD can be associated with LES atrophy and scleroderma, but the LES would be open in GERD, whereas in achalasia it would be closed. Remember, the question asks which is *less likely* to occur with achalasia. In achalasia, the LES does not relax and has increased resting tone resulting in diminution of the possibility of

developing GERD. Scleroderma is associated with achalasia. Answer choices (C), (D), and (E) may or may not occur in this patient, but are unrelated to the increased resting tone often observed in achalasia.

2. C. Hirschsprung (congenital megacolon) and achalasia both lack ganglion cells. In achalasia the cells are missing from the myenteric plexus; in Hirschsprung they are missing from the Meissner and myenteric plexus. In both instances, patients have dilation of the respective portion of the GI tract: the colon in Hirschsprung (resulting in loss of bowel function and inability to pass stool) and the esophagus in achalasia. Collagen vascular disease and squamous cell carcinoma rates are increased in patients with achalasia.

3. A. Answers (B), (C), (D), and (E) are all possible sequelae of achalasia. Collagen vascular disease is associated with achalasia but does not result from the disorder.

4. C. Congenital megacolon is not a component of CREST syndrome, which is characterized by *c*alcinosis, *R*aynaud phenomenon, *e*sophageal dysfunction, *s*clerodactyly, and *t*elangiectasia.

CASE 4-2

1. C. Cimetidine, although effective, has various side effects listed in the question stem as well as gynecomastia, which is an enlargement of the breast tissue in the male, or other anti-androgenic effects. Stevens-Johnson syndrome (skin rash, fever, and multiple lesions of the oral conjunctival and vaginal mucous membranes) is often caused by sulfa-based drugs or ethosuximide. Agranulocytosis is a reaction to the antipsychotic clozapine or the antiepileptic carbamazepine. Microcytic anemia is a type of anemia with a low MCV. Depression is an adverse effect of some beta$_2$-blockers like propranolol.

2. B. NSAIDs are theorized to promote ulceration formation by suppression of mucosal prostaglandins. Ischemia may also impair mucosal defense; however, this is common in the setting of hypovolemic shock. Answers (C) and (D) are theorized as mechanisms for ulceration of the carcinoid tumor Zollinger-Ellison syndrome or other conditions of hyperacidity. Increased gastric emptying occurs in dumping syndrome.

3. E. Gastric ulcers and chronic gastritis increase the patient's risk of gastric carcinoma. Duodenal ulceration is not known to increase a patient's risk of duodenal carcinoma. Answers (A), (B), and (D) are not known complications of ulcers.

4. D. This patient has evidence of gastric ulcer perforation as indicated by the free air shown in the KUB. Commonly, performed ulcers are repaired with an omental patch (Graham patch). This patient is not a candidate for outpatient pharmacologic management (answers B and C). Barium swallow is contraindicated in a patient with a perforated ulcer. Admission with serial abdominal exams is employed in a patient with an acute (surgical) abdomen of unknown etiology but does not offer definitive treatment in this patient.

CASE 4-3

1. D. A deficiency of vitamin K results in a prolonged PT and aPTT that can result in increased bleeding (anticoagulation). Vitamin A deficiency causes night blindness and dermatitis, whereas an excess may result in the listed symptoms. Vitamin D deficiency leads to rickets in children and osteopenia in adults, whereas excess results in elevated calcium levels and anorexia. Vitamin E deficiency causes increased fragility of erythrocytes, not dermatitis. Finally, folic acid deficiency leads to anemia but it is a water-soluble vitamin, not a fat-soluble one.

2. A. This patient exhibits several physical signs of not absorbing enough vitamin K and is consequently bleeding. A PT and aPTT should be checked and vitamin K should be administered in an IM injection. Small intestinal biopsy is important in making the diagnosis of celiac sprue and in determining if a gluten-free diet will be effective. Because this patient is not adhering to her diet, a biopsy would not yield additional information. Likewise, a stool specimen for fecal fat is commonly used to make an initial diagnosis but not to guide treatment. Screening other family members is warranted because there is an increased familial incidence.

CASE 4-4

1. E. In alcoholic liver hepatitis, you would expect an increase in AST and ALT, but usually the AST is approximately twice as high. The conjugated bilirubin is usually increased by 50% of the total.

2. C. Palmar erythema, gynecomastia, skin telangiectasias, and hypogonadism result from the altered metabolism of estrogens and resultant hyperestrinism. Patients with alcoholic cirrhosis have coagulopathy secondary to poor production of clotting factors. Hematemesis and hemorrhoids are a result of increased pressure in the portal venous system.

CASE 4-5

1. D. Rotor and Dubin-Johnson are both types of conjugated hyperbilirubinemias. The defect in Dubin-Johnson is in the bile canalicular membrane, affecting transport of the conjugated bilirubin. Rotor, also a type of conjugated jaundice, is differentiated from Dubin-Johnson pathologically in that it has no black pigment in the liver. Gilbert, ABO incompatibility, Crigler-Najjar, breast milk, and physiologic jaundice are all unconjugated types. Severe hemolytic disease and Crigler-Najjar type I often cause kernicterus.

2. E. Reviewing the production and breakdown of bilirubin is the key to answering this question correctly. An excess of heme resulting in too much bilirubin, decreased hepatic uptake of bilirubin, and decreased conjugation all give predominantly unconjugated bilirubinemia. If the conjugated bilirubin is not excreted or bile flow is decreased secondary to obstruction, then a conjugated hyperbilirubinemia exists.

3. B. In Crigler-Najjar type I, the gene that codes for the enzyme—UDP glucuronyl transferase—is absent, which results in an unconjugated hyperbilirubinemia. Gilbert also gives an unconjugated hyperbilirubinemia secondary to decrease bilirubin UGT. Dubin-Johnson syndrome is an autosomal recessive disorder of conjugated hyperbilirubinemia with a canalicular membrane defect that results in a pigmented liver. Rotor is a conjugated type with defective uptake by the hepatocyte.

CASE 4-6

1. A. Risk factors for stone formation are decreased bile acids or bile salts with or without increased cholesterol solubilized in bile. Simply stated, solubilizing bile acids and lecithin are overwhelmed by an increase in the levels of cholesterol. The stone itself is not enough to cause disease because over 80% of gallstones do not cause pain or other complications. In approximately 90% of cases, acute cholecystitis is precipitated by an obstruction of the gallbladder neck or proximal cystic duct. Bacterial infection may follow these events; however, it is not an inciting event. Enzyme degradation and schistosomes are not known to cause cholecystitis.

2. C. Both (C) and (E) are correct but (C) is the current treatment of choice. The extended spectrum penicillins cover relevant bacteria; also, third-generation cephalosporins plus metronidazole or clindamycin kill the anaerobe (*Clostridium* and *Bacteroides*).

3. D. The likely diagnosis based on the information provided is gallstone ileus. Rarely can a large stone erode through the wall of the gallbladder and into an adjacent loop of small intestine. Please see Key Points in Case 4-6 for differentiation of acute cholecystitis and gallstone pancreatitis. Ascending cholangitis is an infection of the bile ducts secondary to obstruction and is characterized by fever, RUQ pain, jaundice, shock, and neurologic symptoms known as Reynold pentad. Cystic fibrosis is an autosomal recessive disorder characterized by respiratory, pancreatic, and urogenital disease.

4. B. Unlike the rest of the GI tract, the gallbladder does not contain a submucosal or muscularis mucosa. It does contain the other layers listed in this question's choices.

CASE 4-7

1. B. All of the listed illnesses are in the differential diagnosis, and laboratory evaluation is necessary to prioritize this list. PID is likely based on the patient's risk factors—3 days of pain, nausea, vomiting, multiple sexual partners—and physical exam. Although an ectopic pregnancy is also possible, it is unlikely based on her last period. A urine or blood pregnancy test would help. Gastroenteritis is usually a diagnosis of exclusion. This patient denies urinary symptoms and has normal bowel movements, thus renal stones or Crohn disease is unlikely.

2. E. Diverticulitis and acute appendicitis are similar in that they both involve obstruction, often by a fecalith. Lymphoid hyperplasia as an obstructive source for appendicitis is a factor only in adolescents and young adults. The Western diet is proposed as the reason for diverticula to form and it is due to *decreased* not increased fiber in the diet. Bacterial invasion takes part in both appendicitis and diverticulitis; however, this is secondary, not primary.

CASE 4-8

1. D. Pseudopolyps are a common finding in areas where the mucosa is regenerating and bulges. This is uncommon in Crohn disease. However, skip lesions, transmural involvement of the bowel wall, entire alimentary tract involvement, and fistula formation are common features or complications of Crohn disease.

2. A. Patients with Crohn disease are at risk for general or specific malabsorption, including protein-losing enteropathy (low albumin) as well as electrolyte abnormalities. Low calcium levels result in tetany, whereas decreased absorption of vitamin D results in osteopenia. A low hematocrit and microcytosis results from iron deficiency anemia, among other sequelae. This question describes a pernicious anemia of malabsorption that is so severe that the patient has neurologic sequelae, namely, a B12 deficiency.

3. C. Toxic megacolon is more common in patients who suffer from UC secondary to chronic cases of active disease that heal and attenuate the bowel wall, leading to a thinned and weakened structure. The other choices—fistulas, aphthous ulcers, granulomas, and malabsorption—are characteristics or complications of Crohn disease.

PART V: HEMATOLOGY

CASE 5-1

1. C. Blood loss is the most common cause of iron deficiency anemia. The GI tract is the most common source of blood loss for men and postmenopausal women. Malignancy, ulcers, gastritis, hemorrhoids, and vascular abnormalities are all potential causes. You certainly don't want to miss a colon cancer! (A digital rectal exam and guaiac stool test would be a good thing to do in the office.) If this work-up is negative, then you would give iron supplementation and follow up the Hct in 6 weeks.

2. D. Plummer–Vinson syndrome is characterized by the classic findings of iron deficiency (anemia, glossitis, koilonychia) and upper esophageal webs. It is most prevalent in woman; typical age range at diagnosis is 40−70 years. This syndrome is associated with a higher incidence of squamous cell carcinoma of the esophagus. **Fanconi anemia** is an inherited disease leading to bone marrow failure (aplastic anemia). Patients are usually diagnosed by age 12 years and often die of AML by adulthood. **Lead poisoning** directly inhibits heme synthesis and is characterized by gingival lines, GI colic, and renal lesions. **Porphyria** is associated with abdominal pain, neuropsychiatric complaints, and sometimes photosensitivity. It is caused by buildup of toxic intermediates in the heme synthesis pathway, caused by various enzyme deficiencies.

CASE 5-2

1. D. The question stem correctly describes part 1 of the Shilling test. A low urinary excretion of vitamin B12 suggests malabsorption in a broad sense, but calls for part 2. Here the test is repeated and intrinsic factor is given. If excretion improves (therefore absorption has improved), the patient must be deficient in IF (pernicious anemia). If excretion (hence, absorption) does not improve with the administration of IF, then malabsorption is due to a problem with the bowel (e.g., resection, Crohn disease, celiac sprue, bacterial overgrowth, etc.).

2. C. Vitamin B12 levels should be checked in every patient with a suspected macrocytic anemia, even if folate levels are low. It is important **not** to give folate to a patient with vitamin B12 deficiency. This may improve the anemia but may actually worsen the neurologic problems. The early diagnosis of vitamin B12 deficiency is extremely important, as chronic neurologic deficits (e.g., >1 year) are often irreversible despite treatment. It would

	- α	αα
- α	- α / - α (α trait)	- α / α α (silent)
α α	α α / - α (silent)	α α/ α α (normal)

TABLE A-1 α-Trait Genotype

be wise to check iron studies, as many patients have a combination of deficiencies.

CASE 5-3

1. C. Silent carriers 50%; also note that 25% will have α-trait genotype and 25% will be normal (Table A-1). It is useful to draw out the Punnett square for these types of questions.

2. D. β-Thalassemia major is an autosomal recessive disease. Using the **Hardy-Weinberg equation**: $p^2 + 2pq + q^2$; p^2 (normal genotype, β/β), q^2 (homozygous disease genotype, β°/β°), and $2pq$ (heterozygous genotype β/β°). Therefore, $q^2 = 1/1600$, $q = 1/40$ (or 0.025). Using the fact that $p + q = 1$; $p = 0.975$. The probability for heterozygosity is $2pq$ or 2 (0.975) (0.025) = 1/20.

CASE 5-4

1. C. This correctly describes the direct Coombs test. Choice (A) describes the indirect Coombs test, which is the procedure used for blood "type and screening" before a transfusion.

2. A. RhoGAM is given to all Rh-negative pregnant women at 28 weeks' gestation and when they undergo any procedures during which fetal cells may be introduced into maternal circulation (e.g., amniocentesis). It is given again postpartum to any Rh-negative women who have delivered an Rh-positive baby. RhoGAM prevents the formation of anti-D (Rh) IgG antibodies, which could potentially cross the placenta during a subsequent pregnancy and which might otherwise cause hemolytic anemia of an Rh-positive fetus. IgM antibodies do not cross the placenta. Because RhoGAM (IgG anti-O antibodies) is given in a small quantity, it does not cause hemolytic disease of the newborn. Rh-positive women do not need RhoGAM because they will not mount an antibody response to the anti-D antigen.

CASE 5-5

1. B. FXII deficiency is unique in its ability to increase a patient's PTT yet not lead to clinical bleeding episodes. The current recommendation with FXII deficiency is to proceed with any planned surgeries and inform the family that it is unlikely the patient will ever express a bleeding disorder. It is important to inform the patient in case the lab work is repeated later in life.

2. E. The transmission of HIV and other infectious organisms to hemophiliacs is a highly sensitive issue that has involved the medical, legal, and government arenas. Severe hemophiliacs have received purified blood products for over a decade, and new technology has produced recombinant FVIII, which involves in some cases little, and in others no, human blood derivatives. Many parents and patients who lived through the 1980s will be concerned about their own or their child's safety on replacement therapy. This issue should be discussed when patients with severe hemophilia start a prophylactic treatment program.

3. A. Patients with mild hemophilia A rarely present with bleeding unless it is due to trauma or surgery. Following significant trauma, bleeding is a concern for any patient with factor levels less than 30%, and in very severe cases, less than 50%. Labs on this patient indicate a FVIII activity of 14%, a prolonged PTT, and a normal PT. Recombinant FVIII replacement therapy was provided to a 100% correction due to the possibility of brain trauma and hemorrhage.

4. E. Briefly following birth, some children experience decreased vitamin K levels and thus slightly elevated PT and PTT values. In this case description, the repeated times are normal following this dip, indicating no suspected coagulopathy. The presentation of repeated bruising with rib fractures that have continued over time is highly suspect of child abuse. While domestic abuse, by law, does not require reporting to protective services, in abuse of children and the elderly reporting is required, and it is an offense if it is not done within strict time guidelines. It is important to know the state's and specific hospital's policies on reporting suspected child/elder abuse.

CASE 5-6

1. D. Fanconi anemia is unlikely the cause of AA's aplastic anemia as defined by his peripheral pancytopenia with hypocellular bone marrow. Such congenital anomalies are more likely to present earlier in life rather than at the advanced age of 68 years. Other clues in the history make possible several etiologies of aplastic anemia. His recent viral infection after visiting his granddaughter who had been ill with a fever and rash suggests parvovirus B19 infection as a possible cause. Children with this infection may present with fever and the "slapped cheek" rash, while adults may present with nonspecific pharyngitis, abdominal discomfort, and arthralgias from immune complex deposition. His history of hepatitis with negative serologies in fact may be from the as-yet-unidentified hepatitis virus thought to precede many cases of aplastic anemia. The mechanism of this disease is thought to arise from a cross-reactivity of the immune response to the virus causing autoimmunity to hematopoietic precursors. Benzene exposure (from working in a petroleum plant) is also related to aplastic anemias. Lastly, even subclinical deficiencies in hematopoiesis, as in sickle cell trait, can predispose one to fulminant aplastic anemia if newly infected with a hematopoietic cell-tropic virus, such as CMV or EBV.

2. C. Parvovirus B19 is the most unlikely cause of her pancytopenia, as this is usually accompanied by a significant but transient hypocellular bone marrow. Poor nutrition is a common cause of pancytopenia among the elderly, especially those with comorbid conditions and poor social structure. Such patients are susceptible to vitamin B12 and folate deficiency from poor food intake. Otherwise, older patients can develop an autoimmune condition that targets **intrinsic factor,** a protein that binds to vitamin B12 and aids its absorption in the terminal ileum. Loss of this protein's function can cause pernicious anemia, a condition in which normal hematopoiesis is inhibited by the absence of a

necessary substrate for nucleic acid synthesis, vitamin B12. Lastly, both drugs and alcohol cause pancytopenia by ill-defined mechanisms. The diseases mentioned above are often associated with a cellular bone marrow.

CASE 5-7

1. E. This African American male fits the demographic for G6PD deficiency. The antimalarial quinine drug has precipitated a bout of hemolysis by causing an increase in free radicals. You would also expect to see Heinz bodies within RBCs on the peripheral smear. Answer (A) describes warm-reacting antibody hemolysis, and answers (B) and (D) describe cold-reacting antibody hemolysis. Answer (C) is the mechanism for microangiopathic hemolytic anemia.

2. B. This woman has the classic symptoms of TTP: fever, anemia, thrombocytopenia, and renal and neurologic abnormalities. TTP is one of the causes of microangiopathic hemolytic anemia, which is characterized by schistocytes on the blood smear (fragmentation due to damage over microthrombi in small vessels). Bite cells are seen in G6PD deficiency; target cells in thalassemias; spherocytes in autoimmune hemolytic anemias and hereditary spherocytosis; hypersegmented PMNs in folate and vitamin B12 deficiencies.

PART VI: ONCOLOGY

CASE 6-1

1. B. Anemia, bone pain, and blurry vision are most likely due to multiple myeloma. Anemia is almost universal in multiple myeloma. Bone pain occurs from bone marrow replacement with neoplastic plasmacytic cells. Blurry vision is associated with blood hyperviscosity due to elevated paraprotein (or IgM produced by the malignancy). Waldenstrom macroglobulinemia is not usually associated with bone pain. The other lymphomas listed primarily involve lymph nodes and lymphoid tissue and only later spread to bone marrow. They would least likely present with bone pain and anemia. Therefore, answers (A), (C), (D), and (E) are incorrect.

2. B. The identification of Reed-Sternberg (RS) cells first classifies the lymphoma as HD. Staging is then the next most important predictor of prognosis. Single-node involvement is classified as stage 1, multiple nodes on the same side of the diaphragm as stage 2, nodal involvement traversing the diaphragm as stage 3, and diffuse involvement as stage 4. The patient also does not have fever, night sweats, or weight loss and thus is considered category A. Overall, she is expected to have a good outcome, with high likelihood of cure. Thus, she does not have stage IIA or IB HD. Also, given the fact that RS cells were identified, she does not have NHL, such as follicular lymphoma or large, diffuse B-cell lymphoma.

3. C. The lymphomas associated with HIV are HD, diffuse large B-cell lymphoma, and Burkitt lymphoma. Anergy due to T-cell dysfunction can be due to advanced HIV or HD. Impaired T-cell function can predispose one to fungal and mycobacterial disease and may cause the recrudescence of previous mycobacterial infection. B symptoms can result from the lymphoma or mycobacterial infection. Multiple myeloma is the least possible etiology of this clinical presentation, as it is a B-cell disorder and less likely associated with T-cell dysfunction and more so with anemia, bone pain, and hyperviscosity; therefore, (C) is the least likely to explain her symptoms.

CASE 6-2

1. B. Actinic keratosis is only a precursor lesion for squamous cell carcinoma. Excessive sunlight exposure and chronic inflammatory skin conditions predispose to both squamous cell and basal cell carcinomas. Tanning salons use equipment that emit ultraviolet A and B radiation, which are just as damaging to the skin as sunlight, and increase the risk of both squamous cell and basal cell malignancies. Dysplastic nevi are precursors of melanoma.

2. C. Keratin pearls (circular whorls of keratinization) are the histologic hallmark of squamous cell cancer. Acanthosis is abnormal epidermal thickening often seen in chronic inflammatory conditions. Basal cell carcinoma cells are "basaloid" in appearance with palisading nuclei. Basal cell carcinoma is histologically most similar to follicular cells.

3. A. The majority of basal cell carcinomas arise on the structures of the head and neck, most prominently the nose and ears. However, remember that there are no hard-and-fast rules; any location may potentially give rise to skin malignancy, so be sure to biopsy all suspicious lesions!

CASE 6-3

1. C. Neurofibromatosis type 2 (NF2) is a multisystem genetic disorder associated with bilateral vestibular schwannomas, spinal cord schwannomas, meningiomas, gliomas, and juvenile cataracts. The manifestations of NF2 result from mutations in (or, rarely, deletion of) the *NF2* tumor suppressor gene located on the long arm of chromosome 22. Half of affected individuals have NF2 as a result of a new (de novo) gene mutation. Neurofibromatosis type 1 (NF1) is a multisystem genetic disorder that commonly is associated with cutaneous (café-au-lait spots), neurologic (optic nerve gliomas), and orthopedic (arthroses or dysplasias) manifestations. Li-Fraumeni syndrome (LFS) is a cancer predisposition syndrome associated with soft tissue sarcoma, breast cancer, leukemia, osteosarcoma, melanoma, and cancer of the colon, pancreas, adrenal cortex, and brain (medulloblastoma, gliomas). The combination of parathyroid tumors, pancreatic islet cell tumors, and pituitary hyperplasia or tumor formation is called MEN-I. MEN-III (or IIB) includes pheochromocytoma, medullary carcinoma, and multiple mucocutaneous neuromas.

2. E. The multiple lesions spanning both cerebral hemispheres is a tip-off for metastatic disease. Statistically, this answer is your best bet because metastatic brain tumors account for over 50% of all intracranial tumors. Pilocytic astrocytomas are often well-circumscribed, localized lesions. Meningiomas are external to the brain and most frequently occur in the convexities of the cerebral hemispheres. Medulloblastomas are found in the cerebellum and are found mostly in children.

CASE 6-4

1. D. Benign tumors are expected to have normal cellular morphology as well as good adherence to normal tissue architecture. High nucleus-to-cytoplasm ratio, frequent mitotic spindles, loss of

glandular structure, and anaplasia suggest poorly differentiated malignant cells. Thus, answers (A), (B), (C), and (E) are incorrect.

2. B. It would be inappropriate to do a fine-needle aspiration for this woman given the fact that she has no palpable breast mass. Normally, one would use radiographically guided needle biopsy directed toward the clustering of microcalcification. For the most part, microcalcifications are highly specific for ductal carcinoma, which warrants open biopsy with sentinel node dissection. The sentinel node is the draining lymph node of the breast tissue suspected to be involved and would be detected using dye or radioisotope injected into the tumor site preoperatively, which is subsequently detected intraoperatively and then removed. Prior to these invasive diagnostic procedures, it would also be appropriate to perform a breast ultrasound to look for masses.

CASE 6-5

1. A. Hyperplastic glands arranged back to back are histologic patterns expected in well-differentiated tumors. LS has a high-grade, poorly differentiated tumor. Frequent bizarre mitotic spindles suggest cytogenetic instability that may arise from *as well as* lead to genetic rearrangements that give rise to greater anaplasia. High nucleus-to-cytoplasm ratio and hyperchromatic nucleus also appear in high-grade tumors. Lastly, as the tumor proliferates rapidly, outgrowing its vascular supply, unless adequate neovascularization occurs to keep up with the rate of tumor growth, there may be central areas of necrosis, representing tumor cells that have died due to lack of oxygen and nutrients.

2. D. The development of a second primary prostatic tumor is a highly unlikely event, especially under the pressure of antiandrogen therapy. Tumor cells that normally respond to the growth-stimulating signal of endogenous testosterone are deprived of this stimulus via antiandrogen therapy. A random mutation may give rise to an androgen-independent clone. Such a cell will necessarily outgrow those cells that require androgen stimulation. Eventually, these finasteride-resistant cells will make up the majority of the tumor, and the tumor will grow despite this therapy. Thus, (A) and (C) are incorrect answers. The likelihood of this random mutation occurring may have increased secondary to the loss of the DNA repair function of p53. Thus, (B) is incorrect. Lastly, any genetic mutation can give a cell and its progenitors a selective advantage over other cells. Such phenotypes include any phenotype yielding rapid, perhaps uncontrolled, cell proliferation. Thus, (E) is incorrect.

CASE 6-6

1. D. A defect in a DNA repair gene does not directly transform a cell toward unregulated proliferation. Instead, these defects increase the likelihood that cells will develop such genetic mutations. In the case of the familial disease of HNPCC, family members must undergo routine screening for colon cancer, as they have inherited one defective DNA mismatch repair gene in all their somatic cells (the first "hit") in a way that puts all their colonic epithelial cells at risk for developing into a cell homozygous for the defect. Loss of both genes will lead to a cell that is impaired in its abilities to maintain the integrity of the genome. This increases the likelihood of developing errors in many growth- and cell cycle-regulating genes that can subsequently transform the cell into a rapidly proliferating cell. Answers (A), (B), (C), and (E) are included in the pathogenesis of HNPCC, and these are incorrect answers.

2. D. Overabundance of *bcl-2* expression does NOT lead to uncontrolled cellular proliferation. Instead, *bcl-2* provides an *antiapoptotic signal*, which promotes *cell survival* rather than cell division. This is a very important distinction. This illustrates that even the persistence of a cell beyond its programmed lifespan is also a cancer-promoting event, as it defies the normal cycle of cell death and regeneration. It can be overexpressed in the case of Burkitt lymphoma, wherein the *bcl-2* open reading frame is translocated to a sort of "promoter" region of the immunoglobulin heavy chain, which, if stimulated to produce heavy chain, will produce *bcl-2* transcripts instead. Thus, (A), (B), and (C) are incorrect. The abundance of *bcl-2*, which eventually forms *bcl-2* homodimers, mediates signaling that favors cell survival. Thus, (E) is incorrect. There are many more steps in the development of Burkitt lymphoma. However, for the purpose of the board exam, it is important to understand the concept of apoptosis regulation as a step in the pathogenesis of cancer.

CASE 6-7

1. E. Ewing sarcoma is characterized by small, round blue-staining cells. This patient fits the demographic of patients affected by the disease. Multiple myeloma is a plasma cell disorder that causes lytic lesions in the bones, but is extremely rare in children. Giant cell tumors are characterized by multinucleated giant cells and most commonly affect young to middle-aged women. Metastatic bone disease is rare in children. Osteosarcoma consists of spindle cells and osteoid formation.

2. D. Lung metastases are common in both osteosarcoma and Ewing sarcoma. Giant cell tumors have aggressive growth but are considered benign; they do not spread outside of the bone.

CASE 6-8

1. C. Most childhood ALL is of the L1 subtype, which morphologically consists of small, uniform blast cells. Initial cytologic screening would reveal TdT+ blast cells but no Auer rods, myeloperoxidase, or nonspecific esterase activity. Once lymphoid lineage is determined, it is further subtyped to B- versus T-cell leukemias. The primitive B-cell leukemia is common, staining with surface antigens CD10, CD19, CD20, CD21, CD22. CD7 falls under the category of T-cell leukemias whose surface antigens consist of CD2, 3, 5, and 7 (Hint: CD—prime numbers under 10), as well as CD4 and CD8 in more mature T cells.

2. E. All of the above are possible explanations for different aspects of the clinical case. Hyperuricemia occurs from the rapid lysis of a large cell load as found in acute leukemia as a breakdown product of nucleic acids. This can induce an acute exacerbation of gouty arthritis, which is caused by the deposition of uric acid crystals in joints, causing inflammation and pain. Bone pain can be caused by the rapid expansion of leukemic cells in the bone marrow. The femur is a common site of bone pain from leukemia. Recent ingestion of meat can also cause exacerbation of gouty arthritis by introducing a large nucleic acid load into the body, thereby causing hyperuricemia. If the meat were contaminated, this may explain her fever and leukocytosis. Lastly,

people taking corticosteroids chronically are immunocompromised and are susceptible to serious infections like osteomyelitis, an infection of the joint, which can be fatal if untreated. This would explain her knee pain, fever, and leukocytosis as well.

PART VII: ENDOCRINOLOGY

CASE 7-1

1. D. Elevated blood keto acids are responsible for the increased anion gap metabolic acidosis seen in DKA. These acids are utilized by the brain for energy when glucose is unavailable, as in a low insulin state. Anion gap is calculated using the following formula:

$$AG = (Na^+ + K^+) - (Cl^- + HCO_3^-)$$

Normal anion gap values are usually 8 to 12. In this case, the anion gap is elevated at 35. Other causes of anion gap acidosis include methanol ingestion, uremia from chronic renal failure, lactic acidosis, and ethanol intoxication.

2. B. In endogenous pancreatic insulin production, the insulin molecule is first produced in its precursor form, a molecule known as proinsulin. This proinsulin molecule consists of an α and a β chain linked by two disulfide bonds and a C-peptide region. This C-peptide must be cleaved off the proinsulin molecule before it becomes insulin. Serum C-peptide levels can thus be used as a marker for endogenous insulin production. With exogenously administered insulin, the insulin is injected in its active form, without the C-peptide portion. Measurement of C-peptide levels in the blood of patients who are on exogenous insulin therapy will be decreased compared with people who are not on insulin.

CASE 7-2

1. C. The HbA1c test documents the average blood glucose levels in the 3 months immediately prior to testing. The reported value is directly proportional to the average blood glucose concentration over the lifespan of the patient's circulating RBCs (120 days). The glucose tolerance test, fasting serum glucose, and urinalysis can all be used to help diagnose DM and may reflect immediate glycemic status but are not indicative of long-term diabetic control. CBC is also not indicated for this purpose.

2. B. Insulin may be required for treatment of type 2 DM but is usually considered a second-line agent, after several of the other diabetes medications have failed to achieve glucose homeostasis. Because type 2 diabetics have some insulin secretion, but not enough to overcome their resistance, pharmacologic treatment of type 2 DM aims to change insulin secretion/action or alter the absorption of glucose. Glyburide is a sulfonylurea that lowers blood glucose by stimulating insulin secretion from the pancreas and increasing tissue sensitivity to insulin. The most common side effect of the sulfonylureas is hypoglycemia. Metformin is a biguanide drug often used in combination with the sulfonylureas. Its actions are to decrease hepatic gluconeogenesis and increase peripheral glucose utilization. While metformin does not induce hypoglycemia, it does inhibit lactate metabolism and can cause rare lactic acidosis. Acarbose is an β-glucosidase inhibitor that delays the digestion and absorption of complex carbohydrates in the small intestine. This class of medications is primarily used as an adjunct in type 2 patients, but many patients complain of increased GI effects such as nausea, diarrhea, bloating, and flatulence. Pioglitazone is a thiazolidinedione that decreases peripheral insulin resistance in skeletal muscle and adipose tissue without increasing insulin secretion. Because of concerns for hepatitis and liver failure, these medications have currently been removed from the market. At the very least, patients must have liver function tests measured regularly, because increased liver transaminases are a common occurrence.

3. D. All of the choices except smoking are risk factors for the development of type 2 diabetes. Diabetes results from a combination of genetic and environmental factors. While genetic factors cannot be altered, environmental influences are modifiable and should be altered toward the prevention and treatment of diabetes. In this case, the patient should be encouraged to exercise, lose weight, and eat sensibly. Smoking cessation is not a bad idea either, since smoking is a known risk factor for other multiple conditions. Since these recommendations require major lifestyle changes, the patient should receive as much lifestyle support and diabetes education as possible. This may include diabetes classes for the patient and encouraging family members to assist with her health management.

CASE 7-3

1. C. Levothyroxine is used to treat lifelong hypothyroidism, not hyperthyroidism. All of the other methods are potential treatments for hyperthyroidism. The thioamides (PTU and methimazole) are drugs that decrease thyroid hormone synthesis by binding to and inhibiting all steps of thyroid hormone synthesis catalyzed by thyroid peroxidase. Skin rash is a common side effect of these medications. Aplastic anemia and agranulocytosis can also occur on rare occasions. Beta-blockers such as propranolol are sometimes used as symptomatic therapy to decrease the peripheral manifestations of hyperthyroidism, such as increased heart rate, arrhythmias, and excess sweating. Surgery is the definitive therapy for all patients with thyrotoxicosis, but patients must be supplemented with exogenous thyroid hormone for the rest of their lives.

2. E. TSH is the best test for assessing thyroid function because changes in TSH can be detected before alterations in the levels of T_4. Free T_4 is a more accurate measurement than total T_4 because total T_4 includes all the T_4 that is bound to thyroid-binding proteins. Although the total T_4 may rise or fall secondary to changes in serum-binding protein levels, the free T_4 value remains normal if the patient is healthy. A pattern of increased TSH and low free T_4 and T_3 is consistent with hypothyroidism, while decreased TSH and increased free T_4 and T_3 suggest a hyperthyroid state.

CASE 7-4

1. B. The most specific test to screen for glucocorticoid excess is **24-hour urinary cortisol** production. The patient's urine is collected over a 24-hour period and tested for the amount of cortisol. Levels higher than 50–100 µg a day in an adult suggest Cushing syndrome. An elevated urinary cortisol confirms excess cortisol production; however, it does not distinguish one cause from another. Subsequent evaluation to localize the source of

ACTH or cortisol is usually required. Pituitary MRI can be used if a pituitary adenoma is suspected; the pituitary fossa will be enlarged or the tumor may be visualized. CT scan can be used to evaluate the possibility of adrenal adenoma or carcinoma; the CT scan may show a mass in the affected gland. Low- and high-dose dexamethasone suppression tests help distinguish patients with excess production of ACTH due to pituitary adenomas from those with ectopic ACTH-producing tumors. Dexamethasone is a synthetic glucocorticoid that should suppress endogenous cortisol and ACTH secretion. Ectopic ACTH production will not respond to dexamethasone suppression. Low doses are given first to confirm Cushing syndrome. A high dose can subsequently be given to localize the etiology to the pituitary or adrenal gland. A drop in blood and urine cortisol levels is consistent with Cushing syndrome, but the dexamethasone suppression test can produce false-positive results in patients with depression, alcohol abuse, high estrogen levels, acute illness, and stress. Conversely, drugs such as phenytoin and phenobarbital may cause false-negative results in response to dexamethasone suppression (Fig. A-2).

2. E. All of the choices provided are actions of cortisol, but it is cortisol's anti-inflammatory properties that decrease airway edema and inflammation in asthma. This anti-inflammatory action is mediated through the inhibition of prostaglandin formation. Specifically, glucocorticoids inhibit phospholipase A2, the enzyme that liberates arachidonic acid from cell membranes. Arachidonic acid is the precursor to prostaglandin, prostacyclin (PGI_2), thromboxane, and leukotriene synthesis. Without prostaglandins, prostacyclins, and leukotrienes, the inflammatory response that accompanies airway hyperreactivity in asthma is blunted. Although quite effective in controlling inflammation, chronic oral steroid therapy is associated with numerous side effects that must be weighed against the benefits of treatment. Specifically, patients can develop cushingoid features, including

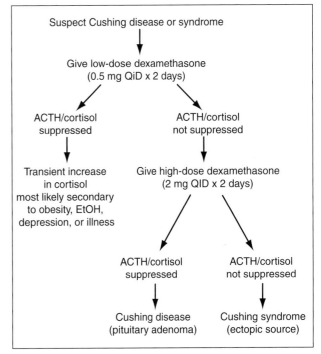

● **Figure A-2.** Algorithm for the dexamethasone suppression test.

excess fat deposition, moon facies, and striae. Chronic complications from glucocorticoid excess can also develop, such as osteoporosis, hypertension, and diabetes. Interestingly, exogenous steroid intake is the most common cause of Cushing syndrome.

CASE 7-5

1. B. **Craniopharyngiomas** are pituitary gland tumors derived from remnants of Rathke pouch oral ectoderm. Craniopharyngiomas are the most common cause of panhypopituitarism in adolescents. With panhypopituitarism, patients are deficient in LH, FSH, TRH, PRL, ACTH, and GH. The lack of gonadotropins and GH explains this patient's delayed puberty and short stature. In addition, secondary adrenal insufficiency will result from the lack of ACTH stimulation to the adrenal cortex. Because ACTH regulates secretion from the zona fasciculata and the zona reticularis, cortisol and androgen production will be decreased. Aldosterone secretion from the zona glomerulosa will not be affected. Secondary insufficiency differs in presentation from primary insufficiency (Addison disease) in that the patients do not present with hypotension or hyperpigmentation.

2. A. Autoimmune adrenalitis is the most common cause of primary adrenal insufficiency in the United States. An autoimmune cause is also most likely in this patient because she has a history of Graves disease, an autoimmune-mediated thyroiditis. Patients with autoimmune diseases tend to have other simultaneous autoimmune-mediated conditions. Although skin hyperpigmentation is characteristic of Addison disease secondary to increased MSH, this patient presents with patches of depigmentation. This depigmentation is known as vitiligo and is also common in patients with autoimmune disease. The vitiligo occurs through an autoimmune-mediated attack on melanocytes. The diagnosis of Addison disease can be confirmed with laboratory findings of low morning cortisol levels (<3 μg/dL) and high plasma ACTH levels ($\geq$100 pg/mL).

CASE 7-6

1. A. Metabolic alkalosis, not acidosis, is a primary feature of Conn syndrome, occurring as a result of elevated aldosterone levels stimulating H^+ secretion from the renal distal tubule. In addition, the excess aldosterone increases K^+ excretion and Na^+ reabsorption. The sodium and water retention elevates systemic BP, which usually is not responsive to antihypertensive medications. Plasma renin levels are low in primary hyperaldosteronism because the elevated aldosterone feeds back upon the RAS in the form of increased Na^+ to the JGA. The JGA senses increased renal perfusion and decreases renin secretion from the JG cells.

2. E. Both spironolactone and ACE inhibitors can be used for medical treatment of primary hyperaldosteronism due to bilateral adrenocortical hyperplasia. This is the most common cause of primary hyperaldosteronism in children, although the cause of hyperplasia remains unknown. The adrenal glands start to grow excessively to produce nodules, either large (macronodular) or small (micronodular), that secrete aldosterone. Since these nodules are usually responsive to angiotensin II, ACE inhibitors have been effective in decreasing aldosterone secretion from the nodules. In addition, spironolactone, an aldosterone antagonist, can be used to block aldosterone's actions. In high doses, however, spironolactone can inhibit testosterone production, causing

gynecomastia, reduced libido, and impotence in men or irregular menstrual cycles in women. To improve the hypokalemia associated with hyperaldosteronism, potassium-sparing diuretics such as amiloride can be used. Loop diuretics are actually contraindicated with hyperaldosteronism because they cause potassium wasting from the loop of Henle and can aggravate the hypokalemia. Surgery is the definitive therapy for hyperaldosteronism due to discreet lesions such as an adrenal adenoma or carcinoma, but not for bilateral zona glomerulosa hyperplasia.

CASE 7-7

1. C. DHEA levels are most likely elevated in this young girl who presents with hirsutism and growth abnormalities secondary to a mild form of CAH. DHEA is a mild androgen that can cause virilization in a female infant if present in excess amounts. Patients with nonclassical CAH have enough enzyme function to spare them from virilization and salt wasting, but they can present later in life with evidence of androgen excess from the shunting of cortisol and aldosterone precursors. In this case, androgen excess has resulted in an abnormal growth pattern, delayed menarche, obesity, and hirsutism. Women with unrecognized CAH often present with infertility. The most commonly involved enzyme deficiency in CAH is 21-hydroxylase, followed by 11β-hydroxylase. These enzymes are necessary for the biosynthesis of cortisol and aldosterone from cholesterol. Patients with CAH will have decreased levels of serum cortisol and aldosterone, which can lead to secondary electrolyte abnormalities and an inability to mount an appropriate stress response. ACTH levels will be increased in these patients as well due to the loss of negative feedback on the pituitary gland. These patients may complain of increased skin pigmentation secondary to the chronically elevated levels of ACTH.

2. B. Of the choices listed, the hormone most likely to account for this child's symptoms is aldosterone. Aldosterone is a mineralocorticoid produced by the zona glomerulosa of the adrenal cortex. Aldosterone functions to maintain BP by increasing renal tubular absorption of sodium and thus facilitating excretion of potassium. Aldosterone secretion is regulated by the RAS; angiotensin II directly stimulates its secretion from the adrenal cortex. Patients classically CAH present with both cortisol and aldosterone deficiency at birth. In female infants, it is often recognized early because of the presence of ambiguous genitalia secondary to androgen excess. Male infants, however, usually present a few weeks after birth because their external genitalia appear normal. These infants are diagnosed with CAH after they present with acute symptoms of glucocorticoid and mineralocorticoid deficiency, including failure to thrive, dehydration, vomiting, and severe hyponatremia with hyperkalemia. Lifelong treatment with exogenous mineralocorticoid and glucocorticoid therapy is required for these infants to survive. Deficiencies in the other hormones listed would not present in the first few weeks of life with dehydration and failure to thrive.

CASE 7-8

1. B. Autosomal dominant mutations in the *menin* tumor suppressor gene on chromosome 11 are responsible for MEN type I, described in this patient's mother. MEN I consists of parathyroid hyperplasia, pituitary adenoma, and pancreatic islet cell neoplasm. The history of DM implies hyperglycemia secondary to a

pancreatic glucagonoma, while kidney stones suggest symptomatic hypercalcemia. In addition, the presence of a pituitary neoplasm is a likely explanation for her mother's chronic headaches. Parathyroid hyperplasia is the most common finding in MEN I, consistent in up to 90% of patients. It is also present in MEN IIa. While the other choices are helpful screening tests for the diagnosis of MEN II syndromes, they would not contribute to the diagnosis of MEN I. Serum Ca and intact PTH measurement may be helpful for both MEN I and MEN IIa, but only *menin* germline mutation evaluation is specific for MEN I.

2. E. This patient most likely has MEN IIb, as suggested by attacks of paroxysmal hypertension secondary to pheochromocytoma and a distinctive marfanoid appearance. Because MEN IIb consists of medullary thyroid carcinoma, pheochromocytoma, and mucosal neuromas, this patient is most at risk for thyroid carcinoma. Derived from C cells within the thyroid gland, medullary carcinoma often causes elevated calcitonin levels. In MEN IIb patients, this type of cancer is extremely aggressive and is responsible for the major morbidity and mortality arising from the syndrome. PUD, osteoporosis, and galactorrhea are features of MEN I. Hyperthyroidism is not associated with the multiple endocrine neoplasias.

PART VIII: RHEUMATOLOGY

CASE 8-1

1. E. It is possible that this patient has SLE like her sister. Familial occurrence of SLE has been documented and it is known that family members have an increased risk of developing the disorder. Moreover, it has been shown that unaffected first-degree relatives have higher levels of autoantibodies and immunoregulatory abnormalities. However, an important part of the patient's sister's history that cannot be overlooked is the fact that she has been taking hydralazine for her elevated BP. A lupus-like syndrome can be caused by this drug as well as by the drugs procainamide, isoniazid, chlorpromazine, quinidine, and methyldopa. The clinical features of this drug-induced syndrome are similar to those of SLE and include positive ANA titers. However, important differences do exist. First, the gender prevalence of this disorder is equal, as opposed to predominantly female. Second, renal and CNS involvement are not typical. Third, although these patients are positive for ANA, they are neither usually positive for anti-dsDNA antibodies nor are their complement levels markedly decreased. Finally, the symptoms of the drug-induced, lupus-like syndrome are milder and resolve once the drug is discontinued. Discoid lupus is characterized primarily by characteristic skin lesions that begin as erythematous papules or plaques with scaling that may become thick and adherent with a hypopigmented central area. Other symptoms, such as arthritis, are usually absent in this disorder.

2. D. Unfortunately, at this point in time, a perfect diagnostic test for SLE does not exist. All of the answer choices can be positive in patients with this disease. The most sensitive test for screening is ANAs. Nearly all patients with SLE have these antibodies. However, this test is not specific and is elevated in a number of other disorders: systemic sclerosis, scleroderma, Sjögren syndrome, rheumatoid arthritis, polymyositis/dermatomyositis, mixed connective tissue disorder, Wegener granulomatosis, leprosy, infectious mononucleosis, liver disease, primary pulmonary

fibrosis, and vasculitis. Moreover, approximately 5–15% of normal individuals have low titers of these antibodies. In contrast, antibodies to dsDNA are found in only 50% of patients with SLE, but are rarely found in any other disorders. ESR is typically elevated in SLE but is seen in a wide variety of inflammatory processes. Rheumatoid factor is observed in only 20% of patients with lupus. Lupus anticoagulant is an antiphospholipid antibody seen in 7% of lupus patients, which, contrary to its name, is actually associated with venous and arterial thrombosis as well as to placental infarction. Unlike the other antibodies that are tested for by actually measuring the amount of antibody present in serum through titers, lupus anticoagulant is identified by looking at coagulation tests like prolongation of the activated PTT and the Russel viper venom test.

3. D. This patient most likely has SLE—an autoimmune disorder characterized by the production of autoantibodies. The loss of tolerance leading to this immune dysfunction is likely due to abnormalities in clonal anergy. Clonal anergy is the process that occurs in the peripheral blood circulation whereby lymphocytes that react with self antigens are inactivated. Clonal deletion occurs in the thymus and bone marrow as lymphocytes mature. In this process, self-reactive T cells and B cells are eliminated and self tolerance results. Release of sequestered antigens and molecular mimicry are two other mechanisms postulated to be involved in the development of autoimmune phenomenon. However, these are not believed to play a role in SLE. Enzyme deficiency can play a role in other arthritides such as gout, but has no role in this lupus.

4. A. Systemic lupus erythematosus is by definition a multiorgan system disorder. Systemic manifestations include fever, anorexia, weight loss, fatigue, and malaise. Skin and mucocutaneous features include a malar rash, discoid rash, alopecia, and oral ulcers. The eyes can also be affected with conjunctivitis, photophobia, transient blindness, and blurry vision. Pulmonary involvement can be seen as pleurisy, pleural effusion, bronchopneumonia, and pneumonitis. Pericarditis, cardiac arrhythmias, and cardiac failure secondary to myocarditis and hypertension are all possible heart manifestations. Also, Libman-Sacs endocarditis, characterized by small, single or multiple irregular verrucous lesions on any valve of the heart on either surface of the valve leaflets, can be seen. Neurologic symptoms include psychosis, organic brain syndrome, seizures, neuropathies, and depression. GN is the main renal manifestation. Hematologic abnormalities seen in SLE include hemolytic anemia, thrombocytopenia, lymphopenia, and leukopenia. Finally, arterial and venous thrombosis as well as vasculitis characterized by "onion skin lesions" of the central arteries of the spleen can complicate the disease. Although joint involvement is a key feature of SLE, the arthritis seen rarely leads to joint destruction and deformities.

CASE 8-2

1. B. Synovial fluid in early RA reveals evidence of the severe noninfectious inflammatory process occurring in the joints. It is typically turbid with elevated levels of WBCs, the majority of which are neutrophils. This type of fluid can also be seen in gout and pseudogout, both of which are also characterized by noninfectious inflammation of the joints. In septic/infectious arthritis, synovial fluid is also turbid, but levels of WBCs are even greater than that seen with noninfectious arthritis. Fragments of C. trachomatis can be found in the synovial fluid of patients with Reiter syndrome (reactive arthritis). Bloody fluid can be seen whenever the arthrocentesis is traumatic, regardless of the type of joint pathology. Birefringent crystals seen under polarized light microscopy is characteristic of gout. Although levels of rheumatoid factor can be elevated in RA, these antibodies are tested for primarily in the blood.

2. C. The patient was most likely started on methotrexate, which is commonly used in patients with severe RA unresponsive to NSAIDs and other slow-acting agents, such as gold salts, chloroquine, and D-penicillamine. Methotrexate is an immunosuppressant medication that is often used in the treatment of cancer. This chemotherapeutic agent is structurally similar to folic acid and acts by inhibiting dihydrofolate reductase, leading to decreased DNA and RNA production and eventually decreased protein synthesis and cell death. The doses given for patients with RA are significantly lower than those given for chemotherapy. However, the side effects of oral ulcers and nausea are still commonly seen. More importantly, methotrexate can lead to decreased WBC production and subsequent immunosuppression, which places these patients at increased risk for infection. Aplastic anemia is not typically seen with methotrexate but can be associated with use of gold salts and penicillamine. Renal damage can be seen with methotrexate but usually occurs only with high-dose therapy. Hepatic function can also be impaired, but this occurs only with long-term use. Decreased rheumatoid factor is seen with the use of penicillamine.

3. F. Severe, long-standing RA with chronic inflammation of the joint space leads to destruction of the cartilage and underlying bone. On radiographs this is seen as joint space narrowing and bony erosions. Joint space narrowing is initially observed at the juxta-articular margin, which is not protected by cartilage. However, with continued inflammation and destruction of the cartilage, erosions can be seen in the remainder of the bony articular surfaces of the joint. Demineralization of bone and decreased bone density are seen with osteoporosis. Increased bony cortex of increased density is seen in Paget disease and is characterized by excessive bone turnover. Joint space narrowing, osteophytes, and dense subchondral bone are seen in osteoarthritis. A "bamboo spine," characterized by calcification of the anterior and lateral spinal ligaments with squaring and demineralization of the vertebral bodies, is seen in late-stage ankylosing spondylitis. "Punched-out" osteolytic lesions of the skull and long bones is characteristic of multiple myeloma.

4. C. This patient's reaction is an example of a type I hypersensitivity reaction. This immediate/anaphylactic hypersensitivity occurs when an antigen—in this case something in the shellfish—binds to and cross-links IgE on the surface of mast cells, causing mast cell degranulation. Mediators such as histamine, eosinophil chemotactic factor of anaphylaxis, leukotrienes, prostaglandins, and thromboxanes are thus released. This release leads to swelling, vasodilation, and increased capillary permeability, which, in turn, can manifest as urticaria, angioedema, allergic rhinitis, and bronchospasm. IgA is found mostly in the mucus membranes and serves *primarily* to prevent attachment of bacteria and viruses. It is not involved with mast cell degranulation and release of histamine. IgG-mediated immune complexes deposited in the skin is an example of type III hypersensitivity that occurs when immune complexes are deposited in tissues and subsequently activate complement. The onset of this type of reaction is delayed and usually occurs from a few days to a couple of weeks following exposure to the antigen. Serum sickness is an example

of such a reaction. IgG-mediated complement lysis is an example of type II hypersensitivity that occurs when IgG antibodies directed at antigens of the cell membrane activate complement and leads to cell membrane destruction through the membrane-attack complex. Rh hemolytic disease is an example of this kind of hypersensitivity reaction.

CASE 8-3

1. C. Reiter syndrome is characterized by arthritis, conjunctivitis, and urethritis. It often follows chlamydial urethritis or dysentery caused by salmonella, shigella, *Yersinia*, or *Campylobacter*. Skin manifestations are not typically a part of this syndrome. Psoriatic arthritis is, however, characterized by arthritis conjunctivitis and a psoriatic rash that is usually macular papular in nature with scaling.

2. B. Reiter syndrome is associated with HLA-B27 and often follows chlamydial, not gonococcal, infection. Urethral cultures are therefore often positive for *Chlamydia*. This infection is believed to cause inflammatory symptoms through molecular mimicry whereby portions of the infectious agent are homologous to self proteins and thus—when infected—the resulting immune response leads not just to resolution of the infection but also to inflammation of self tissues. The infection itself is not responsible for the arthritis. Examination of synovial fluid reveals the presence of chlamydial peptides, but cultures are negative for the organism. HLA-D4 is associated with rheumatoid arthritis and insulin-dependent diabetes.

3. D. Class I MHC molecules are found on all cells and present antigen to CD8 cells, leading to cytotoxic T-cell destruction by the CD8 cells. Class II MHC molecules are found only on B cells and macrophages and present antigen to CD4 cells, which, in turn, can lead to a T-cell—mediated humoral response that triggers the complement cascade. HLA-DR3 and HLA-DR4 are examples of class II MHC molecules. HLA-B27 is a class I HLA molecule.

CASE 8-4

1. A. Blood vessels are composed of an outer adventitia layer, inner media, and innermost intima. The intima is composed of endothelium, basal lamina, and subendothelial connective tissue. Arteries contain an internal elastic lamina separating the intima from the media. Muscular arteries also have an external elastic lamina to facilitate diameter changes. As the innermost layer with maximal exposure to foreign antigens and immunosurveillance, the endothelium is the most effected in Kawasaki disease.

2. D. The ESR has been the most widely used and studied index of the acute-phase response of inflammatory disease. Elevations in the speed of sedimentation in anticoagulated blood was known to ancient Greeks. Increased acute-phase proteins—particularly fibrinogen and immunoglobulins—cause increased aggregation of erythrocytes (rouleaux formation or stacking). This is facilitated by the decreased natural tendency of erythrocytes to repel each other with negatively charged polysaccharide surface molecules.

3. D. This patient most likely has Takayasu arteritis—a chronic vasculitis of the aorta and its branches—most commonly seen in young women of Asian descent. Initial symptoms include malaise and arthralgias. As the disease progresses and there is increasing fibrosis and narrowing of the aorta, headaches, visual changes, and angina pectoris may develop. On exam, peripheral pulses are noted to be asymmetrically decreased and hypertension can be seen. Patients with this disorder are noted to have an elevated ESR. However, this is not specific for the disease and is seen in numerous other systemic inflammatory disorders. An EKG may reveal ischemic disease if the aortitis affects the coronary artery ostia. Renal disease is rare in this disease and is usually related to ischemia or hypertensive changes. Thus, a renal biopsy is not useful in diagnosis. Arteriography is the best test for confirming the diagnosis. An aortogram usually reveals the narrowing of the great vessels. P-ANCA is associated with polyarteritis nodosa, not Takayasu arteritis.

4. B. Pneumonia can cause an acute asthma exacerbation. However, it is an unlikely diagnosis in this patient who has chronic symptoms and evidence of systemic inflammatory disease. In pneumonia, one would most likely see an elevated WBC count with increased neutrophils and a left shift, and chest x ray would reveal focal consolidation as opposed to patchy or nodular infiltrates. Churg-Strauss syndrome, polyarteritis nodosa, and Goodpasture disease are all systemic vasculitides that can affect the respiratory tract. In polyarteritis nodosa, patients have constitutional symptoms, such as fever and malaise. Joint pains and skin manifestations are also common. Lungs may be affected, but this occurs only rarely. Goodpasture disease is characterized by a necrotizing hemorrhagic interstitial pneumonitis with concomitant proliferative GN. The primary pulmonary symptom is not an asthma exacerbation but hemoptysis. Chest x-ray in these patients usually reveals focal pulmonary consolidation. Churg-Strauss syndrome is often seen in people who have a history of asthma or allergic disease. Patients have symptoms of systemic inflammatory disease, fever, arthralgias, myalgias, and weight loss. Eosinophilia is characteristic of this disease. Diagnosis is confirmed by biopsy of involved vascular or renal tissue, which would reveal inflammation and necrotizing microgranulomas with eosinophilic infiltrates. Buerger disease is seen in heavy smokers and is characterized by acute and chronic inflammation of medium and small arteries of the extremities in conjunction with segmental thrombosis. Usually it does not affect the vessels of the lungs.

CASE 8-5

1. C. This patient has had progressive joint destruction and most likely has developed osteophytes, or bone spurs in the joints of her hands, that are limiting the range of motion in these joints and causing increased pain. When these bony enlargements are found in the PIP joints they are called Bouchard nodes. When they affect the DIP joints they are called Heberden nodes. Acute inflammation characterized by swelling, erythema, warmth, and tenderness is not commonly seen in osteoarthritis; it is more characteristic of the inflammatory arthritides, such as rheumatoid arthritis, gout, and septic arthritis. The metatarsophalangeal joints are found in the feet, not in the hands. Rheumatoid nodules are subcutaneous nodules seen in rheumatoid arthritis. Hyperextension of the PIP joints, otherwise known as "swan neck" deformities, are seen in advanced rheumatoid arthritis.

2. D. Articular cartilage is composed primarily of hyaline cartilage that is formed by a framework of type II collagen, proteoglycan aggregates that make up most of the extracellular matrix,

and chondrocytes. It is the hydrophilic proteoglycan aggregates that bind to water and give this type of cartilage its elasticity. The collagen provides tensile strength and resilience. Chondrocytes produce the extracellular matrix and collagen but do not themselves contribute to any supportive properties of cartilage. *Osteoclasts* are found in bone and are involved primarily with bone reabsorption and remodeling. Synovial fluid is found in the joint space and acts as a lubricant as well as providing nutrition for the cartilage.

3. E. In advanced osteoarthritis such as this patient has, there has been destruction of the cartilage and extensive bony remodeling. Osteoblasts are likely to be the most active cells in the joint at this point because these are involved in laying down more bone in response to the increased stress on the joint with the loss of the articular cartilage. In advanced disease, chondrocyte activity is likely low because most of the cartilage has been destroyed. Neutrophils are involved in acute bacterial infection of the joint and unlikely to be seen in osteoarthritis. CD8 T cells play a key role in cell-mediated immunity. These are not likely to be found in osteoarthritis, which is a degenerative—not autoimmune-mediated—arthritis. Osteophytes are not cells but the bony spurs formed late in the disease as a result of bony remodeling.

PART IX: REPRODUCTION

CASE 9-1

1. E. In testicular feminization syndrome, also known as androgen insensitivity, genetically male fetuses (46,XY) develop phenotypically female external genitalia due to an intrinsic inability to respond to testicular androgens. This is an example of male pseudohermaphroditism. The presence of a Y chromosome in these individuals leads to development of testes as well as MIS. Thus, these individuals do not develop female internal genitalia despite their outward appearance. In addition, the testes are often undescended and should be surgically removed because they have an increased rate of malignancy.

True hermaphroditism occurs very rarely and is the simultaneous presence of both ovarian and testicular tissue in an individual. The external genitalia are often ambiguous. As above, pseudohermaphroditism occurs when the phenotypic sex does not correspond to the genotypic sex. Female pseudohermaphroditism is usually due to abnormalities in adrenal steroid synthesis, resulting in the development of clitoromegaly and hypertrophied labia majora that may be partially fused and resemble a scrotum in genetic females. Turner syndrome occurs when an X chromosome is either absent or abnormal (45,XO or mosaicism in 46,XX or 46,XY), resulting in rudimentary or streak gonads. These individuals are phenotypically female and possess characteristic features that are discussed in the Turner syndrome case. Klinefelter syndrome is another disorder of gonadal development resulting from an XXY karyotype. Clinically, it is characterized by small, firm testes, azoospermia, gynecomastia, and mental retardation.

2. B. The wolffian ducts give rise to the epididymis, vas deferens, and seminal vesicles. The müllerian ducts give rise to the fallopian tubes, uterus, and upper one third of the vagina. The gubernaculum is a mesenchymal condensation attached to the caudal portion of each testis and assists in testicular descent. Bartholin glands are mucous glands that form at the base of the labia majora.

CASE 9-2

1. A. Estrogen leads to a number of changes, including effects on the secondary sexual characteristics, bone growth, and an increase in hepatic enzymes. This can be seen in pregnancy when the increased levels of estrogen lead to greater release of hepatically produced binding proteins and clotting factors. While DHEAS does lead to axillary and pubic hair production in females, it is generally converted to DHT in males. LH and FSH act primarily on the gonads to both foster maturation and produce hormones and gametes. GnRH's effects are mediated in part because of its pulsatile effect. If it is released in a continuous fashion, its receptors are down-regulated and its effect is minimized.

2. B. The most common order of the stages of puberty is adrenarche, gonadarche, thelarche, pubarche, and menarche. Of note, the latter three events can vary in timing with respect to one another. In fact, some girls will start menstruating prior to thelarche.

CASE 9-3

1. E. Because most women have two functioning ovaries, the loss of one does not generally disrupt the onset of puberty in any significant way. Patients with the surgical removal of one ovary may have the onset of menopause approximately 1 year sooner. However, this has never been addressed in a prospective, randomized trial. Intense physical activity can lead to hypogonadotropic hypogonadism. Disruptions in the genital tract, such as transverse vaginal septum and imperforate hymen, result in the collection of menses behind these obstructions and backflow of menses into the pelvis. These patients often have monthly menstrual symptoms and can develop severe endometriosis. Patients with testicular feminization are actually genetically male but because of a failure to respond to testosterone, they are phenotypically female. However, they lack a uterus, fallopian tubes, and ovaries.

2. B. In this patient with excessive weight gain during college making her morbidly obese, the most likely etiology of her secondary amenorrhea is elevated estrogen disrupting her hypothalamic-pituitary-ovarian feedback loop, resulting in anovulation. These patients will often have breakdown of their endometrium, leading to heavy menses every few months (anovulatory bleeding), but they can also present with frank amenorrhea. The weight loss and exercise since college are unlikely to lead to amenorrhea since the weight loss is bringing her back to her optimal weight and the exercise is not particularly excessive. While pregnancy is the leading cause of secondary amenorrhea and should be ruled out in this patient, it is less likely given another etiology and complaints of amenorrhea for 2 years. Because this patient had normal menses throughout adolescence, testicular feminization is not a feasible diagnosis.

3. D. This patient has premature ovarian failure. A lack of response to progestin-only challenge in a previously menstruating woman indicates that she is now estrogen deficient. This is confirmed when she has a withdrawal bleed to estrogen/progestin challenge. The differential diagnosis is now dependent on an FSH level, which, if elevated, will indicate a diagnosis of hypergonadotropic hypogonadism or premature ovarian failure. If the FSH level is low, the patient has hypogonadotropic hypogonadism as a result of either severe hypothalamic dysfunction or brain lesion (e.g., empty sella syndrome, Sheehan syndrome). These can be distinguished by clinical findings as well as head MRI. Asherman syndrome (development of

intrauterine synechiae) is usually the result of intrauterine instrumentation or infection. This is unlikely in this patient who has never been pregnant. Additionally, a patient with Asherman would not have a response to progestin or estrogen/progestin challenge because the abnormality is not hormonal in nature but rather outflow obstruction. Patients with PCOS will often have a withdrawal bleed to progestin alone because they are not estrogen deficient. Additionally, patients with PCOS will have other clinical findings consistent with the syndrome, such as abnormal hair growth or insulin resistance. Patients with testicular feminization syndrome will present with primary rather than secondary amenorrhea.

CASE 9-4

1. B. Cardiac output increases 30–50% in pregnancy. SVR decreases secondary to the increased levels of progesterone that lead to relaxation of smooth muscle. The decrease in SVR leads to decreased blood pressures, which persist until term in the normal patient. Because of the blood volume expansion that outpaces production, both erythrocytes and platelets are more dilute, leading to a decreased hematocrit and platelet count.

2. D. BUN and serum creatinine both decrease in pregnancy as a result of increased GFR. Tidal volume and minute ventilation both increase, while respiratory rate remains unchanged. This increased minute ventilation actually leads to a decrease in P_{CO_2} and an increase in pH.

CASE 9-5

1. B. Not all Rh D-negative women need to receive RhoGAM (anti-D immune globulin) after delivery. If the fetus is found to be Rh D-negative following delivery, administration of anti-D immune globulin is not indicated. However, if determination of fetal Rh status is delayed for any reason, RhoGAM should be administered to all nonimmunized mothers within 72 hours of delivery. Women who are Rh D-negative are given prophylactic RhoGAM in the setting of a spontaneous or elective termination of pregnancy, ectopic pregnancy, invasive procedure such as amniocentesis or CVS, routinely at approximately 28 weeks' gestation, and any time in the third trimester when the antibody screen is negative despite having already received a prophylactic dose.

2. B. When following ΔOD_{450} values for fetal hemolysis, Liley zone 1 is reassuring, but fetuses with values in zone 3 and high zone 2 are at risk for fetal anemia. Once these values are attained, direct fetal blood sampling via PUBS to determine fetal hematocrit and transfuse cross-matched Rh-negative blood is necessary. Because of the risk for delivery either shortly after or during the PUBS, patients are often given a course of antenatal corticosteroids. If the measurement were just in the middle to low area of zone 2, it would be reasonable to continue fetal assessment with ultrasound and more frequent amniocentesis every 7–10 days.

3. E. While ultrasonography is not the most sensitive test for fetal hemolysis, the presence of ascites and pleural and pericardial effusions is particularly specific for fetal hemolysis in Rh-positive fetuses with Rh-negative moms. The Liley curve is used to predict severity of fetal disease. Values in zone 3 are suggestive of severe fetal disease.

4. C. The various fetal structures allow maximum fetal oxygenation. The foramen ovale is located between the two atria and shunts blood from the RA to the LA to bypass the pulmonary circulation. The ductus arteriosus also bypasses the pulmonary system by shunting blood from the pulmonary artery to the aorta. Blood is shunted from the liver by the ductus venosus. The umbilical vein transports oxygenated blood to the fetus while the umbilical arteries transport deoxygenated blood back to the placenta.

CASE 9-6

1. C. Recurrent urinary tract infections have not been shown to increase the risk for cervical dysplasia or cancer. However, HPV and HIV infection, early age at onset of sexual activity, large number of sexual partners, history of sexually transmitted infections, and cigarette smoking are all risk factors for cervical dysplasia and cancer.

2. B. Cervical cancer is clinically staged. As such, physical exam, including pelvic exam under anesthesia, is the main staging modality. MRI is not used, but occasionally CT scan is used to assess for hydronephrosis. Because cervical cancer is not surgically staged, hysterectomy specimen and lymph node dissection are not used to assign stage of disease.

3. E. All of the answer choices would be appropriate treatment for CIN II except for radiation, which is reserved for early to advanced cervical cancer. Although cryotherapy and laser surgery could both be used, cold knife conization and loop electrosurgical excision procedure (LEEP) are preferable because they would provide a specimen for evaluation of margins. Of note, conization must be performed in the operating room, and thus is more costly than LEEP.

4. A. Serum tumor markers can be useful aids in determining response to therapy with germ cell tumors. Dysgerminomas produce LDH and CA-125. Embryonal carcinomas produce hCG, AFP, and CA-125. Endodermal sinus tumors produce AFP. Immature teratomas produce CA-125. Choriocarcinomas produce hCG.

5. B. There are approximately 182,800 new cases of breast cancer diagnosed annually in the United States. This exceeds the total incidence of lung, endometrial, ovarian, and cervical cancers combined. The incidence of lung cancer is 74,600; endometrial cancer, 36,100; ovarian cancer, 23,100; and cervical cancer, 12,800.

6. D. Lung cancer accounts for approximately 67,600 deaths annually in the United States. Breast cancer follows with 40,800 deaths annually. Of the gynecologic cancers, ovarian cancer tends to be diagnosed in later stages and thus accounts for 14,000 deaths per year. Endometrial cancer causes 6,500 deaths and cervical cancer causes 4,600 deaths per year.

7. E. The differential diagnosis for postmenopausal bleeding includes endometrial cancer, endometrial hyperplasia or atrophy, endometrial polyps, exogenous estrogens, cervical polyps or cancer, uterine sarcoma, and trauma.

8. D. Factors that increase exposure to estrogen, particularly unopposed estrogen, are risk factors for endometrial cancer. These include nulliparity, chronic anovulation, late menopause, and exogenous estrogen use. Additionally, obesity increases peripheral conversion of adrenal androgens to estrogens by aromatase activity in adipose tissue. Combined with the lower concentration of sex hormone-binding globulin found in obese women, these factors account for the increased bioavailability of estrogen and make obesity an important risk factor for endometrial cancer. Early age of first intercourse is not associated with endometrial cancer but is associated with cervical cancer.

CASE 9-7

1. A. Eighty percent of GTD is molar pregnancy, with 90% of molar pregnancies being complete moles. Invasive moles account for 10–15% of GTD, while choriocarcinoma accounts for 2–5%. Placental site trophoblastic tumors are exceedingly rare.

2. E. Choriocarcinoma can metastasize to many locations. In fact, it often presents as metastatic disease and is known as the great imitator because its signs and symptoms are very similar to other diseases. Given this potentially confusing presentation and the fact that it can arise weeks to years after any gestation, diagnosis of choriocarcinoma is often delayed.

3. D. Choriocarcinoma consists of cytotrophoblasts and syncytiotrophoblasts only. There are no chorionic villi present. PSTTs also lack chorionic villi. Complete moles have a 46,XY or 46,XX karyotype, while partial moles are either 69,XXY or 69,XXX. Invasive moles contain chorionic villi and trophoblasts.

4. E. Reported risk factors for GTD vary but include all of the following: maternal age younger than 20 or older than 40 years; history of prior molar pregnancy or miscarriage; diets low in beta-carotene, folic acid, and vitamin A; women with blood type A married to men with blood type O; and use of oral contraceptives.

PART X: NEUROSCIENCE

CASE 10-1

1. B. This patient is exhibiting "echolalia," the automatic repetition of auditory input. In extreme examples, the patient may also mimic other perceived sounds. This is often seen in the setting of transcortical sensory aphasia. Essentially this is receptive (Wernicke-like) aphasia with intact repetition. Given his ability to repeat, the perisylvian structure must all be spared. The dominant (left) hemisphere would be affected in this right-handed patient. Note that this patient also makes paraphasic errors. In **semantic paraphasic errors,** words with related meanings are substituted, such as saying "bus" instead of "train." In **phonemic paraphasic errors,** parts of words are substituted, such as saying "bar" instead of "car." **Neologisms** are novel nonsense words.

2. D. Again, language deficits would be associated with the dominant left hemisphere. The perisylvian language structures are primarily supplied by the MCA. Compromise of the MCA-PCA border zone would be most likely to result in a transcortical aphasia. Compromise of the PCA would be associated with a visual fields deficit, although language impairment could also occur. Compromise of the MCA-ACA territory would be associated with a transcortical motor aphasia.

3. A. This patient has alexia (he cannot read, not even his own handwriting) without agraphia (he can still write). Patients with this problem usually have a lesion involving the dominant visual cortex and the splenium of the corpus callosum. Their nondominant visual cortex is able to "read," but that information cannot get to the dominant side for language processing. The frontal cortex and therefore the ability to plan and execute written language are preserved. These patients are able to write but cannot read their own writing (many physicians seem to have this problem).

4. E. This patient does not have aphasia. Dysarthria is often confused for a primary language problem. Note, however, that he has normal language production, comprehension, and repetition. The information provided does not strictly localize his problem. Dysarthria is a manifestation of lower cranial nerve dysfunction but can also be seen in various global and metabolic processes. Given the apparently new confusion, one might suspect a more global hypoperfusion. Given the history, a cardiac event is most likely.

CASE 10-2

1. D. The combination of bilateral leg weakness and incontinence localizes the lesion to the medial aspect of the frontal and prefrontal cortex. A meningioma arising from the falx cerebri in this area could explain the described symptoms. A lateralized lesion would not be expected to cause bilateral disease. Dorsolateral and orbitofrontal prefrontal lesions have more profound clinical manifestations, as discussed previously. A lesion in the area of the pineal gland would not be expected to manifest in this way. An important clinical correlation for pineal tumors is compression of the tectum causing Parinaud syndrome (limitation of upgaze, near-light pupillary dissociation, convergence-retraction nystagmus).

2. B. The dorsomedial nucleus is the main thalamic relay station for limbic information on its way to the frontal and prefrontal cortex. This pathway used to be lesioned deliberately in cases of psychosis and chronic pain to take advantage of the associated apathy as a means of pain control. The anterior nucleus of the thalamus is involved in limbic pathways but does not have a major projection to the frontal lobe. The ventral posterior nucleus of the thalamus relays somatosensory information to the primary somatosensory cortex. The ventral lateral nucleus of the thalamus relays information from the basal ganglia and cerebellum to the motor cortex. The MGN of the thalamus relays auditory information to the primary auditory cortex in the transverse gyrus of Heschl.

3. D. Gait disturbance, incontinence, and confusion are the three principle features of NPH. Remember that these patients are wacky, wobbly, and wet. The frontal release signs listed in the other choices may also be seen, but they are not part of the classic triad.

4. B. Orbitofrontal lesions tend to be associated with impulsive behavior and disruption of normal mood and affect. The other behavioral problems are associated with dorsolateral prefrontal lesions.

CASE 10-3

1. C. Homonymous visual field defects (field cuts) are localized posterior to the optic chiasm. Lesions involving the optic tracts, LGN, or occipital cortex result in homonymous hemianopias. However, the optic radiations are much more diffuse and difficult to disrupt with a single lesion. Lesions of the optic radiations cause homonymous quadrantanopia. Temporal lobe lesions can injure the fibers of the Meyer loop, which carry information corresponding to the upper portion of the visual field (and lower retina), resulting in a homonymous superior quadrantanopia. The Meyer loop can extend almost all the way to the temporal pole. The optic radiations that carry information from the lower portion of the visual field (and upper retina) project directly posterior from the LGN to the visual cortex, passing through the parietal cortex. Parietal cortex lesions can be associated with homonymous inferior quadrantanopia. Quadrantanopia can also be seen with partial lesions of the visual cortex.

2. B. The inferior temporal cortex is associated with the analysis of form and color. Stimulation of this area, as with a seizure, can be associated with visual hallucinations. The posterior parietal cortex is involved in the processing of depth perception and motion. The occipitotemporal junction is involved in face recognition. The angular gyrus is involved with the visual recognition of objects. The calcarine cortex contains the primary visual cortex. Stimulation of this area is associated with flashes of light, not formed images.

3. D. V1 corresponds to the primary visual cortex. Stimulation of this area is perceived as flashes of light. V2 and V3 correspond to secondary visual cortex and the processing of simple forms. V3 is associated with the processing of complex forms. V4 is associated with the processing of color information. V5 is involved in processing information regarding the motion of objects. Lesions in this area can be associated with illusions of motion.

4. E. Discussed with the previous answer.

CASE 10-4

1. C. Altered mentation in the setting of alcoholism should always raise concern for the possibility of Wernicke-Korsakoff syndrome. This is a syndrome resulting from thiamine deficiency in the diet, most commonly seen in the setting of alcoholism. Atrophy of the mammillary bodies is the most commonly sited anatomic finding. Hypertrophy of the pituitary gland would be associated with hormonal abnormalities. The most common clinical association for an enlarged pituitary gland is pregnancy. This can be so prominent as to cause visual field deficits related to compression of the optic chiasm (bitemporal visual field deficits). The other choices are not commonly encountered.

2. B. The syndrome that is described is gelastic epilepsy. It is most commonly associated with bouts of uncontrolled and mirthless laughter. The most commonly encountered anatomic disturbance in these cases is a hamartoma in the hypothalamus. These seizures can be difficult to treat, and surgical resection is controversial. The remaining structures are more commonly associated with seizures but less likely to be associated with this kind of seizure.

3. D. Temperature regulation is mediated by the posterior hypothalamus. The other functions are all mediated by the anterior hypothalamus and would be expected to be disrupted by lesions in this area.

4. A. The control of appetite has been associated with the middle hypothalamic regions, including the tuberal and lateral areas. All of the other processes are associated with the posterior hypothalamus and would be expected to be disrupted by lesions in this area.

CASE 10-5

1. D. Ischemic damage would cause a decrease in all the hormones released from the anterior pituitary, including ACTH, FSH, LH, TSH, and prolactin. Decreased ACTH would manifest as a decrease in cortisol, whereas lowered TSH levels would cause decreased T_4 secretion. ADH is released by the posterior pituitary and would not be affected in Sheehan syndrome.

2. D. The patient has a pituitary adenoma composed of acidophilic cells, so the tumor must have arisen from lactotrophs or somatotrophs. A GH-secreting adenoma would cause symptoms of acromegaly and glucose intolerance (answer D). Basophilic cells in ACTH-secreting adenoma would cause symptoms of hypercortisolism, such as altered fat distribution, diabetes, and hypertension (answer A). A TSH-secreting adenoma could cause symptoms of hyperthyroidism and appear basophilic on histology (answer B). Although prolactinoma does consist of acidophilic cells and can cause headache, it would be expected to cause galactorrhea and amenorrhea, not impairment of lactation or menorrhagia (answer C). Finally, inability to concentrate urine would be seen in diabetes insipidus, caused by decreased ADH secretion from the posterior pituitary (answer E).

3. A. TSH, LH, and FSH all share the same (subunit. ACTH and MSH have a similar precursor, pro-opiomelanocortin (POMC), but are not related structurally to TSH, LH, and FSH (answers B through E).

4. D. Vasopressin is another name for ADH. ADH is normally secreted by cells of the posterior lobe receiving projections from the supraoptic hypothalamus. It regulates fluid balance and urine concentration. Acidophilic cells of the anterior lobe secrete prolactin and GH (answer A). Basophilic cells of the anterior lobe secrete FSH, LH, ACTH, and TSH (answer B). The region of the posterior lobe with inputs from the paraventricular hypothalamus secretes oxytocin (answer C). No part of the posterior lobe receives signals through the portal venous system (answer E).

CASE 10-6

1. E. Postganglionic sympathetic innervation to the head enters the skull along the carotid arteries. Any carotid artery injury can be associated with ipsilateral sympathetic dysfunction. Elimination of the sympathetic tone on the left, as in this case, would result in unopposed parasympathetic function and relative pupillary constriction on the same side (miosis on the left). A carotid artery dissection can be associated with an ipsilateral Horner syndrome (miosis, anhydrosis, ptosis).

2. B. Postganglionic parasympathetic innervation to the eye travels along the surface of the third cranial nerve. Compression of this nerve by an extrinsic mass would be associated with ipsilateral parasympathetic dysfunction. Elimination of the parasympathetic tone, as in this case, would result in unopposed sympathetic function and relative pupillary dilation on the same side (mydriasis on the right).

3. B. The syndrome described in this case is Hirschsprung disease, or congenital megacolon. It is associated with a lack of parasympathetic neurons within the enteric ganglia of a segment of colon. This results in hypomotility of that segment of colon and associated fecal retention. Colostomy and resection or bypass of the affected segment are potential therapies.

4. E. Of the given choices, the most likely neurons to have been affected are preganglionic parasympathetic neurons in the sacral spinal cord. These neurons help mediate erectile function. The cranial portion of the parasympathetic system does not innervate the reproductive organs. The sympathetic system mediates ejaculatory function and uterine relaxation in females rather than erectile function.

CASE 10-7

1. D. Dorsal horn lesions affect all sensory systems within the corresponding ipsilateral dermatome, because dorsal column, spinothalamic, and spinocerebellar fibers all enter at the dorsal horn. Thus, this patient should have complete loss of sensation, including fine touch, vibration, pain, temperature, and proprioception (conscious and unconscious). This is suggested by the case presentation, in which ipsilateral pain/temperature loss is noted at the site of the lesion at the left T10 dermatome.

2. C. This patient's diffuse loss of sensation, particularly a sensory ataxia (difficulty walking due to inability to sense joint position) and positive Romberg sign, suggests dorsal column dysfunction with apparent sparing of the motor and spinothalamic systems. In addition, absent pupillary response to light suggests an Argyll-Robertson pupil (sometimes remembered as "like a prostitute, the pupil accommodates but does not respond to light") consistent with neurosyphilis. Overall, the sensory ataxia is suggestive of tabes dorsalis. Peripheral neuropathies generally are not this dramatic, although syringomyelia should present with pain or lack of sensation to pain with intact proprioception. Subacute combined systems degeneration may cause weakness and should not affect pupillary reflexes; Brown-Séquard syndrome would cause unilateral plegia and fine sensory loss.

3. B. This patient's presentation is suggestive of syringomyelia, with a "cape-like" distribution of lack of sensation to pain and characteristic burning pain in the arms. She is also shown to have an Arnold-Chiari malformation with downward-displaced cerebellar tonsils, which is not a prerequisite for a syrinx. Foraminal stenosis would be expected to give shooting radicular pain, which would not affect the torso in the cervical spine. Diffuse demyelination (MS) would be expected to have more widespread symptoms, and cord compression would give sensory loss and weakness below the level of the lesion with possible bowel/bladder incontinence. A normal scan is possible for peripheral neuropathies, which usually affect the feet and hands before affecting the torso.

4. A. This patient's lack of sensation appears to fit a "glove and stocking" distribution most consistent with peripheral neuropathy. A homeless patient with a possible history of alcohol abuse may develop neuropathy secondary to alcohol abuse itself, as well as nutritional deficiencies such as folate, B12, or B vitamins deficiency, in addition to other possibilities such as diabetes. Subacute combined systems degeneration would be expected to have motor involvement and be more widespread. Syringomyelia usually affects the cervical cord, which does not localize to the distal extremities. Tabes dorsalis should be more widespread and potentially more profound. MS should also have a more diffuse, unpredictable pattern and may cause weakness.

CASE 10-8

1. C. This patient has LMN findings in the upper extremity and UMN findings in the lower extremity. This pattern implicates the cervical spinal cord, where the LMNs for the upper extremity are located. UMNs destined for the lower extremity pass through this area and are affected. Potential causes include traumatic, vascular, neoplastic, infectious, and inflammatory causes.

2. E. This patient's clinical picture is consistent with motor neuron disease, such as ALS. In its classic form, this is a motor neuron disease that affects both LMNs and UMNs. The remaining options would be associated with diminished reflexes.

3. E. A previous history of demyelinating disease in another CNS region supports the diagnosis of MS. A clinical history of optic neuritis, however, should raise the suspicion for Devic disease. This inflammatory condition is localized to the spinal cord and optic nerves. It is considered a distinct entity rather than a subtype of MS, because the mechanism of injury does not remain limited to white matter. These lesions involve both gray and white matter very aggressively. This is thought to be mediated via involvement of CNS vasculature. These patients generally respond poorly to conventional steroid management, and early aggressive intervention, such as plasma exchange, has been advocated by some.

4. D. Brisk reflexes, pathologic reflexes (such as the Babinski response), and eventual spasticity are the results of injury to UMNs and associated descending pathways. There is relative increase of sensory impact on alpha motor neuron function and increased alpha motor neuron activity, but these effects are secondary to the lack of regulatory input from higher centers.

CASE 10-9

1. B. The constellation of neck pain and pain radiating in a dermatomal pattern is typical for a radiculopathy, with both C7 and C8 radiculopathies (C7 is more common) being likely to affect the fingers (C6 might affect the thumb, but dermatomes vary slightly among different individuals). Patients with stenosis of the spinal canal are more likely to develop radiculopathies as well. Triceps involvement also suggests C7 or C8 radicular involvement. Radial nerve injury could cause triceps weakness but is unlikely to cause neck pain. C6 will not involve the triceps, and neither will the musculocutaneous nerve. Cord compression may cause pain but it is less likely to be shooting pain; it might also cause weakness of the arm(s) and leg(s) and possible bowel/bladder incontinence.

2. E. It appears that only a dorsal nerve root is affected, as the patient only has a sensory deficit, making a peripheral nerve injury or ventral nerve root injury unlikely. The sole of the foot is generally confined to the S1 dermatome. The S1 dermatome generally also involves the lateral aspect of the foot and may involve part of the back of the lower extremity.

3. B. EHL involvement is specific to the L5 myotome, which makes it a useful physical finding. In addition, the L5 dermatome usually involves the dorsal foot, as seen with this patient, and the shooting leg pain may be consistent with a radiculopathy (sciatica, which is discussed later, often involves the back of the leg). An L4 radiculopathy would not involve the EHL, and neither would S1

or S2 (these would be expected to affect the ankle jerk and ankle plantar flexion). A lumbar myelopathy would likely involve more myotomes/dermatomes throughout the lower lumbar and sacral nerves and might present with bowel or bladder symptoms.

4. E. Myelopathy is the best explanation due to the stool incontinence seen with this patient. The stool incontinence seen with jarring impact is particularly worrisome for unstable spine fracture with loose bone compressing the cord with each bump, making stable transport and immediate surgery crucial to minimize permanent spinal cord injury. Bowel incontinence may arise from compression at any point above the sacral cord, and the reduced pinprick at and below the kneecaps suggests cord compression/myelopathy localized to L4 with some preservation of spinal cord function (otherwise complete anesthesia would result). Radiculopathy or lumbar spinal nerve transection alone would not cause bowel incontinence, and L4 nerve transection would cause total anesthesia over the L4 dermatome (over the kneecaps). High cervical cord transection would result in quadriplegia and, possibly, respiratory paralysis.

5. C. With such a confusing array of findings, it is worthwhile to take each physical finding one at a time to find certain things that you can "hang your hat on"—that is, that definitively demonstrate a particular type of injury. The inability to extend the wrist (waiter's tip) is consistent only with radial nerve injury, which is associated with fractures of the humeral shaft, presumably by shearing the radial nerve as it courses around the humerus. Ulnar nerve injury is associated with elbow dislocation and is the cause of this patient's ulnar claw. Finally, the presence of thenar atrophy can only be consistent with *chronic* carpal tunnel syndrome, as muscular atrophy takes weeks to develop.

6. B. Elderly patients with neck pain and degenerative changes in the spine often develop cervical radiculopathy secondary to compression of nerve roots from bone spurs and flattening of the intervertebral discs. This results in dermatomal anesthesia (the C6 dermatome runs along the anterolateral arm toward the thumb), frequent neck pain due to the arthritic changes, and myotomal weakness (biceps and deltoids are innervated by C5, C6). C5 radiculopathies are also known to cause referred pain to the scapular region (perhaps similar to how diaphragmatic pain also refers to this area, which is also innervated by C5). The median nerve does none of these things. The axillary nerve does not serve the biceps. Musculocutaneous injury could cause biceps weakness, and possibly anterior arm anesthesia, but not deltoid weakness. An upper brachial plexus injury could present in similar fashion but would be likely to involve more widespread weakness and/or anesthesia; it is also unlikely to present spontaneously without any trauma.

CASE 10-10

1. E. The obturator nerve, which governs adductor function and the ability to cross one's leg, is susceptible to compression against the bony pelvis during vaginal delivery. Inability to dorsiflex the foot is the hallmark of a foot drop. Foot drop may be seen after general or epidural anesthesia, usually due to compression of the common peroneal nerve against a bed rail or other part of the bed. Sciatica would possibly involve the hamstrings but not the thigh adductors; it generally does not result in foot drop. The femoral nerve innervates the quadriceps and would cause weakness of knee extension.

2. B. S1 radiculopathy is suggested by the pain along the back of the leg (S1 dermatome) in conjunction with absent ankle jerk and weakness of plantar flexion. Sciatica could present in a similar pattern; however, the onset of symptoms after lifting is more likely to precipitate radiculopathy, often via disc herniation. Common peroneal nerve injury would present with foot drop (dorsiflexor weakness), not plantar flexion weakness. Tarsal tunnel syndrome involves only the sole of the foot. Femoral nerve palsy would be restricted to the thigh and quadriceps muscles.

3. E. Traumatic injury to the head of the fibula causes compression injury to the common peroneal nerve, which may result in a transient foot drop, a fact known and exploited by police and other personnel when necessary. The common peroneal nerve passes over the head of the fibula, making it susceptible to compression injury. Tibial nerve injury does not cause foot drop. Sciatica is not generally caused by trauma, and neither does it cause isolated foot drop. A fibular head fracture alone would not cause a foot drop but would cause localized pain lasting more than a few hours. The femoral nerve is nowhere near the fibular head, and nor would it cause foot drop.

4. E. The pattern of thigh anesthesia, hip flexor weakness, and quadriceps weakness is suggestive of femoral nerve dysfunction. The femoral nerve is particularly susceptible to compression from retroperitoneal processes because it runs along the bony pelvis near the iliopsoas muscle, which affords little space to move. The sciatic nerve is not susceptible to retroperitoneal compression and does not innervate the hip flexors. The obturator nerve may be compressed within the pelvis, but it would cause thigh adductor weakness. Hematomas generally do not cause radiculopathies because the nerve root is surrounded by the bony spine, which is protective in this case.

CASE 10-11

1. C. A single lesion cannot explain all of the clinical findings. Monocular involvement in this case implicates the left optic nerve or globe. The abnormal reflex findings suggest a UMN lesion involving either the left side of the spinal cord or a right-sided lesion above the pyramidal decussation. A midbrain lesion would not cause a visual field defect. Neurologic symptoms separated by space and time are a clinical hallmark of MS. This diagnosis could be confirmed by evidence of demyelinating white matter lesions on MRI of the brain and spinal cord. Demyelination also could be confirmed by laboratory analysis of the CSF.

2. D. Meyer loop describes the inferior-most optic radiations, which carry information from the upper quadrant of the contralateral visual field. On leaving the LGN, these fibers course anteriorly and superiorly around the temporal horn of the lateral ventricle, passing within a few centimeters of the temporal pole before turning toward the visual cortex. Contralateral quadrantanopia is a potential complication of temporal lobectomy.

3. D. The pituitary gland can become significantly enlarged during pregnancy. This can sometimes result in compression of the optic chiasm, which would be expected to cause bitemporal (peripheral) visual symptoms. Pituitary tumor would be an important consideration. An electrical disturbance of the visual cortex could present in this manner, although there is no history of either seizure or migraine. Also, a large portion of the visual cortex is devoted to central vision. An electrical disturbance originating in

the visual cortex would be less likely to remain isolated in the peripheral visual field. An optic tract lesion on one side would produce contralateral symptoms. Simultaneous bilateral optic tract lesions would be unusual.

4. A. The patient has described amaurosis fugax, transient obstruction of blood flow through the ophthalmic artery. This is often an embolic event, which would be consistent with his medical history. Retinal ischemia is usually hemispheric, rather than involving the whole eye. Optic chiasm lesions cause heteronymous (bitemporal) visual disturbance. Optic tract and visual cortex deficits cause homonymous defects (perceived similarly in both eyes).

CASE 10-12

1. B. This patient most likely has SUNCT (short-lasting, unilateral, neuralgiform headaches with conjunctival injection and tearing). This syndrome is often associated with rhinorrhea and forehead sweating. The ophthalmic division of the trigeminal nerve is most commonly involved. Attacks last only seconds to a few minutes but can occur multiple times per day or even multiple times per hour. The syndrome is less responsive to treatment than is trigeminal neuralgia. Sinus disease would not relapse and remit so abruptly. Involvement of the trigeminal ganglion would likely not be restricted to only one division of the trigeminal nerve. Involvement of the ophthalmic artery would compromise vision. Involvement of the ciliary ganglion would likely involve pupillary abnormalities.

2. C. Right facial sensory disturbance localizes to the right trigeminal nerve, nucleus or tract. Left extremity sensory disturbance localizes to the ascending spinothalamic systems, which decussate in the medulla. The findings are consistent with a small lesion, likely a lacunar infarction, in the right dorsal pontine tegmentum involving the trigeminal nucleus and nearby medial lemniscus.

3. D. This patient has a Bell palsy on the left. The seventh cranial nerve (facial) is affected. This nerve mediates motor control to the face. Innervation to the upper face has bihemispheric representation. The fact that both the upper and lower face are affected suggests an LMN lesion. This is likely a peripheral lesion. A central lesion would spare motor function in the upper face. Branches of the trigeminal nerve briefly carry taste from the anterior two thirds of the tongue, but these fibers pass to the facial nerve via the chorda tympani nerve. The facial nerve does not mediate any other sensory function. However, patients with Bell palsy often complain of subjectively altered sensation on the affected side. The physiologic basis for this is not clear.

4. C. This patient also has Bell palsy. The masseter muscle is spared, as are all of the muscles of mastication. These muscles are innervated by the trigeminal nerve, not the facial nerve. The levator palpebrae muscle also is spared because it is innervated by the third cranial nerve (oculomotor). Patients with peripheral seventh nerve palsies have facial weakness and difficulty closing their eyes (instead of ptosis).

CASE 10-13

1. A. This constellation of symptoms is the precise deficiency that would occur with complete compromise of CN VII. This would involve the motor, sensory, and secretory fibers, resulting in hemifacial palsy, loss of taste (from the fibers coming from the chorda tympani), hyperacusis (from loss of stapedius function), and loss of the sensory and secretory functions. All of these findings will be ipsilateral to the involved facial nerve. Lower facial palsy occurs when the UMNs (corticobulbar fibers) are compromised, such as in the case of stroke.

2. D. The taste of the anterior two thirds of the tongue is governed by fibers that run along CN V, then diverge to form the chorda tympani (which runs in the middle ear), joins CN VII in the facial canal, and then diverge to the nucleus solitarius in the brainstem. The chorda tympani is thus susceptible to middle ear processes, and otitis media may result in chorda tympani dysfunction. Stroke, which involves the motor cortex without involving sensation, would not be expected to involve taste. The areas of the cortex that are associated with taste are not entirely clear. Bell palsy is unlikely in a patient with only a left-sided *lower* facial droop.

3. D. Ablation of the motor fibers of the facial nerve within the parotid gland will result in hemifacial palsy only, because the other fibers of the facial nerve have already diverged at that point. In contrast, a Bell palsy involves the facial nerve within the facial canal, affecting autonomic fibers governing salivation, taste fibers, and the nerve to the stapedius, whose compromise leads to hyperacusis. Facial sensation is governed by the trigeminal nerve and should not be affected by the facial nerve in any circumstance.

4. A. Lacrimation during a salivary stimulus in a patient with previous facial nerve injury (due to Bell palsy or other causes) is the syndrome of crocodile tears. This is believed to occur because of inappropriate regeneration of facial nerve fibers along the wrong tracts, so fibers that should innervate salivary glands grow into the lacrimal glands. This may also occur with motor fibers, leading to facial twitching or hemifacial spasm when the patient attempts to smile or otherwise use the face, known as *synkinesis*. A recurrent Bell palsy would not necessarily be different from a first episode of Bell palsy, and conjunctivitis will give persistent lacrimation, as would a hyperlacrimation syndrome. Crocodile tears and synkinesis are considered abnormal outcomes, so they are not a prodrome of normal recoveries.

CASE 10-14

1. D. In a patient with known MS, one would have to assume the symptoms are related to demyelination until proven otherwise. Although large demyelinating lesions can impinge on adjacent gray matter, this patient does not seem to have a large brainstem lesion, which would likely be associated with other symptoms. Thus, involvement of the cochlear or superior olivary nuclei is not likely. Lesions in the lateral lemniscus or trapezoid body are central to the cochlear nuclei in the auditory pathways and thus would not be associated with unilateral hearing loss. A demyelinating lesion in the lateral pons could involve fascicles of the eighth nerve before they reach the cochlear nuclei.

2. A. This patient has a conductive hearing loss. Excessive buildup of cerumen can cause conductive hearing loss. All of the other choices are more likely to be associated with sensorineural hearing loss.

3. E. Ménière disease is associated with attacks of severe vertigo and decreased hearing. Vomiting, tinnitus, and fullness in the ears are also common associations. Symptoms are usually more

prominent on one side. This condition is associated with increased endolymph pressure and distended semicircular canals. The cause of this syndrome is not known, but altered ionic flow is suspected and supported by the benefit some patients derive from dietary salt restriction. Shunting of the endolymphatic space can spare hearing in some cases.

4. D. This patient has the classic features of Bell palsy (seventh CN palsy). Hyperacusis can be seen in this condition because of involvement of the nerve to the stapedius muscle on the affected side. A slow-growing lesion would be less likely to cause an abrupt onset of symptoms.

CASE 10-15

1. C. Of the given choices, a left-sided Horner syndrome caused by involvement of the ipsilateral sympathetic pathways projecting from the hypothalamus to the intermediolateral cell columns of the spinal cord is most likely. This is a lateral pontine syndrome, most likely caused by infarction of the left AICA or other long circumferential branches. The relatively ventromedial corticospinal tract is spared. Tongue deviation would require involvement of either the corticospinal tract or the hypoglossal nucleus or nerve in the medulla. "Down and out" eye deviation implicates the oculomotor nerve or nucleus in the midbrain. Furthermore, all of these motor structures are close to the midline and would most likely be spared in a lateral syndrome.

2. D. A right one-and-a-half syndrome is described. Involvement of the right sixth nerve nucleus disrupts function of the right lateral rectus. The left lateral rectus is intact, so the left sixth nerve nucleus cannot be involved. Both eyes have impaired adduction on horizontal gaze with intact adduction on vergence (reading). In this syndrome, a single lesion has to affect the ipsilateral sixth nerve nucleus, fibers from that nucleus destined for the contralateral MLF and the ipsilateral MLF. The only horizontal gaze movement left intact is lateral gaze in the eye contralateral to the lesion.

3. A. Pontine lacunar infarctions are most likely to be the result of thrombosis of small pontine penetrating branches from the basilar artery. The basilar artery runs along the inferior surface of the pons.

4. D. The trochlear nerve is located at the junction of the midbrain and the pons. Its fibers do not pass through the body of the pons before exiting the brainstem. The remaining nerves either have their nuclei contained within the pons or have fascicles passing through the body of the pons.

CASE 10-16

1. A. This patient's symptoms appear to localize to Wernicke area and the left motor strip. The patient is able to produce speech that is not understandable (word salad) and is unable to understand speech (receptive aphasia). The right-sided lower facial droop and arm weakness are consistent with left motor strip involvement. A brainstem infarct would not cause aphasia; facial nucleus involvement causes **lower** and **upper** facial droop and dysarthria. Broca area infarct would cause a Broca aphasia, with inability to form words. Left ACA infarct would affect the leg and spare the face and arm. Finally, right-sided lesions would cause left-sided symptoms and, very rarely, aphasias.

2. B. Although the process causing this patient's expressive aphasia is not inherently clear, this is the only answer that localizes the infarct to Broca area in the posterior frontal lobe of the dominant hemisphere, the correct location. A stroke such as this one in an otherwise healthy patient is often from a paradoxical embolus of some kind in the presence of a patent foramen ovale, with oral contraceptives use and smoking as risk factors A temporal lobe infarct might cause a receptive, not an expressive, aphasia. A frontal lobe hemorrhage or carotid occlusion is possible in the setting of paradoxical thromboembolus in this patient, but her symptoms localize to the left side, not to the right. Septic emboli are not likely, and parietal lesions are not generally associated with aphasias.

3. B. This gentleman appears to be experiencing acute retinal artery occlusion, with abrupt and total inability to see out of the affected eye due to retinal ischemia. A pale retina due to absence of blood flow confirms the diagnosis. If this spontaneously remits, then it is **amaurosis fugax** (transient monocular blindness caused by temporary retinal artery occlusion), which signifies unstable carotid atherosclerotic disease and possible impending stroke. A disrupted plaque fragment from the ICA temporarily occludes the ophthalmic artery, causing retinal ischemia. Ocular migraines are controversial and are associated with monocular visual disturbances, not total visual loss. Occipital lobe infarcts will affect one visual **field,** but not the vision of one eye. Elevated ICP may cause papilledema but will not cause abrupt monocular blindness.

4. A. Diffuse weakness affecting the entire leg without respect to peripheral nerve territories is best explained by medial frontal lobe infarct, which would be caused by ACA occlusion (and not the MCA, which serves the motor strip of the face and arm). The ACoA joins the two anterior cerebral arteries and would not cause a stroke unless the ACA relied on it for blood flow due to more proximal occlusion. A pelvic mass would usually affect one nerve, would likely affect sensation, and would likely cause edema. Deep venous thrombosis should not cause weakness per se.

CASE 10-17

1. B. Weakness is not a prominent feature of the lateral medullary (Wallenberg) syndrome. The motor pathways are spared because they are supplied by paramedian branches from both vertebral arteries. One would expect to see an ipsilateral Horner syndrome in the context of a lateral medullary infarction. Loss of pain and temperature would, on the other hand, be seen contralateral to the lesion. Additional findings would include ipsilateral ataxia from involvement of the cerebellar peduncles, dysarthria and dysphagia from involvement of the lower cranial nerves, vertigo and nystagmus from involvement of the vestibular nuclei, ipsilateral altered facial sensation from involvement of the trigeminal nucleus, and impaired taste from involvement of the solitary nucleus. Most commonly, the clinical picture does not include all of the features of the classic syndrome.

2. B. Complete sensory loss to all modalities in half of the body usually can be localized above the brainstem, or in the rostral brainstem. More caudal lesions are likely to result in crossed sensory findings involving the face on one side and the contralateral body. They are also likely to be seen in association with other findings. Isolated thalamic injury can result in complete sensory loss with no other associated findings. Most of

the thalamus derives its blood supply from branches of the PCA and PCoA. Cortical involvement would be less likely to lead to this because the vascular territory for the regions representing the face and arm is different from that representing the leg. Involvement of the internal capsule often results in hemiparesis.

3. D. A hemianopia, or "field cut," is associated with disruption of the visual pathway posterior to the optic chiasm. A complete hemianopia, as opposed to involvement of just one quadrant, indicates that the visual cortex is affected contralateral to the perceived deficit. In this case, the vascular territory most likely to have been affected is that of the PCA on the left.

4. B. The only objective finding on exam implicates the cerebellum. The lesion would have to be on the same side as the deficit. The right PICA is the only choice that could affect the cerebellum in isolation on that side. Although one would not expect prominent weakness with a lateral medullary or cerebellar process (for the reasons outlined earlier), subtle weakness can be associated with cerebellar lesions. It is also not unusual for large cerebellar lesions to manifest with relatively mild clinical symptoms. The MCA is also a good choice here but would be expected to result in some degree of objective weakness and language impairment because we are told the stroke is large.

CASE 10-18

1. C. Thrombosis of the transverse sinus can extend inferiorly to involve the sigmoid sinus and vessels that empty into it. The labyrinthine structures are drained by the labyrinthine vein. Blood flows from this vein into the inferior petrosal sinus, then into the sigmoid sinus. The neurologic deficits associated with sinus thrombosis depend on the region being drained. Although this patient's headache is relatively nonspecific, new onset of vertigo and hearing loss need to be evaluated. The combination of vertigo and hearing loss suggests a peripheral lesion involving the eighth cranial nerve or the labyrinthine structures. Thrombosis of the other vessels listed would not be expected to produce vertigo or hearing deficits.

2. D. Because of its location in the midline, thrombosis of the superior sagittal sinus can present with bilateral motor cortex deficits involving the legs. Remember that the motor cortex is topographically organized as a homunculus. The regions of the cortex controlling lower extremity function are located medially, along the midline, whereas the regions controlling the upper extremities and face are more lateral. Thus, a single midline lesion can cause bilateral lower extremity deficits. The other vessels listed are paired vessels, located on either side of the midline. Involvement of any one of these vessels would not be expected to cause bilateral deficits. This question, together with the case at the beginning of this chapter, highlights the broad clinical range with which sinus thrombosis can present.

3. D. Cavernous sinus thrombosis is associated with proptosis and pain involving the eye, the orbit, and the head on one side. It often presents unilaterally but can spread to involve both sides. Diabetic patients are relatively immunocompromised and susceptible to fungal infections. The combination of fungal infection, diabetes, and cavernous sinus thrombosis is a clinical emergency. Outcome without treatment is often poor. It is frequently tested for this reason.

4. A. Hemorrhage resulting from venous occlusion occurs with the brain parenchyma first. Extension into the subarachnoid space can be seen with superficial parenchymal bleeding as a secondary event. Venous hemorrhage would not be as commonly associated with bleeding in the other spaces listed.

CASE 10-19

1. C. Immediate initiation of appropriate antibiotic therapy is paramount when the diagnosis of bacterial meningitis is considered, because a few hours may make the difference between complete cure and death. Antibiotics should be given before head CT or lumbar puncture are obtained; head CT should precede lumbar puncture in the setting of an abnormality on neurologic exam to rule out obstructing masses. Ampicillin should be added to any young or elderly patient with suspected bacterial meningitis for coverage of *Listeria*. Bony cause of neck stiffness is much less likely than meningismus in this setting, making plain neck films of little use.

2. B. A change in mental status after a fall in an elderly person should raise concerns for subdural hematoma. These will often attain a size that exhibits enough mass effect to cause confusion and possible focal neurologic signs without progressing further, whereas an epidural hematoma is at greater risk of a mass effect because of the higher arterial pressure. Meningioma could create similar symptoms after a slow progression, not abruptly after a fall. Fungal meningitis is unlikely in a patient who is not immunocompromised and it is less likely to be abrupt; Alzheimer disease also does not have abrupt onset. Viral meningitis should not persist for 3 months, and it generally does not cause confusion (unless accompanied by encephalitis).

3. B. This is a setup for an epidural hematoma, which is trauma to the temple with skull fracture, which may result in middle meningeal artery rupture. Her presentation is consistent with the "lucid interval" seen before the mass effect from the expanding hematoma compromises consciousness. A cerebral contusion alone should not cause coma, and a subdural hematoma (answer B, crescentic mass) is less likely in a young person, particularly with such aggressive mass effect. No acute traumatic event results in a calcified mass (calcification is a chronic process), and cerebral edema, although a possibility, is also unlikely to cause such rapid deterioration of consciousness.

4. D. This patient's clinical course is most consistent with viral meningitis because it has resolved spontaneously without treatment, now allowing an essentially normal exam without mental status changes. A bacterial, mycobacterial, or fungal meningitis, which are the most worrisome concerns, would not improve without treatment, and if he presented when his symptoms were acute he would have deserved full empiric treatment for bacterial meningitis until the diagnosis could be made. Syphilitic meningitis is a theoretical possibility that may be addressed via a simple blood test. Therefore, antibiotics and head CT/MRI are not required, and a lumbar puncture is unlikely to give additional information (a resolving lymphocytic pleocytosis is anticipated) and runs the risk of complications. Should his symptoms worsen, he should return immediately for another evaluation.

CASE 10-20

1. E. MS is a demyelinating disease of the CNS. Because oligodendrocytes are responsible for myelin in the CNS, their structure and function are expected to be impaired (answer A). The resulting deficit in conduction can result in faulty "UMN" input to the extremities, which is demonstrated as weakness or hyperreflexia (answers B and C). The optic nerve is a part of the CNS and thus can also cause impaired vision in MS (answer D). Schwann cells provide myelin to the PNS, which is not a primary source of pathology in MS.

2. D. Conduction velocity is the speed at which the action potential travels down the axon. It increases with ion channel density, degree of myelination, and axon diameter. Of these factors, myelination is the most critical. Although the length of an axon may affect the absolute time required for a signal to travel from one nerve to another, this does not affect the conduction velocity of the signal.

3. B. As discussed in the Clinical Correlate section, gliosis, or glial scar formation, impairs neuronal signaling. Glial scars replace myelin and act as barriers to the transmission of action potentials. Myelin is the substance that would insulate the axonal membrane, not glial tissue (answer A). Although axons of larger diameter do have faster conduction velocities, glial deposition would not make the axon itself larger (answer C). Glial scars replace oligodendrocytes in the CNS; oligodendrocytes normally provide myelin to increase conduction velocity (answer D). Finally, glial scars do not increase the density of ion channels (answer E).

4. E. This patient has a classic presentation of Guillain-Barré syndrome: After a viral illness, she subsequently developed weakness of the lower extremities, which is spreading upward. The finding of areflexia is particularly important, indicating that there is a problem at the level of the PNS (reflexes remain present and are often heightened in upper motor lesions). Schwann cells provide myelin in the PNS, which is affected in Guillain-Barré syndrome. The axon hillock is the junction between the neuronal cell body and the axon in both the CNS and the PNS; it is not affected in Guillain-Barré (answer A). Likewise, nodes of Ranvier are present in myelinated axons in both the CNS and the PNS and are not the target of demyelinating disease (answer B). Axonal ion channels can be subject to autoimmune attack, but the presentation of such diseases is usually generalized and does not follow the "distal upward" pattern described here (answer C). Oligodendrocytes are solely in the CNS and are not affected in PNS disease (answer E).

CASE 10-21

1. D. The dopamine in the striatum and the cortex is identical; the receptors determine the postsynaptic response. Which ion channels are opened or closed by a given receptor determines whether the postsynaptic effect is excitatory or inhibitory. Therefore, varying levels of dopamine release or degradation are not responsible for the different types of effects (answers A and E); they only determine the degree of effect. Ionotropic receptors are those that directly open ligand-gated ion channels; metabotropic receptors are those that act through a second messenger.

Although these are different receptor types, both have excitatory and inhibitory subtypes. Whether a second messenger is involved does not determine what type of response a receptor evokes (answer B). (Furthermore, all dopaminergic receptors act through G-protein receptors; there are no known ionotropic dopamine receptors.) Likewise, the affinity of the receptors for their neurotransmitter ligand is unrelated to the type of effect it evokes (answer C).

2. D. The spinal neuron in the question has both glutamate and glycine receptors on its membrane. While the glutamate receptors open Na^+ channels, which cause EPSPs, the glycine receptor opens Cl^- channels, which cause IPSPs. Glycine is an important inhibitory neurotransmitter in the spinal cord because activating its receptors causes a hyperpolarization, bringing the postsynaptic membrane far below threshold. Even simultaneous excitation is then insufficient to trigger an action potential. Glycine acts on its own receptors without directly interacting with glutamate at the synapse (answers A and B). Postsynaptic neurotransmitter receptors are specific for their ligand. Therefore, glycine does not act through direct competitive inhibition (answer C). Finally, glycine has no effect on glutamate reuptake mechanisms (answer E).

3. E. ACh esterase is the enzyme that degrades ACh, clearing it from the synapse at the end of signal transmission. ACh esterase inhibitors block this enzyme and thus permit ACh to remain in the synaptic cleft longer. Without the clearing of the cleft between signals, new signals cannot be sent between neurons, and thus neuronal signaling overall is impaired. Although the other mechanisms described would inhibit signaling, none are the targets of ACh esterase inhibitors.

4. E. SSRIs have the net effect of increasing serotonergic activity. They do this by inhibiting reuptake of serotonin from the synaptic cleft back into the presynaptic terminal (not the postsynaptic terminal, as in answer (C). As a result, serotonin remains in the cleft longer and acts on postsynaptic receptors more. (This mechanism has been a USMLE favorite.) Although answers (A), (B), and (D) all describe ways to increase activity at the synapse, none are the targets of SSRIs.

CASE 10-22

1. C. Chlorpromazine and haloperidol are both antipsychotic drugs commonly prescribed for schizophrenia. Both selectively block D_2 receptors and are generally not used together because they have the same mechanism of action. In a subset of patients, particularly those using a high dose of these drugs, early in the course of treatment, a parkinsonism can arise. Most often this is reversible by either decreasing the antipsychotic or adding an antiparkinsonism agent. Symptoms can resolve over a few months. Even if you were unfamiliar with this syndrome, this question only requires you to know which of the listed enzymes directly acts on L-dopa. (C) is the only possible correct answer. Phenylalanine hydroxylase (A) acts to convert phenylalanine to tyrosine and is deficient in PKU. Tyrosine hydroxylase (B) is the rate-limiting step in natural dopamine synthesis, converting tyrosine to dopa. However, administering exogenous dopa bypasses this enzyme. MAO-A (D) metabolizes NE and serotonin; it is a target of antidepressants and not involved in dopamine synthesis. MAO-B (E) metabolizes dopamine in the brain, which would

have the opposite of the desired effect. In fact, selegiline is an example of an MAO-B inhibitor, which has been used with some success in treating parkinsonism.

2. D. Parkinsonism results when dopaminergic cells of the substantia nigra compacta are lost. The cells of the substantia nigra reticulata are not dopaminergic; they primarily transmit GABA. As shown in Figure 10-16, the loss of dopamine from the substantia nigra compacta directly results in decreased activity in the putamen and caudate, collectively known as the *striatum*. Quieting the striatum has the effect of disinhibiting the internal segment of the globus pallidus, which subsequently "over-inhibits" the ventrolateral thalamus. The result is decreased activity in motor cortex. Lesions to the cerebellum can result in movement disorders, such as in cerebellar stroke, but the cerebellum is not directly affected in PD.

3. D. *Parkinsonism* refers to the syndrome of motor deficits such as rigidity, tremor, and bradykinesia associated with damage to the substantia nigra. Although most cases are idiopathic (of unclear etiology), anything that damages the substantia nigra or its connections can lead to parkinsonism. This includes viral encephalitis, trauma (as in dementia pugilistica, or boxer's dementia), or local ischemia.

4. A. (See Figure 10-17) The substantia nigra separates the cerebral peduncles from the tegmentum of the midbrain. It is not directly adjacent to the red nucleus, which lies dorsally, nor the cerebral aqueduct, also dorsal in the midbrain (B and C).

CASE 10-23

1. A. The serotonergic projections of the descending analgesia circuit inhibit pain signals in the spinal cord. The receptor must have an inhibitory effect on the postsynaptic membrane. Of the answers listed, only one would have an inhibitory effect: Opening K^+ channels to increase K^+ efflux from the cell hyperpolarizes the cell, which inhibits action potential generation at the postsynaptic membrane. Closing K^+ "leak" channels would depolarize the cell, creating an excitatory potential (B). Likewise, opening Na^+ channels would cause an influx of cations and thus an excitatory depolarization (C). Chlorine channels must be opened to produce an inhibitory potential; closing them would not hyperpolarize the cell (D). Finally, increasing presynaptic Ca^{2+} conduction would increase neurotransmitter release from primary afferent neurons, which would not have the desired effect of inhibiting signaling (E).

2. D. Although the enterochromaffin cells of the GI tract do contain large amounts of serotonin, the intestine has no direct innervation from the nucleus raphe. The other structures listed receive serotonergic inputs from the raphe.

3. D. The area postrema is also known as the *medullary vomiting center*; serotonin acting at $5-HT_3$ induces nausea and vomiting. Increased functional serotonin levels may have an antidepressant effect, but not through the area postrema (A). Serotonin normally causes vasoconstriction in cerebral and meningeal vessels, not vasodilation (B). Mimicking this effect is the mechanism of action of certain antimigraine drugs, such as sumatriptan. In this way, serotonin agonists relieve headache, rather than cause headache (C). Finally, although serotonin is involved in the descending analgesia circuit, this does not include the area postrema (E).

4. B. The reticular formation is a dispersed network of neurons regulating sleep through inputs to the thalamus. The periaqueductal gray is a component of the descending analgesia circuit (A). The nucleus raphe in the pons and upper midbrain contains most of the serotonergic neurons in the brain and is a component of the reticular formation but does not receive the inputs controlling sleep (C). The hippocampus is generally associated with memory formation, not sleep patterns (D). The reticular formation indirectly affects cortical activity, but not through direct inputs to the cortex (E).

INDEX

Note: Page numbers referencing figures are italicized and followed by an "f". Page numbers referencing tables are italicized and followed by a "t".